*C*ardiopulmonary

ANATOMY *and* PHYSIOLOGY

Visit our website at **www.mosby.com**

Cardiopulmonary
ANATOMY *and* PHYSIOLOGY

GEORGE H. HICKS, M.S., R.R.T.

Program Director of Respiratory Care and
Instructor in Human Anatomy and Physiology
Mt. Hood Community College
Gresham, Oregon

W.B. SAUNDERS COMPANY

A Harcourt Health Sciences Company
Philadelphia   London   New York   St. Louis   Sydney   Toronto

W.B. SAUNDERS COMPANY
A Harcourt Health Sciences Company

The Curtis Center
Independence Square West
Philadelphia, Pennsylvania 19106

Acquisitions Editor: Karen Fabiano
Developmental Editor: Mindy Copeland
Project Manager: Patricia Tannian
Project Specialist: Suzanne C. Fannin
Book Design Manager: Gail Morey Hudson
Cover Designer: Teresa Breckwoldt

CARDIOPULMONARY ANATOMY AND PHYSIOLOGY   ISBN 0-7216-5199-2

Printed in the United States of America

Last digit is the print number: 9   8   7   6   5   4   3   2   1

Contributors

MARK L. SIMMONS, MSEd, RRT, RPFT
Program Director
School of Respiratory Therapy
York Hospital
York, Pennsylvania

ROBERT L. WILKINS, PhD, RRT
Professor and Chairman
Department of Cardiopulmonary Sciences
School of Allied Health Professions
Loma Linda University
Loma Linda, California

Reviewers

ALAN BARKER, MD
Pulmonary and Critical Care Medicine
Oregon Health Sciences University
Portland, Oregon

ANDREAS FREITAG, BSc, MD, FRCP(CC)
Associate Professor of Medicine and
    Pediatrics
McMaster University
Department of Medicine
Division of Respirology
Hamilton, Ontario
Canada

TERRY KRIDER, BS, RRT
Respiratory Care Program
Mt. San Antonio College
Walnut, California

PAUL J. MATHEWS, EdS, RRT, FCCM
Associate Professor
The University of Kansas Medical Center
School of Allied Health
Department of Respiratory Care Education
Kansas City, Kansas

ANNA W. PARKMAN
Program Director
Respiratory Therapist Program
University of Charleston
Charleston, West Virginia

YVONNE ROBBINS, MEd, RRT
Program Director, Respiratory Therapist
Bryn Mawr Hospital
West Chester University
Bryn Mawr, Pennsylvania

For

Christopher, Julia, and **Kevin**

because you continue to teach me about life

Preface

Cardiopulmonary Anatomy and Physiology was written with the Allied Health student, in particular, the Respiratory Care and Nursing students, in mind. It is intended to support the teaching and learning of basic information about the form and function of the heart and lungs as they are applied in clinical practice. The book was developed to better fill the space beyond the general anatomy and physiology texts. Attention was paid to developing straightforward and modern descriptions of the major topics. These topics are supported by relevant clinical information and cases throughout to help the student understand why the topics are important and how the information can be used. In addition, modern bedside and laboratory tests are described along with their normal values to better equip students with useful information about assessment as well as to prepare them for future discussions about various disease states and interventions.

This book is organized into three sections. The first section is an overview of important topics in physics, chemistry, and biology that are useful in the understanding of heart and lung function. This first section is intended to support those readers who have little or distant experience with these subjects. The second section is a complete description of the cardiovascular system including a chapter on blood. Practical chapters on electrocardiography and hemodynamics are included along with an extensive description of regional circulation and cardiovascular control. The third section focuses on the pulmonary system. Included in this section is a modern description of acid-base balance that utilizes Stewart's approach and an up-to-date and practical description of the control of breathing. Care has been taken to integrate the two systems along with their response to sleep, stress, exercise, and disease, as the discussion unfolds. Relevant information about embryological development, the nervous system, urinary system, immune system, and metabolism are also woven into the discussion rather than appearing as separate chapters.

George H. Hicks

Acknowledgments

I want to express my appreciation to Robert Wilkins, PhD, RRT, Department of Respiratory Therapy, Loma Linda University, for his contribution to Chapter 4 and to Mark Simmons, RRT, School of Respiratory Therapy, York Hospital, for his contributions to Chapters 11, 12, and 13.

I am grateful to Alan Barker, MD, Professor of Medicine, Pulmonary and Critical Care Medicine, Oregon Health Sciences University, for his consistent support, review, and gentle queries about how the book was going.

My thanks also go to the following for their reviews and useful suggestions for making the book more accurate, readable, and useful: Andreas Freitag, MD, Department of Medicine, Division of Respirology, McMaster University; Terry Krider, BS, RRT, Respiratory Care Program, Mt. San Antonio College; Paul J. Mathews, EdS, RRT, Department of Respiratory Care Education, The University of Kansas Medical Center; Anna W. Parkman, RRT, Respiratory Therapist Program, University of Charleston; and Yvonne Robbins, MEd, RRT, Respiratory Therapist training program, Bryn Mawr Hospital and West Chester University.

My appreciation is also extended to the editors, specialists, and administrative assistants at W.B. Saunders Company and Mosby, Inc. for all of their encouragement and support. Without them this book would surely be incomplete.

With the greatest appreciation, I want to thank all my students over the years. They helped me see the need for this book and how to organize it.

Contents

CHAPTER 1

Fundamental Concepts

CHAPTER OBJECTIVES

Upon completing this chapter, you will be able to:

1 Describe the units of measurement commonly used in cardiopulmonary science.
2 Describe the kinetic molecular theory of gas behavior.
3 Define gas density.
4 Describe the composition of the atmosphere.
5 Define barometric pressure and Dalton's law of partial pressure.
6 Define and utilize Boyle's, Charles', Gay-Lussac's, and the combined gas laws.
7 Describe humidity and how it is quantified.
8 Define the standardized conditions for reporting gas volume and pressure.
9 Describe the physical properties of liquids.
10 Define surface tension and Laplace's law.
11 Define diffusion, osmosis, osmotic pressure, active transport, and filtration.
12 Define Fick's first law of diffusion.
13 Describe bulk flow and the factors that influence bulk flow.
14 Define and utilize Hagen-Poiseuille's law of bulk flow.
15 Compare and contrast laminar and turbulent flow.
16 Compare and contrast bulk flow through rigid and distensible tubes.

Cardiovascular and pulmonary function play a central role in the maintenance of the body's internal environment. These systems support exchange of molecules and ions between cells and the external environment. The understanding of how these systems function requires a solid understanding of those factors that influence the behavior of gases and liquids. This chapter explores important aspects of cardiopulmonary measurements and the biophysical behavior of gases and liquids. The essential concepts presented in this chapter are intended to form a foundation upon which you will be better prepared to master the following chapters.

UNITS OF MEASUREMENT COMMONLY USED IN CARDIOPULMONARY SCIENCE

One of the biggest impacts the scientific revolution had on medicine was the introduction of standardized measurements. This is entirely logical when you look at researchers or clinicians who, in distant cities or countries, are trying to share information. For their collaboration to be successful, a common system of terms and measurements would be needed. Over time, however, various systems have been developed and adopted in different parts of the world.

The major systems listed in Table 1-1 have their origins in Europe. The British, or Imperial, system utilizes the foot, pound, and second (FPS) system whereas the continental European metric system uses the centimeter, gram, and second (CGS) system. In 1960 worldwide efforts to adopt a common system resulted in the development of Le Système International d'Unités, or the SI system, which is a derivative of the metric system. The SI system measures length in meters, volume in cubic meters, mass in kilograms, and time in seconds (MKS system). The measurement of other variables such as frequency, velocity, force, pressure, work, power, and surface tension are all derived from the basic units of length, mass, and time. Many of these variables are named in honor of the work done by famous scientists of the past.

Medical practice in the United States has not made a complete conversion to the SI sys-

Table 1-1   Measurement Systems used in Science and Medicine

Variable	SI Units	CGS Metric Units	Imperial Units
Length	meter (m)	centimeter (cm)	foot (ft)
Area	square meter (m^2)	square centimeter (cm^2)	square foot (ft^2)
Volume	cubic meter (m^3)	cubic centimeter (cm^3)	cubic foot (ft^3)
Mass	kilogram (kg)	gram (g)	slug
Time	second (s)	second (s)	second (s)
Frequency	hertz (Hz = 1 cycle/s)	cycle/s	cycle/s
Temperature	kelvin (K)	Celsius (° C)	Fahrenheit (° F)
Velocity	m/s	cm/s	ft/s
Force	newton (N = kg m/s^2)	dyne (g cm/s^2)	pound (lb = slug ft/s^2)
Pressure	pascal (Pa = N/m^2)	dyne/cm^2	lb/ft^2
Work or energy	joule (J = N m)	erg (dyne cm)	ft lb
Power	watt (W = J/s)	erg/s	ft lb/s
Electric potential	volt (V)	volt (V)	volt (V)
Surface tension	Pa m	dyne/cm	ft/lb

tem. The most common measurements made in clinical practice include length, volume, time, frequency, flow, pressure, temperature, and voltage.

Length, Mass, Area, and Volume

Length is measured in meters, centimeters, and millimeters. The conversion from SI units to Imperial units is easily carried out with the following relationships:

$$1\ m = 100\ cm = 1000\ mm = 3.28\ feet = 39.37\ inches$$

Microscopic measurements are commonly made in micrometers (μm), nanometers (nm), or angstroms (Å):

$$1\ m = 1 \times 10^6\ \mu m = 1 \times 10^9\ nm = 1 \times 10^{10}\ \overset{\circ}{A}$$

or

$$1\ mm = 1 \times 10^3\ \mu m = 1 \times 10^6\ nm = 1 \times 10^7\ \overset{\circ}{A}$$

Mass or weight is frequently measured in grams (g) and kilograms (kg). Very small amounts of chemicals or drugs dissolved in solution are frequently expressed in milligrams (mg).

For some physiologic measurements, the body surface area is needed and is expressed in square meters. For example, cardiac performance is frequently adjusted for body size to make more meaningful comparisons between measured and normal values. The typical adult body surface area is approximately 1.6 m^2. For a more precise determination, the **DuBois'** **formula** can be used:

$$BSA = H^{0.725} \times W^{0.425} \times 0.007148$$

where BSA is body surface area of the subject in square meters, H is the subject's height in centimeters (1 inch = 2.54 cm), and W is the subject's weight in kilograms (1 pound = 0.455 kg).

To calculate the BSA for someone who is 6 feet 1 inch tall and weighs 180 pounds, the dimensions must first be converted from Imperial units to metric units:

Height = 6 feet 1 inch = 73 inches = 73 inches $\times$ 2.54 cm/in = 185 cm

Weight = 180 pounds = 180 pounds $\times$ 0.455 kg/lb = 82 kg

Now apply the metric values to the DuBois' formula and determine the body surface area:

$$\begin{aligned} BSA &= 185^{0.725} \times 82^{0.425} \times 0.007148 \\ &= 44.025 \times 6.507 \times 0.007148 \\ &= 2.05\ m^2 \end{aligned}$$

Volume of gas and liquids is measured in liters (L), deciliters (dl), and milliliters (ml). Another unit of small volume measurement is the cubic centimeter (cm^3), or cc, which is the volume of 1 ml of water at 4° C. The conversion factors of volume are as follows:

$$1\ m^3 = 1000\ L = 1 \times 10^6\ cm^3 = 35.315\ ft^3 = 1057\ quarts = 264.3\ gallons$$

or

$$1\ L = 10\ dl = 1000\ ml = 1000\ cc = 1.057\ quarts = 0.264\ gallons$$

Time and Frequency

Physiologic events are frequently timed and expressed in seconds. High-speed events are frequently measured in milliseconds (ms). Repetitive events such as heart rate and breathing frequency are expressed in events or cycles per minute (cycles/min). High-frequency events are often expressed in cycles per second (cycles/s), or **hertz** (Hz).

$$1\ cycle/s = 60\ cycles/min = 1\ Hz$$

Flow

Flow measures the volume of gas or liquid passing a fixed point during a fixed amount of time. Flows of blood and gas are commonly measured in liters per minute (L/min) or liters per second (L/s):

1 L/min = 0.017 L/s = 1000 ml/min = 16.667 ml/s

or

1 L/s = 60 L/min = 10 dl/s = 1000 ml/s

Pressure

Pressure is the amount of force applied to a unit of surface area. In the Imperial system, pounds per square inch (lb/in²) expresses the pressure exerted by the atmosphere where 1 atmosphere exerts 14.7 lb/in². Medical and industrial tanks containing compressed gases use pounds per square inch to express the internal pressure of the tank. Blood pressure is commonly measured in terms of millimeters of mercury (mm Hg) or its equivalent, the *torr* (which honors the famous physicist Torricelli). Gas pressure is expressed in both millimeters of mercury and centimeters of water (cm H_2O), both of which are based on the force exerted by these two liquids as they fill a vertical column of known height. Pressure, in the SI system, is expressed in units of the **pascal** (Pa), which equals a force of 1 newton/m² where 1 newton equals 1 kg m/s². The kilopascal (kPa) is the preferred SI unit of pressure used in medicine. The conversion from millimeters of mercury to centimeters of water or kilopascals is relatively simple with the following conversion factors:

1 mm Hg = 1.359 cm H_2O = 0.133 kPa

What would the pressure be in cm H_2O and kPa in a subject whose arterial blood pressure is 120/80 mm Hg?

120 mm Hg × 1.359 cm H_2O/mm Hg = 163.1 cm H_2O
80 mm Hg × 1.359 cm H_2O/mm Hg = 108.7 cm H_2O
120 mm Hg × 0.133 kPa/mm Hg = 16.0 kPa
80 mm Hg × 0.133 kPa/mm Hg = 10.6 kPa

The subject's blood pressure is 163/109 cm H_2O or 16.0/10.6 kPa

Work

Mechanical work exists when a force causes a body with known mass to move a given distance. Mechanical work is determined by taking the product of the force and the distance a body is moved:

W = Fd

where W is the value of work, F is the amount of force applied, and d is the distance the body is moved. In the Imperial system the foot pound describes the work done on an object when a force causes a body weighing 1 pound to move 1 foot. In the CGS system the dyne cm or **erg** is used. In the MKS system the kilogram meter (kg m) is used, and the **joule** (J) is the unit of work in the SI system. They can be converted through the following relationships:

1 J = 1.02 × 10⁴ ergs = 0.102 kg m = 0.738 ft lb

Work can be determined for each event or the amount performed over time. For example, a 1-kg body can be moved 10 m/min, resulting in a work value of 10 kg m/min.

The measurement of work done by the cardiac and pulmonary systems is an important measurement for determining the ability of the heart to pump blood and the ventilation muscles to move air. In this situation, work is the product of pressure needed to move a volume of blood or gas. The cardiovascular and respiratory systems perform large amounts of work over time but can become limited during various disease states. These limitations can lead to decreased exercise tolerance, disability, and even death.

Temperature

The temperature of an object is a measurement of its internal kinetic energy. The higher the temperature, the faster the molecules that comprise the object are moving. The temperature where no molecular movement exists is a logical starting point for an absolute temperature scale. In the SI system the kelvin (K) scale is used, and that point where no molecular motion exists is 0 K. In a centigrade (C) scale there is a span of 100° C between the freezing and boiling points of water. In the kelvin scale water freezes at 273 K and boils at 373 K.

The Celsius (C) scale is also a centigrade scale, which parallels the kelvin scale. However, the Celsius scale does not start at conditions of absolute zero kinetic energy. The freezing point of water is 0° C and the boiling point of water is 100° C. Use the following formulas to convert between the Celsius and kelvin scales:

$$K = °C + 273$$
$$°C = K - 273$$

In clinical practice, body, blood, or gas temperature is measured in degrees Celsius or degrees Fahrenheit (F). The Fahrenheit scale is part of the Imperial system of measurements. The Celsius scale is becoming the preferred unit of measurement. The clinician can easily convert from one scale to another using the following formulas:

$$°C = 5/9 \ (°F - 32) \qquad °F = (9/5 \times C) + 32$$

Convert the following temperatures:

°F = 98.6	°C = 30
°C = 5/9 (98.6 − 32)	°F = (9/5 × 30) + 32
°C = 5/9 (66.6)	°F = (54) + 32
°C = 37	°F = 86

⬭ PHYSICAL CHARACTERISTICS OF GASES

Kinetic Molecular Theory

The **kinetic molecular theory of gas** classically describes the physical properties of a gas. First, this theory describes a gas as being comprised of atoms and molecules in motion with a great deal of space between them. Second, the gas molecules travel in straight lines (at velocities of almost 1000 mph at room tem-

perature) until they collide with an object or the wall of the container. Third, the collisions are completely elastic and do not result in any loss of kinetic energy. Fourth, no attraction or repulsion exists between the gas molecules. And fifth, the kinetic energy or motion of the molecules is directly proportional to the temperature. This description explains why a gas takes on the shape of its container, exerts and maintains a given pressure in a container, and changes volume or pressure when heated or cooled. However, the kinetic molecular theory describes the behavior of an *ideal* gas. Real gases behave differently under conditions of extreme temperature and pressure. Under less extreme conditions, such as in the body, real gases behave like an ideal gas.

Gas Density

The density of an object is generally defined by the number of atoms or molecules of the object that fills a given space or volume. Gas density is commonly described on the basis of the weight of molecules present in a given volume with the following relationship:

$$\rho = \frac{m}{V}$$

where ρ is the density of the gas, m is the mass of the gas, and V is the volume occupied by the gas.

A standard approach used to describe the density of gas utilizes the weight of 1 mole of gas molecules (6.02×10^{23} molecules) that occupies a volume at standard conditions of 0° C and 1 atmosphere of pressure. Under these conditions a standard volume of 22.4 L is occupied by an ideal gas and is commonly referred to as the **molar volume** (mv). Gas density is determined by taking the weight of 1 mole (**gram molecular weight** [gmw]) and dividing it by the molar volume, or 22.4 L.

Determine the density of O_2:

$$O_2 = \frac{gmw}{mv}$$

$$O_2 = \frac{32 \text{ g/mole}}{22.4 \text{ L/mole}}$$

$$= 1.43 \text{ g/L}$$

In SI units, density is expressed in kilograms per cubic meter (kg/m^3). Because there are 1000 g in 1 kg and 1000 L in a 1 m^3, the value for the density of O_2 is 1.43 kg/m^3.

Atmosphere and its Pressure

The earth is wrapped, like an onion, in a series of gaseous atmospheric layers that have evolved over time. This gaseous envelope extends out over 1000 km from the earth's surface. The outermost layer, the **exosphere,** begins at an altitude of 300 km and the few gases present (primarily ozone, nitrogen, helium, and hydrogen) gradually thin out to the vacuum of space with increasing altitude. Two-thirds of the earth's atmosphere lies in the first layer, the **troposphere,** which rises to an altitude of 8 to 10 km. The summit of Mt. Everest (29,028 ft [8848 m]) and the cruising altitude of commercial jets (35,000 ft [10,700 m]) place them at the upper edge of the troposphere.

The gas mixture of the troposphere is commonly called **air.** The composition of air is 78.084% N_2 and 20.946% O_2 with the remaining 1% comprised of a long list of organic and inorganic compounds (Table 1-2). Gas molecules are concentrated in the troposphere because of gravity. Gas atoms and molecules have mass, which, when acted upon by the force of gravity, results in an atmospheric weight, or pressure. This pressure is exerted equally over the surface of objects that are "immersed" in the atmosphere. At sea level the pressure exerted is termed 1 atmosphere (atm) of pressure. This pressure can be easily measured with a device called a **barometer.** Pressure in the amount of 1 atm forces mercury up into an evacuated glass column of a barometer 760 mm (Fig. 1-1). Thus 1 atm of pressure is 760 mm Hg, which is equivalent

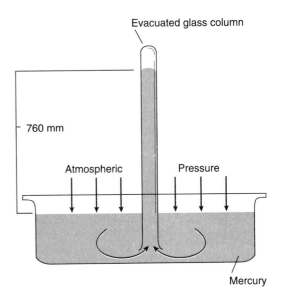

FIG. 1-1 Mercury barometer is an instrument that allows direct observation of the total "weight," or pressure, of the atmosphere. At sea level the atmosphere forces mercury 760 mm up into an evacuated glass column.

to 1034 cm H_2O, 101.3 kPa, and 14.7 lb/in^2. While ascending through the troposphere, gas density, pressure, and temperature drop at a uniform rate. For example, at an altitude of 10,000 m the barometric pressure drops to approximately 200 mm Hg and air temperature drops to $-40°$ C.

Partial Pressure

The total pressure of air or any gas mixture is the product of all the partial pressures exerted by the various gases in the mixture. This relationship was first described by Dalton and bares his name. **Dalton's law** with regard to air would be written as follows:

$$P_B = P_{N_2} + P_{O_2} + P_{H_2O} + P_{Ar} + P_{CO_2} + P_{gases}$$

where P_B is the total barometric pressure, P_{N_2} is the partial pressure of N_2, P_{O_2} is the partial pressure of O_2, P_{H_2O} is the partial pressure of water vapor, P_{Ar} is the partial pressure of

Table 1-2   Composition of Dry Air at Sea Level

			Partial Pressure	
Gas	Percentage	Parts Per Million	mm Hg	kPa
Nitrogen	78.084	78.084×10^4	593.44	79.13
Oxygen	20.946	20.946×10^4	159.19	21.23
Argon	0.934	9340	7.10	0.95
Carbon dioxide	0.032	320	0.24	0.032
Other gases*	0.004	40	0.03	0.004
Water vapor	0	0	0	0
Total	100	1×10^6	760.00	101.33

*Helium, neon, krypton, methane, hydrogen, ozone, carbon monoxide, and nitrous oxide.
10,000 parts per million = 1%.

Argon, P_{CO_2} is the partial pressure of CO_2, and P_{gases} is the partial pressure of all the other gases present.

To determine the partial pressure of a particular gas in a dry gas mixture, the following formula is used:

$$P_{gas} = F_{gas} \times P_{baro}$$

where P_{gas} is the partial pressure of the gas in question, F_{gas} is the concentration as a decimal fraction (e.g., 0.1, not 10%), and P_{baro} is the total atmospheric or barometric pressure. For example, the partial pressure of O_2 in the atmosphere is as follows:

$$P_{O_2} = F_{O_2} \times P_{baro}$$
$$= 0.20946 \times 760 \text{ mm Hg}$$
$$= 159 \text{ mm Hg}$$

Table 1-2 lists the composition and partial pressure of gases throughout the troposphere. As one ascends into the atmosphere, total gas pressure declines but gas concentration remains constant to an altitude of approximately 10 km. This results in a declining partial pressure of each gas. Fig. 1-2 illustrates the barometric pressure and partial pressure of O_2 found when ascending from sea level to Denver, Colorado, and then to the summit of Mt. Everest.

DESCRIPTION OF IDEAL GAS LAWS

Boyle's Law

During the seventeenth century, Boyle discovered that the volume of a gas varies inversely with pressure when temperature and mass or gas molecule number are held constant. In other words, Boyle's law describes that if pressure is increased, the volume occupied by the gas decreases or if the gas volume increases, the pressure exerted by the gas molecules decreases. Fig. 1-3 illustrates Boyle's law as gas volume is decreased or increased. By decreasing the volume, a greater number of molecular collisions can occur per unit time, which results in increased pressure. Boyle's law also describes the compressible nature of gas. By holding temperature and mass constant, Boyle's law can be written as follows:

$$P_1V_1 = P_2V_2$$

where P_1 represents the initial pressure of the gas, V_1 is the initial volume of the gas, P_2 is the new pressure of the gas, and V_2 is the new volume of the gas.

For example, if you fill your lungs with 6 L of gas, close your airway, and bear down with your chest and abdominal muscles (Valsalva's

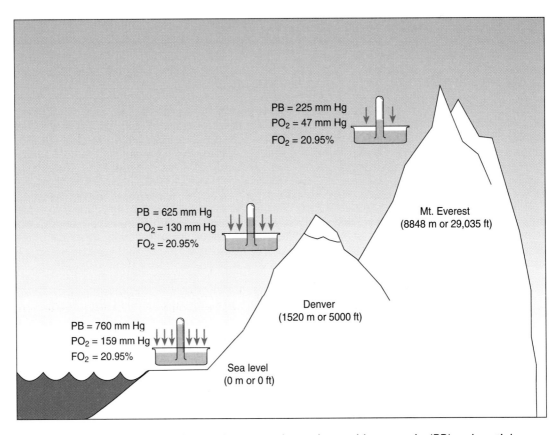

PB = 225 mm Hg
PO_2 = 47 mm Hg
FO_2 = 20.95%

PB = 625 mm Hg
PO_2 = 130 mm Hg
FO_2 = 20.95%

Mt. Everest
(8848 m or 29,035 ft)

PB = 760 mm Hg
PO_2 = 159 mm Hg
FO_2 = 20.95%

Denver
(1520 m or 5000 ft)

Sea level
(0 m or 0 ft)

FIG. 1-2 As one ascends into the atmosphere, the total barometric *(PB)* and partial *(PO$_2$)* pressures of gases decline whereas the fractional concentration *(FO$_2$)* remains constant.

maneuver) with enough force to bring the pressure inside the lungs from 760 mm Hg (1 atm) to 860 mm Hg, what would be the volume of gas in your lungs? By rearranging Boyle's law to solve for the new volume, the equation would appear as follows:

$$V_2 = \frac{P_1V_1}{P_2}$$

$$= \frac{760 \text{ mm Hg} \times 6 \text{ L}}{860 \text{ mm Hg}}$$

$$= 5.3 \text{ L}$$

V_1 = 6 L
P_1 = 760 mm Hg
P_2 = 860 mm Hg

Note that the lung volume has been compressed from 6 L to 5.3 L by the force generated during the breath hold maneuver.

Charles' Law

In the early nineteenth century, Jacques Charles discovered that the volume of a gas varies directly with temperature changes while mass and pressure are held constant. Fig. 1-4 illustrates Charles' law of increasing volume as a gas at constant pressure is heated. At the molecular level, heating the gas molecules increases the kinetic energy, which results in greater molecular speed. This would result in greater pressure, but the pressure is held constant. This could only occur if the volume is allowed to increase so that the number of molecular collisions with the container is held constant. Conversely, when a gas is cooled the molecular speed is reduced and volume will decrease.

$$P_1V_1 = P_2V_2$$

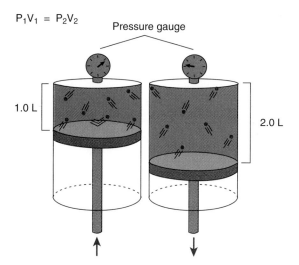

$$\frac{V_1}{T_1} = \frac{V_2}{T_2}$$

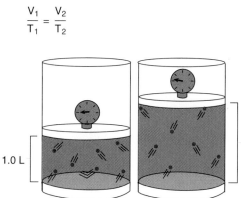

FIG. 1-3 Boyle's law describes that gas pressure increases with decreasing volume and pressure decreases with increasing volume while holding the temperature and number of gas molecules constant.

FIG. 1-4 Charles' law describes that gas volume decreases with cooling and increases with heating while holding the pressure and number of gas molecules constant.

By holding pressure and mass constant, Charles' law can be written as follows:

$$\frac{V_1}{T_1} = \frac{V_2}{T_2}$$

where V_1 is the initial volume of the gas, T_1 represents the initial kelvin temperature of the gas, V_2 is the new volume of the gas, and T_2 is the new temperature of the gas.

The following is an example problem. A subject exhales 6 L of gas at body temperature (37° C [310 K]) into a volume-measuring device called a spirometer that is at room temperature (20° C [293 K]). What would be the new volume in the spirometer at the new temperature assuming the pressure remains at 1 atm? Rearrange Charles' law to solve for the new volume, and convert the temperature to the kelvin scale:

$$V_2 = \frac{T_2V_1}{T_1}$$

$$= \frac{293 \text{ K} \times 6 \text{ L}}{310 \text{ K}}$$

$$= 5.67 \text{ L}$$

$V_1 = 6 \text{ L}$
$T_1 = 310 \text{ K}$
$T_2 = 293 \text{ K}$

This illustrates that gas volume can be significantly altered when exposed to different temperatures.

Gay-Lussac's Law

In the early nineteenth century, Gay-Lussac demonstrated that gas pressure is directly related to kelvin temperature when volume and mass remain constant. Fig. 1-5 illustrates Gay-Lussac's law as a fixed volume of gas that is heated. The additional kinetic energy increases molecular collisions per unit time. This results in greater pressure. The reverse would be true if the temperature was decreased. Gay-Lussac's law can be represented with the following equation:

$$\frac{P_1}{T_1} = \frac{P_2}{T_2}$$

where P_1 is the initial pressure of the gas, T_1 is the initial kelvin temperature of the gas, P_2 is the new pressure of the gas, and T_2 is the new kelvin temperature of the gas.

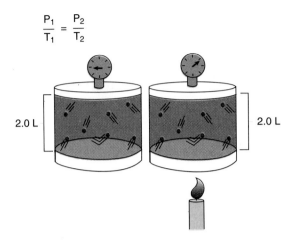

$$\frac{P_1}{T_1} = \frac{P_2}{T_2}$$

2.0 L   2.0 L

FIG. 1-5 Gay-Lussac's law describes that gas pressure decreases with cooling and increases with heating while holding the volume and number of gas molecules constant.

The following example illustrates how Gay-Lussac's law works. The partial pressure of O_2 in a sample of gas in a sealed container is 100 mm Hg. The sample is cooled from body temperature (37° C [310 K]) down to 2° C (275 K) by immersion in an ice bath. What would be the new partial pressure of O_2 at the new temperature? Gay-Lussac's law can be rearranged to solve for the new pressure:

$$P_2 = \frac{P_1 T_2}{T_1}$$

$$= \frac{100 \text{ mm Hg} \times 275 \text{ K}}{310 \text{ K}}$$

$$= 89 \text{ mm Hg}$$

$P_1 = 100$ mm Hg
$P_1 = 100$ mm Hg
$T_2 = 275$ K

Note the drop in pressure from 100 mm Hg to 89 mm Hg. This demonstrates how gas pressure can be influenced by temperature changes.

Combined Gas Law

Boyle's, Charles', and Gay-Lussac's laws can be brought together into a combined gas law when the mass of gas is held constant. This equation allows the calculation of a resulting new volume, pressure, and temperature when mixed changes in gas condition occur.

$$\frac{P_1 V_1}{T_1} = \frac{P_2 V_2}{T_2}$$

Rarely can all the factors that influence gas volume, pressure, and temperature be held constant. The combined gas law can be written to include other factors:

$$V = \frac{nRT}{P}$$

or

$$P = \frac{nRT}{V}$$

where V is the volume of gas in liters, P is the pressure of gas in millimeters of mercury, T is the kelvin temperature, n is the number of gas molecules in moles, and R is the universal gas constant (0.0821). Note that in the first equation the volume of a gas is directly related to the number of gas molecules and the kelvin temperature and inversely related to the pressure. The second equation demonstrates that gas pressure is also directly related to the number of gas molecules and kelvin temperature and inversely related to volume. This equation combines all the factors that influence gas volume, pressure, and temperature.

The gas laws, the constants, and the major relationships are summarized in Table 1-3.

● HUMIDITY AND HOW IT IS QUANTIFIED

The air we breathe is rarely dry or free of water. In fact, one of the important functions of the upper part of the respiratory tract is the action of adding water to the air inhaled to prevent injury to the delicate structures of the lungs. Water **evaporation** occurs when water, in the liquid state, receives sufficient kinetic energy to change it into a gas. **Humidification**

Table 1-3 Gas Law Constants, Relationships, and Examples

Gas Law	Constant	Relationship	Example
Boyle's law	T and molec number	$P \approx 1/V$	$\uparrow P \rightarrow \downarrow V$
Charles' law	P and molec number	$V \approx T$	$\uparrow T \rightarrow \uparrow V$
Gay-Lussac's law	V and molec number	$T \approx P$	$\uparrow T \rightarrow \uparrow P$
Combined law	R	$V \approx nT/P$	$\uparrow P, \downarrow T$ and $\downarrow n \rightarrow \downarrow V$

T, Temperature (in kelvins); *P*, gas pressure; *V*, gas volume; *R*, universal gas constant; *n*, number of gas molecules in moles.

Table 1-4 Maximum Water Vapor Pressure and Content in Air at Various Temperatures

Temperature (° C)	Water Vapor Pressure (mm Hg)	Absolute Humidity Content (mg/L)
20	17.50	17.30
21	18.62	18.35
22	19.80	19.42
23	21.10	20.58
24	22.40	21.78
25	23.80	23.04
26	25.20	24.36
27	26.70	25.75
28	28.30	27.22
29	30.00	28.75
30	31.80	30.35
31	33.70	32.01
32	35.70	39.60
36	44.60	41.70
37	47.00	43.80

refers to the addition of water vapor to a gas through evaporation. **Water vapor** is the term used to describe water when it is in a gaseous state. Like any other gas, water vapor has mass and exerts a partial pressure. Water vapor pressure can be quantified as a partial pressure and expressed in millimeters of mer-cury or kilopascals. Table 1-4 lists the maximal water vapor pressure at various temperatures. With the addition of water vapor to a gas mixture, the partial pressure of water vapor becomes part of the total pressure of the gas mixture. Thus the addition of water vapor reduces the partial pressure of all the other gases in the mixture.

Correcting Gas Pressure for Humidity Content

To determine the partial pressure of a gas in a humidified gas mixture, the total pressure of the gas mixture must be corrected by subtract-ing the water vapor pressure. Following that, the partial pressure of a certain gas can be determined if the concentration of the gas under study is known. Humidity content cor-rection is carried out by using the following equation:

$$P_{gas} = F_{gas} (P_{total} - P_{H_2O})$$

where P_{gas} is the partial pressure of the gas being evaluated, F_{gas} is the decimal concentra-tion of the gas being evaluated, P_{total} is the total pressure of the gas mixture (usually baromet-ric pressure), and P_{H_2O} is the partial pressure of water vapor pressure.

The following is a sample problem. A sub-ject exhales gas at body temperature (37° C) with an O_2 concentration of 15% or a decimal concentration of 0.15. The gas has a total pres-sure of 1 atm (760 mm Hg) and has a maximal water vapor pressure. Table 1-4 shows that the maximal water vapor pressure at 37° C is 47 mm Hg. What is the partial pressure of O_2 in the gas being exhaled? Using the equation described previously, the partial pressure of O_2 can be determined as follows:

$$P_{O_2} = 0.15 \ (760 \text{ mm Hg} - 47 \text{ mm Hg})$$
$$= 0.15 \times 713 \text{ mm Hg}$$
$$= 107 \text{ mm Hg}$$

Humidity Content

The **humidity content** describes the actual amount of water per liter of gas. The amount of water vapor in a gas mixture is a function of temperature. At any given temperature between the freezing and boiling points of water, there is a maximal amount of water that evaporates and then exists as a gas. It can be expressed in units of either vapor pressure or milligrams of water per liter of gas (mg/L).

Absolute Humidity

Absolute humidity is the maximal amount of water content in a given volume of gas. Table 1-4 lists the values of absolute humidity content at different temperatures. When a gas mixture has a maximal amount of water vapor, it is referred to as being saturated.

Relative Humidity

A gas may not be completely saturated with water vapor. For example, at room temperature (20° C) a gas will be saturated when it contains 17.30 mg of water per liter of gas (see Table 1-4). If it contained 8.65 mg/L, the gas would be described as being 50% saturated. The use of percentage enables the humidity content to be described in relative terms. **Relative humidity** (RH) expresses humidity content of a gas as a percentage of the maximal or absolute humidity possible at a given temperature. RH can be calculated with the following equation:

$$\% \ RH = \frac{\text{Actual humidity content}}{\text{Absolute humidity content}} \times 100\%$$

What is the percent RH of a gas at 25° C with an actual humidity content of 5 mg/L? Table 1-4 shows that the absolute humidity content is 23.04 mg/L. The RH is easily determined by using the relationship described previously:

$$\% \ RH = \frac{5 \text{ mg/L}}{23.04 \text{ mg/L}} \times 100\%$$
$$= 0.217 \times 100\%$$
$$= 21.7\%$$

The percent RH is determined daily by meteorologists with an instrument called a **hygrometer.** By knowing the percent RH and the temperature of the gas, the equation could be rearranged, the actual content could be calculated, and the water vapor pressure could be determined with the use of Table 1-4.

One of the phenomena frequently observed in nature and in clinical cardiopulmonary practice is **condensation.** Condensation refers to the change of state of water from a vapor to a liquid that occurs when a gas at a certain temperature and with a relatively high humidity is cooled to a lower temperature. As the gas temperature drops, it reaches a point where the actual humidity content equals or surpasses the absolute humidity content possible. When this occurs, the excess water vapor changes its state into liquid water and forms droplets on the surface of cool objects. The temperature, when this occurs, is known as the **dew point.** Thus a drop in gas temperature results in condensation and reduced humidity content in a gas.

Relative Body Humidity

In clinical practice the humidity content of inhaled gas is expressed as the **relative body** humidity (RBH), which is also expressed as a percent saturation but is always referenced to normal body temperature (37° C) rather than ambient temperature. The absolute humidity content of gas at body temperature is 43.8 mg/L (see Table 1-4). RBH can be calculated with the following equation:

$$\% \text{ RBH} = \frac{\textbf{Actual humidity content}}{\textbf{43.8 mg/L}} \times \textbf{100\%}$$

For example, determine the percent RBH. What is the % RBH of a gas at 25°C with an actual humidity content of 5 mg/L? The percent RBH is easily determined by using the relationship described previously:

$$\% \text{ RBH} = \frac{5 \text{ mg/L}}{43.8 \text{ mg/L}} \times 100\%$$
$$= 0.114 \times 100\%$$
$$= 11.4\%$$

This gas is relatively dry when compared with the gas in the lung that is maintained at 100% RBH. If this relatively dry gas came into direct contact with the delicate microscopic airways of the lungs, these structures would be dehydrated and injured and would fail to function properly.

 ## STANDARDIZED CONDITIONS FOR REPORTING GAS VOLUME AND PRESSURE

We have seen how gas volume and partial pressure can be changed by variations in barometric pressure (Dalton's law and Boyle's law), gas temperature (Charles' law), and humidity content (water vapor pressure). This introduces a problem when reporting the value of a gas volume or partial pressure. If the conditions of the gas at the time of measurement were not defined, erroneous conclusions could be made about the health of an individual. Standardized conditions have been defined to clarify the way gas volume and partial pressure are reported.

Ambient Temperature and Pressure, Saturated Conditions

A starting point for reporting gas volume and pressure is the determination of the current conditions of a gas when saturated with water vapor. It is defined by the **ambient temperature** and barometric **pressure, saturated** with water vapor (ATPS). An example of ATPS conditions follows:

Volume	= 6 L
Temperature	= 20°C (293 K)
Pressure	= 760 mm Hg
Relative humidity	= 100%
Water vapor pressure	= 17.50 mm Hg
Corrected pressure	= 760 − 17.50 = 742.5 mm Hg

Body Temperature and Ambient Pressure, Saturated Conditions

A common standard condition used in clinical practice is **body temperature** and ambient barometric **pressure,** and **saturated** with water vapor (BTPS). An example of BTPS conditions for the same gas described previously following correction to BTPS conditions would be as follows:

Volume	= 6.61 L
Temperature	= 37° C (293 K)
Pressure	= 760 mm Hg
Relative humidity	= 100%
Water vapor pressure	= 47.00 mm Hg
Corrected pressure	= 760 − 47 = 713 mm Hg

Note that volume, temperature, and water vapor pressure have increased because of the increase in temperature to a standard body temperature of 37° C. The ambient barometric pressure does not change, but the corrected pressure decreases because of the greater water vapor pressure at body temperature.

Standard Temperature and Pressure, Dry Conditions

Another condition to report gas volume is at **standard temperature and** barometric **pressure,** and **dry** (STPD). Standard temperature

Table 1-5 Factors* to Convert Volume from ATPS to BTPS and ATPS to STPD Condition

Ambient Temperature (° C)	ATPS to BTPS	ATPS to STPD
20	1.102	0.907
21	1.096	0.902
22	1.091	0.898
23	1.085	0.893
24	1.080	0.888
25	1.075	0.883
26	1.068	0.879
27	1.063	0.874
28	1.057	0.869
29	1.051	0.864
30	1.045	0.859
31	1.039	0.854
32	1.032	0.848
33	1.026	0.843
34	1.020	0.838
35	1.014	0.832
36	1.007	0.826
37	1.000	0.820

*At a barometric pressure of 760 mm Hg.

is 0° C, standard pressure is 1 atm, and the gas has no humidity. An example of STPD conditions for the same gas described previously following correction would be as follows:

Volume	= 4.92 L
Temperature	= 0° C (273 K)
Pressure	= 760 mm Hg
Relative humidity	= 0%
Water vapor pressure	= 0 mm Hg
Corrected pressure	= 760 − 0 = 760 mm Hg

Note that the gas volume is significantly less than both the ambient and body temperature values found previously. This is because of the much lower temperature and absence of water vapor at STPD conditions. In addition, the corrected pressure is higher as a result of a lack of vapor pressure.

When gases are measured under ATPS conditions, they can be converted to BTPS or STPD conditions through the use of the combined gas law and corrected barometric pressure. However, an easier method is to use conversion factors. Table 1-5 lists the factors for converting gas volume at various temperatures. The following formula is used to correct a volume of gas from ATPS to either BTPS or STPD conditions:

Corrected volume = Volume$_{ATPS}$ × Conversion factor

The ATPS conditions of a gas just collected are as follows:

Volume = 5 L
Temperature = 25° C
Pressure = 760 mm Hg

What is the volume when corrected to BTPS conditions?

ATPS to BTPS conversion factor = 1.075
Volume$_{BTPS}$ = 5 L × 1.075
= 5.38 L

What is the volume when corrected to STPD conditions?

ATPS to STPD conversion factor = 0.883
Volume$_{STPD}$ = 5 L × 0.883
= 4.42 L

PHYSICAL CHARACTERISTICS OF LIQUIDS

Liquid water is the base **solvent** for the various transport mediums that are used by the body for molecular exchange between cells of the internal environment and exchange with the external environment. The various types of molecules and ions dissolved in the solvent are **solutes.** The fluid behavior of liquids and gases has helped sculpt the structure and function of both the cardiovascular and pulmonary systems. Understanding the physical properties of liquids is very important in the practice of cardiopulmonary medicine.

Measuring Pulmonary Function to Better Understand Dyspnea

Mr. N, a 73-year-old man, began to complain of increasing shortness of breath (dyspnea) during his morning walk. His physician ordered a pulmonary function screening test to determine his ability to breathe. The clinician recorded the following pulmonary function variables:

Test	Predicted Value (for Age, Height, Sex)	Uncorrected Values (Measured at 20° C)	Corrected Values (Corrected to BTPS)
Peak expiratory flow rate	7.30 L/s	5.10 L/s	5.62 L/s
Forced vital capacity	4.85 L/s	3.50 L/s	3.86 L/s

Mr. N's peak expiratory flow rate, an indicator of the ability to cough and give an adequate effort during the test, is 70% of the predicted value and is considered below normal when measured at 20° C. The uncorrected forced vital capacity, the maximal amount of gas that can be forced out following a maximal inspiration, is 72% of the predicted value and is also below normal when measured at 20° C. These low values are consistent with an obstructive defect of the respiratory tract and may help explain the dyspnea Mr. N. is having.

However, the appropriate comparison should be made between values measured at 37° C and predicted values. Predicted values are based on BTPS (at body temperature and ambient pressure, and saturated with water vapor) conditions. Failure to correct flow and volume values to BTPS conditions results in falsely low comparisons. In this case the peak expired flow and forced vital capacity are actually 77% and 80%, respectively, and are normal and not consistent with obstructive pulmonary disease. Mr. N was further evaluated and found to have coronary artery disease, which is the true source of his dyspnea.

Liquid Density

The molecules and ions of a liquid solution are not held together in a tight or rigid geometric structure like that of a solid. Although molecules are close together, they can move past one another. This allows a liquid to flow and possess a volume that has no definite shape. Like gases, liquids take on the shape of the container. But unlike gases, they settle to the bottom of the container because of the force of gravity. These properties are the result of a liquid's much greater density. The density of a liquid, like that of a gas, is defined as its mass per unit volume:

$$\rho = \frac{m}{V}$$

where ρ is the density, m is the mass, and V is the volume of the liquid. For example, the density of water is 1000 kg/m³ at 4° C whereas mercury has a density of 13,600 kg/m³ at room temperature. These densities are much greater than that of a gas such as air, which has a density of only 1.29 kg/m³; this is 775 and 10,540 times less dense than that of water and mercury, respectively.

Compressibility

The higher the density of a liquid, the lower the compressibility. When compared with gases, liquids can be treated as though they are incompressible in the pressure ranges that are commonly encountered in the body. This is an important property in cardiovascular function. For example, when the heart muscle contracts, it generates pressure that forces blood out of the heart rather than compressing blood within the heart. If blood were highly compressible, the amount of force the heart would need to exert to maintain the same blood flow would greatly increase.

Pressure

A fundamental property of any liquid is its ability to exert pressure, which is caused by a liquid's density, the force of gravity, and very low compressibility. The ability of liquids to exert pressure is essentially the same concept described earlier in the discussion of the pressure exerted by the atmosphere on the surface of the earth. The pressure exerted by a liquid

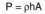

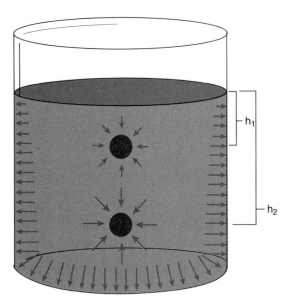

FIG. 1-6 Pressure (*P*) exerted on the walls and surface of an object immersed in a liquid increases with increasing liquid density (ρ), depth (or height) of the water column (*h*), and the surface area (*A*) of the object exposed to the liquid. The object immersed to a depth of h_2 has considerably greater pressure exerted on it when compared with the object at a depth of h_1.

on the walls of a container and the surface of an object immersed in it increases with depth (Fig. 1-6). The following equation describes this relationship:

$$P = \rho hA$$

where P is the pressure exerted by the liquid, ρ is the density of the liquid, h is the depth or the height of the liquid column, and A is the surface area exposed to the liquid. Increasing liquid density, depth, and surface area results in greater pressure exerted by a fluid. For example, a diver descends into water. Greater pressure is exerted on all of the external surfaces of the diver's body. In fact, for every 33 feet of depth, an additional atmosphere of pressure is added.

In clinical practice the effects of liquids under pressure caused by gravity can be seen. Take, for example, the swollen ankles of a patient experiencing heart failure. Heart failure results in reduced blood flow and pooling of blood and lymphatic fluid in the dependent regions of the body. While the patient is in an upright position, the blood pressure in these vessels is significantly higher than those in the upper torso as a result of gravity. This higher pressure results in fluid leakage into the space between the tissues, which results in swollen, or **edematous,** ankles.

Viscosity

The movement of a liquid or gas is opposed by the frictional forces between the molecules of the mixture and the surface over which they are flowing. The frictional forces between the molecules of a liquid are largely a result of the cohesive forces that attract molecules to one another. The greater the cohesive forces, the greater the viscosity of the liquid and the greater the opposition to movement. Increasing the temperature of a fluid reduces the cohesive forces and thus reduces the viscosity. Compare the viscosity with that of air and water. Water is significantly more viscous than air. This is because of the much greater density and cohesive properties of water.

The viscosity of moving fluids and gases causes these materials to have different speeds or velocities in different parts of a tube through which they are moving. Fig. 1-7 shows the velocity profile of matter (gas or liquid) as it moves through a tube in a **laminar** pattern. At the edges of the tube the velocity is lower because of greater friction. In the center the velocity is greatest because of lower friction. During this type of flow the friction between different fluid layers results in the shearing of fluid into regions with different velocities. Increasing viscosity causes increased shearing of the fluid into layers with different velocities as it moves through the tube. Thus the viscosity of a fluid is quantitatively defined as the ratio of the pressure needed to move it (shearing force) to the relative velocity of adjacent fluid layers (shearing rate). Viscosity of a fluid is shown in the following relationship:

$$\eta \approx \frac{P}{SR}$$

where η is the viscosity, P is the driving pressure or shear force, and SR is the shear rate of the liquid or gas. The viscosity of the material is directly proportional to the driving pressure needed to move it and inversely proportional to its shear rate. High viscosity fluids, such as molasses, have very low shear rates as a result of very high molecular cohesion; thus greater pressure is required to move it. Heating molasses reduces molecular cohesion and increases the shear rate, which reduces its viscosity.

Viscosity is measured in poise (P). One poise is equal to an amount of pressure or force exerted on an area over a period of time—1 dyne s/cm^2. It is not measured in clinical practice but is useful to describe the physical properties of fluids. Of more practical use is the relative comparison of the viscosity of various fluids with a standard such as water. It can be easily determined by comparing the flow rate (shear rate) of different fluids while driving them through the same tube with the same driving pressure (shear force) and temperature. For example, blood plasma is 1.8 times more viscous than water, whereas whole blood is four times more viscous. Thus blood requires approximately four times more force to move it compared with water.

Surface Tension

The surface of a liquid behaves as if it were an elastic skin that is constantly attempting to contract the liquid's surface area. This force of contraction is called **surface tension.** Surface tension is generated by uneven cohesive forces that are applied to the molecules at the surface of a liquid (Fig. 1-8). Molecules deeper in the liquid have equal cohesive forces applied to them in all directions. The molecules at the surface have cohesive forces applied to them from the sides and from below. Gas molecules exert little or no cohesive force. This uneven force causes the surface molecules to be drawn into the liquid. Thus a droplet of water takes on a unique shape as the surface tension forces are applied over its entire surface, causing it to form a structure with the lowest possible surface area—a sphere.

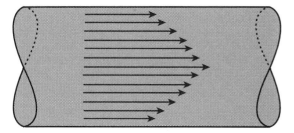

FIG. 1-7 Liquids and gas flowing through a tube develop a parabolic velocity profile during laminar flow. The interaction of friction and viscosity of flowing liquid or gas causes the molecules to separate or shear into regions of slower and faster velocities. Those at the center move faster whereas those along the wall of the tube move slower.

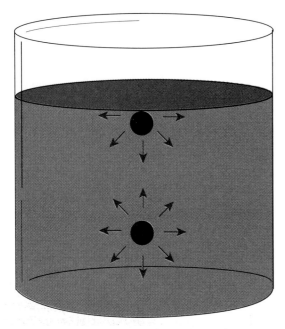

FIG. 1-8 Molecules at the surface of a liquid experience lateral and downward cohesive attraction to surround molecules whereas those molecules below the surface experience equal attraction in all directions. The unequal attraction on the surface molecules results in the development of surface tension.

The force or pressure generated within a droplet as a result of surface tension was first described by Laplace. **Laplace's law** shows this relationship:

$$P = 2 \times \frac{ST}{r}$$

where P is the collapsing pressure generated within the droplet, ST is the surface tension, and r is the radius of the droplet. This equation demonstrates that, as the surface tension of the liquid increases, the internal pressure increases twice as much. It also shows that as the droplet becomes smaller and the radius decreases, the pressure within also increases rapidly.

Liquid bubbles are highly influenced by surface tension because they have two sur-

CASE STUDY FOCUS

Respiratory Distress in a Premature Infant

A male infant who is 9 weeks premature was breathing at a rate of 78 breaths per minute with poor air exchange shortly after birth. A chest x-ray showed poor lung inflation and confirmed the diagnosis of respiratory distress syndrome (RDS) of the newborn. The basic problem in RDS is a poorly developed lung that has elevated surface tension in the terminal portions of the microscopic airways that carry out gas exchange. The elevated surface tension is caused by a deficiency in the production of the chemical mixture known as surfactant. When this occurs, it is difficult for the immature lung to inflate, and the lung is unable to exchange oxygen and carbon dioxide between the air and blood. It was decided to start continuous ventilatory support with oxygen to improve the infant's gas exchange. After several hours of support, the infant was more stable with moderately improved gas exchange, and a second chest x-ray revealed poor lung expansion. To improve lung expansion and reduce the level of mechanical ventilation that was needed, the infant was given several small doses of artificial surfactant (Survanta). The artificial surfactant was injected into his airways. He tolerated this and responded very well with improved lung expansion and oxygenation. He was gradually weaned from ventilatory support over the next several days. He recovered from RDS without significant complications and was discharged home 18 days after birth.

faces (inner and outer) that are experiencing surface tension. A bubble is a volume of gas that is within a liquid container. Because the bubble has two liquid surfaces, it generates twice the amount of surface tension and thus twice the collapsing pressure. Laplace's law is easily modified to describe the pressures generated within a bubble:

$$P = 4 \times \frac{ST}{r}$$

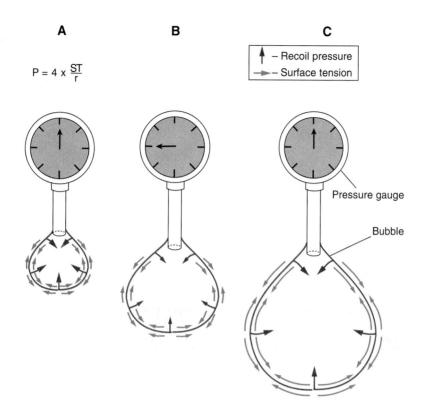

FIG. 1-9 Laplace's law describes the pressure *(P)* generated within a bubble of a given radius *(r)*, and surface tension *(ST)*. The collapsing pressure increases when the bubble is reduced in size (**B** to **A**) or when the chemical composition of the bubble results in increased surface tension (**B** to **C**).

This results in much greater pressures as surface tension is increased or as the size decreases. Fig. 1-9 illustrates the collapsing pressure generated by various bubbles. Smaller bubbles (Fig. 1-9, *A*) and bubbles comprised of liquids with greater surface tension (Fig. 1-9, *C*) generate greater collapsing pressures.

The small alveoli of the lung are spherical structures that are coated with water. This type of structure closely resembles a cluster of tiny bubbles. Laplace's law reveals that this type of structure requires a certain amount of pressure to inflate the alveoli as a result of surface tension. Interestingly, the lung can reduce the surface tension of alveoli by the production of a complex surface tension reducing chemical mixture—**surfactant.** It can be seen how a surfactant deficiency could lead to increased alve-

olar surface tension, which would, in turn, lead to greater effort needed to expand the lung and a greater propensity for lung collapse.

Capillary Action

Surface tension is also responsible for the movement of fluid in a capillary tube. **Capillary action,** the vertical movement of a liquid with sufficient cohesive and adhesive properties into a capillary tube of small diameter, is produced by the cohesive action of the liquid molecules and the adhesive attraction between the liquid molecules and the capillary tube's inner surface. The adhesive properties allow the liquid to cling to the capillary tube wall. The cohesive forces at the surface of the liquid pull the liquid up to the point where the liquid is clinging to the capillary tube wall.

Capillary tubes with a smaller diameter allow the liquid to climb higher because there is less mass being pulled up the tube. Thus a liquid with higher cohesive and adhesive properties and low density climbs further up into a small diameter tube when compared with a liquid with low cohesive and adhesive properties and higher density in a larger diameter tube (e.g., water vs. mercury). Capillary tubes are commonly used in clinical practice for the collection of blood for analysis.

MIXTURE AND MOVEMENT IN BIOLOGICAL SYSTEMS

The physical conditions and phenomena that cause ions, molecules, gases, and liquids to mix and move form the core of cardiopulmonary physiology.

Diffusion

The molecules and ions in a solution are in constant motion (**Brownian motion).** The velocity of these particles is primarily a function of temperature and the degree of cohesive attraction between particles. **Diffusion** describes the movement of molecules or ions from one location to another. Particles will move by diffusion through space in a random fashion. However, when a concentration of particles is higher in one location relative to another, the particles move from the point of highest concentration toward regions of lower concentration. This results in a net diffusion of particles from one region to another (Fig. 1-10). This continues until equilibrium in concentration occurs. When an equal concentration exists, particles continue to move randomly but now there is no net movement of particles toward any particular location. Thus a net diffusion of particles from one point to another occurs from a region of higher concentration to a region of lower concentration.

Many important factors influence the rate of diffusion across a membrane. The more important factors include the size and chemical composition of the ion or molecule that is diffusing, the concentration gradient, the chemical composition of the medium through which diffusion occurs, the distance of diffusion, and the temperature. In the late nineteenth century, Fick described the major factors that influence diffusion through a membrane. **Fick's first law of diffusion** relates these factors:

$$J = \frac{DA(C_1 - C_2)}{d}$$

where J is the net movement or flux of molecules moving by diffusion through a membrane, D is the diffusion coefficient of a given molecule with a certain size at a given temperature (D ≈ molecular solubility in the membrane divided by the square root of the molecular weight), A is the surface area of the membrane, $(C_1 - C_2)$ is the concentration gradient across the membrane, and d is the thickness of the membrane. Fick's equation demonstrates that diffusion of molecules through a membrane is directly related to the concentration gradient of molecules across the membrane, the surface area of the membrane, and the diffusion coefficient. The rate of molecular diffusion is inversely related to the thickness of the membrane. Generally, diffusion occurs most rapidly for small ions or molecules that have high concentration gradients across thin

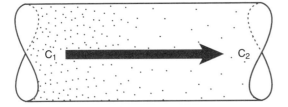

FIG. 1-10 Net migration of particles will move by diffusion from a region of higher concentration *(C₁)* to a region of lower concentration *(C₂)*.

membranes with a relatively large surface area and at elevated temperatures.

Diffusion is a critically important process in the exchange of material across the cell membrane and between different compartments within the body. The movement of O_2 and CO_2 in the lung and between cells is a diffusive process regulated by adjusting the concentrations of gas molecules in various compartments. The cell membrane is best described to be **selectively permeable** because it allows some molecules to move easily (e.g., CO_2) whereas others move poorly (e.g., proteins) through it. This property is both a function of the chemical composition of the cell membrane and the permeability of channels that exist in it. The movement of glucose into or out of the cell is a process of **facilitated diffusion** that utilizes concentration gradients and is facilitated by the actions of hormones (insulin and glucagon) and cell membrane channel proteins.

Osmosis

Water molecules also move by a diffusive process called **osmosis.** The osmotic movement of water generally refers to the movement of water molecules across a water-permeable membrane, which results in equalizing the concentration of water on either side of the membrane.

Fig. 1-11 illustrates a U-shaped container that has a water-permeable membrane separating each limb of the tube. Pure water is placed on one side and a water and protein (e.g., albumin) solution is placed on the other side. The membrane has pores that are large enough for the water molecules to cross through but too small for the much larger protein molecules to cross. As a result of the imbalance in concentration across the membrane, water molecules move into the protein solution side to equalize the concentration. The concentration of the protein solution does decrease, but protein molecules are always

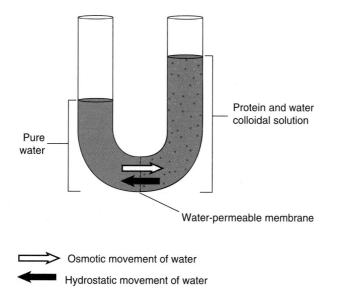

Pure water

Protein and water colloidal solution

Water-permeable membrane

➪ Osmotic movement of water

➧ Hydrostatic movement of water

FIG. 1-11 Water is osmotically attracted across the membrane from the pure water side of the U-shaped tube into the protein and water colloidal solution. Eventually the hydrostatic pressure developed by the height of the colloidal solution will force an equal amount of water back across the membrane. The hydrostatic pressure that offsets the osmotic "pull" of water across the membrane is termed the *oncotic pressure.*

present. The net movement of water does not go on indefinitely. Eventually the movement of water molecules moving across under the influence of osmosis will be equal to the number moving back as a result of building hydrostatic pressure that is produced by the height of the protein solution column. At this point the volume of water in each side stabilizes as the osmotic force is equalized by the hydrostatic pressure generated. The amount of hydrostatic pressure that equalizes the osmotic force is called **osmotic pressure.** In this example the osmotic pressure was generated by a colloidal solution of protein and is, therefore, referred to as a **colloidal oncotic pressure.**

The osmotic pressure generated in an experiment like that depicted in Fig. 1-11 can be determined by using the formula for osmotic pressure:

$$\pi = kC_{\text{solution}} T$$

where π is the osmotic pressure, k is a constant of proportionality (0.0827 L atm/degree K mole), C is the concentration of osmotically active particles, and T is the kelvin temperature. Osmotic pressure increases with increasing concentration of osmotically active particles and the temperature.

Solutions can be compared by the ability to generate osmotic pressure. Two solutions are termed **isosmotic,** or **isotonic,** when they have the same number of particles dissolved. If these solutions were separated by a semipermeable barrier, there would be no net movement of water from one to the other as a result of equal osmotic forces. A 0.9% sodium chloride (saline) solution is isotonic with blood. A solution that has a greater concentration of solutes dissolved in it is **hyperosmotic,** or **hypertonic,** whereas a solution with a lower concentration is **hypoosmotic,** or **hypotonic.** These concepts are important in clinical practice when solutions are given to patients by intravenous infusion. The solutions should be isosmotic with blood to avoid osmotic movement of water into or out of cells. Mixing a hypertonic solution with blood results in the

movement of water out of cells whereas mixing a hypoosmotic solution results in the movement of water into cells. The movement of water into or out of cells could lead to cellular dysfunction or even death.

Active Transport

The net movement of ions and molecules by diffusion and osmosis is from regions of higher concentration to regions of lower concentration. However, many molecules and ions move across cell membranes from regions of lower concentration to regions of higher concentration. In effect these ions and molecules are defying the natural process of diffusion and osmosis. This "up hill" movement of ions and molecules across the cell membrane is a process that requires energy called **active transport.**

Active transport across the cell membrane requires a specific carrier protein that is mounted in the cell membrane. The carrier protein has an active binding site for a specific ion or molecule. When the ion or molecule binds to the site, the carrier protein uses energy from adenosine triphosphate (ATP) to alter its shape and move the ion or molecule to the opposite side of the membrane. Once on the other side, the ion or molecule is released and the carrier protein resumes its low energy shape and is ready to repeat the process. All living cells have thousands of these ion "pumps" in their membranes and carry out this remarkable process. It is estimated that 40% of the cell's entire metabolism supports this activity.

The net result of active transport is the maintenance of different concentrations of ions or molecules in compartments outside and inside the cell. For example, the carrier protein sodium-potassium ATPase moves Na^+ out and K^+ into the cell. The activity of this pump results in a Na^+ concentration that is 14 times higher on the outside and a K^+ concentration that is 28 times higher on the inside of the cell. If this process failed as the result of inadequate ATP production, the cell would accumulate Na^+, thus water would move into the cell osmotically until the cell ruptured. Active transport is critical for the maintenance of life.

Filtration and Reabsorption

The heart's pumping action causes blood to be pressurized within the elastic blood vessels. The blood pressure within microscopic vessels, called *capillaries,* forces water and solutes through the thin cell membrane of the capillary. This form of transport moves water and solute molecules into the interstitial fluid surrounding the capillary. This process of mass movement is called **filtration.** Filtration results in the separation of components in a solution. Separation of the solution results from the hydrostatic pressure exerted on a solution while it is in contact with a semipermeable membrane. Water molecules and small particles such as ions and molecules like glucose are easily forced through the capillary wall by filtration. Larger protein molecules and cells are not capable of moving through the capillary membrane under normal conditions. Filtration is a normal process for the movement of water and small solutes from the vascular system to the cells. Water and solutes are **reabsorbed** back into the vascular system through osmosis and diffusion, respectively. The kidney uses large-scale filtration and reabsorption to regulate the fluid and electrolyte balance of blood. Injuries to the capillary can occur through exposure to toxins or abnormally high blood pressure, which causes the capillary to leak at faster rates than normal and to reabsorb poorly. This may allow proteins and cells to pass through, and edema can occur as a result of excessive filtration and poor reabsorption.

Bulk Flow

The molecules of a gas or liquid can be forced to move in one direction through a certain dis-

tance over a given amount of time. This process of moving a volume of matter from one point to another is termed **bulk flow.** Bulk flow of either gas or liquid depends on unequal force or pressure being applied to it.

Pressure Gradients and the Generation of Flow

If a region of gas or liquid is exposed to higher pressure, the molecules in that region move in mass toward a region of lower pressure. The difference in pressure from one point to another is called a **pressure gradient.** A pressure gradient is necessary for the development of bulk flow.

Fig. 1-12, *A*, shows a reservoir and a system of vertical manometer tubes that holds a volume of liquid. The height of the liquid is equal throughout the system. This illustrates that the system has equal amounts of pressure at any given height in the system. Thus the pressure in the horizontal pipe at the bottom is equal along its entire length. When the liquid is allowed to escape through one end of the horizontal pipe (Fig. 1-12, *B*), the height of the liquid in the various manometer tubes decreases with increasing distance from the reservoir. This demonstrates a uniform pressure drop from the reservoir to the opening of the horizontal pipe. The pressure drop from the top of the reservoir to the opening in the horizontal pipe equals the pressure gradient that is forcing the liquid to flow out through the opening.

The pressure drop shown in Fig. 1-12, *B*, illustrates that the potential energy in the static liquid filled reservoir is being converted to the kinetic energy of a bulk-flowing liquid. In addition, a decrease in potential energy, shown by the uniform drop in the height of liquid in each of the manometer tubes, can be seen as the fluid moves along the horizontal pipe toward the opening. This drop in potential energy or pressure is caused by friction. Friction occurs as a result of the cohesive forces within the liquid (viscosity), the adhesive properties between the liquid and the

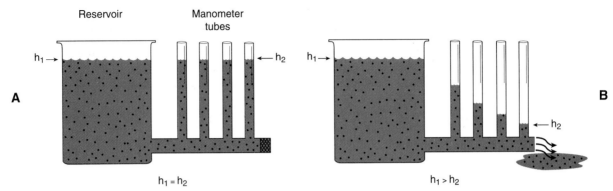

FIG. 1-12 A, Reservoir is filled with liquid to an equal height throughout the system, which generates an equal hydrostatic pressure along the length of the horizontal tube. **B,** When liquid is allowed to flow out of the horizontal tube, a uniform pressure drop occurs as shown by the height of liquid in each of the manometer tubes. The pressure drop indicates the driving pressure and resistance of flow out of the horizontal tube.

wall of the pipe, and the degree of swirling or turbulence in the liquid as it moves through the pipe. Thus the flow rate out of the horizontal pipe is the result of the amount of **driving pressure** applied by the height of the fluid in the reservoir and the amount of **frictional** resistance to flow.

The relationship of flow through a tube, driving pressure, and resistance to flow are united in the following relationship:

$$\dot{V} \text{ or } \dot{Q} = \frac{P_1 - P_2}{R}$$

where $\dot{V}$ is the flow rate of a gas (e.g., air) or $\dot{Q}$ is the flow rate of a liquid (e.g., blood) through the tube, $(P_1 - P_2)$ is the driving pressure or pressure drop across the length of the tube, and R is the resistance to flow. This relationship demonstrates that flow is directly related to the driving pressure and inversely related to the resistance (Fig. 1-13). Increasing the pressure gradient increases flow whereas decreasing the pressure gradient results in decreased flow. Also, an increase in resistance reduces flow whereas reduced resistance results in greater flow.

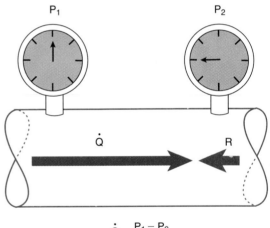

$$\dot{Q} = \frac{P_1 - P_2}{R}$$

FIG. 1-13 Flow $(\dot{Q})$ through a tube is generated by a pressure gradient $(P_1 - P_2)$ and opposed by resistance (R).

For example, what would be the flow of blood through the aorta (a large-diameter artery carrying blood from the heart) if the upstream average or mean pressure is 90 mm Hg, the downstream pressure is 5 mm Hg, and the vascular resistance is 15 mm Hg/L/min?

Table 1-6 Relationships in Hagen-Poiseuille's Law

Flow	Driving Pressure	Tube Radius	Tube Length	Viscosity
↑	↑	Constant	Constant	Constant
↑↑	Constant	↑	Constant	Constant
↑	Constant	Constant	↑	Constant
↑	Constant	Constant	Constant	↓

$$\dot{Q} = \frac{90 - 5 \text{ mm Hg}}{15 \text{ mm Hg/L/min}}$$

$$= \frac{85 \text{ mm Hg}}{15 \text{ mm Hg/L/min}}$$

$$= 5.6 \text{ L/min}$$

Pressure gradient = 90 − 5 mm Hg
Resistance = 15 mm Hg

This flow of blood through the aorta is a normal value in an adult.

Hagen-Poiseuille's Law

The relationship between flow, driving pressure, tube dimension, and viscosity (Fig. 1-14) was independently described by both Hagen and Poiseuille in the middle of the nineteenth century. **Hagen-Poiseuille's law** is as follows:

$$\dot{Q} = \frac{\Delta P \pi r^4}{8 l \eta}$$

where $\dot{Q}$ is the flow rate, ΔP is the driving pressure or pressure gradient ($P_1 - P_2$), r is the radius of the tube, l is the length of the tube, η is the viscosity of the gas or liquid, and 8 and π are constants. This law demonstrates that flow is directly proportional to the driving pressure and to the radius of the tube to the fourth power. This means that if the driving pressure were doubled, the flow would double. Also, the size of the tube, as represented by the radius dimension, has a dramatic effect on flow. Doubling the tube's radius would result in a **sixteenfold** increase in flow. On the

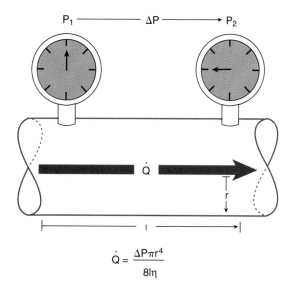

$$\dot{Q} = \frac{\Delta P \pi r^4}{8 \eta}$$

FIG. 1-14 Hagen-Poiseuille's law. Flow $(\dot{Q})$ through a tube is directly proportional to the driving pressure (ΔP) and radius (r) to the fourth power. Flow is inversely proportional to the length (l) and the viscosity of the flowing liquid or gas (η). The constants, π and 8, proportion the equation.

other hand, flow is inversely related to the length of the tube and the viscosity of the liquid or gas. If the tube length increases or the viscosity of the gas or liquid increases, flow decreases. These relationships are summarized in Table 1-6.

Resistance to Flow

The resistance to bulk flow through a tube can be determined by rearranging the general flow equation:

$$R = \frac{P_1 - P_2}{\dot{Q}}$$

This relationship demonstrates that the resistance to flow is directly proportional to the pressure drop across the tube and inversely related to the flow. Greater resistance is present if a given flow requires a high driving pressure.

Calculate the resistance to blood flow in the following example. The average pressure in the pulmonary artery is 20 mm Hg whereas downstream the pressure in the pulmonary vein is 5 mm Hg, yielding a pressure drop or gradient of 15 mm Hg. The flow rate of blood through this network is 5 L/min. What is the pulmonary vascular resistance (R_{pv})?

$$R_{pv} = \frac{20 \text{ mm Hg} - 5 \text{ mm Hg}}{5 \text{ L/min}}$$
$$= \frac{15 \text{ mm Hg}}{5 \text{ L/min}}$$
$$= 3 \text{ mm Hg/L/min}$$

Pressure gradient = $20 - 5$ mm Hg
Flow = 5 L/min

This example demonstrates that for each liter per minute of blood flow through the pulmonary vessels there is a resistance of 3 mm Hg. Or, in other words, for each liter per minute pressure drops 3 mm Hg because of resistance.

The simplified flow equation and the Hagen-Poiseuille's law allows us to see the major elements of resistance:

$$\dot{Q} = \frac{P_1 - P_2}{R} \qquad \dot{Q} = \frac{(P_1 - P_2)\pi r^4}{8l\eta}$$

or $\qquad R = \dfrac{P_1 - P_2}{\dot{Q}} \qquad \dfrac{8l\eta}{\pi r^4} = \dfrac{P_1 - P_2}{\dot{Q}}$

or $\qquad R = \dfrac{8l\eta}{\pi r^4}$

Resistance is directly related to the length of the tube and the viscosity of the gas or liquid. Resistance is also inversely related to the radius of the tube to the fourth power. Accordingly, resistance to flow increases with increased tube length and fluid viscosity and dramatically increases with a decrease in the radius or diameter of the tube.

These relationships help understand the flow, resistance, and pressure drop relationships when comparing blood flow through medium-sized arteries with blood flow through microscopic capillaries. Why is there a significant pressure drop of almost 60 mm Hg across medium-sized arteries when there is virtually no drop across the microscopic capillaries? The higher blood flow through the few medium-sized arteries meets with significant resistance, which results in a significant pressure drop. On the other hand, the much lower flow through billions of microscopic capillaries results in little or no pressure drop. The cross-sectional area of all the capillaries is many more times greater than the relatively few arteries. Therefore flow through a smaller cross-sectional area of arteries results in a greater pressure drop because of the greater resistance to flow.

Laminar and Turbulent Flow

The Hagen-Poiseuille's law describes the behavior of ideal liquid or gas flow that is moving in a laminar flow pattern. Laminar flow is the condition in which all the molecules and ions are moving through a tube in the same direction. As was described earlier, they move in a bullet or parabolic velocity profile (see Fig. 1-7). This pattern results from frictional forces in the liquid and between the liquid and the wall of the tube.

The flow pattern becomes more chaotic at higher flows as the molecules begin to swirl, eddy, and form vortices that generate a **turbulent** flow pattern. Fig. 1-15 shows the relationship between driving pressure and flow. As the driving pressure increases, flow increases

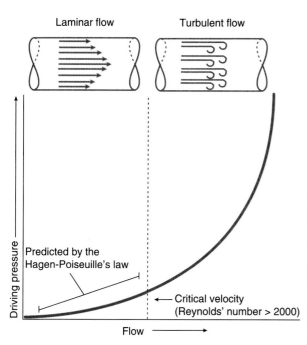

Laminar flow   Turbulent flow

Driving pressure

Predicted by the
Hagen-Poiseuille's law

← Critical velocity
(Reynolds' number > 2000)

Flow →

FIG. 1-15 Relationship between flow, velocity, and driving pressure in laminar and turbulent flow states.

and initially moves in a laminar pattern. When the flow rate reaches a critical value, eddying develops and a turbulent pattern forms. During turbulent flow, molecules of a liquid or gas are not all moving in the same direction and the bulk flow front becomes squared off. It should be noted that the driving pressure necessary to maintain flow rapidly increases with the development of turbulence. The increased driving pressure is needed to overcome the increasing resistance to flow as turbulence develops. Thus turbulent flow requires a greater driving pressure and is, therefore, a much less efficient form of bulk flow transport.

In the late nineteenth century, Reynolds described those conditions that influenced the development of turbulent flow and a method of predicting the point when the flow of a liquid or gas changes from laminar to turbulent flow. **Reynolds' number** describes the flow state and is calculated with the following formula:

$$R_e = \frac{2rv\rho}{\eta}$$

where R_e is Reynolds' number (a dimensionless term), r is the radius of the tube, v is the average velocity of gas or liquid molecules, ρ is the density of the gas or liquid, and η is the viscosity of the gas or liquid. In straight smooth tubes, turbulence occurs when the value of Reynolds' number exceeds 2000. The equation demonstrates that as velocity and density of flowing matter increases in a large tube, the likelihood of developing turbulent flow increases. It also shows that a higher viscosity fluid is less likely to develop turbulence.

Reynolds' number, however, does not account for geometric changes in the tube or the presence of a partial obstruction. These irregularities in the path of flowing gas or liquid induce the formation of turbulence and increase the resistance to flow.

Flow Through Rigid and Distensible Tubes

So far in the discussion of bulk flow, the focus has been on flow through rigid tubing. The vessels of the cardiovascular system and the airways of the lung are distensible tubes that can expand and contract. For example, when you feel your pulse in your wrist you are feeling the pulsatile distension of the radial artery as blood pressure increases and decreases within it. Laplace described that the pulsatile distension generated in a thin vessel resulted from inner pressure-induced wall tension that occurs at right angles to the axis of the tube (Fig. 1-16). The tension is the product of unequal pressure exerted across the wall of the tube. **Laplace's law of distension** (with Frank's modification for vessel wall thickness) calculates the amount of tension developed in a thin-walled tube:

$$T = \frac{(P_i - P_e)r}{\mu}$$

$$T = \frac{(P_i - P_e)r}{\mu}$$

Normal vessel

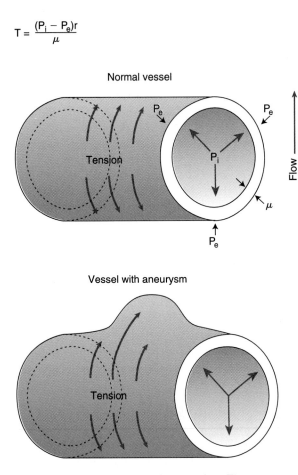

Vessel with aneurysm

FIG. 1-16 Laplace's law of distension. The pressure-tension relationship of a normal blood vessel and a vessel that has weakened and developed an aneurysm. Vessel wall tension is directly proportional to the pressure difference $(P_i - P_e)$ across the wall and the radius *(r)* of the vessel. Tension development is inversely proportional to the vessel wall thickness *(μ)*.

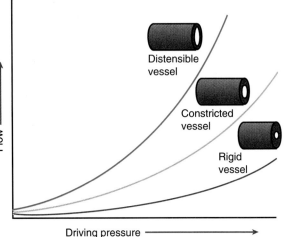

FIG. 1-17 Blood flow and driving pressure relationship in distensible, constricted, and rigid vessels. Note the much greater flow through the more distensible vessels at higher driving pressures.

where T is the circumferential tension generated, $(P_i - P_e)$ (or P_{i-e}) is the pressure difference between the internal and external surfaces of the tube, r is the radius of the tube, and μ is the wall thickness. The amount of tension developed in the wall of the tube increases with the pressure difference and the size or radius of the tube. The tension is reduced with increasing wall thickness. This demonstrates that a large, thin-walled tube (e.g., a large vein) experiences high wall tension with increasing internal pressure that would lead to the distension.

In those people with high blood pressure, the artery wall tension is chronically elevated, which may lead to weakening of the wall. Sections of the wall may thin and balloon outward, further weakening the artery wall. This condition of artery wall ballooning is called an arterial **aneurysm** (see Fig. 1-16). An arterial aneurysm requires surgical repair to avoid a sudden rupture that is often life threatening.

The driving pressure requirements to force a flow of gas or liquid through a distensible tube are different when compared with that of a rigid tube. Fig. 1-17 shows the difference in flows in different types of vessels with increasing driving pressure. The rigid vessel has blood flow that is predicted by Hagen-Poiseuille's law. The distensible vessel has a much greater flow. Greater flow is possible as the diameter of the vessel opens up with increasing driving pressure. The constricted vessel demonstrates intermediate characteristics of both a rigid vessel and a vessel that does allow some distension. These conditions are found in the vascular system such as the thin-walled veins that distend easily, the constricted arteries with thicker walls, and the more rigid diseased arteries that have extensive depositions of calcium and fat in their walls (atherosclerosis). The ability of vessels and airways to distend reduces the work needed to pump blood and air through them.

CHAPTER SELF-TEST QUESTIONS

1. A patient is being high-frequency ventilated at a rate of 300 times per minute. What is the frequency in hertz?
   a. 300.0
   b. 10.0
   c. 5.0
   d. 1.0
2. A sample of gas is found to have a PO_2 of 100 mm Hg. What is the partial pressure in kilopascals?
   a. 137.0
   b. 17.3
   c. 1.3
   d. 13.3
3. The mechanical work done on an object is the mathematical product of _____.
   a. distance ÷ force
   b. force × distance
   c. distance ÷ volume
   d. force ÷ volume
4. What is the equivalent kelvin temperature when the Celsius temperature is 30°?
   a. 273
   b. 243
   c. 303
   d. 310
5. The density of a gas or a liquid is defined by which one of the following relationships?

a. mass × volume
b. volume × mass
c. mass ÷ volume
d. volume ÷ mass
6. 1 atm of pressure is equal to
   a. 76 mm Hg
   b. 10.3 cm H_2O
   c. 14.7 lbs/in
   d. 1000 kPa
7. 3.2 L of gas at 15° C is heated to 37° C. What will the new volume be if the pressure is held constant at 1 atm of pressure?
   a. 7.9 L
   b. 1.3 L
   c. 3.4 L
   d. 2.9 L
8. A sample of gas at 2° C has a pressure of 40 mm Hg. What will the new pressure be if the temperature is raised to 37° C while holding the volume constant?
   a. 36 mm Hg
   b. 45 mm Hg
   c. 74 mm Hg
   d. 22 mm Hg
9. 5.7 L of gas at 1 atm of pressure is exposed to a new pressure of 700 mm Hg. What will the new volume be if the temperature is held constant?
   a. 6.2 L
   b. 3.8 L
   c. 7.8 L
   d. 5.3 L
10. According to the equation used to determine Reynolds' number, which of the three following conditions would increase the likelihood of developing a turbulent flow pattern in a gas flowing through a tube?
    1. increased gas velocity
    2. decreased gas viscosity
    3. increased tube radius
       a. 1 only
       b. 1 and 3
       c. 2 and 3
       d. 1, 2, and 3

For answers, see p. 475.

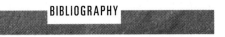
BIBLIOGRAPHY

1. Abbot AF: *Physics,* ed 5, Oxford, 1989, Heinemann Educational.
2. Burton AC: *Physiology and biophysics of the circulation,* Chicago, 1972, Year Book Medical.
3. Cromer AH: *Physics for the life sciences,* ed 2, New York, 1977, McGraw-Hill.
4. Epstein II: *Basic physics in anesthesiology,* Chicago, 1976, Year Book Medical.
5. Green JF: *Fundamental cardiovascular and pulmonary physiology,* ed 2, Philadelphia, 1987, Lea & Febiger.
6. Hewit PG: *Conceptual physics,* ed 7, New York, 1993, Harper Collins.
7. Holland HD: *The chemistry of the atmosphere and oceans,* New York, 1978, John Wiley & Sons.
8. MacDonald SG, Burns DM: *Physics for the life and health sciences,* Menlo Park, Calif, 1975, Addison-Wesley.
9. Nave CR, Nave BC: *Physics for the health science,* ed 2, Philadelphia, 1985, WB Saunders.
10. Serway RA, Faughn JS: *College physics,* ed 4, Philadelphia, 1995, WB Saunders.
11. Weast RC: *Handbook of chemistry and physics,* ed 69, New York, 1988, Chemical Rubber.

Anatomy of the Cardiovascular System

CHAPTER OBJECTIVES

Upon completing this chapter, you will be able to:

1 Describe the general design of the cardiovascular system.
2 List the general functions of the systemic and pulmonary circuits.
3 Describe the embryological development of the heart.
4 Identify the size, location, and structure of the human heart.
5 Describe the pathway for blood flow from the vena cava through the heart and to the aorta.
6 List and locate the major arteries and veins of the coronary circulation.
7 Describe the structure and function of arteries, capillaries, and veins.
8 List and locate the major arteries and veins.
9 Describe the general structure and function of the lymphatic system.

● WHY A CIRCULATORY SYSTEM IS NEEDED

A functioning cardiovascular system is critical to survival through its support of a stable internal environment. The complex structure of the human body requires a circulatory system to provide a continuous flow of blood to each cell. Cellular metabolism is supported by the circulatory system by a supply of nutrients, gas exchange, waste removal, hormone transport, thermoregulation, and tissue defense and repair. If the cardiovascular system were to fail and blood was not circulated for more than 10 minutes, tissues throughout the body would not receive an adequate supply of oxygen. Also, nutrients and waste products such as carbon dioxide and lactic acid would rapidly accumulate. Under these conditions the cells would experience metabolic dysfunction that could lead to widespread organ failure and death.

Vascular Circuit Design

The circulatory system is a closed system of cardiac chambers and blood vessels. In 1628 Harvey described the current concept that blood is continuously pumped in a circular route from the heart, to arteries, through capillaries, into veins, and back to the heart. Our

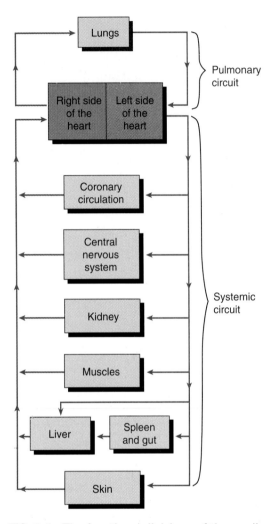

FIG. 2-1   The functional divisions of the cardiovascular system are divided into pulmonary and systemic circuits. Note that blood flows from the pulmonary circuit to the systemic circuit and back to the pulmonary circuit as a "series" system. Within both circuits are "parallel" circuits through various organs.

mammalian cardiovascular system is really two separate systems or circuits (Fig. 2-1). The **systemic circuit** is a large circuit that includes the left side of the heart and vessels that supply blood to and from various systemic organs including the brain, gastrointestinal tract, liver, skeletal and cardiac muscles, bone, skin, kidneys, and various endocrine glands. The **pulmonary circuit** is a smaller circuit that includes the right side of the heart and blood vessels that carry blood to and from the lungs for gas exchange. The two circuits are organized so that blood flow is pumped from one circuit to the other. The two circuits of this typical mammalian design are separated for greater gas exchange efficiency.

HOW AND WHEN THE HEART IS FORMED

Embryologic Development of the Heart

Following fertilization, the developing human undergoes a remarkable series of anatomic and physiologic changes throughout the 266 days, or 38 weeks, of pregnancy. During the first 3 weeks after conception, the embryo develops without a circulatory system and relies on simple diffusion for gas, nutrients, and waste exchange with nearby maternal blood and tissues. As the embryo enlarges and simple diffusion is unable to support development, the cardiovascular system forms before many of the other organ systems. On day 20 after conception, angiogenic cells of the mesodermal layer of the developing embryo form a simple tubular heart within a primitive pericardial cavity (Fig. 2-2). This tubular heart is formed from an inner lining of **endothelial cells,** a loose connective tissue middle layer called **cardiac jelly,** and an outer layer of myoepicardial cells, which gives rise to the heart muscle. On day 21 after conception the primitive heart begins to beat as the myoepicardial cells contract in synchrony. On either end of the heart are primitive arteries and veins. Development of the heart and vessels proceeds while it continues to beat and supply blood to the developing embryo. By day 23 the rapidly growing heart twists into an S-shaped structure as the arterial ends are pulled down and the venous

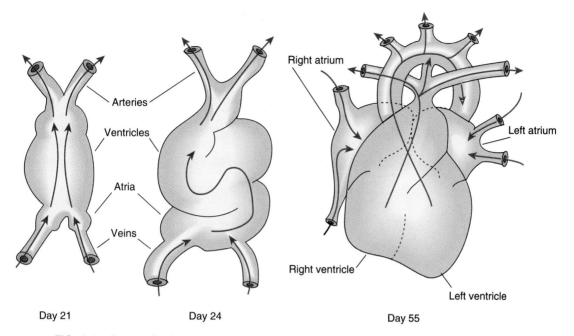

FIG. 2-2 Anatomic changes in the embryonic development of the heart at different points in time following fertilization.

ends are pulled up and behind. Between days 27 and 33 the arteries divide into the **pulmonary trunk,** which supplies blood to the pulmonary circuit, and an **aortic trunk,** which supplies blood to the systemic circuit. During this same period, walls, or septa, begin to form within the atrial and ventricular chambers. When the septa are complete on about day 55, the previously common ventricle (similar to the single ventricle of a frog) separates into right and left chambers. The atrial septum does not completely close until after birth. A septal opening (**foramen ovale**) is maintained throughout gestation for better oxygenated blood returning from the placenta to flow from the right atrium to the left atrium and on into the systemic circuit. The valves of the heart form during this same period of septal development. Between day 55 and the end of pregnancy the heart undergoes little change other than enlargement and refinement.

⬤ STRUCTURE AND LOCATION OF THE HEART

Size and Position of the Heart

The adult human heart is a cone-shaped structure that is about the size of your clenched fist and weighs approximately 310 g in men and 225 g in women. It is located in the center and lower half of the thoracic cavity (Figs. 2-3 and 2-4) and lies within a membrane-bound region called the **mediastinum,** which is a space formed between the lungs. Other structures within the mediastinum include the great vessels of the heart, trachea, esophagus, numerous lymph nodes and vessels, thymus gland, and phrenic and vagus nerves. The heart lies at an oblique angle in the middle of the mediastinum between the sternum and the vertebral column.

The heart has a **base,** an **apex,** and **borders.** The base is located on the superior aspect of

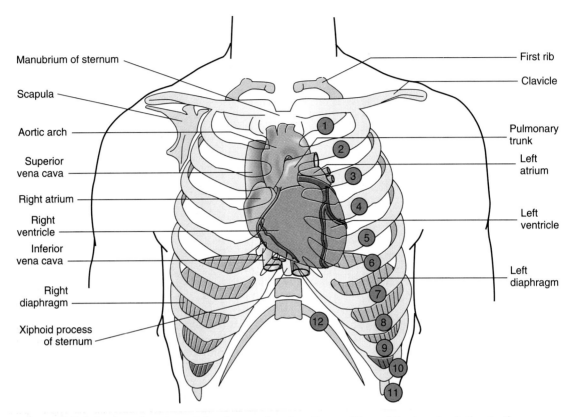

FIG. 2-3 Anterior view of the thorax showing the position of the heart relative to the rib cage, sternum, vertebral column, and diaphragm.

the heart. The heart extends downward from its base, into the left hemithorax, and anteriorly to end in the blunt apex. The apex can be felt thumping the chest wall in a region just below the left nipple at a level between the fifth and sixth ribs (fifth intercostal space). This physical examination landmark is referred to as the **point of maximal impulse (PMI)** and indicates the heart's position within the thorax. On a rare occasion the clinician may encounter an individual who has a heart that lies in the right hemithorax—a condition called **dextrocardia.**

Anatomy of the Heart

To function as a pump, the heart must have vessels to carry blood to it, blood-collecting chambers, pumping chambers, valves to prevent back-flow, and vessels to carry blood away.

External Features of the Heart

On the superior end, or base, of the heart are the trunks of the great vessels that bring blood to and from the heart and the external appendages of the right and left atria (Fig. 2-5). The large muscular region that forms the right

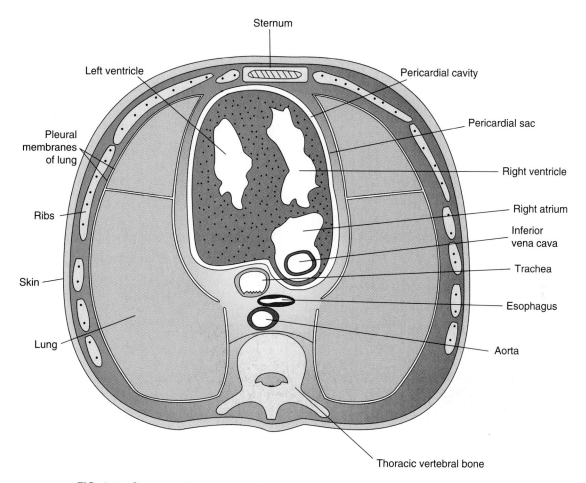

FIG. 2-4 Cross-sectional view of the thorax showing the position of the heart in the mediastinum.

and left **ventricles** lies below the atria. Grooves, or sulci, are found on the surface of the heart. A prominent **atrioventricular sulcus** runs horizontally around the heart between the upper and lower chambers. The **interventricular sulci** run down the anterior and posterior surfaces from the base to the apex. These sulci contain the major coronary arteries and veins, which supply the heart's muscle with blood.

Membranes and Wall of the Heart

The wall of the heart is comprised of three distinct layers: an outer **pericardium,** a thick

muscular myocardium, and an inner **endocardium** (Fig. 2-6).

The pericardium is a saclike structure that contains the heart. It is comprised of tough, white **fibrous pericardium** and a thin **serous pericardium.** The fibrous portion is comprised of collagen fibers that give it a rather inelastic quality. The moist serous pericardium, or parietal pericardium, lines the inner surface of the sac. The two layers form a loose sac that extends down from the great vessels, over the heart, and on to the diaphragm, which separates the thoracic and abdominal cavities. The

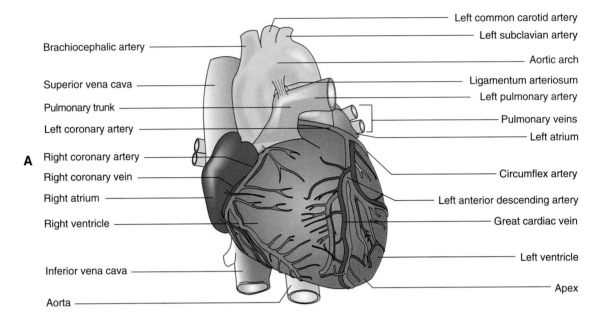

A

Brachiocephalic artery

Superior vena cava

Pulmonary trunk

Left coronary artery

Right coronary artery

Right coronary vein

Right atrium

Right ventricle

Inferior vena cava

Aorta

Left common carotid artery

Left subclavian artery

Aortic arch

Ligamentum arteriosum

Left pulmonary artery

Pulmonary veins

Left atrium

Circumflex artery

Left anterior descending artery

Great cardiac vein

Left ventricle

Apex

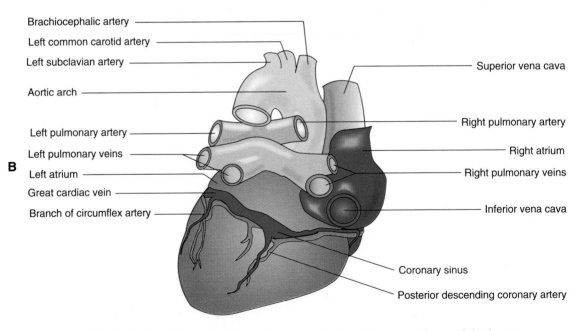

B

Brachiocephalic artery

Left common carotid artery

Left subclavian artery

Aortic arch

Left pulmonary artery

Left pulmonary veins

Left atrium

Great cardiac vein

Branch of circumflex artery

Superior vena cava

Right pulmonary artery

Right atrium

Right pulmonary veins

Inferior vena cava

Coronary sinus

Posterior descending coronary artery

FIG. 2-5 A, Anterior, and **B,** posterior views of the external anatomy of the heart.

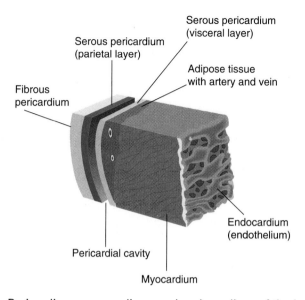

Serous pericardium
(visceral layer)

Serous pericardium
(parietal layer)

Adipose tissue
with artery and vein

Fibrous
pericardium

Endocardium
(endothelium)

Pericardial cavity

Myocardium

FIG. 2-6   Pericardium, myocardium, and endocardium of the heart wall.

serous layer is a continuous layer that lines both the inner surface of the pericardial sac and the outer surface of the heart muscle. The serous lining on the heart's surface is called the **visceral pericardium,** or the **epicardium.** A thin pericardial cavity is formed between the parietal and visceral membranes. This cavity is filled with a small amount of clear **pericardial fluid** that is secreted and reabsorbed by the serous membranes. The pericardial fluid acts to lubricate the moving surfaces of the heart muscle within the pericardial sac.

Although the pericardial sac forms a protective lining around the heart, it can also be a source of problems. Blood coming from the heart or vessels can be trapped and can accumulate within the firm pericardial sac. Collection of as little as 30 ml of blood or fluid can compromise filling of the heart's chambers and result in heart failure. This condition is called a **cardiac tamponade.** Infections of the pericardial sac can lead to inflammation of the pericardial membranes, which is termed **pericarditis.** Pericarditis can result in a roughened

inner sac surface, pain, excess fluid accumulation, and heart failure in extreme cases.

The myocardium is the muscular layer that is responsible for generating the force that propels blood out of the heart. It can vary in thickness in different regions of the heart. The atrial regions are approximately 2 mm thick and are the thinnest myocardiums in the heart. The right ventricle free wall is approximately 4 mm thick whereas that of the left ventricle is approximately 12 mm thick. The myocardial wall of the ventricles is comprised of numerous overlapping and interdigitating layers of cardiac muscle fibers. The various layers originate on the fibrous plate of the cardiac skeleton at the base of the great vessels, twist down around the apex of the heart, and bend back up and insert back on to the fibrous plate. Fig. 2-7 shows the orientation of muscle fibers in the left ventricular myocardium during a contraction. The outer and inner fibers are obliquely oriented at 45-degree angles with respect to the midwall fibers, which are oriented in a circumferential pattern around the

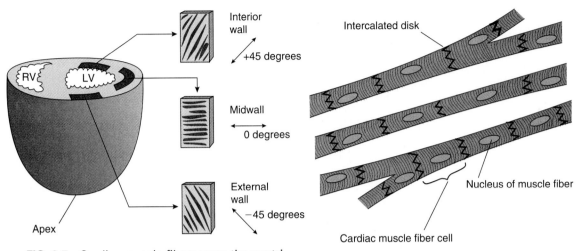

FIG. 2-7 Cardiac muscle fibers wrap the ventricles in various orientations. The internal and external wall fibers are oriented at oblique angles, and the mid-wall fibers wrap the ventricles in a circumferential pattern. (*RV,* Right ventricle; *LV,* left ventricle.)

FIG. 2-8 Cardiac muscle fibers as seen under the microscope.

ventricle. The result of this orientation allows the inner and outer fibers to pull the apex and base of the heart together while the midwall fibers squeeze the apposing walls of the ventricle together. Both actions reduce the volume of the ventricle chambers during the contraction phase of the cardiac cycle. The irregular inner surface (the **trabeculae carneae**) of both ventricles is formed by the folding and bridging of muscle fibers.

A thin endocardium lines the inner surface of the cardiac chambers. It is comprised of a single layer of squamous epithelium and a basement membrane. Extensions and folds of this tissue form the valves of the heart. The epithelial cells of the endocardium are part of the **endothelium,** which lines the entire circulatory system.

Myocardial Cells

Cardiac muscle fibers form the bulk of the myocardium. They are striated fibers that contain numerous contractile filaments of **actin** and **myosin** that are arranged in essentially the same pattern as is found in skeletal muscle fibers (Fig. 2-8). Unlike skeletal muscle fibers, each cardiac muscle fiber is fused to the next one at a connection called the **intercalated disk.** Numerous **gap junctions** are also present within the intercalated disks and function to allow the transfer of material between cells. Cardiac fibers branch and have a single nucleus in each fiber segment. The branching and fusing of these fibers at the intercalated disks enable the entire cardiac muscle to function as a single unit or **syncytium.** The intercalated disks and gap junctions permit the contraction stimulus to pass from one cell to the next. This allows the contraction to proceed throughout the entire cardiac muscle in a uniform manner without the need of nerve fibers to stimulate each cell. Skeletal muscle, on the other hand, requires thousands of motor nerve fibers to send the needed im-

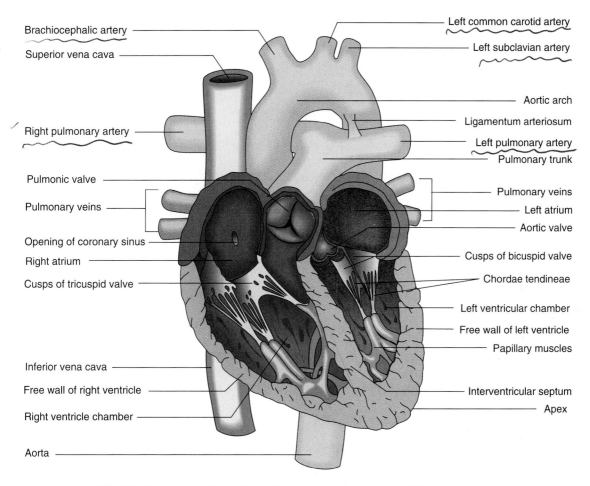

Brachiocephalic artery

Superior vena cava

Right pulmonary artery

Pulmonic valve

Pulmonary veins

Opening of coronary sinus

Right atrium

Cusps of tricuspid valve

Inferior vena cava

Free wall of right ventricle

Right ventricle chamber

Aorta

Left common carotid artery

Left subclavian artery

Aortic arch

Ligamentum arteriosum

Left pulmonary artery

Pulmonary trunk

Pulmonary veins

Left atrium

Aortic valve

Cusps of bicuspid valve

Chordae tendineae

Left ventricular chamber

Free wall of left ventricle

Papillary muscles

Interventricular septum

Apex

FIG. 2-9   Coronal section through the heart showing the interior anatomy.

pulses to each of millions of skeletal muscle fibers within a muscle. Cardiac muscle fibers also contain the red oxygen-carrying pigment **myoglobin** and have numerous mitochondria to support their aerobic metabolism.

Chambers and Valves of the Heart

The heart is actually comprised of two pumps in one (Fig. 2-9). The chambers of the right and left sides of the heart are separated by a vertical septum. Blood enters each side of the heart by way of a chamber called an **atrium.** The right and left atria are thin-walled structures that are located on the superior and posterior parts of the heart. Blood is prevented from mixing between these two chambers by the **interatrial septum.** Blood flows from each atrium through an atrioventricular valve into the **ventricles.** The more muscular ventricles pump blood through a pair of **semilunar valves** to the pulmonary and systemic circuits.

The muscles of both atria and ventricles and the valves are attached to a fibrous plate of connective tissue referred to as the **cardiac**

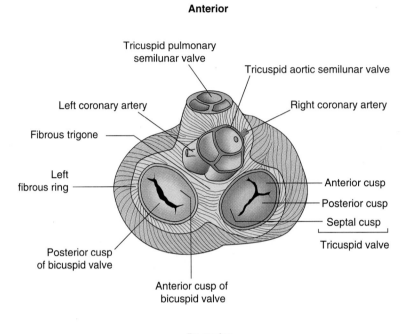

Anterior

Tricuspid pulmonary semilunar valve

Tricuspid aortic semilunar valve

Left coronary artery

Right coronary artery

Fibrous trigone

Left fibrous ring

Anterior cusp

Posterior cusp

Septal cusp

Tricuspid valve

Posterior cusp of bicuspid valve

Anterior cusp of bicuspid valve

Posterior

FIG. 2-10 Looking down on the base of the heart with the atria and great vessels removed. The fibrous skeleton of the heart (annulus fibrosus) is shown with the valves in relative position.

skeleton or **annulus fibrosus** (Fig. 2-10). This plate of connective tissue separates the atrial and ventricular cavities and houses the atrioventricular and semilunar valves.

The **tricuspid** and **bicuspid** atrioventricular **valves** function as in-flow valves for the ventricles. The tricuspid valve is comprised of three leaves, or **cusps,** and functions to direct blood flow from the right atrium to the right ventricle. The bicuspid valve, or **mitral valve,** is formed by two cusps and directs blood flow from the left atrium to the left ventricle (Fig. 2-11). The cusps of both valves are supported from below by inelastic strands of connective tissue called **chordae tendineae** and cone-shaped muscles called **papillary muscles** that are anchored in the walls and floors of the ventricles. The tricuspid and bicuspid

valves act as check valves to prevent blood from flowing backward into the atria when the ventricles contract. The supporting chordae tendineae and papillary muscles prevent the valve cusps from opening as pressure builds in the ventricles during a contraction.

Two semilunar valves function as out-flow valves for the ventricles. The **pulmonary valve,** or **semilunar valve,** is located at the base of the **pulmonary trunk.** It has three cusps and functions to direct blood flow out of the right ventricle into the pulmonary circuit. The **aortic semilunar valve,** located at the base of the **aorta,** also has three cusps and functions to direct blood flow from the left ventricle into the systemic circulatory system (see Fig. 2-11). Both semilunar valves act as check valves to prevent blood from flowing backward into the

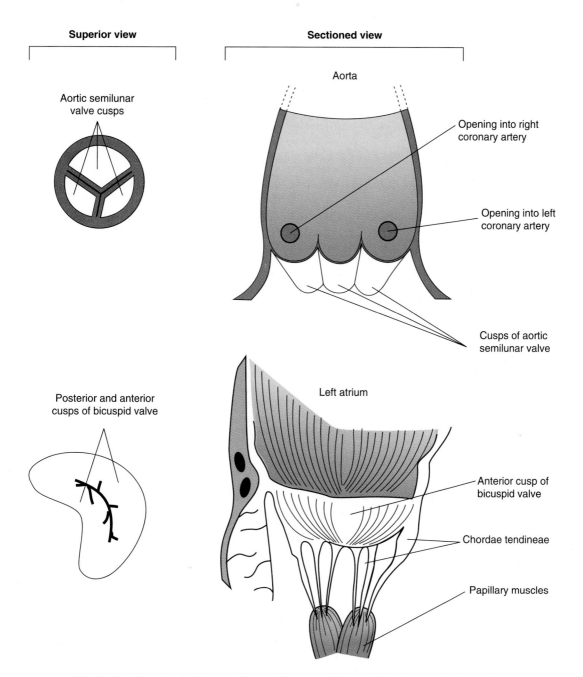

Superior view

Sectioned view

Aortic semilunar
valve cusps

Aorta

Opening into right
coronary artery

Opening into left
coronary artery

Cusps of aortic
semilunar valve

Posterior and anterior
cusps of bicuspid valve

Left atrium

Anterior cusp of
bicuspid valve

Chordae tendineae

Papillary muscles

FIG. 2-11   Structure of the aortic semilunar and bicuspid atrioventricular valves.

Mitral Valve Stenosis and Regurgitation

A 61-year-old woman began to experience increasing shortness of breath (dyspnea) and congested coughing during her work in the garden, and she would occasionally faint. She was seen by her physician who found her to have a systolic murmur over the area of the mitral valve and crackling breath sounds during inspiration over the lower half of both lung fields. The history and physical findings suggested transient congestive heart failure with pulmonary edema possibly from mitral valve stenosis and regurgitation.

Mitral valve stenosis is a condition of narrowing and stiffening of the valve. Regurgitation is a backward flow of blood through the valve that results from incomplete closure of the valve during left ventricular contraction. When this occurs, less blood flows into the systemic circuit and greater amounts remain in the pulmonary circuit. This can result in reduced systemic blood pressure and increased pulmonary blood pressure. The increased pulmonary pressures can lead to fluid leakage and congestion in the lungs. These changes can be intensified during exercise and lead to dyspnea (difficulty breathing) and a congestive cough.

She was referred for resting and for an exercise stress echocardiography. Echocardiography is a noninvasive technique that uses a surface probe to emit and detect the reflections of ultrasonic sound waves. In this type of case it is used to study the structures and blood flow within the heart. At rest her mitral valve was found to be narrowed, some blood flow was seen to flow backward through it (mitral regurgitation), and the right ventricle wall was found to be thickened and enlarged (right ventricular hypertrophy). After exercising on a treadmill for a few minutes to the point of significant dyspnea, the amount of regurgitation was seen to significantly increase, the heart dilated somewhat, and she developed jugular vein distension. Jugular vein distension occurs when the right side of the heart is unable to pump all of the venous blood returning to it. This suggests that the right ventricle is failing as the pulmonary pressures increase.

The physician decided to perform surgery and replace the diseased valve with a Starr-Edwards ball-type prosthetic valve and to place her on anticoagulant therapy. She tolerated the procedure well and recovered.

---

ventricles from the pulmonary trunk and aorta. Neither of these valves is supported by chordae tendineae or papillary muscles. When blood begins to flow backward through these valves, the cusps fill with blood and form a tight seal as they make contact with each other.

◖ BLOOD FLOW PATTERN THROUGH THE HEART

Understanding the normal blood flow pattern through the heart is central to understanding the variations brought on by abnormal devel-opment, disease, and injury. It is traditionally described by tracing flow as blood returns from the systemic veins to the right side of the heart, out to the pulmonary circuit, back to the left side of the heart, and out to the arterial vessels of the systemic circuit. The major components are listed in Fig. 2-12.

Blood Flow Through the Heart

Systemic venous blood returns to the heart by way of the superior vena cava, the inferior vena cava, and the **coronary sinus.** The superior vena cava returns venous blood from the

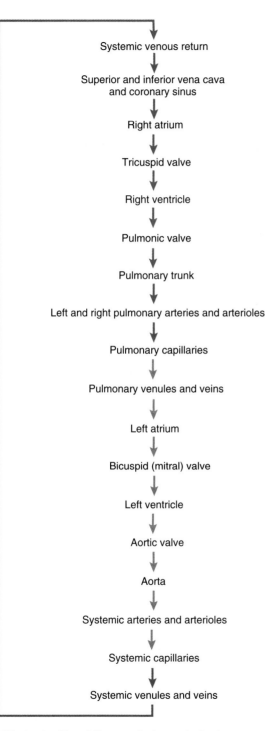

Systemic venous return

↓

Superior and inferior vena cava
and coronary sinus

↓

Right atrium

↓

Tricuspid valve

↓

Right ventricle

↓

Pulmonic valve

↓

Pulmonary trunk

↓

Left and right pulmonary arteries and arterioles

↓

Pulmonary capillaries

↓

Pulmonary venules and veins

↓

Left atrium

↓

Bicuspid (mitral) valve

↓

Left ventricle

↓

Aortic valve

↓

Aorta

↓

Systemic arteries and arterioles

↓

Systemic capillaries

↓

Systemic venules and veins

FIG. 2-12   Blood flow path through the heart.

head, upper extremities, and chest wall. The inferior vena cava is returning venous blood from the trunk, abdominal organs, and lower extremities. The coronary sinus returns venous blood from the myocardium. Blood from these veins is emptied into the right atrium. The right atrium is a reservoir for returning venous blood. The pressure exerted by the returning venous blood coupled with right atrial contraction directs blood through the tricuspid valve. For the valve to open and blood to flow through it, blood pressures must be greater on the atrial side of the valve. Blood flow through the tricuspid valve is directed into the right ventricle.

During right ventricular contraction, blood pressure increases within the chamber, the tricuspid valve closes, and blood is forced through the pulmonary semilunar valve into the trunk of the pulmonary artery and on to the pulmonary circuit. The blood flows through the left and right pulmonary arteries and into each corresponding lung. Flow continues through pulmonary capillaries, where gas exchange occurs. Blood drains from the pulmonary circuit back to the heart by way of four pulmonary veins.

Highly oxygenated blood returns to the left atrium from the pulmonary veins. The left atrium also functions as a reservoir for blood returning to the heart. In addition to being slightly smaller than the right atrium, the left atrium is less distensible. This property enhances pulmonary venous flow through the bicuspid valve and into the left ventricle.

During contraction of the left ventricle, blood is forced out through the aortic semilunar valve and into the aorta and on into the systemic circuit. After flowing through the systemic arteries and capillaries, blood returns to the heart by way of the two vena cava.

Anatomy of the Coronary Circulation

Blood is supplied to the heart by the right and left coronary arteries from the systemic circuit

(Fig. 2-13). These vessels originate at the base of the aortic trunk in a region called the coronary sinus, which is just above the cusps of the aortic semilunar valve. High-pressure arterial blood flows from the aorta through these arteries to the tissues of the heart.

The right coronary artery arises from the right side of the aorta and extends down the outside of the heart embedded in adipose tissue in the atrioventricular sulcus. It branches in most subjects to give rise to the conus artery, sinus artery, marginal branch arteries, and the posterior descending artery. The conus artery supplies blood to portions of the right ventricle. The sinus artery supplies blood to regions of the right atrium. The branches of the marginal arteries supply blood to most of the right ventricular free wall. The posterior descending artery supplies blood to the interventricular septum and inferior free wall of the left ventricle. In about 70% of normal subjects the posterior descending and atrioventricular branches arise from the right coronary artery. This is occasionally referred to anatomically as being a "right-dominant" system. Dominance in this context is an anatomic reference and does not imply that most of the heart receives blood from the right coronary artery. In fact, the bulk of the myocardium's blood flow normally comes from the left coronary artery system.

The left coronary artery arises from the left side of the aorta and advances out between the pulmonary artery and left atrium. Its major branches include the left anterior descending artery and the **circumflex artery.** The left anterior descending artery is embedded in epicardial adipose tissue and extends down the anterior surface of the heart. In most subjects it supplies blood to the interventricular septum and the anterior free wall of both the left and right ventricles. The circumflex artery extends around toward the posterior and inferior portion of the heart and supplies blood to the left ventricular free wall.

More than half a million people in the United States die each year from coronary disease. Coronary artery disease or **coronary atherosclerosis** is the leading cause. It results in

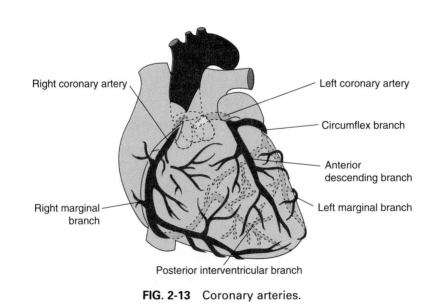

Right coronary artery

Left coronary artery

Circumflex branch

Anterior descending branch

Right marginal branch

Left marginal branch

Posterior interventricular branch

FIG. 2-13 Coronary arteries.

a narrowing of the coronary arteries. Fig. 2-14 shows cross-sectional specimens taken from various individuals that range from less than 15% blockage (grade 0) to 100% blockage (grade 5). This disorder is a chronic and progressive disease that primarily affects the surface of epicardial coronary arteries. The obstructive lesion, or atheroma, is most often a fatty deposition in the wall of the artery that results in luminal narrowing. High cholesterol concentrations in blood (>240 mg/dl) are associated with the disorder. The degree of narrowing generally must exceed 75% obstruction to produce inadequate blood flow in cardiac tissues at rest. If blood flow to regions of the heart is interrupted for a few

seconds, a sharp or heavy pressurelike pain is often felt in the center of the chest and frequently radiates into the left arm and up into the neck as **referred pain.** Chest pain of this nature is called **angina pectoralis.** If blood flow is restricted for more than 10 minutes, adequate supplies of oxygen will not be delivered to cardiac tissues and regions of heart muscle will fail to function correctly and will die. Death of cardiac muscle tissue is commonly referred to as a **myocardial infarction** or more generally as a heart attack.

The right and left coronary artery branches are interconnected or anastomosed by very small arteries that provide the potential for cross flow from one artery to the other.

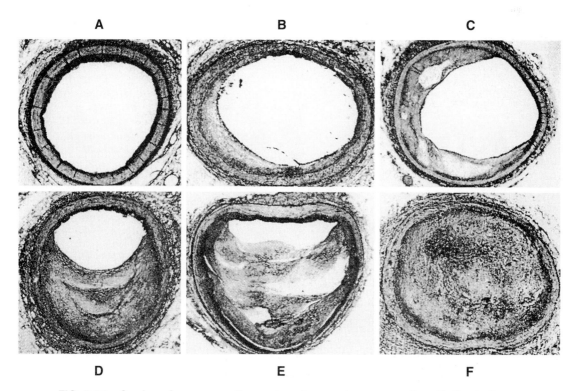

FIG. 2-14 Grades of coronary atherosclerosis seen in cross section. **A,** Grade 0 normal vessel from a 33-year-old woman. **B,** Grade 1 from a 54-year-old woman. **C,** Grade 2 from a 54-year-old woman. **D,** Grade 3 from a 74-year-old woman. **E,** Grade 4 from a 69-year-old man. **F,** Grade 5 (100% occlusion) from a 62-year-old man. (Courtesy of the Mayo Foundation.)

Normally, these **collateral vessels** provide little cross flow of blood. If, however, obstruction occurs in a branch of one or more coronary arteries, the collateral vessels may provide additional blood flow to those regions that have reduced blood supply.

Blood that has passed through the capillaries of the cardiac tissues flows into the coronary venous system. These veins parallel the arteries and are easily located in the coronary sulci. The **cardiac veins** are found on the anterior and posterior surfaces of the heart and drain about 65% to 75% of the blood into the **coronary sinus.** The coronary sinus runs horizontally across the posterior portion of the heart just below the left atrium in the atrioventricular sulcus. It returns blood to the right atrium. The anterior coronary vein carries about 15% to 20% of the blood into the right atrium. A small amount of venous blood is drained by the arteriosinusoidal, arterioluminal, and Thebesian vessels directly into the atrial and ventricular chambers of both hearts. The coronary circulation is summarized in Fig. 2-15.

HOW THE STRUCTURE OF BLOOD VESSELS FACILITATES FUNCTION

Blood leaves and returns to the heart by way of numerous blood vessels that are collectively referred to as the vascular system (Table 2-1). Vessels that carry blood *away* from the heart are termed **arteries.** The major arteries that carry blood away from the heart include the aorta and pulmonary arteries. These vessels branch into hundreds of major arteries, which further branch into approximately one-half million smaller **arterioles** where they branch into billions of microscopic **capillaries.** The capillaries join and blood drains into millions of **venules** that converge into hundreds of major **veins.** The major veins *return* blood to the atria by way of the superior and inferior vena cava and the pulmonary veins.

Form and Function of the Arteries and Veins

Arteries and veins have tubular walls that are comprised of three different layers, or tunics, of tissue (Fig. 2-16). The outermost layer, the **tunica externa,** is composed of elastic and collagenous connective tissue. Vessels such as the aorta have small nutritive blood vessels, the vasa vasorum, which are located in the tunica externa and supply the muscular and outer connective tissue layers with blood. Just below the tunica externa is a thin layer of elastic fibers, or **elastin,** which is called the **external elastic lamina.** The aorta and other large arteries have a thicker layer of elastin in their

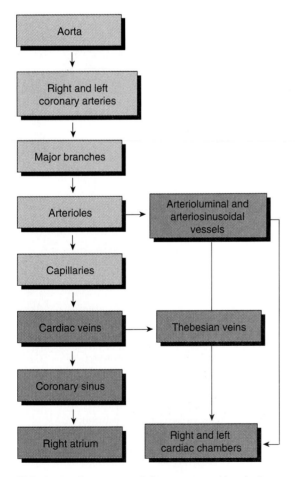

FIG. 2-15 Summary of the coronary circulation.

walls. This greater elastic quality allows these vessels to swell as blood is pumped into them. As they swell (which you feel as a pulse), they store potential energy in the elastic fibers of their wall. When the pressure drops, the artery releases the stored potential energy as it recoils back to its original size which, in turn, forces blood toward the tissues.

The middle layer, the **tunica media,** is comprised largely of smooth muscle fibers. The muscle fibers are primarily organized in a circular orientation. Arteries have a much thicker

● Table 2-1   Types and Dimensions of Various Blood Vessels

Type	Number	Wall Thickness	Internal Diameter	Total Cross-Sectional Area*
Aorta	1	3 mm	2.5 cm	4.5 cm²
Arteries	200	1 mm	0.5 cm	20 cm²
Arterioles	500×10^3	20 μm	30 μm	400 cm²
Capillaries	10×10^9	1 μm	8 μm	6000 cm²
Venules	500×10^3	20 μm	30 μm	400 cm²
Veins	250	0.5 mm	1 cm	40 cm²
Vena cava	2	1.5 mm	6 cm	18 cm²

*Total cross-sectional area of all vessels of this type.

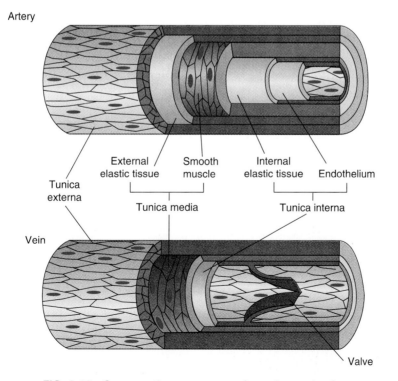

FIG. 2-16   Comparative structures of arteries and veins.

and well-developed tunica media when compared with veins of similar size. The smooth muscle tension developed in the tunica media is referred to as **blood vessel tone.** Vessels with increased tone cause a narrowing of the vessel diameter, which is termed **vasoconstriction.** Vasoconstriction of an artery results in increased resistance to blood flow. When smooth muscle tension decreases and the muscle relaxes, the vessels dilate as a result of internal blood pressure. **Vasodilation** produces less resistance and greater blood flow.

Small arteries and arterioles have a proportionally greater concentration of smooth muscle in their walls when compared with larger arteries. These vessels, which have a greater ability to effect blood pressure and flow, are sometimes referred to as "resistance" vessels. On the other hand, veins, which have a much thinner layer of smooth muscle, are largely unable to produce vasoconstriction when compared with arteries of similar size.

The **tunica interna,** the innermost layer of a vessel, is formed by a single-cell, thick-layered, simple squamous epithelium. These cells are commonly called **endothelium.** The tunica interna also includes a thin layer of elastic connective tissue called the **internal elastic lamina.** Endothelium, the only layer common to all blood vessels, forms an unbroken surface throughout the cardiovascular system over which blood flows. Injury to the endothelium and exposure of the underlying collagen fibers trigger the formation of a blood clot.

Veins have thin and more compliant walls that are able to swell and hold much more blood at various pressures when compared with arteries of similar size. For this reason, veins are known as "capacitance" vessels and actually house most of the blood in the body. Large veins of the upper and lower extremities have valves that prevent the backward flow of blood through them. These simple bicuspid valves are comprised of folds of endothelium and connective tissue fibers. This feature aids in directing blood flow through the compliant vein. During muscular contraction in a limb, blood is squeezed through the valves toward the heart.

Form and Function of the Capillaries

Capillaries are the smallest blood vessels with an inner diameter of 7 to 8 μm, making them

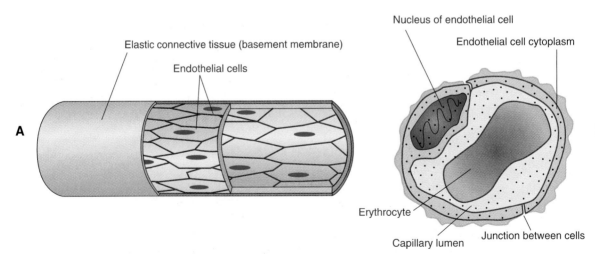

FIG. 2-17 Structure of the capillary. **A,** Longitudinal view. **B,** Cross-sectional view.

not much larger than the size of a red blood cell (Fig. 2-17). Generally, the capillary wall is essentially nothing more than the tunica interna of the arteriole. It is comprised of a single layer of endothelial cells, which forms a "patchworklike" tube. The thin semipermeable wall and the junctions between endothelial cells allow the capillary to carry out its primary function of molecular exchange between blood and the surrounding tissues. Molecular exchange occurs by diffusion and active transport through the endothelial cells and by diffusion through the junctions between cells.

The capillaries found in muscle, connective tissue, pulmonary tissue, and the nervous system are comprised of solid sheets of endothelial tissue. These capillaries have tight junctions with relatively small pores between the endothelial cells. These continuous capillaries normally exchange small quantities of molecules across their walls. Capillaries of the brain have the lowest permeability because they have tight cell junctions and an outer layer of **glial cell** extensions that wrap the capillary to form the **blood-brain barrier.** Low-permeable capillaries in the central nervous system help isolate the neurons from the numerous molecules in blood, which could affect nervous system function.

The capillaries of the liver, spleen, intestine, and kidney are formed by endothelial cells with relatively leaky cell junctions. The larger and more numerous leaky junctions of these fenestrated capillaries allow for greater exchange. Both larger amounts and sizes of molecules are permitted to move across the walls of these capillaries. The glomerular capillaries of the kidney's one million nephrons are the leakiest capillaries in the body. They leak at a phenomenal rate of about 180 L/day as the first step in urine formation.

Capillaries are organized in extensive networks around the cells of tissues to better carry out exchange (Fig. 2-18). Blood flows from the arteriole to the **metarterioles** and true capillaries and then on to the venule. Metarterioles provide blood flow both to the capillary beds and directly to the venule. Capillary networks branch primarily from the metarteriole. Blood flow through a capillary bed is regulated by donut-shaped rings of smooth muscle called **precapillary sphincters** that rap the capillary at its origin. Precapillary sphincters are located at the junction of the capillary bed and the arteriole or metarteriole. Local hormones, respiratory gas, nutrients, waste concentrations, and temperature influence the precapillary sphincter tension, which can be signaled either to relax and open or to constrict and close. This local control of blood flow allows for a proper amount of blood flow to support the local metabolic needs. For example, when the internal temperature increases and the oxygen content decreases in exercising skeletal muscle tissue, the precapillary sphincters dilate. This allows greater blood flow past the muscle fibers, which, in turn, carries away heat and increases the oxygen delivery.

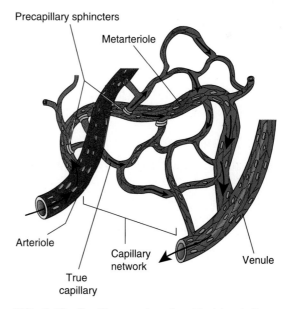

FIG. 2-18 Capillary network with blood flow directed to it from an arteriole.

CASE STUDY FOCUS

Treatment of Coronary Artery Disease

While skiing, a 55-year-old man developed chest pain (angina pectoris) and an unstable blood pressure. He was rushed to the nearby medical center for treatment. The attending physician decided to inject opaque dye into the coronary artery system and take x-rays to see the vessels (coronary angiography). The angiogram revealed that there was 95% occlusion of the anterior descending coronary artery and 90% occlusion of a portion of the circumflex artery.

A number of options are available for the treatment of coronary artery narrowing. They include drug-induced vessel dilation, coronary angioplasty, and coronary artery by-pass grafting (CABG). Oral nitroglycerin causes the smooth muscle of coronary arteries to relax, and this results in dilation and improved blood flow. It is effective in the treatment of coronary artery disease in some patients. Coronary angioplasty is a technique in which a balloon-tipped catheter is threaded from a major peripheral artery, such as the carotid artery, into the coronary artery that is partially occluded. When the catheter is in the area of the narrowed region, the balloon is inflated and the vessel is dilated. The angioplasty technique can also be used to place a stainless steel springlike cylinder called a *stent* within the vessel to help keep it dilated after balloon dilation. CABG is an open-heart surgical procedure that requires the patient to be heavily anesthetized, have their chest opened, and be placed on a heart-lung machine. The CABG surgery is actually several different surgeries. While the chest is being opened and the patient is being placed on the heart-lung machine, the great saphenous vein is collected from the leg. Portions of the vein are attached to the diseased artery above and below the region that is narrowed. This grafting technique acts as a parallel path that allows blood to flow to the regions that the narrowed artery supplies.

The physician decided that a double-vessel CABG would be necessary for long-term treatment of the vessel disease in this patient. The patient underwent the procedure and tolerated the surgery without complication, went home after 3 days, and went through a cardiac rehabilitation program to help ensure the success of the surgery.

LOCATION OF THE MAJOR SYSTEMIC ARTERIES AND VEINS

Major Systemic Arteries

Blood that is pumped to the aorta enters the arterial side of the systemic circuit. The general locations of major arteries are shown in Fig. 2-19.

A succession of arteries branch off the aorta along its ascending arch and descending portions. The ascending aorta exits from the superior and anterior portions of the heart and bends backward over the pulmonary artery. The first arteries to branch off the aorta are the left and right coronary arteries, just above the aortic semilunar valve.

Three major arteries branch off the aortic arch as it leaves the pericardial sac. The **brachiocephalic** (also known as the **innominate**) **artery,** the **left common carotid artery,** and the **left subclavian artery** supply blood to the head, neck, chest wall, and arms (Box 2-1).

The descending aorta is divided at the level of the diaphragm into the thoracic and abdominal portions. Numerous arteries branch off the thoracic aorta to supply blood to the spinal cord, chest wall, mediastinum, large airways, esophagus, and diaphragm. The abdominal aorta gives rise to arteries that supply blood to the diaphragm, abdominal wall, gut, spleen, spine, kidneys, reproductive organs, and legs.

Arteries that are frequently cannulated for measuring blood pressure or for sampling

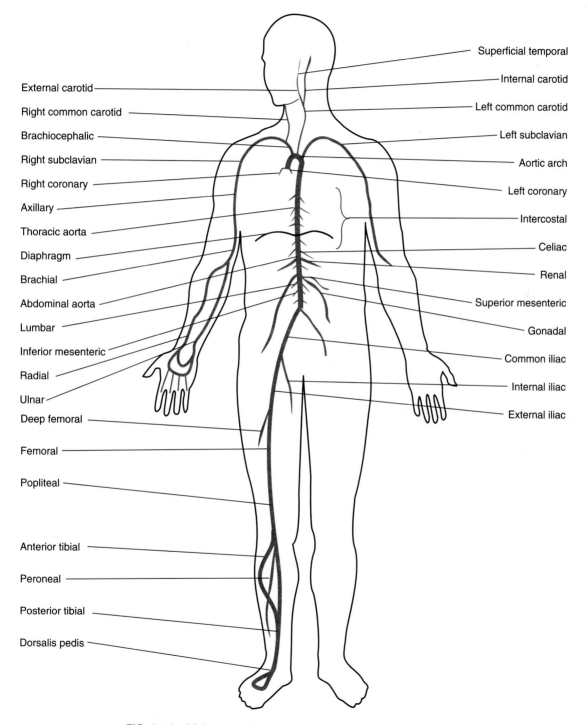

FIG. 2-19 Major arteries of the systemic circulatory system.

BOX 2-1

Major Arteries that Branch from the Aorta and the Regions They Supply

Ascending aorta	
Coronary arteries	Myocardium
Aortic arch	
Brachiocephalic artery	
Right common carotid artery	Head
Right subclavian artery	Right arm
Right vertebral artery	⎫
Right thyrocervical artery	⎬ Head, neck, and chest wall
Right internal thoracic artery	
Right costocervical artery	⎭
Left common carotid artery	Head
Left subclavian artery	Left arm
Left vertebral artery	⎫
Left thyrocervical artery	⎬ Head, neck, and chest
Left internal thoracic artery	
Left costocervical artery	⎭
Descending aorta	
Thoracic aorta	
Intercostal arteries	Chest wall
Pericardial arteries	Cardiac membranes
Mediastinal arteries	Mediastinum
Bronchial arteries	Large airways
Esophageal artery	Esophagus
Subcostal arteries	Chest wall
Superior phrenic arteries	Diaphragm
Abdominal aorta	
Inferior phrenic arteries	Diaphragm
Celiac artery	Liver, gut, and spleen
Superior mesenteric artery	Gut
Lumbar arteries	Spine
Suprarenal arteries	Adrenal gland
Renal arteries	Kidneys
Gonadal artery	Reproductive organs
Inferior mesenteric artery	Gut
Middle sacral artery	Lower spine and sacrum
Common iliac artery	Femoral arteries and legs

blood include the radial, brachial, and dorsalis pedis arteries. Short-term cannulation of the carotid and femoral arteries is done for the injection of dyes to study the blood flow patterns in the heart, brain, aorta, kidneys, and other regions.

Major Systemic Veins

All of the major veins drain either into the superior vena cava or the inferior vena cava. These major vessels, in turn, carry blood back to the right side of the heart. Fig. 2-20 shows the location of major veins found in the body.

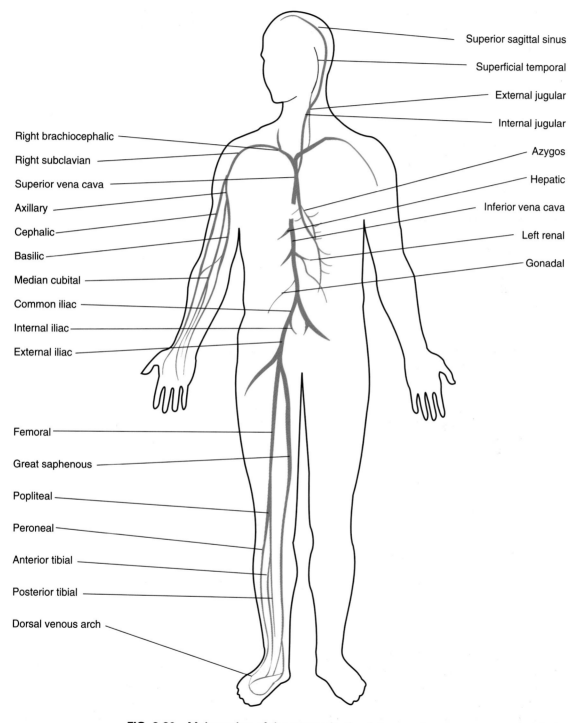

FIG. 2-20   Major veins of the systemic circulatory system.

The superior vena cava receives the great majority of blood from the right and left **brachiocephalic veins.** These veins receive blood from numerous veins that drain the head, chest, and upper limbs. The jugular, subclavian, and median cubital veins are commonly used for the placement of venous catheters for sampling blood or for delivering fluids and drugs.

Venous blood from the abdomen, pelvis, and lower limbs is drained into the inferior vena cava. A major portion of this blood flows from the left and right **hepatic veins.** These veins carry blood from the stomach, intestines, spleen, and pancreas. Veins from these organs combine to form the **hepatic portal vein.** The hepatic portal vein carries blood to the liver, which is then drained into the inferior vena cava after passing through the liver. Most of the rest of the blood entering the inferior vena cava comes from the kidneys, adrenal glands, reproductive organs, and lower limbs (Box 2-2).

● LYMPHATIC SYSTEM

Form and Function of the Lymphatic Vessels

Water and solutes continuously leak from the vascular system. Leakage into the interstitial space of tissues occurs continuously. Most of the fluid is absorbed by the cells of tissue and reabsorbed back into blood before it leaves the capillary bed. But, approximately 2 to 3 L of this leakage from the vascular system is absorbed

---

BOX 2-2

Major Veins that Drain Into Superior and Inferior Vena Cava and Regions They Drain

Superior vena cava	
Left and right brachiocephalic veins	
Internal jugular veins	Brain
Vertebral veins	Spine and head
Internal thoracic veins	Chest wall
Subclavian veins	Arms and head
	⎧ Chest wall
	⎪ Large airways
Azygus and hemiazygus veins	⎨ Esophagus
	⎩ Cardiac membranes
	⎧ Liver
Inferior vena cava	⎨ Hepatic portal vein
Hepatic veins	⎪ Gut
	⎩ Spleen and pancreas
Right suprarenal veins	Adrenal gland
Renal veins	Kidney
Gonadal veins	Reproductive tissues
Lumbar veins	Spine and abdominal wall
Middle sacral vein	Spine
Common iliac veins	Internal and external iliac veins
	Left and right femoral veins
	Saphenous and popliteal veins
	Legs

by the lymphatic system and returned to the circulatory system each day. The lymphatic system, which also plays a major role in absorbing proteins in the liver and lipids in the gastrointestinal tract, filters out foreign substances and houses many of the immune system cells.

The lymphatic system, comprised of a network of lymphatic capillaries, thin-walled **lymph vessels,** and **lymph nodes,** returns absorbed fluid to the venous side of the systemic circulatory system. Generally, the lymphatic system parallels the venous system of vessels.

Lymphatic capillaries are closed on one end and are often referred to as "blind" capillaries (Fig. 2-21). They have a structure that is similar to very porous fenestrated capillaries. These capillaries are anchored between the cells by fine filaments. Fluid and solutes absorbed by lymph capillaries are carried to larger lymph vessels that have a structure similar to that of veins. The lymph vessels are equipped with valves that direct fluid through the system and prevent it from pooling or moving backward.

Lymph vessels drain through lymph nodes (Fig. 2-22). Lymph nodes are bean-shaped structures that range in size from that of a pinhead to as large as a lima bean. Each

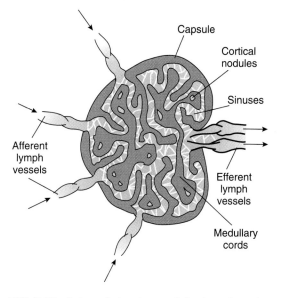

FIG. 2-22 Internal structures of the lymph node.

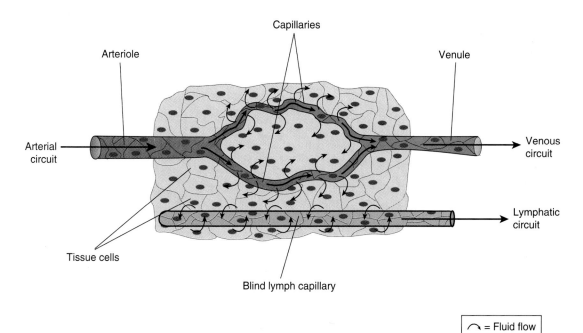

FIG. 2-21 Relationship between vascular capillaries and lymphatic capillaries.

lymph node has an outer capsule and inner sinuses. Within the sinuses are "islands" of cells arranged into cortical nodules and medullary cords. These cellular "islands" are largely comprised of numerous **lymphocytes.** Lymph fluid enters the lymph node from several afferent lymph vessels, moves through the sinuses of the node, and exits through one or two efferent lymph vessels. The numerous lymph nodes in the lymphatic system function as filters for foreign particles, viruses, and cells. Lymphocytes function within the lymph nodes by identifying and eliminating foreign molecules, particles, and cells by various immune mechanisms.

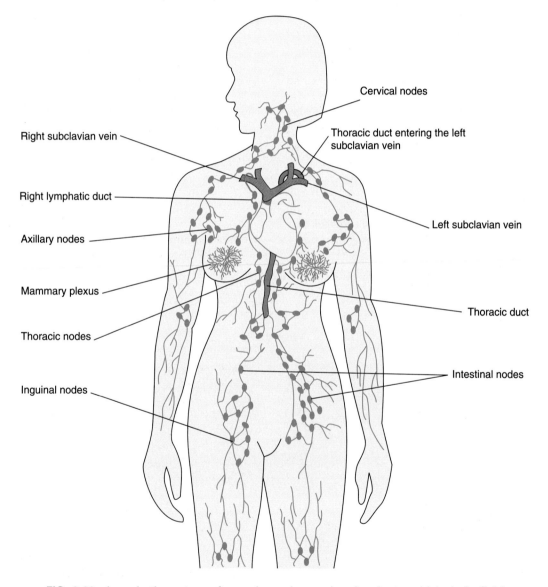

FIG. 2-23 Lymphatic system of vessels, nodes, and major ducts, which drain fluid from the extracellular spaces back to the subclavian veins.

The constant accumulation of fluid within the lymphatic vessels propels the fluid out of the lymphatic capillary bed and into the lymphatic system (Fig. 2-23). The valves of the larger vessels facilitate the movement of lymph fluid through the system. Skeletal muscular contractions squeeze lymph fluid through the lymphatic vessels and propel it through the system. The lymph vessels merge into two major **lymphatic ducts.** The thoracic duct drains lymph fluid from three-quarters of the body into the left subclavian vein. The right lymphatic duct drains lymphatic fluid from the right arm and the right side of the chest and head into the right subclavian vein. The only tissues not drained by the lymphatic system are the central nervous system, epithelia, cartilage, and bone. They rely on the reabsorption of fluid by the vascular capillaries.

CHAPTER SELF-TEST QUESTIONS

1. Which of the following are general functions of the cardiovascular system?
   1. nutrient molecule transport
   2. hormonal molecule synthesis
   3. respiratory gas transport
   4. waste molecule transport
      a. 1 and 3
      b. 2 and 4
      c. 1 and 4
      d. 1, 2, and 3
      e. 1, 3, and 4
2. The atrial and ventricular septa have completed their embryonic development on or about the _____ of gestation.
   a. 40th day
   b. 55th day
   c. 70th day
   d. 85th day
3. The apex of the beating heart makes contact with the chest wall at a location near the fifth rib on the left anterior side. This location is referred to as the
   a. angle of Louis
   b. point of maximal impact

c. suprasternal notch
d. fourth intercostal space

4. The outer membrane of the heart is a tough inelastic membrane of connective tissue called the
   a. ectocardium
   b. endocardium
   c. pericardium
   d. mesocardium
5. The free wall of the left ventricle is generally _____ when compared with the free wall of the right ventricle.
   a. much thinner
   b. about the same thickness
   c. much thicker
6. The bicuspid valve prevents the back flow of blood into the
   a. right atrium
   b. right ventricle
   c. left atrium
   d. left ventricle
7. The _____ and _____ valves are supported by chordae tendineae and papillary muscles which hold the valves closed when pressures below them build.
   1. pulmonic semilunar
   2. tricuspid
   3. aortic semilunar
   4. bicuspid
      a. 1 and 2
      b. 2 and 3
      c. 3 and 4
      d. 1 and 3
      e. 2 and 4
8. The bulk of the myocardium is supplied with blood from the
   a. right coronary artery
   b. Thebesian vessels
   c. collateral vessels
   d. left coronary artery
9. The tunica externa of both veins and arteries is comprised of
   a. smooth muscle
   b. collagenous and elastic connective tissue
   c. simple squamous epithelia with a basement membrane
   d. nonelastic connective tissue

10. The endothelial lining of arteries, veins, and capillaries is formed from an unbroken sheet of
    a. collagenous and elastic connective tissue
    b. smooth muscle
    c. nonelastic connective tissue
    d. simple squamous epithelia

For answers, see p. 475.

BIBLIOGRAPHY

1. Berne RM, Levy MN: *Cardiovascular physiology,* St Louis, 1992, Mosby.
2. Brandenburg RO et al: *Cardiology: fundamentals and practice,* Chicago, 1987, Year Book Medical.
3. Cohn PF: *Clinical cardiovascular physiology,* Philadelphia, 1985, WB Saunders.
4. Ganong WF: *Review of medical physiology,* ed 18, Stamford, Conn, 1997, Appleton & Lange.
5. Guyton AC: *Textbook of medical physiology,* Philadelphia, 1996, WB Saunders.
6. Langman J, Woerdeman MW: *Atlas of medical anatomy,* Philadelphia, 1978, WB Saunders.
7. Little RC: *Physiology of the heart and circulation,* ed 2, Chicago, 1981, Year Book Medical.
8. Martini FH: *Fundamentals of anatomy and physiology,* Upper Saddle River, NJ, 1998, Prentice Hall.
9. McMinn RMH, Hutchings RT: *Color atlas of human anatomy,* Chicago, 1977, Year Book Medical.
10. Netter FH: *The Ciba collection of medical illustrations,* Vol 5, Summitt, NJ, 1969, CIBA Pharmaceutical Products.
11. Rushmer RF: *Cardiovascular dynamics,* Philadelphia, 1978, WB Saunders.
12. Smith JJ, Kampine JP: *Circulatory physiology: the essentials,* ed 3, Baltimore, 1990, Williams & Wilkins.
13. Spence AP, Mason EG: *Human anatomy and physiology,* ed 4, St Paul, Minn, 1992, West.
14. Wilson DB, Wilson WJ: *Human anatomy,* New York, 1978, Oxford University Press.

Blood

CHAPTER OBJECTIVES

Upon completing this chapter, you will be able to:
1 Describe the general functions of blood.
2 Describe the composition of plasma.
3 Describe the formed elements.
4 Define hemopoiesis.
5 Describe the normal blood volume and its distribution in the circulatory system.
6 Describe the form and function of the erythrocytes, leukocytes, and platelets.
7 List the major blood types.
8 Describe the complete blood count.
9 Define hemostasis and the mechanisms that limit blood loss.
10 Describe anticoagulation and fibrinolysis.

⬤ BLOOD: FORM AND FUNCTION

Blood is a complex fluid that the cardiovascular system circulates for the collection and transport of important materials. These materials are transported to and from all the tissues to support their metabolism. Blood supports the tissues indirectly through the constant conditioning of the fluid that surrounds the cells—the **interstitial fluid.** The conditioning of the interstitial fluid is vital to the maintenance of a constant internal environment. All cells need this conditioning for normal function.

Blood carries out various transport functions to maintain the internal environment. One of the more critical functions is the uninterrupted delivery of oxygen to support aerobic metabolism. Blood supplies nutrient molecules such as amino acids, fatty acids, sugars, and a variety of important ions and trace metals. Interaction with blood maintains the necessary concentrations of water, electrolytes, and hydrogen ions in the interstitial fluid. To avoid the toxic effects of waste products produced by cellular metabolism, blood transports carbon dioxide, ammonia, lactic acid, and other waste chemicals away from tissues to excretory organs. Blood plays a role in thermoregulation (the maintenance of body temperature) by transporting heat, another type of waste product of metabolism, from the deeper core tissues to the surface tissues of skin for its release. Blood brings instructions to cells in the form of hormones and vitamins, which regulate various cellular activities. Blood also plays a critical role in body defenses through the actions of its white cells, its role in inflammation, and antibody protein production. Interestingly, blood also has the ability to help prevent its own loss through various mechanisms.

Plasma

Blood is classified as connective tissue because of its composition of cells that are suspended in a nonliving liquid matrix called **plasma.** Blood can be collected in a capillary tube and separated into the plasma and cellular fractions by application of high-speed centrifugation (Fig. 3-1). The straw-colored plasma occupies 55% of the total volume, and the remaining 45% is the packed cellular

elements. The percentage comprised by the cells is almost all red blood cells and is called the **hematocrit.**

Plasma is an aqueous solution of proteins, ions, and various other solutes. Table 3-1 summarizes the major constituents of plasma. By weight, plasma is 91.5% water and 7% protein, and the remaining 1.5% is an assortment of dissolved solutes. The aqueous nature of plasma allows it to transport all types of water-soluble compounds as well as heat. For example, in each 100 ml of plasma there are approximately 7 g of protein, 600 mg of lipid, 100 mg of glucose, and 15 mg of urea dissolved in it. In addition, approximately 300 mEq/L of electrolytes and 2.3 ml of respiratory gases are dissolved in it.

The protein component of plasma includes albumin, fibrinogen, and globulins. Albumin, as well as the other proteins, plays a major role in transporting various molecules and ions. Albumin is also important in the osmotic

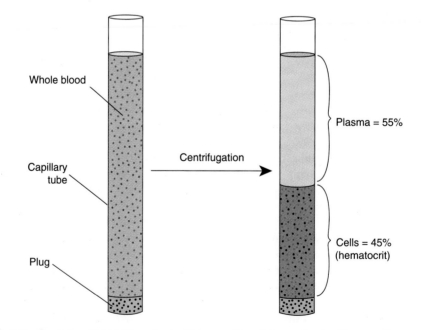

Whole blood

Capillary tube

Plug

Centrifugation

Plasma = 55%

Cells = 45% (hematocrit)

FIG. 3-1 Sample of blood is collected in a capillary tube, mixed with an anticoagulant, and spun in a centrifuge which separates it into the plasma and cellular component.

attraction of water into the vascular compartment. Fibrinogen is an important protein in the clotting process. The various types of antibody proteins present in plasma constitute the globulin fraction.

 Table 3-1 Normal Composition of Plasma

Component	Percentage
Water	91.5%*
Protein	7.0%*
Albumin	3.5-5.0 g/dl
Globulins	2.3-3.5 g/dl
Fibrinogen	0.2-0.35 g/dl
Total protein	6.0-8.0 g/dl
Other solutes	1.5%*
Respiratory gases	
Oxygen	0.3 ml/dl
Carbon dioxide	2.0 ml/dl
Nutrients	
Total lipids	450-1000 mg/dl
Fatty acids	190-420 mg/dl
Cholesterol	150-220 mg/dl
Triglycerides	40-150 mg/dl
Glucose	70-100 mg/dl
Amino acids	30-45 mg/dl
Electrolytes	
Na^+	135-145 mEq/L
K^+	3.5-5.0 mEq/L
Ca^{++}	8.5-10.0 mEq/L
Mg^{++}	1.5-2.5 mEq/L
Cl^-	100-106 mEq/L
HCO_3^-	22-26 mEq/L
PO_4^{3-}	0.5-1.5 mEq/L
SO_4^{2-}	0.3-0.6 mEq/L
Waste products	
Blood urea nitrogen	10-20 mg/dl
Uric acid	2.0-8.0 mg/dl
Creatinine	0.6-1.5 mg/dl
Bilirubin (total)	0.3-1.1 mg/dl
Lactic acid	0.6-1.8 mg/dl
Hormones	
Total less than 70 μg/dl	

*Percent of total weight.

Formed Elements

The cellular components of blood, also referred to as the formed elements (Fig. 3-2), include the **erythrocytes** (red blood cells [RBCs]), **leukocytes** (white blood cells [WBCs]), and **thrombocytes** (platelets). Table 3-2 summarizes the average number and functions of the various formed elements found in blood.

Hemopoiesis

The formed elements of blood, which are produced in the red marrow of bones through a process known as **hemopoiesis**, were, before birth, largely produced in the spleen and liver.

In the adult, red marrow is commonly found in the skull bones, sternum, ribs, vertebral bones, pelvis, and proximal ends of the humerus and femur bones. Blood is carried to the red marrow by the nutritive arteries of bone; the nutritive arteries deliver blood to capillaries and walled spaces called sinusoids. The various blood cells form within the sinusoids. The formed elements gain access to the vascular system through the veins, which drain bone.

The red marrow contains stem cells, or **hemocytoblasts,** the parent cells that form all the cells of blood (Fig. 3-3). Two general lines of cellular development arise from the hemocytoblasts, including the lymphoid line, which produces all the lymphocytic white blood cells, and the myeloid line, which forms the erythrocytes, thrombocytes, and all the other leukocytes. Approximately half of the immature lymphocytes leave the red marrow and finish their development in the thymus gland.

Hemopoiesis occurs at a phenomenal rate. For example, approximately 145 million erythrocytes and 5 million leukocytes form each minute to take the place of those that wear out or die. These rates can increase in response to numerous conditions such as hemorrhage or infection. Different growth factors have been identified that influence blood cell

Table 3-2   Formed Elements

Element	Number per mm³	Life Span	Function
ERYTHROCYTES			
	5,000,000	120 days	Transports respiratory gases
LEUKOCYTES			
	7000		
Granulocytes			
Neutrophils	60%	3 days	Forms phagocytic cells for defense against bacteria
Eosinophils	3%	2 weeks	Destroys various parasitic worms and participates in immune response
Basophils	1%	3 days	Secretes histamine and heparin
Agranulocytes			
Lymphocytes	30%	Years	Produces antibodies
Monocytes	6%	Months	Evolves into phagocytic macrophages in the tissues
THROMBOCYTES			
	300,000	1 week	Forms plugs in damaged vessels and secretes serotonin and thromboxane A_2

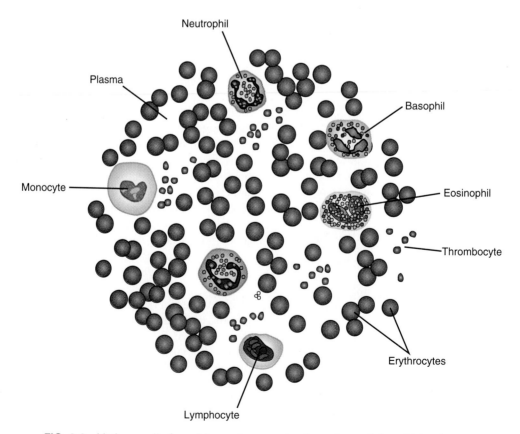

FIG. 3-2   Various cells found in a microscopic view of a peripheral blood smear.

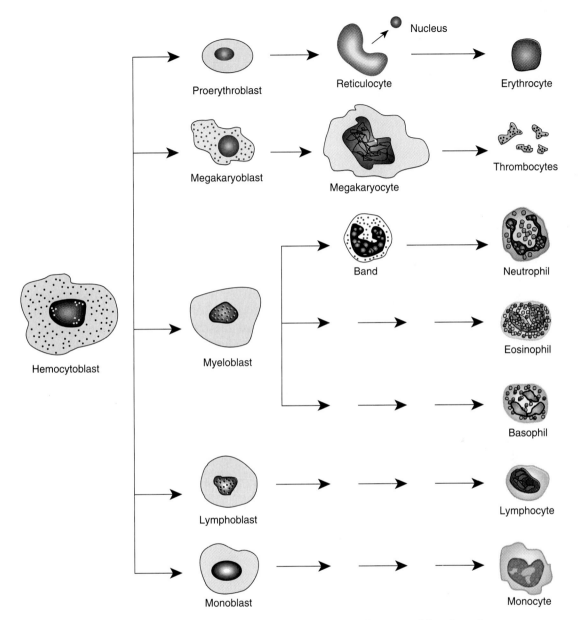

FIG. 3-3 Development of formed elements by the parent hemocytoblast in red marrow.

development in red marrow. A glycoprotein called **erythropoietin** that is formed in the kidney in response to reduced levels of blood oxygen circulates through the red marrow and stimulates erythrocyte production. Various tissues in response to specific conditions (e.g., bacterial infection or allergic reactions) release other glycoproteins called **cytokines** (e.g., **interleukins** and colony-stimulating factors) and stimulate the development of various leukocytes. A glycoprotein called thrombopoietin stimulates platelet formation by the megakaryocyte.

NORMAL BLOOD VOLUME AND DISTRIBUTION

Total Blood Volume

The total blood volume of an adult is about 8% to 9% of lean body mass, which equates to about 75 ml of blood per kilogram or approximately 4 to 6 L. Individual variation depends primarily on age, physical activity, and altitude of residence. Those who are younger, more physically active, and reside at high altitudes (e.g., 3000 m) maintain slightly greater blood volumes. On the other hand, those who are older, those forced to bed rest, and those exposed to weightlessness in space for long periods have reduced blood volume. Pregnancy causes a 20% to 30% increase in blood volume by the end of gestation.

Distribution of Blood Volume

Blood is not evenly distributed throughout the circulatory system. Fig. 3-4 illustrates the percentage of blood volume in various regions of the circulatory system. Approximately two-thirds of total blood volume is "pooled" in the systemic veins whereas only about one-sixth is found in the systemic arterial system. This big difference is caused by the larger and more expansive nature of the thin-walled veins. The thicker-walled arteries (especially the smaller arteries and arterioles) are less distensible and thus less able to "pool" blood. In fact, the more elastic arteries actually help propel blood toward the capillary beds of the tissues by their greater elastic behavior. The more disten-

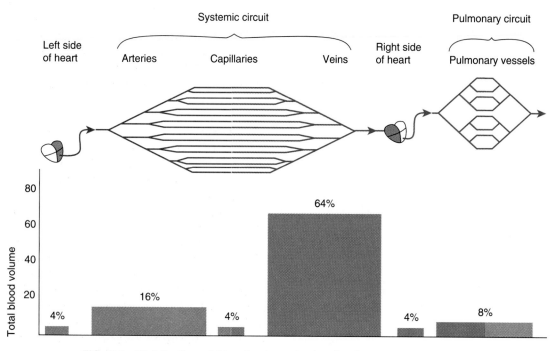

FIG. 3-4 Distribution of blood volume in the circulatory system at rest.

sible veins with their one-way valves enhance blood flow out of the capillary beds toward the heart.

🔴 RED BLOOD CELLS: FORM AND FUNCTION

Erythrocyte

The mature erythrocyte cell, which lacks a nucleus and most other organelles, has a structure commonly described as a flexible biconcave disk (Fig. 3-5). They are 7.5 µm in diameter and 2.5 µm in thickness. This shape allows for a greater surface for gas exchange and the size allows them to squeeze through the capillary in single file. Erythrocytes com-

prise more than 99% of the formed elements. Their average concentration is about 5.4 million per mm^3 of blood in men and 4.8 million per mm^3 in women. Thus they represent the vast majority of the formed elements that comprise the hematocrit. The average hematocrit is about 45% in men and 41% in women. The fetus maintains a greater value of about 55% until shortly after delivery and then drops to about 45% within a week after birth. The primary function of the erythrocyte is the transportation of oxygen and carbon dioxide.

The erythrocyte's role in respiratory gas transport centers around the iron-carrying protein hemoglobin and the enzyme **carbonic anhydrase.** Erythrocytes are essentially cellular sacks of hemoglobin. Each erythrocyte carries approximately 300 million molecules of hemoglobin, which amounts to about 35% of the total erythrocyte weight. A common method of evaluating hemoglobin concentration in blood is to measure the total amount present in 100 ml or 1 dl of blood. The normal value of hemoglobin is about 13.7 g/dl in women and 15 g/dl in men.

The four iron ions of hemoglobin are able to reversibly bond with oxygen whereas the protein portion of the molecule is able to reversibly bond with carbon dioxide. The erythrocyte also carries the enzyme carbonic anhydrase, which plays an important role in catalyzing the reaction of carbon dioxide and water to form carbonic acid, which dissociates into the much more plasma-soluble **bicarbonate** (HCO_3^-) ion. A more detailed description of this process is found in Chapter 13.

The process of erythrocyte formation is called **erythropoiesis** (see Fig. 3-3). The hormone erythropoietin stimulates the hemocytoblast in red marrow to differentiate through a series of divisions until reaching the **normoblast** stage. During this differentiation, that portion of the cell's DNA that carries the genetic coding for hemoglobin is activated and the cell manufactures large quantities of hemoglobin. When the hemoglobin concentration

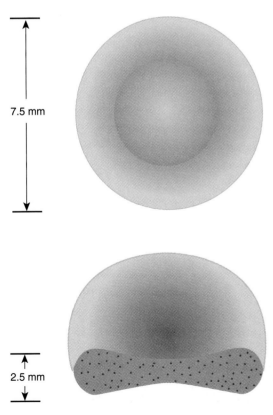

7.5 mm

2.5 mm

FIG. 3-5 The erythrocyte.

in the normoblast reaches 34% of its total mass, the nucleus is ejected and the biconcave reticulocyte is formed. Normally, the reticulocyte count is only 1% to 1.5% of all the circulating erythrocytes. Reticulocytes transform into mature erythrocytes over a 24-hour period after entering the blood. For normal development, the erythrocyte requires sufficient amino acids, iron, and vitamins B_9, B_{12}, and C.

The erythrocyte has a life span of 110 to 120 days. The limited life span is largely a result of the lack of a nucleus, which renders the cell unable to repair itself and replace nec-

essary enzymes. Old, damaged, and abnormal cells are destroyed by phagocytic cells in the spleen, liver, and bone marrow (Fig. 3-6). The hemoglobin is recycled by splitting it into the protein **(globin)** and iron complex **(heme)** portions. The globin portion is broken up into the individual amino acids for reuse. The heme portion is comprised of **porphyrin rings**, which house the ferrous iron ions (Fe^{++}). The porphyrin ring is converted in the liver and spleen into the greenish pigment biliverdin and then into the yellowish pigmented bilirubin. Bilirubin, which is partially responsible

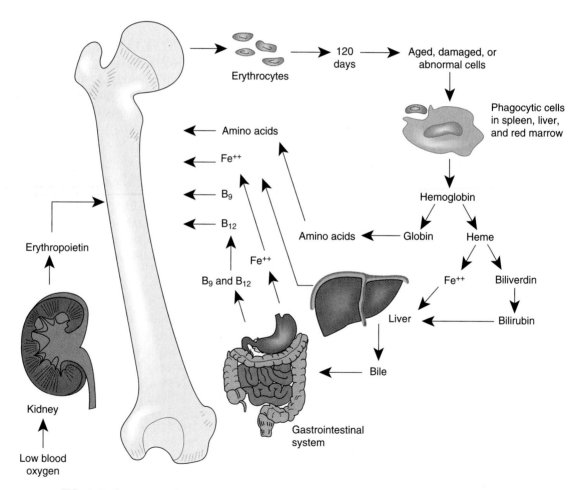

FIG. 3-6 Important factors necessary for the development of the erythrocyte and their destruction and recycling in the spleen and liver.

for the yellow color of plasma, is incorporated into bile in the liver and secreted into the small intestine to aid in the digestion of fats. Bilirubin is further metabolized by intestinal bacteria and excreted in urine and feces. The Fe^{++} is stored in the liver and is reused in the synthesis of hemoglobin in new cells. Virtually all of the Fe^{++} are transported in blood by the plasma protein transferrin.

Anemia

The erythrocyte count, hematocrit, and hemoglobin concentrations drop below normal values during conditions of iron or vitamin B deficiencies or when erythrocytes are being lost at a faster rate than they can be produced. This condition is known as **anemia.**

The most common cause of anemia, **hemorrhagic anemia,** occurs from either acute blood loss following trauma and surgery or chronic loss from a gastrointestinal ulcer.

Various deficiencies are responsible for anemia. **Pernicious anemia** results from a vitamin B_{12} deficiency, which causes the production of fewer, larger, and more fragile erythrocytes. **Folate-deficiency anemia** is the result of a vitamin B_9 deficiency that also results in reduced erythropoiesis. Inadequate amounts of iron in the diet lead to an **iron-deficiency anemia,** resulting in fewer hemoglobin molecules formed in each erythrocyte.

Hemolytic anemias are caused by conditions that produce more fragile or damaged erythrocytes. Infections, toxins, and inherited conditions result in damaged or distorted erythrocytes that are more prone to breakage and phagocytosis in the spleen. **Sickle cell anemia,** an example of an inherited hemolytic anemia, results from the hemoglobin molecule changing shape when exposed to low oxygen levels. The change in hemoglobin shape causes the entire cell to take on a "sickle" shape, which makes the cell less flexible, more likely to get stuck in capillaries, and prone to phagocytosis.

When the bone marrow develops erythrocytes at an accelerated rate to compensate for the loss of cells, the reticulocyte count increases. An increased reticulocyte count indicates appropriate marrow response to an anemic state. If, however, anemia is present with an abnormally low or absent reticulocyte count, it suggests that the bone marrow is failing to produce erythrocytes. This condition is referred to as **aplastic anemia.** One of the more common causes of aplastic anemia is red marrow destruction following exposure to radiation or the use of some chemotherapy agents used in the treatment of certain cancers.

Polycythemia

When more erythrocytes are produced and maintained in circulating blood, as indicated by elevated hematocrit, erythrocyte counts, and hemoglobin concentration, a condition called **polycythemia** occurs. Although uncommon, it does occur as a compensatory response in those who have a chronic hypoxemic (reduced blood oxygen content) condition. Chronic hypoxemia, which stimulates the production of erythropoietin, can develop in those with chronic lung or heart disease or in those who live at high altitudes (>3000 m).

Blood Typing

Numerous situations dictate the need for a blood transfusion. However, care is needed to avoid a transfusion reaction. Transfusion reactions occur when donor blood cells clump together, or **agglutinate,** and eventually rupture or undergo **hemolysis.** The agglutination and hemolysis of a large amount of donor cells plug the microcirculation and cause organ failure and even death of the recipient. To avoid this reaction, blood is tested for compatibility through the typing of blood.

The surface of the erythrocyte contains numerous glycoproteins, some of which cause agglutination; they are therefore called **agglutinogens.** The type of agglutinogens or antigens that are present are genetically determined.

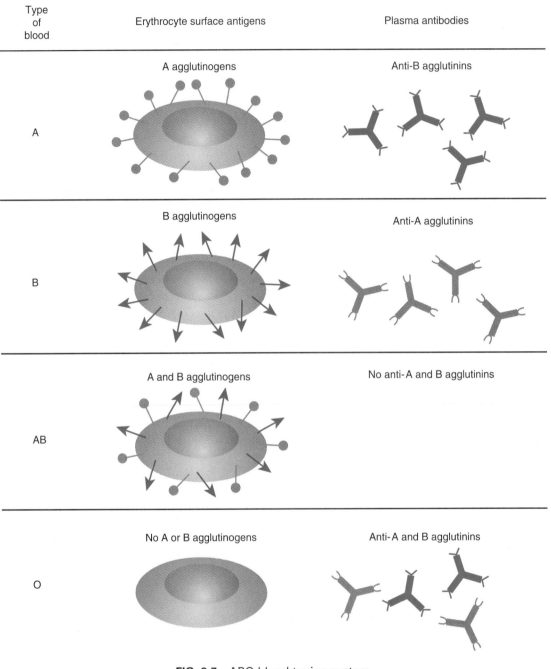

Type of blood	Erythrocyte surface antigens	Plasma antibodies

A

A agglutinogens

Anti-B agglutinins

B

B agglutinogens

Anti-A agglutinins

AB

A and B agglutinogens

No anti-A and B agglutinins

O

No A or B agglutinogens

Anti-A and B agglutinins

FIG. 3-7 ABO blood typing system.

The three most responsive agglutinogens are the A, B, and Rh types.

The plasma may contain antibody or antiagglutinogen proteins called **agglutinins,** which are also genetically determined. The presence of a certain type of agglutinin is responsible for the clumping of cells when a transfusion reaction occurs. The types of agglutinins that may be present include anti-A, anti-B, and anti-Rh.

The presence or absence of a particular agglutinogen on the erythrocytes and agglutinin in the plasma determines the type of blood a person has. The ABO blood types are organized as follows:

Type A blood has erythrocytes with type A agglutinogens on their surface and has anti-B agglutinins in the plasma.

Type B blood has erythrocytes with type B agglutinogens on their surface and has anti-A agglutinins in the plasma.

Type AB blood has erythrocytes with types A and B agglutinogens on their surface and has no anti-A or anti-B agglutinins in the plasma.

Type O blood has *neither* type A nor B agglutinogens on their surface and has both anti-A and anti-B agglutinins in the plasma.

The ABO blood typing system is summarized in Fig. 3-7. In addition, an individual may or may not have another agglutinogen called the Rh factor on their erythrocytes and anti-Rh agglutinins in the plasma:

Rh$^+$ blood has Rh agglutinogens on the surface of its erythrocytes and no anti-Rh agglutinins in the plasma.

Rh$^-$ blood does not have Rh agglutinogens on the surface of its erythrocytes and *can* develop anti-Rh agglutinins in the plasma if exposed to Rh$^+$ blood.

As an example, an individual with type O positive blood means the erythrocytes have neither of the A or B agglutinogens but does have Rh agglutinogens on the surface of the cells. Their plasma contains both anti-A and anti-B agglutinins but does not have the anti-Rh agglutinins.

The transfusion of blood from a donor to a recipient requires the blood to be typed and cross matched to avoid the agglutination and hemolysis that occurs if the ABO and Rh systems are not compatible. Typing is the determination of the ABO and Rh agglutinogens present. Cross matching is the mixing of a small sample of donor blood with a small sample of recipient blood to see if agglutination occurs. Mixing types A and B blood results in a transfusion reaction. Those with type AB blood are universal recipients because they lack the anti-A and anti-B agglutinins whereas those with type O blood are universal donors because their erythrocytes lack the A and B agglutinogens. Generally, the same type of donor blood is given to a needy recipient, or, when possible, the patient anticipating the need for a blood transfusion can bank their blood ahead of time.

⬤ WHITE BLOOD CELLS: FORM AND FUNCTION

Leukocytes

The leukocytes are nucleated cells that are generally larger than erythrocytes; they comprise only 0.1% of the cells in blood. The total leukocytes count is normally between 5000 to 10,000/mm^3 of blood. When the leukocyte count increases above the normal range it is referred to as a **leukocytosis** and is frequently associated with an infection or allergic reactions. **Leukemia,** a type of cancer characterized by a proliferation of a type of leukocyte, results in leukocytosis with white blood cell counts that can easily reach values that are ten times normal. A leukocyte concentration below the normal range is referred to as a **leukopenia.** Leukopenia can be caused by overwhelming infections or red marrow damage from radiation and certain drugs (e.g., steroids or cancer chemotherapy).

Leukocytes are organized into two general classes: the **granulocytes** and the **agranulocytes.** The granulocytes are all formed in the red bone marrow, have multilobed nuclei, and possess granules in their cytoplasm. The agranulocytes do not have granules in their cytoplasm, and many finish their development outside the bone marrow. Individual types of granulocytes and agranulocytes can be counted and the percentage of each type reported as a white blood cell differential count. Generally, the leukocytes function to defend the body against infection, to participate in the inflammatory process, and to clear cellular debris.

Granulocytes

Neutrophils possess large numbers of lysosomes and secretory vesicles in their cytoplasm. They are also known as polymorphonuclear (PMN) leukocytes because they possess prominent nuclei that have multiple lobes. As the most numerous type of leukocyte present in blood, they account for 40% to 70% of all leukocytes. They are capable of both phagocytosis and secretion of destructive enzymes (e.g., trypsin), oxidants (e.g., superoxide, O_2^-), and antimicrobial proteins called defensins. These mobile cells are capable of **diapedesis,** a process of moving from the blood, through the vessel wall, and into tissues. Their principal function is the destruction of bacteria that have invaded tissue. Neutrophils are attracted to injured tissues by a process known as **chemotaxis,** which refers to the movement of cells toward a region that contains certain chemical attractants.

During major infections, the total leukocyte count can double or triple and the number of neutrophils can increase to 80% or 90%. When this occurs, the number of immature neu-

trophils, or **band cells,** which normally total less than 6% of all leukocytes, increases as the bone marrow is stimulated to increase its production of neutrophils. In clinical practice, this increase in band cells, which is often referred to as a left shift, indicates a responsive bone marrow and a sign of a bacterial infection. The neutrophil's life span ranges from a few hours during infections to about 3 days.

Eosinophils, which are less numerous and account for only 0% to 6% of all leukocytes, also have numerous lysosomes and secretory vesicles in their cytoplasm. They are also mobile cells that are capable of diapedesis. Eosinophils function as both phagocytic and secretory cells during parasitic worm infections and during allergic reactions. The central activity of an allergic reaction is the binding of foreign antigen molecules by the antibodies formed by the immune system. Following an allergic reaction, the eosinophils act to clear the antigen-antibody complexes that are formed, triggering inflammatory reactions. In addition, they secrete histaminase, an enzyme that breaks down **histamine,** a potent chemical causing inflammation. Eosinophil counts often increase in response to some types of allergic reactions and appear to play a role in limiting an inflammatory reaction. Their life span averages 10 to 12 days.

Basophils, which are relatively rare, number less than 1% of all leukocytes. They have numerous secretory vesicles in their cytoplasm that carry various chemical mediators of inflammation. They leave the circulatory system and enter the tissues to carry out their secretory activity as **mast cells.** These cells become sensitized to various stimuli and, when triggered, release **histamine, heparin,** and other mediators of inflammation. Histamine causes vasodilation and increased capillary leakage whereas heparin prevents blood coagulation. Both of these agents induce swelling and redness around a wound and help dilute any potential toxins that may be present. The basophil life span in blood ranges from a few hours to 3 days.

Agranulocytes

Lymphocytes, which develop into large- and small-type cells, have a prominent nucleus and a relatively small amount of cytoplasm that lacks cytoplasmic granules. These cells are the second most common white cell in blood, ranging from 20% to 45% of all leukocytes. Actually, many more lymphocytes are found outside of blood in various lymphoid tissues. Lymphocytes are generally classified as **B cells** (those that mature in bone marrow) or **T cells** (those that mature in the thymus gland). Both play major roles in the immune system. The B lymphocytes differentiate into plasma cells and manufacture and secrete specific antibodies, which form a significant portion of the globulin proteins of plasma. The T lymphocytes act as killer, helper, and suppressor cells that act in and modify the immune response. The T-helper lymphocyte is the prime target of the acquired immunodeficiency syndrome (AIDS) virus. Members of both the B and T cells can become memory cells, which carry the genetic information about a specific antibody that is formed in response to exposure to a specific antigen. Most lymphocyte life spans average several months but the memory cells can live for many years and reproduce.

Monocytes, which account for only 2% to 10% of all leukocytes, have relatively large nuclei and lack granules in their cytoplasm. They are able to move out of the circulatory system and into tissue where they develop into **macrophages.** Macrophages are large phagocytic cells that move throughout the tissues and ingest bacteria and other foreign materials. The macrophage also plays a key role in the immune response by presenting the foreign material or antigens it has ingested to the lymphocytes for the production of specific antibodies. The antibodies act to neutralize the antigen when they bind to them. Macrophages have life spans in blood that number into months.

PLATELETS: FORM AND FUNCTION

Thrombocytes

Platelets, or **thrombocytes,** are small cellular fragments about 3 m in diameter that lack nuclei. They are relatively numerous with concentrations of 250,000 to 400,000/mm^3 of blood. Platelets are formed in red marrow from a parent cell called a **megakaryocyte.** The megakaryocyte develops from the hemocytoblast. The individual platelets form as a cellular extension of the megakaryocyte pinches off. The platelets contain numerous secretory vesicles and primarily function to help prevent blood loss. When triggered, they have the ability to stick to damaged sites of the blood vessel wall and to each other to form a **platelet plug.** In addition, they can release a variety of substances such as the lipid **thromboxane A$_2$,** which enhances their stickiness, and **serotonin,** which is a potent vasoconstrictor. Their life span in blood averages about 1 week but can be much less when vessels are damaged or when the clotting mechanism is triggered.

COMPLETE BLOOD COUNT

Counting the various cells present in 1 mm^3 of blood is a common laboratory test called the **complete blood count (CBC).** This test determines erythrocyte count, hematocrit, hemoglobin concentration, leukocyte count, and platelet count. The erythrocytes are further evaluated by determining the percentage of cells that are immature reticulocytes and various average dimensions or indices of the erythrocyte. The erythrocyte indices

Table 3-3 Normal Complete Blood Count

Component	Count
ERYTHROCYTE COUNT	
Men	4.6-6.2 million/mm³
Women	4.2-5.4 million/mm³
RETICULOCYTE COUNT	1.0%-1.5%
HEMATOCRIT	
Men	40%-54%
Women	38%-47%
HEMOGLOBIN	
Men	13.5-16.5 g/dl
Women	12.0-15.0 g/dl
ERYTHROCYTE INDICES	
Mean cell volume	80-96 μm³
Mean cell hemoglobin	27-31 pg
Mean cell hemoglobin concentration	32%-36%
LEUKOCYTE COUNT	5000-10,000/mm³
LEUKOCYTE DIFFERENTIAL	
Neutrophils	40%-75%
Bands	0%-6%
Eosinophils	0%-6%
Basophils	0%-1%
Lymphocytes	20%-45%
Monocytes	2%-10%
THROMBOCYTES	250,000-400,000/mm³

include the **mean cell volume (MCV)** in cubic micrometers, **mean cellular hemoglobin (MCH)** content in picograms, and the **mean cellular hemoglobin concentration (MCHC)** as a percentage of total cellular weight. In addition, the CBC further evaluates the leukocytes by determining the percent of each type present, which is also known as the white blood cell differential count. Table 3-3 lists the components and normal values found in a CBC.

DIAGNOSTIC FOCUS

Hematology Studies Following Traumatic Injury

An 18-year-old man was involved in a motor vehicle accident and suffered blunt force trauma to the abdomen and chest. He ruptured several mesenteric and pulmonary vessels. These vessels bled into the abdominal and thoracic cavities. On admission to the emergency department, his blood pressure was found to be 90/55 mm Hg. The physician decided to collect a sample of blood to quickly determine the status of the patient's blood, given the injuries he sustained, and the possible need for a transfusion. Blood was rapidly collected from a peripheral vein in the left arm and carried to the laboratory for an immediate complete blood count (CBC) and blood type. The CBC showed the following:

Hematocrit	27%
Hemoglobin	9.2 g
Erythrocyte count	3.2 million/mm³
Leukocyte count	4400/mm³
Blood type	O negative

These results, coupled with the physical findings, indicate significant anemia and blood loss. The patient's blood type was cross matched with several units of stored blood that was given intravenously. He was then taken to the operating room for exploratory surgery to determine the location of bleeding and to have it repaired.

HOW BLOOD LOSS IS MINIMIZED

Hemostasis

Blood vessels can be damaged and blood can be lost from the vascular system into spaces between tissues, into body cavities, as well as to the outside of the body. A variety of mechanisms are present to minimize blood loss.

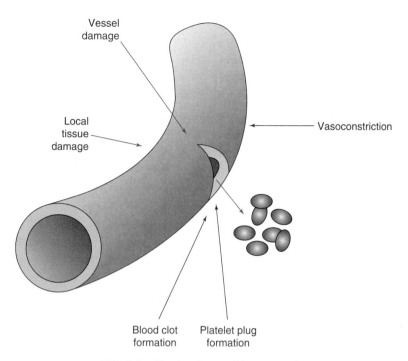

FIG. 3-8 Mechanisms of hemostasis.

Hemostasis, which refers to the mechanisms that work toward the prevention of blood loss, is most effective following small-vessel and capillary injuries. Large- and medium-sized artery lacerations often overwhelm the hemostatic mechanisms and require medical assistance to stop their bleeding. Hemostatic mechanisms include vessel constriction, platelet plugging, and blood clotting (Fig. 3-8).

Vasoconstriction

Vessels that are lacerated or ruptured can constrict through the activation of the smooth muscle in the tunica media. Vasoconstriction is most effective in small arteries, arterioles, and venules. The mechanism that triggers this reflex action is thought to be caused by direct injury to the smooth muscle, irritation of the nearby nerves that stimulate vasoconstriction, and the release of various vasoconstrictive chemical mediators (e.g., epinephrine, thromboxane A_2, and serotonin).

Platelet Aggregation

Platelets normally circulate freely and do not stick to the endothelium or to one another. If the endothelium is injured and the underlying connective tissue is exposed, platelets will stick to the exposed collagen fibers of the connective tissue. This adherence is facilitated by a plasma protein secreted by the endothelium called the **von Willebrand's factor.** As the platelets adhere to the wall of the injured vessel, they release mediators (adenosine diphosphate and thromboxane A_2) that trigger other platelets to change their shape and become sticky and adhere to the injury site as well as to one another. A growing mass of platelets forms. This process, known as **platelet aggregation,** results in the formation of a platelet plug that reduces or prevents further blood loss from the damaged vessel. In addition, platelets play a role in the clotting process by supplying certain phospholipids and stimulating vasoconstriction by secretion of serotonin and thromboxane A$_2$.

Platelet activation and subsequent aggregation is inhibited in normal vessels by the secretion of the lipid **prostacyclin** from the endothelial cells of an uninjured vessel wall. The use of **aspirin** and eating a diet rich in certain fish oils are known to reduce the development of thromboxane A$_2$ and thus the responsiveness of the platelets. Individuals who are at risk for developing coronary artery occlusion are often advised to take low doses of aspirin and to adjust their diets to reduce platelet aggregation in their damaged vessels.

Blood Clotting

Blood has the unique ability to change from a liquid to a jellylike state in just a matter of seconds. This property of being able to clot not only is important in the prevention of blood loss but also represents a potential threat if triggered and occlusion of the circulatory system occurs. This rather complex process involves some 13 different factors, many of which are plasma proteins produced by the liver (Table 3-4). For these factors to be produced, the liver needs to be healthy and have stable supplies of amino acids and vitamin K. When triggered, the factors interact through a series of reactions often referred to as a **clotting cascade** (Fig. 3-9). The clotting cascade culminates in the formation of an insoluble plasma protein called **fibrin** (Fig. 3-10). Fibrin filaments stabilize to form an interlinking network that traps erythrocytes, plasma, and platelets in a growing mass called a blood clot. The clot plugs the injured vessel and limits blood loss.

The first stage of clotting cascade begins with activation of either the **extrinsic** or **intrinsic** clotting pathway. The extrinsic pathway is activated when tissues are injured. Injured tissues release a complex lipoprotein called **tis-**

Table 3-4 Clotting Factors

International Designation	Factor Name
I	Fibrinogen
II	Prothrombin
III	Thromboplastin
IV	Ca^{++}
V	Proaccelerin or Labile factor
VI	No longer in use
VII	Serum prothrombin conversion accelerator
VIII	Antihemophilic factor
IX	Plasma thromboplastin component or Christmas factor
X	Stuart factor
XI	Plasma thromboplastin antecedent
XII	Hageman factor
XIII	Fibrin-stabilizing factor

sue thromboplastin, which begins the extrinsic clotting cascade. The intrinsic pathway is triggered when blood is exposed to injured vessels or to foreign surfaces outside the body such as the glass walls of a container. The intrinsic cascade begins with the activation of the **Hageman factor** when it is exposed to collagen fibers in the wall of an injured vessel, activated platelets, and foreign surfaces. In addition, the Hageman factor can be activated during times of stress such as anxiety, fear, and anger. Both the extrinsic and intrinsic pathways converge at the step where **prothrombin activator** is formed.

The second stage of the cascade proceeds with the enzymatic action of prothrombin activator on the conversion of **prothrombin** to **thrombin.**

The third stage continues the cascade with thrombin converting the plasma-soluble **fibrinogen** to the insoluble **fibrin** filaments of a clot. The fibrin filaments are stabilized by the presence of Ca^{++}, **fibrin stabilizing factor,** and thrombin. This process continues at the

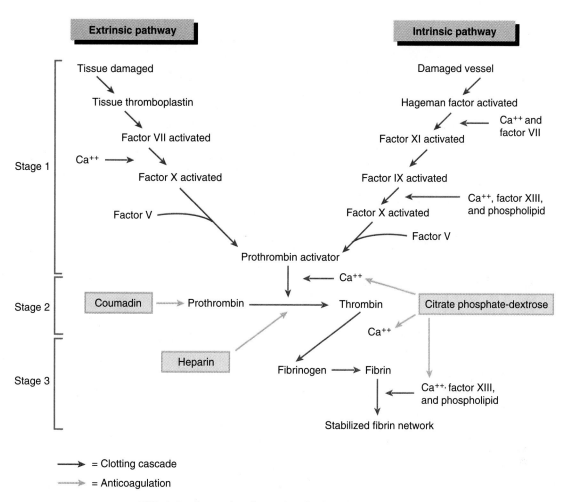

FIG. 3-9 Cascade of reaction in the clotting process.

location of the injury until the local concentration of one or more of the clotting factors is exhausted.

Clotting Disturbances and Disorders

A thrombus is a clot that forms in a vessel at the site of an injury. A thrombus that occludes or partially occludes a vessel is referred to as a **thrombosis.** A thrombosis can be life saving when it forms in a ruptured and bleeding vessel, or it can be life threatening when it forms in a vessel that is supplying blood to critical tissues (e.g., cerebral thrombosis). A clot that forms in one area of the body and moves through the circulatory system to another area is called an **embolus.** When an embolus occludes or partially occludes a vessel, the condition is known as an **embolism** (e.g., pulmonary embolism) and is often associated with complications from the disruption of blood flow to various tissues.

A variety of substances can prevent the clotting process by blocking the activity of one or more factors. The drugs that act to block the formation of clots are called **anticoagulants.** This group includes **aspirin, heparin, warfarin**

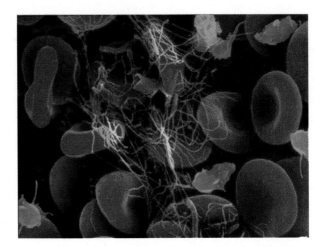

FIG. 3-10   Scanning electron micrograph of a fibrin network that has entrapped erythrocytes. (From Thibodeau GA, Patton KT: *Anatomy and physiology,* ed 4, St Louis, 1999, Mosby.)

(Coumadin), and **citrate phosphate-dextrose (CPD).** At low doses, aspirin inhibits the aggregation of platelets and at higher doses inhibits the production of prothrombin. Heparin acts by blocking the conversion of prothrombin to thrombin. Coumadin works indirectly by inhibiting the liver's ability to use vitamin K and by preventing the synthesis of several factors including prothrombin. These drugs are used to prevent clot formation in those patients who are prone to clotting and who will experience circulatory problems as a result (e.g., a patient who is to have open-heart surgery for a valve replacement). CPD is used in blood banking to block donor blood coagulation by removing Ca^{++} from plasma.

Liver and kidney failure commonly disturb the clotting mechanism. Liver failure (e.g., cirrhosis) results in an inability to produce necessary clotting factors. Kidney failure leads to an accumulation of various toxic substances (e.g., urea and ammonia) that causes the liver to malfunction. In both cases the ability of the blood to coagulate is impaired, which can result in spontaneous hemorrhaging.

Hemophilia, a hereditary condition of impaired clotting resulting in spontaneous bleeding or excessive bleeding following injuries, is caused by a gene deficiency for factor VIII (type A hemophilia) or factor IX (type B hemophilia). Treatment for hemophilia consists of isolating these factors from numerous units of donor blood, concentrating them, and providing regular transfusions of this concentrated plasma fraction that contain the needed factors.

Disseminated intravascular coagulation (DIC) is a condition where an obstetric complication, widespread tissue trauma, an infection, or a toxin triggers the coagulation system to start clotting. Microscopic clots begin to fill various regional capillary beds, which, in severe cases, can result in multiple organ failure. To further compound the problem, various clotting factors and platelets are consumed during the process, which can then lead to spontaneous bleeding.

A number of coagulation tests are frequently employed to determine the blood's clotting ability when questions arise about why a patient is bleeding or how well anticoagulant therapy is working. The **bleeding time** is a simple screening test that determines how long a puncture site on the ear lobe takes to

Treatment of Transient Ischemic Attacks

A 68-year-old woman began to experience intermittent confusion and loss of muscle control on the left side of her body. Her family brought her to the medical center where it was determined that she had a sudden and short-term reduction of blood flow in the right hemisphere of her brain known as transient ischemic attack (TIA). TIA is brought about by injury of the blood vessels from atherosclerosis. Vessel spasm, platelet aggregation, and blood coagulation are triggered by the release of the fatty acid thromboxane A_2 from injured cells in the vessel wall. This leads to a reduction in local blood flow and can lead to a stroke.

To prevent blood vessel spasm and to reduce the coagulability of her blood, she was prescribed a low dose of aspirin, which reduces the incidence of TIA, stroke, and heart attack by inhibiting the synthesis of thromboxane A_2. She recovered and went home.

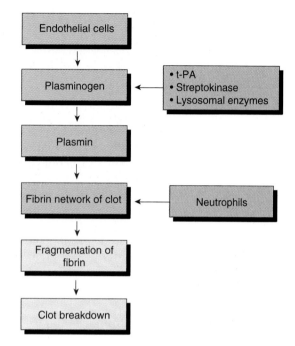

FIG. 3-11 Simplified sequence of fibrinolysis (tissue plasminogen activator [t-PA]).

stop bleeding. A normal bleeding time is between 1 and 6 minutes; a greater time indicates a coagulation defect. The **prothrombin time (PT)** is a test of how long it takes for blood to clot in a test tube following the addition of a large amount of thromboplastin and Ca^{++}. An average value of 11 to 16 seconds indicates that the second stage of clotting is normal. Another test of the second stage of clotting is the **partial thromboplastin time (PTT),** which is the amount of time it takes to form a clot in a test tube following the addition of activated partial thromboplastin. A normal value is about 60 to 85 seconds; longer times indicate defects in the intrinsic clotting pathway. The **platelet count** is another important indicator of the ability for blood to clot. Values less than $150,000/mm^3$, which indicate a **thrombocytopenia,** indicate the potential for spontaneous or excessive bleeding.

Fibrinolysis

Blood is constantly forming blood clots as the two pathways of the clotting cascades are activated. To prevent the accumulation of clot material and promote healing, the body has a mechanism to break down clots (Fig. 3-11). The fibrin network that holds the clot together can be decomposed by the enzyme **plasmin,** which circulates in the blood in an inactive form called **plasminogen.** Plasminogen is converted to plasmin by various factors called **plasminogen activators** (e.g., **tissue plasminogen activator [t-PA],** thrombin, and the Hageman factor), which are released by the liver, the endothelial cells of the vessel wall, and local tissues. In addition, neutrophils become active and break down the clot by phagocytosis and enzyme action. Soon after a clot forms, plasminogen activators begin to accumulate and neutrophils move into the area over a period of about 48 to 72 hours. As the local plasmin concentration climbs and neutrophils begin their phagocytosis, the clot begins to dissolve while, simultaneously, the vessel wall and local tissues heal.

A clot formation in the coronary arteries can be triggered by an atherosclerotic injury forming in the vessel wall. The production of a clot in an already narrowed vessel can lead to a coronary thrombosis and reduction of coronary blood flow. **Ischemia** (the reduction of blood flow) to the myocardium can result in tissue dysfunction and **necrosis** (death). When the tissues die, it is known as a **myocardial infarction.** Clot-"busting" drugs are available to treat this and other thrombotic or embolic events. **Streptokinase,** a bacterial enzyme, is a common **thrombolytic** agent used for the emergency removal of blood clots. It works indirectly by converting plasminogen to plasmin. In addition, tissue plasminogen activator has been produced through genetic engineering and has been used for emergency clot removal.

CHAPTER SELF-TEST QUESTIONS

1. Blood is _____% water.
   a. 99
   b. 95
   c. 91
   d. 85
   e. 55

Match the following ion types with its normal blood plasma concentration:
2. Na^+
3. Cl^-
4. K^+
   a. 140 mEq/L
   b. 100 mEq/L
   c. 25 mEq/L
   d. 10 mEq/L
   e. 4 mEq/L

Match the following components of the complete blood count with its normal value
5. erythrocyte count
6. leukocyte count
7. platelet count
   a. 300,000/mm³
   b. 10,000/mm³
   c. 2000/mm³
   d. 5,000,000/mm³
   e. 10,000,000/mm³
8. The hematocrit is the percentage of blood that is comprised of
   a. water
   b. plasma
   c. leukocytes
   d. formed elements
   e. platelets
9. Which one of the following is known to stimulate bone marrow to increase red blood cell production
   a. erythropoietin
   b. cytokines
   c. plasminogen
   d. thromboxane
10. Type O blood has
    a. no A or B surface agglutinogens and types a and b agglutinins
    b. type A surface agglutinogens and type b agglutinins
    c. type B surface agglutinogens and type a agglutinins
    d. type A and B surface agglutinogens and neither type a nor b agglutinins

For answers, see p. 475.

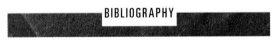

BIBLIOGRAPHY

1. Babior BM, Stossel TP: *Hematology: a pathophysiological approach,* New York, 1984, Churchill Livingstone.
2. Cummins RO et al: *Advanced cardiac life support,* Dallas, 1997, American Heart Association.
3. Ganong WF: *Review of medical physiology,* ed 18, Stamford, Conn, 1997, Appleton & Lange.
4. Guyton AC: *Textbook of medical physiology,* Philadelphia, 1996, WB Saunders.

5. Martini FH: *Fundamentals of anatomy and physiology,* Upper Saddle River, NJ, 1998, Prentice Hall.
6. Miale JB: *Laboratory medicine: hematology,* ed 6, St Louis, 1982, Mosby.
7. Mountcastle VB et al: *Medical physiology,* ed 14, St Louis, 1980, Mosby.
8. Shoemaker WC et al: *Textbook of critical care,* ed 2, Philadelphia, 1989, WB Saunders.
9. Tortora GJ, Grabowski SR: *Principles of anatomy and physiology,* ed 7, New York, 1993, Harper Collins College.
10. West JB et al: *Best and Taylor's physiological basis of medical practice,* ed 11, Baltimore, 1985, Williams & Wilkins.
11. Williams DO: Intravenous recombinant tissue type plasminogen activator (r-tPA) in acute myocardial infarction, *J Am Coll Cardiol* 5:6191, 1985.
12. Wintrobe MM et al: *Clinical hematology,* ed 7, Philadelphia, 1974, Lea & Febiger.

Electrophysiology of the Heart

⬭ ELECTROPHYSIOLOGY

The circulatory system provides the vital function of moving blood throughout the body to meet the needs of cellular metabolism. The force needed to circulate the blood is provided by the coordinated pumping action of the heart chambers. The orderly sequence of atrial and ventricular contraction is only possible when a healthy electrical conduction system is present. Heart disease that disturbs the electrical conduction system can lead to a serious dysrhythmia that may be life threatening. This chapter provides a description of the bioelectrical system of the healthy heart and its role in circulation. In addition, this chapter describes how the electrical activity of the heart is recorded and how to recognize abnormal rhythms.

⬭ BIOELECTRICAL PROPERTIES OF CARDIAC CELLS

In a resting state, cardiac cells have an interior electrical charge of approximately 60 to 90 mV lower than that outside the cell membrane (Fig. 4-1). This intracellular electronegativity is typical of smooth muscle, nerves, and skeletal muscle and virtually all cells throughout the body including the cardiac cells. The creation of electrical polarity across the cell membrane and the changes in polarity that occur in response to electrical stimulus are crucial to the contractile abilities of muscle fibers, especially in the myocardium.

Generation of the Resting Membrane Potential

Creation of cardiac cell polarity is a complex activity that involves the movement of ions across the membrane. Changes in cell membrane permeability alter the speed at which ions, such as calcium, sodium, and potassium, travel across the membrane. Alterations in the permeability of the membrane are created by the opening and closing of voltage-sensitive ion channels specific for each ion.

Healthy cardiac cells, similar to other cells of the body, have a K^+ concentration much higher on the inside as compared with that of the outside of the cells. The concentration of Na^+ and Ca^{++} outside the cell greatly exceeds that of inside the cell (Fig. 4-2).

Ion channels for K^+ are significantly more permeable compared with the channels for Ca^{++} and Na^+. The higher concentration of K^+ inside the cells and the greater permeability of the K^+ channels combine to cause a net movement of K^+ out of the cell. The diffusion of K^+ out of the cell leaves a deficiency of cations and causes the interior of the cardiac cell to become electronegative.

The negative intracellular charge and higher extracellular concentration of Na^+ force

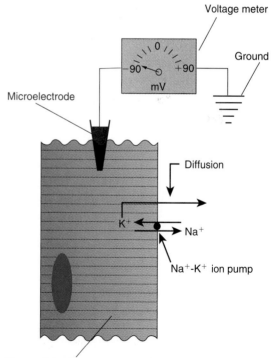

FIG. 4-1 Measurement of a cardiac cell resting potential with a microelectrode.

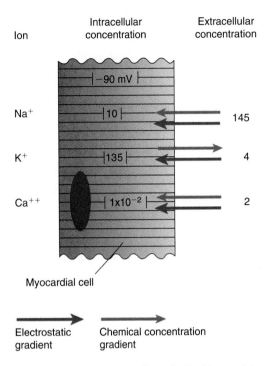

Ion | Intracellular concentration | Extracellular concentration

−90 mV

Na⁺ ... 10 ... 145

K⁺ ... 135 ... 4

Ca⁺⁺ ... 1×10⁻² ... 2

Myocardial cell

Electrostatic gradient   Chemical concentration gradient

FIG. 4-2 Ion concentrations (mEq/L) on either side of the cardiac cell membrane. Ion movement is driven by concentration and electrostatic gradients. The electrostatic gradient attracts the cations into the cell as a result of an intracellular charge or resting potential of −90 mV.

moves more Na⁺ out than it moves K⁺ in at a ratio of about 3:2. This further contributes to the development of an electrical polarity. Cardiac disease, such as coronary artery disease, can reduce the supply of energy to the myocardium and inhibit the Na⁺-K⁺ pump from contributing to the polarization of cardiac cells.

The presence of numerous intracellular proteins also helps create a negative intracellular charge. Proteins are negatively charged at a normal intracellular pH of 7.0. These large molecules remain inside the cell and contribute to the voltage polarity.

The combination of selective ion channel permeability, transmembrane ion gradients, the activity of the Na⁺-K⁺ pump, and the presence of intracellular protein acts to create a normal intracellular electrical potential of −60 to −90 mV. This electrical gradient, normally occurring at rest across the cardiac cell membrane, is known as the **resting membrane potential.**

Action Potential

The application of a sufficient chemical or electrical stimulus to the polarized cardiac cell causes the cell to rapidly lose its intracellular negative charge. This loss of polarization is termed **depolarization.** The stimulus has to be sufficient to cause cellular depolarization. The minimum amount of stimulus that just causes the cell to depolarize is known as the threshold stimulus. The typical cardiac cell has a threshold stimulus level that produces an internal voltage of about −55 mV. Fig. 4-3 shows the electrical and ionic changes in a cardiac cell following a threshold stimulus.

The early phase of depolarization occurs primarily as a result of Na⁺ ions rushing through ion specific channels across the cell membrane and inside the cell (Fig. 4-3, *phase 0*). At the same time, K⁺ ion channels close in response to the positive voltage and slow the movement of K⁺ ions out of the cell. Closure of the K⁺ channels allows the Na⁺ ions to

Na⁺ inside the cell. Significant movement of Na⁺ into the cell would counteract the negative charge created by the outward movement of K⁺. However, the permeability of the cardiac cell membrane to sodium is very low, which results in low influx of Na⁺ ions. In addition, an ion pump, a protein complex located in numerous cites in the cell membrane, continuously moves Na⁺ out of the cell and K⁺ into the cell. This Na⁺-K⁺ pump removes the small amount of Na⁺ that leaks in and replaces the small amount of K⁺ that leaks out of the cell. The pump moves Na⁺ and K⁺ simultaneously through the membrane against chemical concentrations and electrostatic gradients by utilizing energy in the form of adenosine triphosphate to perform this action. This pump

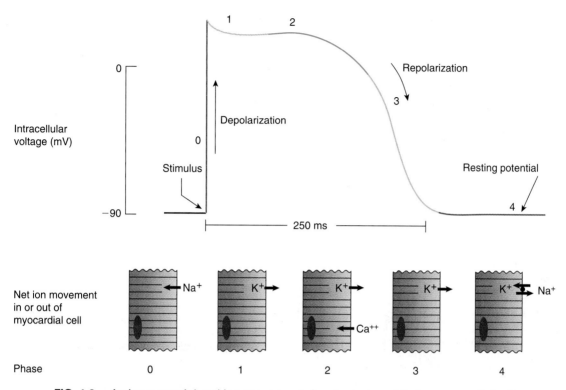

FIG. 4-3 Action potential and ion movements in a typical ventricular myocardial cell (see text for description).

enter the cell much faster, which is essential for depolarization. This is termed the fast response. The fast response phase of depolarization depends on an appropriate concentration of extracellular Na⁺. The amplitude of depolarization may be suppressed when significant reductions in extracellular Na⁺ concentrations **(hyponatremia)** occur.

The cardiac cell rapidly begins to return to normal polarity after depolarization. This is known as **repolarization** and is the result of several different ions passing through the cardiac cell membrane. Once the normal internal electronegativity returns, the cycle is complete and the cell is again ready to depolarize if stimulated.

Just after the fast response and when reaching a depolarization voltage of about 30 mV, K⁺ begins to move out of the cell (Fig. 4-3, *phase 1*). This brings about a transient dip in voltage, which is then retarded by a slow inward movement of Ca⁺⁺ through Ca⁺⁺ channels (Fig. 4-3, *phase 2*). The plateau in voltage is referred to as the slow response. The inward movement of Ca⁺⁺ not only prolongs depolarization, but also assists in the contraction process of myocardial cells. Calcium ions are necessary for proper function of contractile proteins within the cell and for a forceful contraction by the heart muscle. Predictably, depletion of extracellular Ca⁺⁺ **(hypocalcemia)** can cause a significant reduction in the contractile forces of the heart.

Repolarization continues as the outward movement of K⁺ exceeds the slowing inward movement of Na⁺ and Ca⁺⁺; this is complete when the intracellular voltage returns to the resting potential (Fig. 4-3, *phase 3*). At this point, the voltage-sensitive ion channels return to their pre-depolarization permeability. The excess Na^+ that entered the cell during depolarization and the K^+ lost from the cell during repolarization are both offset by the activity of the Na^+-K^+ ion pump (Fig. 4-3, *phase 4*). Another ion pump, a Na^+-Ca^{++} pump, rapidly removes the small excess of Ca^{++} that entered the cell. Repolarization is retarded when conditions of increased extracellular concentrations of K^+ **(hyperkalemia)** exist.

The early phase of repolarization is known as the absolute refractory period because during this time the cardiac cell is unresponsive to any stimuli. In the later phase of depolarization, the cardiac cell responds only to a strong stimulus; this phase is known as the relative refractory period. Stimulus of the cardiac cell during the relative refractory period, at best, results in a weak response of the myocardial cell.

The entire depolarization-repolarization cycle is known as the **action potential,** which normally takes about 250 to 300 ms.

The myocardium is a functional syncytium of many heart muscle cells. The myocardial muscle fibers are made up of many different cells connected to each other by a porous junction. This allows the action potential to rapidly pass from one cell to another and on to all other myocardial cells following the initial stimulus (Fig. 4-4). The propagation of the action potential through the heart stimulates the myocardium to contract.

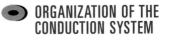 **ORGANIZATION OF THE CONDUCTION SYSTEM**

The heart possesses a specialized group of myocardial cells that spontaneously triggers an action potential and forms a pathway or channel for the action potential to travel through the heart. This specialized group of cells, known as the cardiac conduction system, is responsible for the heart's ability to continue beating even after being removed from the body.

Sinoatrial Node and Atrial Conduction

The region of the mammalian heart responsible for triggering or pacing the heart normally is the **sinoatrial (SA) node.** The SA node is

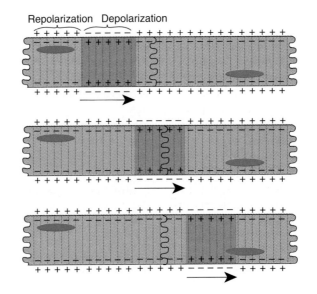

FIG. 4-4 Propagation of depolarization and repolarization from cardiac cell to cardiac cell.

about 8 mm × 2 mm and lies in the groove where the superior vena cava attaches to the right atrium (Fig. 4-5). The SA node normally serves as the pacemaker of the heart because it is comprised of cells that have the ability to spontaneously depolarize. These cells spontaneously depolarize because of a greater leakage of Na^+ and Ca^{++} across the cell membrane, which, in turn, causes the intracellular voltage to reach the threshold stimulus level of about −55 mV. Cells that can spontaneously depolarize are said to have **automaticity** and are located at various points along the electrical conduction system. The SA node generates action potentials at a frequency of about 60 to 80 times per minute and normally paces the heart.

Near the SA node lie other cells with a high degree of automaticity that also can serve as the pacemaker for the heart. These cells along with the SA node make up the **atrial pacemaker complex.** Frequently all the cells of the atrial pacemaker complex initiate impulses simultaneously.

The electrical impulse generated by the atrial pacemaker complex travels over the right and left atria in a wavelike fashion at a conduction velocity of about 1 m/s. The impulse spreads over the right atrium along ordinary myocardial fibers but travels to the left atrium

through special pathways. The anterior interatrial myocardial band or internodal pathway, which has three tracts, rapidly conducts the impulse from the SA node directly to the left atrium. Rapid passage of the cardiac impulse from the SA node to the left atrium is needed to allow near simultaneous contraction of both atria and thus better filling of the ventricles before contraction.

Atrioventricular Node and Atrioventricular Conduction

The cardiac impulse passes through the atria and quickly reaches the **atrioventricular (AV) node.** The anterior interatrial myocardial band probably plays a key role in passing the impulse from the SA node to the AV node. The AV node represents the only path for the cardiac impulse to pass from the atria to the ventricles normally. This node lies posteriorly on the right side of the interatrial septum and is approximately 22 mm long, 10 mm wide, and 3 mm thick.

The AV node, similar to the SA node, is made of special cardiac cells that have automaticity capabilities. The cells of the AV node spontaneously depolarize normally at a rate slower than the SA node. This allows the AV node to serve as a backup pacemaker rather

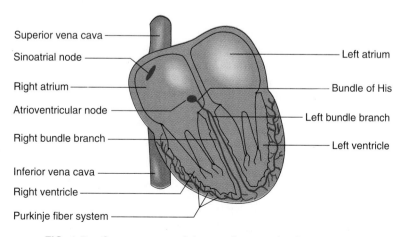

Superior vena cava

Sinoatrial node

Right atrium

Atrioventricular node

Right bundle branch

Inferior vena cava

Right ventricle

Purkinje fiber system

Left atrium

Bundle of His

Left bundle branch

Left ventricle

FIG. 4-5 Components of the cardiac conduction system.

than a primary pacemaker. The AV node paces the ventricles if the SA node fails.

The cardiac impulse passes through the AV node at about 0.05 m/s, which is much slower than through other parts of the electrical conduction system. This delay of the cardiac impulse at the AV node permits more optimal filling of the ventricles before ventricular contraction. The AV node also serves to protect the ventricles from extremely rapid impulse rates arising from the atria. The AV node does not allow excessive impulse rates to pass through to the ventricles if the SA node or atria develop excessive excitation rates. This protective function of the AV node helps preserve cardiac function by allowing adequate time for filling. At heart rates of more than 200 bpm the amount of blood pumped per minute actually declines because of inadequate filling.

Ventricular Conduction

Once the cardiac impulse exits the AV node, the goal of the electrical conduction system is to rapidly deliver the trigger for systole throughout both ventricles. This is the function of the specialized ventricular conduction system made up of the **bundle of His, left and right bundle branches,** and the **Purkinje fibers.**

The bundle of His, located just distal to the AV node, passes subendocardially down the right side of the interventricular septum for approximately 1 cm where it then divides into the right and left bundle branches (see Fig. 4-5).

The right bundle branch, a direct extension of the bundle of His, proceeds down the right side of the interventricular septum. The left bundle branch, which is much thicker than the right bundle branch, penetrates the interventricular septum and quickly branches into the left **anterior division** and left **posterior division.** The left anterior division conducts the impulse to the anterior and superior portions of the left ventricle. The left posterior division provides the posterior and inferior sections of

the left ventricle with cardiac impulses. The right bundle branch and the anterior and posterior divisions of the left bundle branch subdivide into many Purkinje fibers. The Purkinje fibers terminate in the myocardium throughout the left and right ventricles. Conduction of the cardiac impulse throughout the Purkinje fibers is the fastest of any tissue in the conduction system with velocities that range from 1 to 4 m/s. This rapid movement of the action potential by the Purkinje fibers is needed so that near-simultaneous contraction of right and left ventricles occurs.

Fig. 4-6 summarizes the components of the cardiac conduction system and the order in which an impulse travels through it.

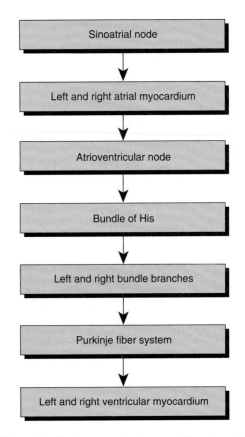

FIG. 4-6 Pathway of the cardiac impulse through the cardiac conduction system.

● FACTORS THAT INFLUENCE THE CONDUCTION SYSTEM

Extrinsic Influences on the Conduction System

The conduction system of the heart is capable of maintaining an effective heart rhythm without any input from the nervous system. The autonomic nervous system, however, plays an important role in heart function by adjusting the rate and strength of myocardial contraction when needed (Table 4-1). For example, exercise increases the demand for circulation to meet the increased metabolic needs of the muscles involved with the activity. This increase in circulation is accomplished through activation of the sympathetic portion of the autonomic nervous system. Activation of the sympathetic system causes a release of norepinephrine from the sympathetic nerve endings in the heart, which causes an increase in the rate and strength of heart contraction. Excessive stimulation of the sympathetic system is likely to cause fast heart rates that can exceed 100 bpm **(tachycardia)** and abnormal rhythms such as premature contractions.

Parasympathetic impulses reach the heart through the vagus nerve. Branches of the vagus nerve release the neurotransmitter **acetylcholine,** which stimulates cholinergic receptors on the cardiac cells. This causes the cells to change their cell membrane ion permeability. The K^+ channels are stimulated to open and the Na^+ and Ca^{++} channels are closed. This results in greater K^+ leakage from the cell and less Na^+ and Ca^{++} movement into the cell. The intracellular voltage becomes more negative making it more difficult for the SA node cells to reach their threshold stimulus voltage and to spontaneously depolarize. The lower intracellular concentration of Ca^{++} causes the contractile proteins to interact less. These effects result in a slower heart rate and a weaker myocardial contraction. Significant stimulation of the vagus nerve can cause an abnormally slow heart rate of less than 60 bpm **(bradycardia)** and even temporary blockage of the cardiac impulse through the AV node.

Other external factors, such as temperature and abnormal ion concentrations, can influence the cardiac conduction system. Warming the heart causes the SA node to spontaneously

● **Table 4-1**   Influence of the Autonomic Nervous System on the Cardiac Conduction and Heart Function

Autonomic Branch	Neurotransmitter	Receptor Type	Myocardial Response
Sympathetic	Norepinephrine	Beta-1	↑ Ca^{++} and Na^+ membrane permeability Cause slow depolarization toward threshold ↑ Automaticity ↑ SA and AV node activity ↑ Heart rate ↑ Contractility
Parasympathetic	Acetylcholine	Cholinergic	↑ K^+ membrane permeability Cause hyperpolarization away from threshold ↓ Automaticity ↓ SA and AV node activity ↓ Heart rate ↓ Contractility

depolarize at a faster rate whereas cooling has the opposite effect. Numerous ions are crucial to cardiac function but K^+ and Ca^{++} are the most important ones. The concentrations of these ions are very low outside the cell, and any change causes disturbances of ion movement across the cell membrane. An increase or decrease in the extracellular concentration of these electrolytes can disturb the conduction system and the contraction capabilities of the myocardium. Severe electrolyte abnormalities can result in serious dysrhythmias.

Alterations in extracellular K^+ concentrations cause changes in the leakage rates of K^+ out of the cell. Plasma K^+ concentrations of greater than 5 mEq/L (hyperkalemia) cause a decrease and lengthening of depolarization and a lengthening of repolarization. This generally causes the heart rate to decrease. Concentrations of less than 3.5 mEq/L **(hypokalemia)** cause enhanced depolarization, increased cardiac cell irritability, and retarded repolarization. This promotes premature beats and increased heart rate.

Altered extracellular concentrations of Ca^{++} generally cause changes in the movement of Ca^{++} into the cell. Elevated plasma concentrations of greater than 3 mEq/L **(hypercalcemia)** increase cardiac irritability and enhance rapid repolarization. These effects promote a rapid heart rate and premature beats. Concentrations of less than 1 mEq/L (hypocalcemia) cause prolonged repolarization and a reduced heart rate.

Numerous pharmacologic agents can affect the membrane conductance rate of the ions mentioned previously. **Catecholamines,** such as **epinephrine, norepinephrine,** and **isoproterenol,** activate β-adrenergic receptors on cardiac cells causing Ca^{++} channels to open and allowing intracellular Ca^{++} concentrations to increase. This lowers the threshold stimulus needed to trigger an action potential, increases the slow response, and provides more Ca^{++} to the contractile proteins of the myocardial cell. Catecholamines are used to increase heart rate

and strengthen contraction. **Verapamil** and **nifedipine** are Ca^{++} channel blockers that reduce the movement of Ca^{++} into the cell. This alteration in Ca^{++} channel function primarily affects the slow response phase and

CASE STUDY FOCUS

Crushing Chest Pain and Shortness of Breath

A 48-year-old male was brought to the emergency department complaining of the sudden onset of "crushing" substernal chest pain and shortness of breath. He has a history of smoking two packs of cigarettes per day for the past 22 years and is 100 pounds overweight. His vital signs were as follows:

Respiratory rate	26/min
Heart rate	52 bpm
Blood pressure	66/40 mm Hg
Temperature	97° F

His skin was cold and clammy and his lung sounds were clear, bilaterally.

The patient was given supplemental oxygen to breathe, and an intravenous line was started in the median cubital vein in his left arm. An immediate electrocardiogram (ECG) showed a complete (third-degree) heart block that resulted in ventricular bradycardia and reduced blood pressure. Some ST segment and Q wave changes were also noted, all of which are consistent with a myocardial infarction. The physician decided to give him atropine to block the parasympathetic nervous system, which should have resulted in a faster heart rate and improved blood pressure. This improved his heart rate to 60 bpm but failed to improve his blood pressure. The patient was then given dobutamine to stimulate the sympathetic receptors of the heart. The ECG converted to a sinus rhythm with a heart rate of 83 bpm, and his blood pressure increased to 128/78 mm Hg. He was then given morphine sulfate to reduce pain, anxiety, and cardiac workload by dilating the blood vessels. He was then transferred to the coronary care unit for further evaluation.

increases the threshold stimulus necessary to start an action potential. In addition, Ca^{++} channel blockers reduce the strength of contraction. They are useful in slowing down abnormally rapid heart rate rhythms. **Digitalis** inhibits the Na^+-K^+ ion pump, which results in a reduction in the concentration of intracellular K^+. As the concentration of K^+ decreases, a net increase in the intracellular Ca^{++} concentration occurs and the stimulus necessary to trigger an action potential increases. Both of these actions combine to cause the heart to slow down and beat with greater strength. This makes digitalis ideal for the treatment of a heart that is beating rapidly and losing its strength of contraction.

HOW CARDIAC BIOELECTRICAL ACTIVITY IS MEASURED AND MONITORED

The electrical activity of the heart is conducted by the surrounding tissues and fluids to the surface of the body. These weak electrical impulses can be detected, amplified, and recorded by placing electrodes on the patient's skin. The instrument used to create a recording of the heart's electrical activity is called an electrocardiograph, and the resulting tracing is known as an **electrocardiogram (ECG).** The tracing is useful for detecting abnormalities in the cardiac rhythm. The following discussion presents the fundamentals related to creating and interpreting the ECG.

Principles of Electrocardiography
Lead Placement

The standard ECG calls for placement of electrodes, or leads, on the limbs and on the surface of the chest wall over the heart. By placing positive electrodes in various positions relative to negative and ground electrodes, the electrical activity of the heart's conduction system can be recorded and analyzed from a variety of vantage points. The standard 12-lead ECG utilizes four limb electrodes and six chest

electrodes to position positive and negative electrodes in 12 different configurations.

The six limb lead configurations are known as leads I, II, III, aVR, aVL, and aVF (Fig. 4-7). Leads I, II, and III detect activity by

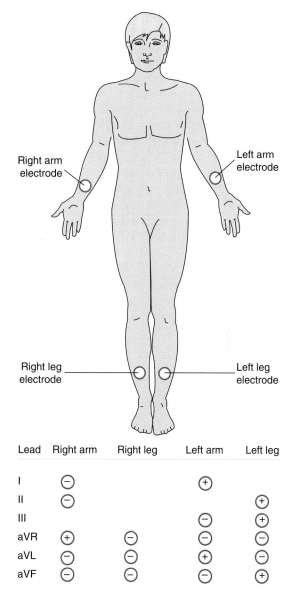

Lead	Right arm	Right leg	Left arm	Left leg
I	$\ominus$		$\oplus$	
II	$\ominus$			$\oplus$
III			$\ominus$	$\oplus$
aVR	$\oplus$	$\ominus$	$\ominus$	$\ominus$
aVL	$\ominus$	$\ominus$	$\oplus$	$\ominus$
aVF	$\ominus$	$\ominus$	$\ominus$	$\oplus$

FIG. 4-7 Location of electrodes and their charge for the six types of limb leads used for recording an electrocardiogram.

comparing the difference in electrical voltage between two electrodes and are known as bipolar leads. For example, in lead I the electrocardiograph temporarily designates the left arm electrode as a positive lead and the right arm electrode as a negative lead. The voltage difference between these two leads creates the lead I tracing. Lead II is created by designating the left leg lead as positive while the right arm lead remains negative. Lead III calls for the left arm electrode to become negative and the left leg lead to become positive. The electrode on the right leg serves as a ground.

The other limb leads, aVR, aVL, and aVF, are unipolar and are created by the ECG machine amplifying the voltage detected at each limb to obtain an adequate tracing (see Fig. 4-7). The positive voltage recorded at the right arm, left arm, and left foot is amplified and recorded to create the tracing for leads aVR, aVL, and aVF, respectively.

The chest leads are also unipolar and are known as V1, V2, V3, V4, V5, and V6 (Fig. 4-8). Some refer to the chest leads as the precordial leads. These leads are useful in measuring the electrical impulses that travel in the transverse or horizontal plane and that move anteriorly or posteriorly in the patient. Leads V1 and V2 are designed to measure activity over the right ventricle, leads V3 and V4 measure activity over the anterior surface of the heart, and V5 and V6 measure activity over the left ventricle.

To allow a more complete view of the electrical activity occurring in the heart, 12 leads are needed. The limb leads measure activity in the vertical plane whereas the chest leads view the horizontal plane. Defects in conduction system that affect a select portion of the heart may go undetected if the ECG tracing does not provide a view of the heart from many different angles.

Frequently, the patient admitted to the intensive care unit needs continuous ECG monitoring. In such cases one or two leads are frequently used such as lead II or a modified chest lead 1 (MCL1) as shown in Fig. 4-9. Continuous monitoring of the ECG allows immediate recognition of serious dysrhythmias that may occur in the critically ill patient.

Normal ECG

Recording the electrical activity of the heart is useful in detecting abnormalities in the conduction system, the extent and location of ischemic myocardial damage, the effects of therapy, and the anatomical orientation of the heart. However, the ECG recording does *not* measure the pumping ability of the heart. A normal ECG tracing may be obtained from the patient in shock with a poor cardiac output. In addition, the ECG cannot predict the onset of myocardial ischemic problems. A normal ECG may be present just moments before an ischemic event.

The waves of depolarization and repolarization occurring across the atria and ventricles of the heart are detected and recorded with the leads described previously. A wave of depolarization moving toward a positive lead produces a positive (upward) deflection on the ECG recording (Fig. 4-10). Depolarization

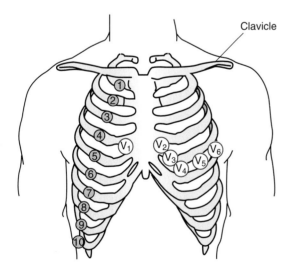

FIG. 4-8 Location of chest electrodes used for recording the six different chest leads of an electrocardiogram.

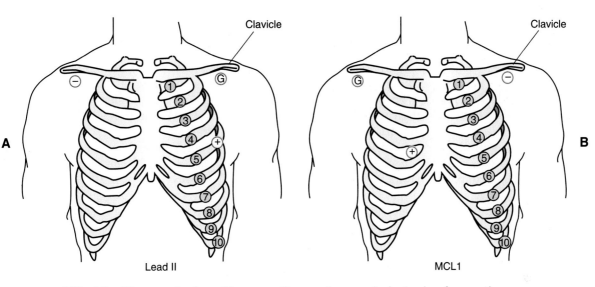

FIG. 4-9   Placement of positive, negative, and ground electrodes for continuous electrocardiogram monitoring with **(A)**, *lead II,* and **(B)**, modified chest lead 1 *(MCL1).*

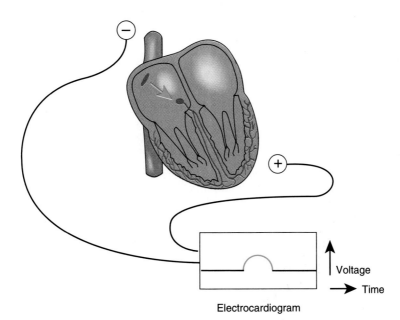

FIG. 4-10   Depolarization wave that moves toward a positive electrode causes a positive deflection of the voltage recorded on an electrocardiogram. Movement of the depolarization away from the positive electrode causes a negative deflection.

moving away from a positive lead causes a downward deflection on the ECG.

The normal cycle of electrical activity in the heart begins with spontaneous depolarization of the SA node and depolarization of the atria. This is recorded on the ECG as a small wave of electrical activity known as the **P wave** (Fig. 4-11, *A*). Repolarization of the atria is not typically seen on an ECG tracing because it occurs simultaneously with ventricular depolarization, which dominates the electrical recording.

Normally the P wave is followed by a slight pause while the electrical impulse passes slowly through the AV node. This is seen as a short isoelectric flat line on the ECG recording (Fig. 4-11, *B*). An isoelectric line represents time during the cardiac cycle in which no significant depolarization or repolarization of myocardium is occurring or the movement is at right angles to the electrodes. The length of the P wave and the isoelectric period is known as the **P-R interval.**

Next, depolarization of the ventricles is seen on the ECG as a **QRS complex** (Fig. 4-11, *C* and *D*). The QRS complex is normally much taller than the P wave because the muscle mass of the ventricles is greater than that of the atria.

After a slight pause, ventricular repolarization is recorded on the ECG as the **T wave**

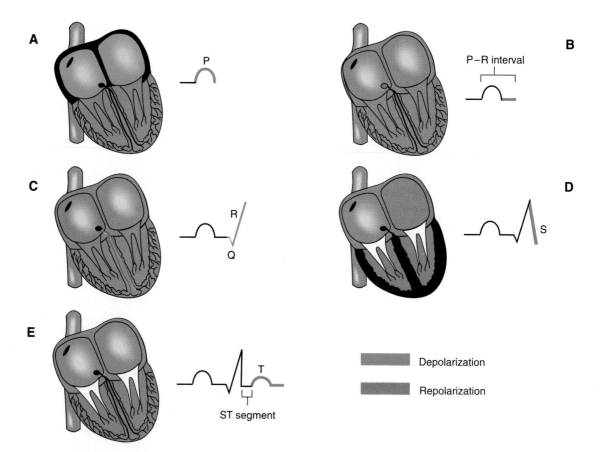

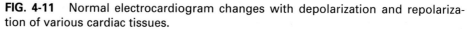

FIG. 4-11 Normal electrocardiogram changes with depolarization and repolarization of various cardiac tissues.

(Fig. 40-11, *E*). Normally the T wave is upright and slightly rounded. The slight pause before the T wave is referred to as the **ST segment** and is normally seen as a short isoelectric line. The cycle of electrical activity concludes with the T wave. The cycle starts over again with a P wave that emanates from the SA node.

Occasionally, a U wave may be recorded just after a T wave. This small positive deflection in lead II represents late repolarization of some cardiac tissues such as the cardiac valves. It is not considered to be an abnormal finding.

Fig. 4-12 shows a single cardiac electrical cycle with all the normal elements and a summary of what they represent.

ECG Paper and Measurements

The standard ECG paper has gridlike boxes with light and dark lines running in vertical and horizontal directions to record the electrical activity (Fig. 4-13). The lighter lines define boxes 1 mm square and the darker ones outline 5 mm square boxes.

The horizontal axis represents time as the electrical events are recorded at a rate of 25 mm/s. Therefore each small box represents 0.04 second and each larger and darker box represents 0.20 second. Five large boxes represent 1 second.

The vertical axis records the voltage change or amplitude of the electrical signals. The standard electrocardiograph is calibrated to produce a vertical deflection of 10 mm when 1 mV is recorded. As a result each vertical small box represents 0.1 mV and each vertical dark line represents 0.5 mV. Amplitude of the ECG wave is measured in a vertical direction from the isoelectric baseline. Larger myocardial muscle mass is expected to cause a more significant deflection from the isoelectric baseline.

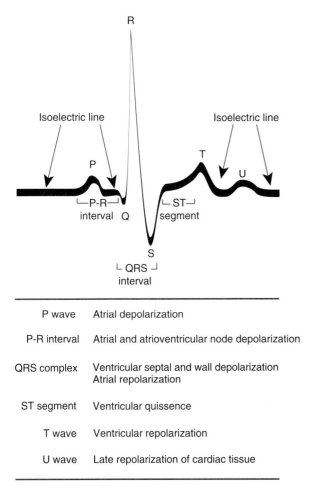

P wave	Atrial depolarization
P-R interval	Atrial and atrioventricular node depolarization
QRS complex	Ventricular septal and wall depolarization Atrial repolarization
ST segment	Ventricular quissence
T wave	Ventricular repolarization
U wave	Late repolarization of cardiac tissue

FIG. 4-12   Normal components of the electrocardiogram and the events that cause them.

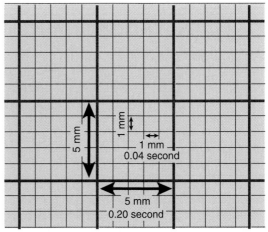

FIG. 4-13   Dimensions of electrocardiographic recording paper.

The normal P wave is no more than 2.5 mm in height and no more than 3 mm in length. Taller P waves imply that one or both atria have become hypertrophied.

The P-R interval, measured as the time from the beginning of the P wave to the beginning of the QRS complex, represents the time the electrical impulse takes to pass from the SA node through the atria and through the AV node. Normally it is between 0.12 and 0.2 second. Excessive slowing of the impulse through the AV node causes the P-R interval to exceed 0.20 second, or one large box. This is known as **AV block.**

The time of ventricular depolarization is normally less than 0.12 second. Therefore the QRS complex should be no wider than three small boxes or 0.12 second. QRS complexes wider than 0.12 second suggest that a conduction defect is present in one of the bundle branches.

The configuration of the ST segment is important to appreciate. Normally the ST segment is isoelectric. Significant deviation of the ST segment from the isoelectric baseline most often occurs with myocardial ischemia or infarction. In such cases the ST segment becomes significantly depressed or elevated.

HOW THE ECG RECORDING IS EVALUATED

A standardized process of evaluating an ECG includes the analyses of rate, rhythm, atrial activity, ventricular activity, mean electrical axis, and signs of hypertrophy, ischemia, and infarction.

Heart Rate

The initial parameter to assess on the ECG recording is the atrial and ventricular rates of contraction. Usually the atrial and ventricular rates will be the same. However, when an AV block is present, they may be contracting at different rates. The most important rate to evaluate is the ventricular rate since the ventricles represent the primary force for the circulation of blood.

Ventricular rate can be evaluated by determining the number of large (0.2-second) boxes between two successive QRS complexes. The number of boxes is then divided into 300. For example, suppose there are three large boxes between two successive QRS complexes. By dividing 3 into 300, a rate of 100/min is calculated (Fig. 4-14). Table 4-2 shows the estimated heart rate for different numbers of squares between QRS complexes. This approach should only be used when the ventricular rhythm is regular.

This method for evaluating ventricular rate becomes inaccurate with irregular rhythms because the distance between QRS complexes varies from beat to beat. In such cases an average heart rate can be determined by counting the number of QRS complexes in a 6-second interval and multiplying this number by 10. The top of the standard ECG paper has small vertical dashes every 3 seconds. For example, if six QRS complexes are present in two 3-second intervals (6 seconds), the ventricular rate is approximately 6 x 10, or 60, bpm (Fig. 4-15).

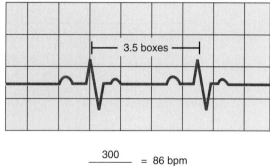

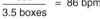

$$\frac{300}{3.5 \text{ boxes}} = 86 \text{ bpm}$$

FIG. 4-14 Estimating cardiac rate by counting the number of large boxes between QRS complexes.

Table 4-2 Estimating Heart Rate by Counting the Number of Large Boxes Between QRS Complexes

Number of Large Squares	Interval Between Beats	Rate Per Minute	
1	0.2 sec	300	
2	0.4 sec	150	
3	0.6 sec	100	Normal
4	0.8 sec	75	sinus
5	1.0 sec	60	rhythm
6	1.2 sec	50	
7	1.4 sec	43	
8	1.6 sec	37	
9	1.8 sec	33	
10	2.0 sec	30	

From Davis D: *Differential diagnosis of arrhythmias*, Philadelphia, 1992, WB Saunders.

A normal heart rate is 60 to 100 bpm. Heart rates less than 60 are classified as being **bradycardia** and rates greater than 100 bpm are considered to be **tachycardia.**

Rhythmicity, Atrial Activity, and Ventricular Activity

The overall rhythm of the ECG is easily evaluated by looking at the distance between QRS complexes. In a normal rhythm the distance is equal. During **dysrhythmias** the distance varies between QRS complexes. Early or premature beats and late beats show changes in the QRS-to-QRS distance.

The next step is to evaluate the atrial activity by analyzing the P wave and P-R interval. A normal P wave should be seen and should precede each QRS complex, and the P-R interval should be less than 0.2 second (one large box). This indicates normal pacing of the

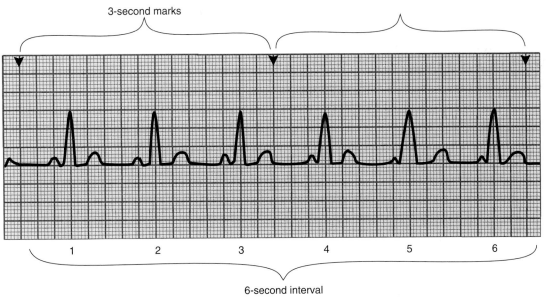

3-second marks

6-second interval

Heart rate = 6 × 10 = 60 bpm

FIG. 4-15 Estimating heart rate by counting the number of QRS complexes in a 6-second interval.

heart and conduction of the impulse through the atria and AV node.

Ventricular activity is evaluated by analyzing the QRS complex, ST segment, and T wave. Normal ventricular conduction is indicated by a normal QRS complex and interval of less than 0.12 second (three small boxes). The ST segment should be on the isoelectric baseline and followed by a normal T wave, which indicates normal ventricular repolarization.

Mean Electrical Axis

The average, or mean, path of electrical transmission through the heart is termed the mean electrical axis of the heart. It can be determined by viewing the 12 leads and the direction of the deflections in each lead. Normally the mean axis orientation is located at about 60 degrees in the vertical plane (Fig. 4-16). However, the axis can deviate to the right or left if the heart changes position or if impulse conduction is altered by substantial injury to the myocardium following an infarction. By analyzing the QRS complex in leads I and aVF, the axis can be determined. The QRS complex deflects in a positive direction in both leads I and aVF with a normal electrical axis. If a negative deflection exists in either lead, an axis deviation exists.

Signs of Ischemia, Infarction, and Hypertrophy

Reduced blood supply to a portion of the myocardium results in ischemia. This results in metabolic changes in the region of the myocardium affected. Conduction defects occur in these regions and cause ECG changes. Ischemia typically shows on the ECG as an inverted T wave (Fig. 4-17, *A*).

A myocardial infarction is an injury and death of myocardial tissue. The most common cause is a sudden loss of blood supply to a particular region secondary to coronary artery disease. These changes lead to depolarization changes in the QRS complex. The most common findings include ST segment elevation or suppression or the presence of prominent Q waves that deflect downward (Fig. 4-17, *B*). The shape and degree of ST segment changes and Q waves in various leads help pinpoint the location of the infarction. For example, prominent Q waves and ST segment elevation in V1, V2, V3, and V4 indicate an infarction in the anterior and septal wall of the heart.

Myocardial enlargement of a particular region of the heart is known as cardiac hypertrophy. Greater myocardial mass causes an increase in the size of the depolarization

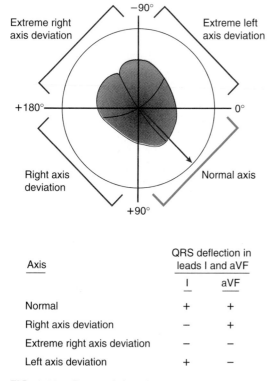

Axis	QRS deflection in leads I and aVF	
	I	aVF
Normal	+	+
Right axis deviation	−	+
Extreme right axis deviation	−	−
Left axis deviation	+	−

FIG. 4-16   Determining the mean electrical axis of the heart by analyzing the deflections of the QRS complexes in leads I and aVF.

recording. Atrial hypertrophy causes diphasic changes and enlargement in the P waves (Fig. 4-17, *C*). Ventricular hypertrophy produces greater deflections of the QRS complex (Fig. 4-17, *D*). In left ventricular hypertrophy, the S portion is enlarged in V1 and the R portion is enlarged in V5. Right ventricular hypertrophy produces large R waves in V1 and progressively smaller waves in V2, V3, and V4.

⬤ A NORMAL ECG

A normal rhythm is termed a **normal sinus rhythm (NSR).** An example of an NSR, recorded with lead II, is shown in Fig. 4-18, *A*. An NSR has a rate between 60 and 100 bpm and atrial and ventricular rhythms that are essentially regular during a resting state. The P waves are normal and consistent from one cycle to the next in configuration. This indicates that the SA node is originating each heartbeat. The P-R interval is less than 0.2 second with normal sinus rhythm, and the R-R intervals are equal or vary only slightly. The QRS complexes are less than 0.12 second and consistent in configuration from one complex to the next in the same ECG lead. Fig. 4-18, *B*, shows a 12-lead ECG recording of a patient with an NSR. Remember, an NSR does not provide information related to the pumping ability of the heart.

⬤ TYPES OF CARDIAC DYSRHYTHMIAS

Dysrhythmias are present when an abnormality occurs during impulse generation or

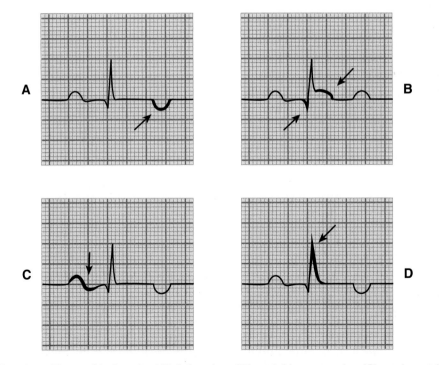

FIG. 4-17   Signs of ischemia, **(A)**, infarction, **(B)**, atrial hypertrophy, **(C)**, and ventricular hypertrophy, **(D)** in the electrocardiogram.

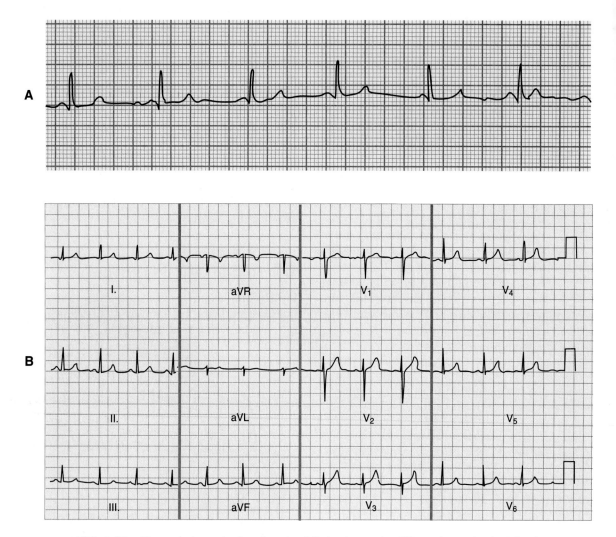

FIG. 4-18   Normal sinus rhythm in a lead II rhythm strip, **(A)**, and standard 12-lead electrocardiogram, **(B)**. (From Davis D: *Differential diagnosis of arrhythmias,* Philadelphia, 1992, WB Saunders.)

when impulse conduction causes an abnormal rhythm. The term **arrhythmia** is synonymous with dysrhythmia but is not popular with some clinicians because it implies a total lack of rhythm. In some cases an abnormal rhythm may be occurring on a regular basis, thus the term *dysrhythmia* may be more appropriate.

Ectopic beats are said to be present when the impulse causing the rhythm recorded on the ECG originates outside the SA node. Ectopic activity can occur in the atria or the ventricles and is usually the result of failure of the SA node to fire or of excessive excitation of tissue outside the SA node.

Sinoatrial Dysrhythmias

The most common form of sinus dysrhythmia is one in which the heart rate is normal but the spacing between cardiac cycles varies. This is referred to as sinus arrhythmia and is believed to be most often caused by the effects of breathing on the heart (Fig. 4-19). Typically the heart rate increases during inspiration and decreases during expiration. Sinus arrhythmia may also occur as a side effect of certain medications such as digitalis. The P wave, P-R interval, QRS complex, and ST segment are within normal limits. Sinus arrhythmia is not clinically significant unless it causes variation in blood pressure that results in symptoms such as dizziness or syncope.

Another common sinus dysrhythmia, sinus tachycardia (Fig. 4-20), is recognized by identifying the heart rate to be more than 100 bpm. The rhythm is regular with the P wave and QRS complexes identical from one cycle to the next in the same lead. The P-R interval, QRS complex, ST segment, and T wave are normal in configuration and length. Sinus tachycardia is commonly seen in a patient who is suffering from some acute lung disease with hypoxemia, acute cardiac problems, severe pain, and anxiety and as a side effect of many medications. Other causes of sinus tachycardia include exercise, fever, anemia, and hypotension. Sinus tachycardia is often the result of the sympathetic nervous system stimulating

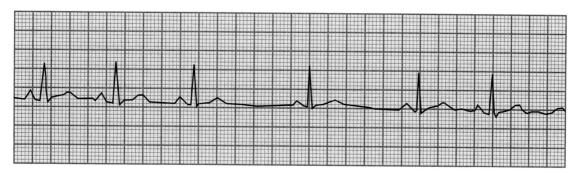

FIG. 4-19 Sinus arrhythmia. (From Davis D: *Differential diagnosis of arrhythmias,* Philadelphia, 1992, WB Saunders.)

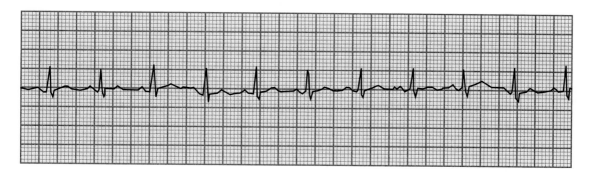

FIG. 4-20 Sinus tachycardia. (From Davis D: *Differential diagnosis of arrhythmias,* Philadelphia, 1992, WB Saunders.)

the heart to increase cardiac output to compensate for a defect in the tissue oxygen delivery system.

Sinus bradycardia is present when the heart rate is less than 60 bpm and the SA node is the source of every heart beat (Fig. 4-21). Sinus arrhythmia may also be present and cause the rhythm to become irregular. The P-R interval, QRS complex, ST segment, and T waves are normal. Marked bradycardia (<50/min) is likely to cause clinical symptoms such as dizziness and syncope as the blood pressure drops below normal. Significant bradycardia usually is the result of a defect in the SA node or excessive vagal nerve stimulation of the heart. Bradycardia is also seen in the person at rest who exercises regularly.

Atrioventricular Blocks

Conduction of the cardiac impulse from the SA node to the ventricles must pass through the AV node, as mentioned previously. Defects in the AV node or the electrolytes surrounding the AV node can cause the impulse to pass more slowly than normal. **AV block** is present when the cardiac impulse passes through the AV node too slowly, intermittently, or not at all. First-degree AV block exists when each impulse from the atria above passes through to the ventricles but at a slower rate than normal. As a result the P-R interval is prolonged beyond 0.20 second (Fig. 4-22). Each QRS complex is preceded by a single P wave, but the interval between the P wave and the QRS complex is prolonged for each heart beat.

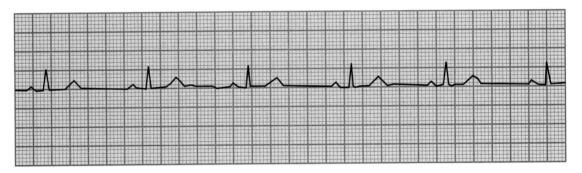

FIG. 4-21   Sinus bradycardia. (From Davis D: *Differential diagnosis of arrhythmias*, Philadelphia, 1992, WB Saunders.)

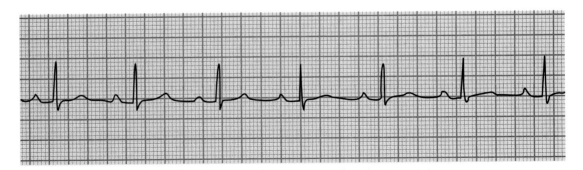

FIG. 4-22   Sinus rhythm with first-degree atrioventricular block. (From Davis D: *Differential diagnosis of arrhythmias*, Philadelphia, 1992, WB Saunders.)

Second-degree AV block is present when the P-R interval becomes progressively longer until one impulse from the SA node is blocked completely. The blocked impulse is seen as an isolated P wave with no corresponding QRS complex (Fig. 4-23). Another form of second-degree block occurs when a series of nonconducted SA node impulses (P waves) is followed by one that does pass through to the ventricles.

Third-degree AV block is present when none of the cardiac impulses generated by the SA node or ectopic foci in the atria passes through to the ventricles. The atria and ventricles beat independently in such cases. Third-degree block is recognized by a slow ventricular rate that is very regular. In addition, the P waves occur very regularly but usually more often than the QRS complexes. As a result, the P to P intervals and the R to R intervals are very regular with third-degree block (Fig. 4-24). Third-degree block is often treated by placement of an artificial pacemaker to pace the heart.

Premature Contractions and Ectopic Rhythms

All cardiac tissue is capable of becoming a pacemaker for the heart. Ischemia, injury caused by infarction or trauma, or heightened excitability of an area of the heart can lead to ectopic beats. Ectopic rhythms may originate in the atria or ventricles and may occur within or outside the normal conduction system. Ectopic beats may be conducted in a retrograde direction resulting in an odd-shaped

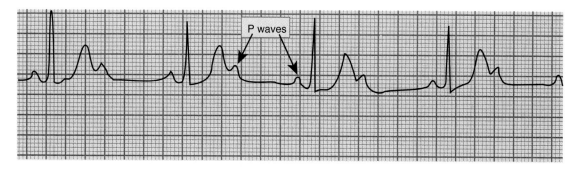

FIG. 4-23   Sinus rhythm with second-degree atrioventricular block. (From Davis D: *Differential diagnosis of arrhythmias,* Philadelphia, 1992, WB Saunders.)

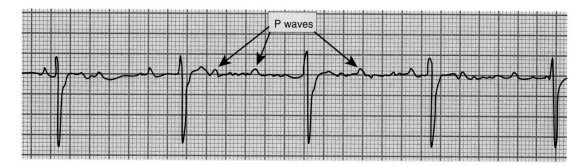

FIG. 4-24   Third-degree, or complete, atrioventricular block. Atrial activity and ventricular activity are completely disassociated. (From Davis D: *Differential diagnosis of arrhythmias,* Philadelphia, 1992, WB Saunders.)

P wave or QRS complex. The resulting ECG tracing provides clues to identify the location of any ectopic beats.

Premature ectopic beats are frequently followed by a compensatory pause because the ectopic beat results in depolarization of the SA and AV nodes as well as the surrounding myocardial tissue. The pacemaker cells cannot generate an impulse until repolarization is complete. The compensatory pause has an advantage in that it allows more complete filling of the ventricles and the subsequent ventricular contraction should produce an increased stroke volume.

A variety of premature ectopic rhythms can occur in the atria. **Premature atrial contractions (PACs),** one of the more common dysrhythmias seen under the category of ectopic rhythms, occur when atrial tissue outside the SA node becomes excessively excited and prematurely depolarizes. PACs are recognized by the premature timing of a heartbeat and the often different configuration of the P wave in the premature beat (Fig. 4-25). The PAC may not conduct through to the ventricles in normal fashion if it occurs before repolarization of the AV node. The impulse of the PAC may be conducted slowly or not at all by the AV node. The PAC will not be followed by a QRS complex when it occurs during the absolute refrac-tory period of the AV node. As a result, the impulse of the PAC is not conducted through to the ventricles in this situation.

PACs are caused by increased sympathetic activity, ingestion of stimulants (e.g., caffeine, nicotine), the side effects of sympathomimetic drugs (e.g., epinephrine, isoproterenol), electrolyte imbalance, cardiac hypoxia, or digitalis toxicity. In some cases PACs occur without any apparent cause and are insignificant when they occur infrequently. In patients with heart disease, however, frequent PACs may be an early warning sign of more serious impending dysrhythmias such as atrial flutter or atrial fibrillation.

Atrial flutter occurs when the atria depolarize at a very rapid rate of 240 to 300 bpm (Fig. 4-26). Usually an ectopic pacemaker outside the SA node is responsible for atrial flutter. The atrial contraction rate is often too fast to result in effective movement of blood although coordinated contractions are possible. In many cases of atrial flutter a 2:1 block is present that results in a ventricular rate that is half of the atrial rate. This AV block is useful in allowing the ventricles adequate filling time between contractions. Atrial flutter may cause excessive ventricular rates that cause cardiac output to fall. For this reason, atrial flutter is a serious dysrhythmia that needs immediate attention.

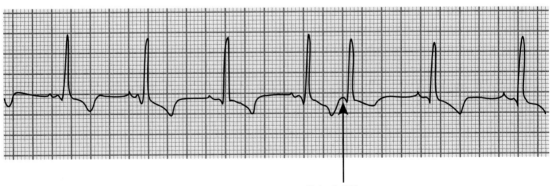

Ectopic "P" wave

FIG. 4-25   Sinus rhythm with one isolated atrial premature contraction. (From Davis D: *Differential diagnosis of arrhythmias,* Philadelphia, 1992, WB Saunders.)

Under certain conditions myocardial tissue undergoes an irregular type of contraction that is incapable of propelling blood. This type of contraction is known as fibrillation. **Atrial fibrillation** occurs in certain heart diseases and does not allow the atria to contribute to ventricular filling. As a result, stroke volume and cardiac output are often reduced when atrial fibrillation occurs. The ECG shows no P waves with atrial fibrillation. The P waves are replaced with continuous fluctuations called **f** waves (Fig. 4-27). The ventricular rate is often 160 to 180 bpm with atrial fibrillation. Ventricular fibrillation may result if the atrial fibrillation is not recognized and treated immediately. For this reason, atrial fibrillation is a serious dysrhythmia.

Premature ventricular contractions (PVCs) are ectopic beats that are caused by one or more pacemaker sites in the ventricles. The ectopic pacemaker sites develop excessive excitation caused by an increase in sympathetic tone, ischemia, acidosis, hypokalemia, or hypoxia of the ventricles. PVCs are easily identified by their five classic signs:

1. The QRS complexes are premature.
2. The QRS complexes are wider than normal and abnormal in configuration.
3. There is no P wave preceding the PVC.
4. The corresponding T wave is deflected in the opposite direction of the QRS complex.
5. There is a full compensatory pause following the PVC.

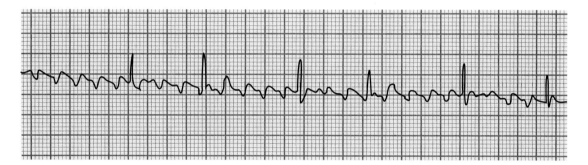

FIG. 4-26 Atrial flutter at 350 bpm with a 2:1 conduction resulting in a ventricular rate of 75 bpm. (From Davis D: *Differential diagnosis of arrhythmias,* Philadelphia, 1992, WB Saunders.)

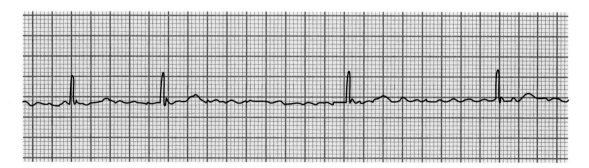

FIG. 4-27 Atrial fibrillation with a slow ventricular response. (From Davis D: *Differential diagnosis of arrhythmias,* Philadelphia, 1992, WB Saunders.)

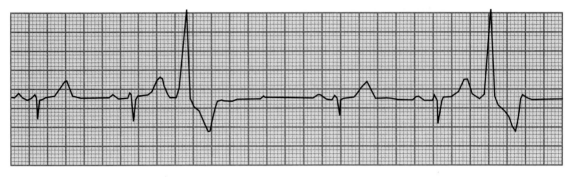

FIG. 4-28   Sinus bradycardia with unifocal premature ventricular contractions. (From Davis D: *Differential diagnosis of arrhythmias,* Philadelphia, 1992, WB Saunders.)

Unifocal PVCs are seen as a consistent configuration of each PVC (Fig. 4-28), suggesting that only one ectopic pacemaker site is present. Multifocal PVCs are present when the QRS complexes of the PVCs have more than one configuration, indicating that multiple ectopic sites are present. Single unifocal PVCs, which occur on a rare basis, are not a serious concern. Multifocal PVCs, PVCs occurring frequently (>6/min), or two or more PVCs in a row usually indicate a serious cardiac problem. Immediate assessment and care are needed.

Ventricular tachycardia represents an ectopic ventricular rhythm that is seen as three or more consecutive PVCs. The ventricular rate is greater than 100 bpm and may be as high as 250 bpm. The rhythm is usually regular and P waves are often absent (Fig. 4-29, *A*). If P waves are present they have no relationship to the QRS complexes and are negative (retrograde). The P waves are retrograde with ventricular tachycardia because the impulse originates in the ventricles and enters the atria from below.

Patients with ventricular tachycardia may be able to maintain adequate perfusion of the vital organs, but cardiac output is usually marginal at best. Ventricular tachycardia is usually an ominous sign that indicates a serious underlying heart problem. The patient with ventricular tachycardia is prone to develop dysrhythmias that pose an even greater threat to life such as ventricular flutter and ventricular fibrillation.

Ventricular flutter represents an advanced form of ventricular tachycardia. Ventricular flutter is seen as a rapid ventricular rate in which the QRS complexes tend to merge with the T waves, producing a continuous, wavy pattern with no clear separation between cardiac cycles (Fig. 4-29, *B*). Ventricular flutter is a serious life-threatening dysrhythmia because the ventricles do not have adequate time for filling between contractions. As a result, the blood flow and pressure produced by the heart fall dramatically.

Ventricular fibrillation, seen on the ECG tracing as abnormal, chaotic waveforms (Fig. 4-30), is the next stage in the progression of dysrhythmias associated with cardiac hypoxia. As with atrial fibrillation, the ventricles in fibrillation cannot pump blood effectively. This represents a serious problem since the ventricles are responsible for the movement of blood throughout the body. Circulation stops and the patient suffers permanent tissue death if cardiac output is not rapidly restored.

Asystole

Ventricular asystole is seen as a "flat line" on the ECG recording. There is no ventricular rate or rhythm. Ventricular asystole, often the final

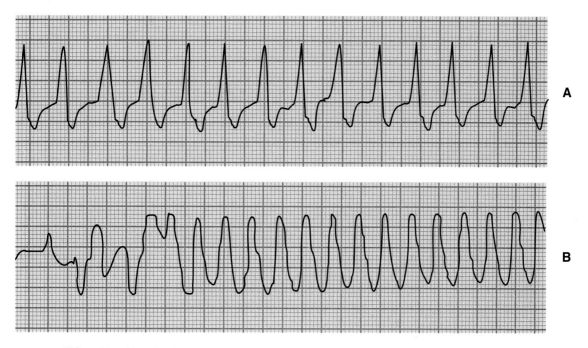

FIG. 4-29 Ventricular tachycardia **(A)** and multifocal ventricular tachycardia escalating into ventricular flutter **(B)**. (From Davis D: *Differential diagnosis of arrhythmias,* Philadelphia, 1992, WB Saunders.)

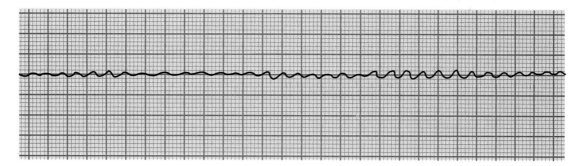

FIG. 4-30 Fine ventricular fibrillation. (From Davis D: *Differential diagnosis of arrhythmias,* Philadelphia, 1992, WB Saunders.)

dysrhythmia following ventricular tachycardia, ventricular flutter, and ventricular fibrillation, is usually the result of a serious heart ailment such as a severe myocardial infarction. The heart is unable to pump blood with ven-

tricular asystole and the patient suddenly loses consciousness. Immediate cardiac life support techniques are necessary, although the heart is often resistive to rescue efforts with ventricular asystole.

CASE STUDY FOCUS

Sudden Loss of Consciousness and Pulse

A 52-year-old man was becoming progressively more excited and angry as he watched his team lose the Superbowl football game. He developed a sudden onset of chest pain and difficulty breathing. He was brought to the emergency department where he lost consciousness, stopped breathing (apnea), and was found to have no pulse. Advanced cardiac life support was started. He was ventilated with 100% oxygen, and cardiac compressions were started immediately to maintain circulation and gas exchange. Monitoring of his electrocardiogram (ECG) was started, and it revealed that he was in ventricular fibrillation, a cardiac dysrhythmia that lacks organized ventricular activity and results in no cardiac pumping. Irreversible organ damage can result if cardiopulmonary resuscitation (CPR) is not instituted and the fibrillation is not returned to a more normal ventricular rhythm within 8 to 10 minutes. Electrical paddles were placed on the right anterior and left lateral portions of his chest, and 200 J of direct current were delivered to defibrillate the heart. A second electrical defibrillation of 300 J was delivered and his ECG converted to a flat line asystole. CPR was continued and 1 mg of epinephrine was given intravenously. The epinephrine is indicated to induce cardiac activity and to improve the response to defibrillation. After several minutes of continued CPR, the ECG showed continuing asystole. The physician decided to give the patient 500 mg of calcium chloride and 1 mg of epinephrine intravenously. The calcium chloride and epinephrine were given to induce cardiac activity. After 30 seconds of continued CPR, the ECG converted to ventricular fibrillation. The paddles were again applied to the chest and 300 J of direct electrical current were delivered. The ventricular fibrillation converted to a sinus tachycardia of 124 per minute and a pulse was detected. The patient continued to be ventilated with 100% oxygen and was transferred to the coronary care unit where he returned to consciousness. Cardiac catheterization revealed three regions of coronary artery narrowing of more than 90%. A coronary artery bypass grafting was successfully performed, and the patient went home 5 days after admission.

CHAPTER SELF-TEST QUESTIONS

1. The resting membrane potential is defined as:
   a. a sudden loss of negative charge within the cell
   b. changes in the transmembrane potential upon stimulation
   c. the electrical gradient occurring at rest across the cell membrane
   d. the return of the cell to normal polarity
2. The fast response phase of depolarization primarily is the result of what ion moving across the cell membrane?
   a. sodium
   b. potassium
   c. calcium
   d. magnesium
3. Which of the following is a correct definition of automaticity?
   a. the automatic response of the cells when stimulated
   b. the sudden loss of electrical charge within the cell
   c. prolongation of the action potential during depolarization
   d. the ability to spontaneously depolarize
4. The primary pacemaker for the heart is the:
   a. SA node
   b. AV node
   c. bundle of His
   d. Purkinje cells

5. Which of the following does parasympathetic stimulation cause?
   1. bradycardia
   2. increased AV node conduction
   3. increased SA node automaticity
      a. 1 only
      b. 1 and 2
      c. 2 and 3
      d. 1 and 3
      e. 1, 2, and 3
6. Which of the following ECG leads is bipolar?
   a. lead II
   b. aVR
   c. aVF
   d. V6
7. Atrial depolarization is seen on the ECG tracing as a:
   a. P wave
   b. QRS complex
   c. T wave
   d. U wave
8. The normal P-R interval is less than:
   a. 0.12 second
   b. 0.20 second
   c. 0.24 second
   d. 0.33 second
9. What dysrhythmia is present when the P-R interval is abnormally prolonged but each impulse passes through to the ventricles?
   a. sinus dysrhythmia
   b. ectopic beats
   c. first-degree AV block
   d. sinus bradycardia
10. What does the term *multifocal PVCs* indicate?
    a. the PVCs are life threatening
    b. the PVCs are from multiple ectopic sites
    c. the PVCs are originating in the bundle branches
    d. the PVCs are originating in the Purkinje fibers

For answers, see p. 475.

BIBLIOGRAPHY

1. Berne RM, Levy MN: *Cardiovascular physiology*, ed 6, St Louis, 1992, Mosby.
2. Cummins RO et al: *Advanced cardiac life support*, Dallas, 1997, American Heart Association.
3. Davis D: *Differential diagnosis of arrhythmias*, Philadelphia, 1992, WB Saunders.
4. Ganong WF: *Review of medical physiology*, ed 18, Stamford, Conn, 1997, Appleton & Lange.
5. Guyton AC: *Textbook of medical physiology*, Philadelphia, 1996, WB Saunders.
6. Huszar RJ: *Basic dysrhythmias: interpretation and management*, St Louis, 1988, Mosby.
7. Martini FH: *Fundamentals of anatomy and physiology*, Upper Saddle River, NJ, 1988, Prentice Hall.
8. Phillips RE, Feeney MK: *The cardiac rhythms: a systematic approach to interpretation*, ed 3, Philadelphia, 1990, WB Saunders.
9. Smith JJ, Kampine JP: *Circulatory physiology: the essentials*, ed 3, Baltimore, 1990, Williams & Wilkins.
10. Wilkins RL, Sheldon RL, Krider SJ, eds: *Clinical assessment in respiratory care*, ed 3, St Louis, 1994, Mosby.

CHAPTER 5

The Cardiac Pump

Upon completing this chapter, you will be able to:

1 Describe the sliding filament theory of the myocyte.
2 Relate the role of Ca^{++} and adenosine triphosphate in the excitation-contraction coupling mechanism of the myocyte.
3 Describe ventricular filling and list the factors that influence it.
4 Describe ventricular compliance.
5 Define inotropic status.
6 Describe the Frank-Starling law of the heart and how this phenomenon is an *intrinsic* property of cardiac autoregulation.
7 Describe atrial and ventricular activity during the cardiac cycle.
8 Describe what causes the four cardiac sounds and the various types of murmurs.
9 Define stroke volume, cardiac output, and cardiac reserve.
10 Define myocardial chronotropic status.
11 Describe what factors influence heart rate and how heart rate influences stroke volume and cardiac output.
12 Define end-diastolic volume, ejection fraction, and end-systolic volume.
13 Define preload, contractility, and afterload and how these factors influence stroke volume.
14 Describe what factors influence venous return and the effect venous return has on cardiac output.
15 Describe the role of venous return pumps.
16 Define central venous pressure and describe its effect on cardiac output.
17 Describe the effect downstream vascular resistance has on cardiac output.
18 Describe the nutrient and oxygen requirements of the heart during rest.
19 Define myocardial work and efficiency.

The heart functions primarily as a pump to propel sufficient blood through the vascular system to sustain life. The heart is capable of adjusting its pump performance to meet various demands and is able to pump an incredible 350 million liters of blood during a lifetime. This chapter explores cardiac pump performance and the various factors that influence it.

⟫ ELASTIC AND CONTRACTILE PROPERTIES OF THE HEART

Activity of the Myocyte

The myocardium of the heart is comprised of millions of interconnected cardiac muscle fibers **(myocytes),** each of which has a cell membrane (sarcolemma) with tubular extensions called transverse tubules, or T tubules, that penetrate deep into the cell (Fig. 5-1). Within the cell are numerous mitochondria and a bundle of myofibrils. The myofibrils are surrounded by cytoplasm and a network of membranous channels called the sarcoplasmic reticulum. Each myofibril is comprised of numerous **myofilaments** of **actin** and **myosin.**

Actin and myosin are fibrous proteins that interact and generate the contractile properties of the myocytes and myocardium.

The functional unit of the myofibril is the **sarcomere,** which is organized from the alignment of thousands of actin and myosin filaments within it. Fig. 5-2 shows that the sarcomere is defined as the actin and myosin between two Z lines. The thin actin filaments are anchored in either end of the sarcomere in the Z lines, which are comprised of a matrix of protein. The actin filaments extend toward each other from each Z line. The heavier myosin filaments are positioned in the center of the sarcomere. Each myosin filament is surrounded by six actin filaments. Each myofibril is comprised of numerous sarcomeres, which are organized into a repeating pattern that gives the myocytes a striated look under the microscope.

Sliding Filament Theory

In the relaxed myocyte the length of the sarcomere is about 1.8 m. Upon contraction, the sarcomere shortens to about 70% of its relaxed length. The basic process of muscle fiber shortening results from activation of the actin and myosin filaments by the presence of Ca^{++} and

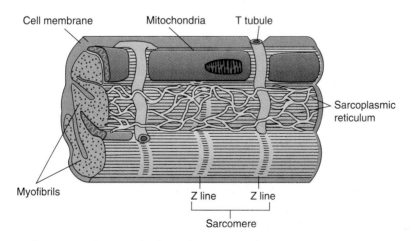

FIG. 5-1   Cutaway microscopic view of a portion of a myocyte showing the enclosed myofibrils, sarcoplasmic reticulum, and the T tubules that penetrate deep into the cell. Myofibrils are comprised of numerous sarcomeres.

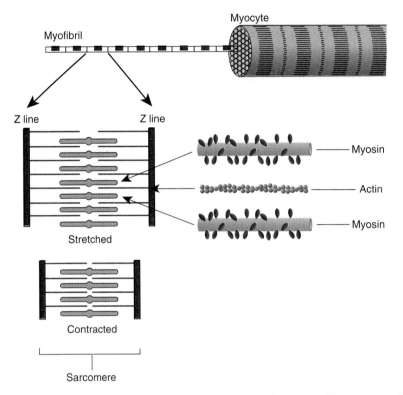

FIG. 5-2 Myofibrils of the myocyte are comprised of the myofilaments actin and myosin. Actin and myosin are organized in an overlapping pattern between Z lines of the sarcomere. When Ca^{++} is released within the myocyte by the sarcoplasmic reticulum, myosin cross bridges bind to actin and pull actin in a sliding process. This results in pulling the Z lines together and shortening the sarcomere.

adenosine triphosphate (ATP). Activation starts with the depolarization of the myocyte and results in the mechanical interaction of myosin and actin. For this interaction to occur, Ca^{++} is released and binds to the regulatory protein troponin, which causes it to change shape. This shape change causes the tropomyosin regulatory protein on actin to move and uncover special binding sites. The cross bridges of myosin reversibly bind to these sites on actin. The cross bridges are maintained in an energized state by sufficient quantities of ATP. When the energized myosin cross bridge binds to actin, it rapidly bends. The bending of the cross bridge utilizes some of the energy in ATP through the process of

hydrolysis. The hydrolysis of ATP results in the production of adenosine diphosphate (ADP) and inorganic phosphate after each cross bridge bend is complete and recycled by cellular metabolism. A rapid series of binding and bending of myosin cross bridges pulls actin past myosin toward the center of the sarcomere. This process is repeated rapidly and causes actin to be pulled past myosin as long as there is sufficient Ca^{++} and ATP present. The Z lines of all the sarcomeres are pulled together causing the myocyte to shorten or contract.

When the intracellular concentration of Ca^{++} decreases, the troponin-tropomyosin complex covers the binding site on actin and the myosin cross bridges are blocked from

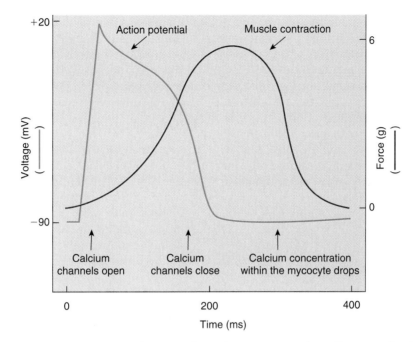

FIG. 5-3 Excitation-contraction coupling phenomenon of cardiac muscle tissue. Voltage changes of the action potential stimulate the force changes generated by contraction of a strip of cardiac muscle.

binding to actin. Actin filaments are pulled back as the myocyte relaxes.

This process of actin and myosin binding and movement is known as the **sliding filament theory.**

Excitation-Contraction Coupling

A sufficient stimulus of the myocyte results in an electrical excitation that is rapidly followed by a mechanical contraction. The excitation is in the form of an action potential, which is discussed in Chapter 4. The action potential is a rapid reversal in cellular voltage from $-90\,\text{mV}$ to $20\,\text{mV}$ (depolarization) and back to $-90\,\text{mV}$ (repolarization), sweeping over the entire cell. The action potential in the myocyte is the product of rapid movement of Na^+ and Ca^{++} into the cell followed by a rapid movement of K^+ out of the cell.

The action potential is carried deep into the cardiac cell by the T tubule system. When the

cell membrane and sarcoplasmic reticulum are depolarized, Ca^{++} channels open and a small amount of Ca^{++} moves into the region of the myofibril. This, in turn, activates the binding and sliding of myosin and actin and the contraction of the myocyte.

During cellular repolarization, the myocyte returns to its resting potential and Ca^{++} channels close. The concentration of Ca^{++} rapidly declines within the cytoplasm of the cell through the action of membrane-bound Ca^{++} pumps that move Ca^{++} out of the cytoplasm of the cell. The reduced intracellular Ca^{++} concentration results in the failure of cross bridge binding, ends sarcomere shortening, and terminates the contraction. As the tension within the myocyte falls, the myocyte returns to its resting length.

Entry of Ca^{++} into the cardiac muscle fiber is critical to the coupling of the electrical and mechanical events. Fig. 5-3 shows a normal excitation-contraction coupling in a papillary muscle. Note that the action potential precedes muscular contraction. The process can be uncoupled when a high dose of a calcium channel-blocking drug such as diltiazem is given. In clinical practice, excitation-contraction uncoupling can occur in an individual who presents with some form of electrocardiogram (ECG) rhythm but has no detectable pulse or blood pressure. This phenomenon is commonly called **electromechanical dissociation (EMD).**

Cardiac Filling

The myocardium has both elastic and contractile properties. The elastic behavior of the heart is the product of the passive nature of the myocytes and the active tension they are capable of developing. The ability of the heart to fill with blood is apposed by the elastic and muscle tension status of the tissue. **Ventricular compliance** is a common method used to describe the overall elastic behavior of the heart. It is defined as an amount of blood volume filling a ventricle for a given amount of distending pressure:

$$\frac{\Delta Q}{\Delta P}$$

where Q is the amount of blood filling the ventricle and P is the distending pressure. A normal left ventricular compliance at the end of filling would be 120 ml/2 mm Hg, or 60 ml/mm Hg. With age or following a myocardial infarction, ventricular compliance falls. This results in a reduced filling of the ventricle at normal filling pressures.

Ventricular filling is influenced by four distinct factors: (1) the pressure driving venous blood to the atrium, (2) the tendency of the ventricle to draw blood in when it relaxes following a contraction, (3) the atrial pressure generated when the atria contracts, and (4) the compliance of the ventricle. The majority of ventricular filling is the product of venous

pressure and ventricular compliance. Greater venous pressure and compliance lead to greater filling whereas lower venous pressure and compliance result in poor filling and cardiac pump failure.

Cardiac Contractility

Contractility of the heart, a concept used to describe myocardial performance during the active phase of pumping, is a measure of the amount of force or tension the myocardium generates over time following stimulation from the conduction system. One method of evaluating contractility is the analysis of the pressure-time plot (dP/dt) recorded in the ventricle during a cardiac catheterization procedure. Fig. 5-4 shows the pressure changes in three different left ventricles. Each ventricle shows a different rise in pressure per unit

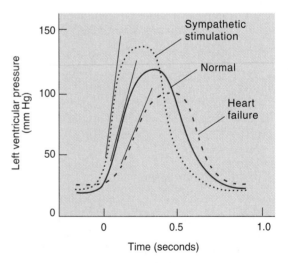

FIG. 5-4 Pressure changes within three different ventricles demonstrates different states of contractility. Tangent lines on the up-stroke of the pressure recording show the different rates of pressure changes generated in a normal heart, a heart stimulated by the sympathetic nervous system, and a heart in failure. (Modified from Berne RM, Levy MN: *Cardiovascular physiology,* St Louis, 1992, Mosby.)

time during the early phase of contraction. By measuring the slope of the dP/dt during the early period of pressure development, the state of contractility, or **inotropy,** can be evaluated. The normal ventricle possesses greater inotropy (greater dP/dt) when compared with the ventricle in failure and less than the ventricle under the influence of a positive inotropic drug such as epinephrine or digitalis. The inotropic state of the heart is most likely caused by the amount of actin and myosin binding, the amount of overlap between actin and myosin, the sensitivity of troponin to Ca^{++}, and the amount of ATP available.

Frank-Starling Law of the Heart

At the beginning of the twentieth century Starling, following the earlier work of Frank, described a fundamental property of cardiac activity that now bears their names. They discovered that the heart generates greater force with greater filling. Fig. 5-5 shows that the peak pressure generated in the ventricle during contraction increases as the blood volume filling the ventricle increases. During the filling phase, intraventricular pressure remains low until the ventricle nears the end of filling and the intraventricular pressure rapidly increases. In the normal human heart the greatest contractile pressures are generated

---

DIAGNOSTIC FOCUS

Abnormal Clinical Findings in Left Side Heart Failure

A variety of systemic and pulmonary changes are associated with left side heart failure:

    Cool and clammy skin
    Weak pulse and low blood pressure
    Weakness, confusion, and coma
    Reduced urine formation
    Distended neck veins and liver
    Dyspnea
    Wheezing and crackling breath sounds

Heart failure on the left side of the heart is most often caused by coronary artery disease or narrowing of the mitral or aortic valve. Coronary artery disease can lead to reduced coronary blood flow and subsequent reductions in myocardial contractility. Mitral or aortic valve narrowing or stenosis leads to poor ventricular filling and elevated outflow resistance, respectively. These conditions result in reduced ability to pump the venous blood returning to the left side of the heart into the aorta. Stroke volume and cardiac output are reduced, and blood being pumped by the right side of the heart builds up and congests the pulmonary circuit. Systemic blood pressure and flow are low, which can lead to renal failure, weakness, confusion, and coma. Because of poor blood flow to the skin, the skin is often cool and clammy. As the blood backs up into the pulmonary circuit, the blood pressures throughout the circuit increase and water can leak into the interstitial spaces and alveolar spaces of the lung. This can result in pulmonary edema that is manifested by difficult breathing (dyspnea), especially when lying flat, expiratory wheezing from congested and narrowed airways, and inspiratory crackling breath sounds from congested and wet small airways that "pop" open during inspiration. The patient may be gray or cyanotic from poor oxygenation of blood and reduced blood flow. With pulmonary circuit congestion and increased pulmonary artery pressures, the right side of the heart often fails and blood pools and congests the venous portion of the systemic circuit. Increased systemic venous pressure results in distended neck (jugular) veins, enlarged liver, and edematous ankles.

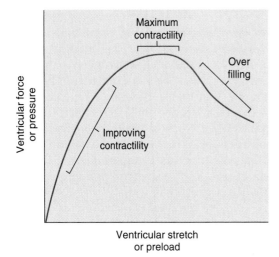

FIG. 5-5 Ventricular pressure vs. volume curve showing the Frank-Starling law of the heart. As myocardial stretch or preload is increased, ventricular force or pressure increases. The ventricle develops less force when it is over filled.

when the relaxed ventricle is filled with approximately 280 ml of blood, which is generated by a filling pressure of about 12 mm Hg.

The Frank-Starling law also implies that contractility is adjusted by the heart as the preload of the ventricle changes. This property of variable performance is observable down to the level of the sarcomere. Maximum contractility is found when the sarcomere is stretched to a length of 2.2 m. The optimal length of the sarcomere is thought to be that length where actin and myosin are able to cycle through the highest number of bindings. When the sarcomere is stretched below this point, fewer binding cycles will occur and the force of contraction is reduced. If the sarcomere is overstretched, myosin is unable to bind to actin effectively and the strength of contraction is lower. These findings demonstrate that the myocardium has *intrinsic* properties of autoregulation, which allow adjustment of the force that is generated according to the amount of stretching it is exposed to during the filling

phase. This intrinsic property of automatic regulation is important to the heart's ability to adjust itself as conditions change.

Starling also demonstrated that the ventricle could be overloaded or stretched beyond an optimum point that would result in decreased peak pressure generation. This indicates that the ventricle could be overloaded into a state of failure where it would be unable to pump all the blood with which it was filled.

⬤ EVENTS OF THE CARDIAC CYCLE

Each heart beat is an elaborate sequence of electrical, muscular, and valvular events. All of the events of one heart beat are referred to as the **cardiac cycle.** Chapter 4 describes the electrical events that sweep over the heart to initiate the mechanical events. The electrical events are recorded on an ECG. The mechanical events can be shown by recording pressure, volume, flow, and sound changes that occur throughout the cycle. By evaluating these various recordings the major events of the cardiac cycle are revealed.

Each cycle is comprised of a contractile phase called **systole** and a relaxation or filling phase called **diastole.** The volume of blood pumped by each ventricle during systolic phase is termed the **stroke volume.** Box 5-1 summarizes the major events of a cardiac cycle.

In a normal resting subject the heart rate is about 75 cycles per minute. At this rate, one cycle would require about 0.8 second or 800 ms. The normal ventricular systolic phase lasts about 300 ms or approximately one third of the cycle. The remaining 500 ms or two thirds of the cycle is the diastolic phase. During tachycardic conditions where the heart rate can reach 150 cycles per minute, the entire cycle only lasts 400 ms. At this high heart rate both systolic and diastolic times are reduced. Most of the reduction occurs during the diastolic phase, which leads to reduced

Major Events of the Cardiac Cycle

SYSTOLIC PHASE

Ventricular depolarization
↓
Ventricular contraction
↓
Ventricular pressures increase (isovolumic contraction period)
↓
Ventricular pressures exceed aortic and pulmonary artery pressures
↓
Aortic and pulmonary valves open and blood flows from the ventricles
↓
Ventricular contraction ends and pressures drop below aortic and pulmonary artery pressures

DIASTOLIC PHASE

Aortic and pulmonary valves close
↓
Ventricular pressures drop below atrial and venous pressures (isovolumic relaxation period)
↓
Tricuspid and bicuspid valves open
↓
Blood flows from the atria into the ventricles (passive rapid-filling phase)
↓
Atria depolarize
↓
Atria contract
↓
Atrial pressures increase and more blood flows into ventricles (active rapid-filling phase)

Fig. 5-6 shows the cardiac cycle as it would be recorded in the left side of the heart from a subject at rest. Pressure, volume, sound, and electrical changes are all recorded simultaneously and show the relationship that each has to one another.

Atrial Activity

During the diastolic phase, the atria act as passive conduits to direct venous blood flow to the ventricles. They passively fill with blood as a result of the low pressure and momentum of returning venous blood. Atrial pressure remains higher than ventricular pressure throughout the diastolic phase, which enables ventricular filling (see Fig. 5-6).

Atrial systole occurs just after atrial depolarization, which is recorded as the P wave on the ECG. Contraction of the atria results in a small increase in intraatrial pressure to about 8 to 10 mm Hg, which forces a small amount of blood into the ventricles. In effect, atrial systole functions to "top off" ventricular end-diastolic volume (EDV).

Ventricular filling and pumping ability are not entirely dependent on atrial systole. The magnitude of atrial contribution to ventricular filling is a function of heart rate and the anatomy of the atrioventricular valves. During a normal heart rate, atrial contraction contributes only 20% to 30% of the total blood volume to the ventricle during the filling phase. Long diastolic times that occur during bradycardia result in better ventricular filling before atrial systole, which results in little or no role for the atria during prolonged diastolic times. During tachycardia in which diastolic time is reduced, the atria can play a greater role in increasing EDV. When narrowing or stenosis occurs in the tricuspid or bicuspid valves, atrial contraction provides additional pressure to force blood flow through the narrowed valve.

Although no valves exist between the atria, the vena cava, and the pulmonary veins, little blood moves backward into these veins during

ventricular filling and subsequently reduced blood volume pumped per contraction. During bradycardic conditions the diastolic time is extended whereas the systolic time remains largely unchanged.

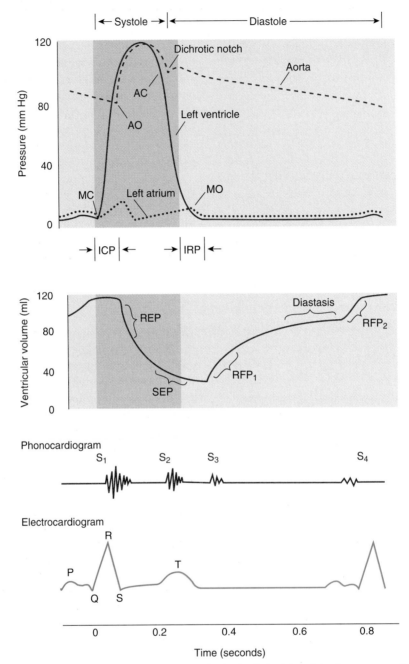

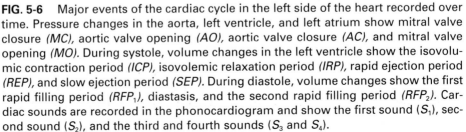

FIG. 5-6 Major events of the cardiac cycle in the left side of the heart recorded over time. Pressure changes in the aorta, left ventricle, and left atrium show mitral valve closure *(MC)*, aortic valve opening *(AO)*, aortic valve closure *(AC)*, and mitral valve opening *(MO)*. During systole, volume changes in the left ventricle show the isovolumic contraction period *(ICP)*, isovolemic relaxation period *(IRP)*, rapid ejection period *(REP)*, and slow ejection period *(SEP)*. During diastole, volume changes show the first rapid filling period *(RFP₁)*, diastasis, and the second rapid filling period *(RFP₂)*. Cardiac sounds are recorded in the phonocardiogram and show the first sound *(S₁)*, second sound *(S₂)*, and the third and fourth sounds *(S₃* and *S₄)*.

atrial systole. This is primarily because of the momentum of venous blood returning to the atria and the low pressures generated by the atria during systole.

Ventricular Activity

Ventricular systole is stimulated during the QRS portion of the ECG. Ventricular pressure builds rapidly, causing the mitral valve to close as pressures within the ventricle exceed those in the atria. Blood flow leaves the ventricle when the aortic valve is forced open at a pressure of about 80 mm Hg. Pressure continues to build in the ventricle to about 120 mm Hg and then declines as the ventricle begins to relax. The aortic valve closes as ventricular pressure drops below aortic vessel pressure at about 90 to 100 mm Hg. Ventricular pressure continues to rapidly decline until it falls below atrial pressure when the mitral valve opens at about 10 mm Hg.

The systolic and diastolic phases of ventricular activity are often described in subphases or periods. These phases are illustrated in the volume recording found in Fig. 5-6.

The systolic phase is composed of three periods. The isovolumic contractile period is the initial period of contraction. During this period the ventricles respond to the stimulation from the cardiac conduction system and develop tension rapidly. As ventricular tension builds, the volume of blood within the intraventricular chamber is squeezed and pressurized rapidly. This causes the atrioventricular valve to close as the intraventricular pressure exceeds atrial pressure and pressure continues to build rapidly against a closed semilunar valve. The isovolumic contractile period is referred to as being isovolumic in nature because the volume of blood within the ventricle remains constant. This period is also described as being an isometric contraction period because the ventricle generates tension while not moving blood. This period ends as the intraventricular pressure exceeds the

blood pressure in the aorta or pulmonary artery. When this occurs, the semilunar valve is forced open and blood flows out of the ventricle. In the left ventricle the isovolumic contractile period produces pressure changes that start at about 5 mm Hg and climb to 80 mm Hg when the aortic valve opens over a duration of 50 msec. It is during this period of systole that pressure changes are the most rapid and best reflect the contractility or inotropic status of the myocardium.

The next phase of systole is the rapid ejection period. During this period two thirds of the stroke volume is pumped out in about one third of the entire systolic time. This period begins with the opening of the semilunar valves and the rapid flow of blood out of the ventricles. Peak blood flow is greater from the left ventricle and occurs earlier in this period of systole when compared with the flow rates generated by the right ventricle. The average flow rate from each ventricle is the same. Aortic and pulmonary artery diameters both expand during this period as blood is pumped into them and they reach their peak systolic pressures. The rapid ejection period ends when the intraventricular and arterial pressures peak and blood flow into the artery declines.

As the myocardium relaxes and the intraventricular pressure begins to decline, the last phase of systole, the slower ejection period, occurs. During this period, blood continues to flow from the ventricles despite a declining intraventricular pressure and the slightly higher pressures in the aorta and pulmonary artery. One would think that flow would stop under these conditions, but it continues largely because of the momentum of the moving blood. The end of the slower ejection period and systole occurs when blood pressure in the ventricles drops low enough for blood flow to reverse and start to flow back into the ventricles. At this point both of the semilunar valves close. Pressure in the ventricles and arteries continues to fall as the diastolic phase of the cardiac cycle begins.

When blood pressure drops low enough in the ventricles and blood flow begins to reverse back through each of the semilunar valves, the valves rapidly close. This closure can be detected on an arterial blood pressure recording as a notching and slight surging of pressure at the end of systole (see Fig. 5-6). This phenomenon, caused by the sudden closure of the semilunar valve and the recoil pressure produced by the distended artery, is referred to as the **dicrotic notch.**

The diastolic phase of the cardiac cycle lasts approximately 500 msec at rest and is dominated by the activity of filling. Ventricular diastole begins with the closure of the aortic and pulmonic semilunar valves. Following closure of these valves there is a rapid fall in intraventricular pressure until the atrioventricular valves open. This early period of diastole is referred to as the isovolumic relaxation period and, like its systolic counterpart, is marked by a large pressure change, in this case a drop, with no change in blood volume since the valves remain closed.

When the intraventricular pressure drops below the atrial pressure, the bicuspid and tricuspid valves open and the filling phase of diastole begins. It is comprised of passive and active filling periods. The first rapid-filling phase is primarily passive in nature and is driven by the recoil of vessels that force venous blood into the atria and ventricle. Two thirds of ventricular filling occurs during this initial rapid-filling phase. Flow into the ventricle slows and then a second rapid-filling phase occurs when the atria contract. The low flow period between the two rapid-filling phases is sometimes termed *diastasis.*

⬤ TYPES OF SOUNDS THE HEART MAKES AND THEIR CAUSE

The heart sounds heard over the left anterior chest are produced by various mechanical events during the cardiac cycle. Listening with

the aid of a stethoscope, termed *cardiac auscultation,* normally reveals not only the low-pitched "lubb-dupp" sounds but others as well. Fig. 5-6 shows these various sounds as they are recorded on a **phonocardiogram** and their relation to other mechanical and electrical events of the cardiac cycle. In fact, there are four sounds that can be heard in some subjects. Each of these sounds is associated with certain events and can be better evaluated by listening over five specific areas of the chest as shown in Fig. 5-7. The origin of these sounds is thought to be the product of sudden deceleration and acceleration of blood flow around various cardiac structures.

"Lubb," the first sound (S_1), is the product of tricuspid and bicuspid valve closure at the beginning of the isovolumic contraction period of systole. S_1 can best be heard over the apex of the heart, which is located under the midclavicular line, at the level of the fifth intercostal space, on the left side of the chest.

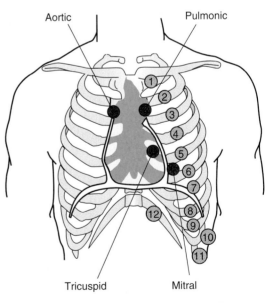

FIG. 5-7   Areas to best hear the sounds generated by the various valves during the cardiac cycle.

Normally, S_1 is a mixture of sounds produced by the near simultaneous closure of both valves. If closure of the two valves occurs at different times, S_1 begins to sound "split." When a split S_1 occurs, the bicuspid valve is usually heard during the first part of the split.

"Dupp," the second sound (S_2), is produced by closure of the aortic and pulmonic semilunar valves and occurs at the end of systole. It is best heard over the second intercostal space on the left and right sides of the sternum. S_2 can change during the breathing cycle and become split during the inspiratory phase. Intrathoracic pressure becomes more negative during inspiration and causes a momentary increase in venous return and increased filling of the right ventricle. The better-filled right ventricle now requires a longer ejection period, causing closure of the pulmonic valve to occur later than that of the aortic valve. This split disappears during the expiratory phase and breath holding.

The third and fourth heart sounds (S_3 and S_4, respectively) are difficult to hear. They occur during diastole and are associated with the passive and active filling phases. S_3 occurs just after S_2 and is produced during the passive rapid-filling phase as the atrioventricular valves open. S_4 occurs toward the end of diastole and is produced by atrial contraction. S_3 and S_4 may be heard in younger individuals but is more often heard in individuals over 40 years of age who have developed abnormal cardiac conditions. For example, a prominent S_3 is associated with increased flow caused by congestive heart failure and bicuspid or tricuspid regurgitation. An audible S_4 is associated with reduced ventricular compliance secondary to fever, hypertension, and coronary artery disease. A pathological S_3 is occasionally called a **ventricular "gallop"** whereas the pathological S_4 is referred to as an **atrial "gallop."**

Murmurs are abnormal sounds that are additional in nature and vary according to their timing, duration, pitch, location, and volume. Generally, they are produced by the formation of turbulent blood flow that accompanies a cardiac pathologic condition. Turbulent flow results from flow over partial obstructions, increased flow through normal structures, swirling in dilated structures, and regurgitation through faulty valves. Murmurs can be classified according to their presence during the systolic and diastolic phases or if they are continuous in nature (Fig. 5-8).

Systolic murmurs vary according to their onset and intensity. Systolic ejection murmurs are sounds that build and fall in intensity and are caused by narrowed semilunar valves (e.g., aortic valve stenosis). Pansystolic murmurs have a continuous intensity between S_1 and S_2 and are caused by atrioventricular valve leakage (e.g., **mitral regurgitation**) or a hole in the ventricular septum (e.g., **ventricular septal defect**). Late systolic murmurs, as their name implies, typically start partway through systole and may start with a "click" sound such as the turbulent sound produced by an unstable and leaky bicuspid valve (e.g., **mitral valve prolapse**) that opens as ventricular pressure builds.

Diastolic murmurs also vary in their nature, but they generally have some degree of decreasing intensity during the diastolic phase. An early diastolic murmur develops as a result of a leaky atrioventricular valve (e.g., **aortic regurgitation**). This condition allows blood to flow backward into the ventricle, causing considerable turbulence, which decreases in intensity as the ventricle fills. Mid-to-late diastolic murmurs occur as a result of turbulent flow that develops through a narrowed atrioventricular valve (e.g., **mitral stenosis**).

Continuous murmurs are heard throughout the cardiac cycle. These murmurs are produced by flow from areas of high pressure to areas of low pressure. An example of this type of murmur is that produced by a **patent ductus arteriosus.** The ductus arteriosus is a vessel that connects the pulmonary artery with the aorta. During fetal development this vessel is kept open to allow blood to flow from

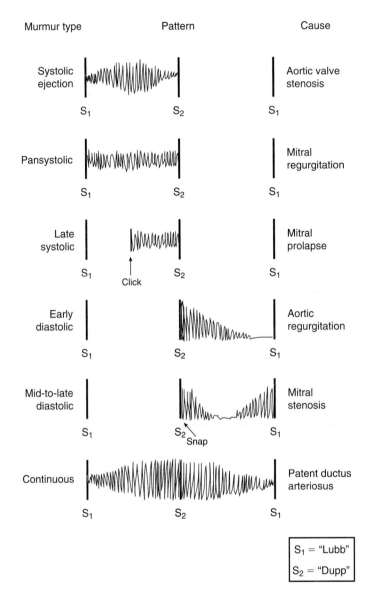

Murmur type	Pattern	Cause

FIG. 5-8 Major types of cardiac murmurs heard before and following the first (S_1) and second (S_2) cardiac sounds are a major cause of this type of murmur.

the right side of the heart to the aorta. After birth this vessel normally closes. The ductus arteriosus may remain open after birth and allows high-pressure blood from either vessel to flow back and forth through it. When the ductus arteriosus is open, it causes a continuous murmur.

CARDIAC OUTPUT AND FACTORS THAT INFLUENCE IT

The most straightforward method used to evaluate cardiac pump performance is the measurement of **cardiac output.** Cardiac output is defined as the amount of blood pumped by one ventricle each minute. Because the amount of blood pumped by each ventricle is virtually identical in the normal subject, the output of either ventricle can be used for the measurement. The method used in the measurement of cardiac output is described in Chapter 6.

Cardiac output is the product of the stroke volume and heart rate per minute:

$$CO = SV \times HR$$

where CO is the cardiac output, SV is the stroke volume, and HR is the heart rate. The normal resting value of cardiac output in an adult is determined as follows:

$$CO = 75 \text{ ml/beat} \times 70 \text{ bpm}$$
$$= 5250 \text{ ml/min or } 5.3 \text{ L/min}$$

Thus alterations in either stroke volume or heart rate offer mechanisms to adjust CO to meet the blood flow and pressure requirements of the vascular system.

A resting cardiac output of 5 to 6 L/min results in circulating the entire blood volume each minute. As an individual's metabolic rate increases with exercise, the cardiac output is increased to meet the metabolic needs. In a healthy individual the cardiac output can be increased about fivefold to a maximum value of about 25 L/min. This upper limit is reached when the heart is stimulated to beat at its maximum rate and stroke volume. The difference between the resting cardiac output and the maximum value achievable is known as the **cardiac reserve.** The normal value in a subject is determined using the following equation:

$$CR = CO_{max} - CO_{rest}$$
$$= 27 \text{ L/min} - 5.3 \text{ L/min}$$
$$= 21.7 \text{ L/min}$$

where CR is the cardiac reserve, CO_{max} is the maximum cardiac output, and CO_{rest} is the resting cardiac output. In this example the subject was able to increase cardiac output by an additional 21.7 L/min, or about 5 times the resting value. Patients with severe heart failure may have reserves as low as 1 or 2 L/min.

 Table 5-1   Factors that Influence Cardiac Output

Factors	Effect on Cardiac Output
↑ Heart rate	↑
↑ Stroke volume	↑
↑ Metabolic rate	↑
↑ Body size	↑
↑ Age	↓ Maximum output

This results in a limited ability to exercise or even carry out everyday living activities without becoming symptomatic (e.g., tachycardia and shortness of breath) for a condition of poor blood flow.

The major factors that influence cardiac output are listed in Table 5-1. Cardiac output is adjusted to support the metabolic rate (e.g., respiratory gas and nutrient-waste exchange) of an individual. Exercise and body temperature are two examples when the metabolic rate is increased and cardiac output is increased proportionately. Body size also influences the resting cardiac output. Larger individuals have greater mass and thus have greater resting metabolic rates, which require a greater cardiac output. The normal value for healthy adults at rest is approximately 80 ml/kg/min. Thus the normal resting cardiac output for a 75-kg adult with a normal body surface area would be as follows:

$$CO = 80 \text{ ml/kg/min} \times 75 \text{ kg} =$$
$$6000 \text{ ml/min} = 6.0 \text{ L/min}$$

Age also has a profound effect on cardiac output. Neonatal and pediatric subjects have resting cardiac outputs that tend to scale with their body size. Healthy adults have approximately the same cardiac output at rest throughout their life. What changes is the maximum output reached during maximum exercise. The maximum cardiac output declines with aging at a rate of about 1% per year after the age of 25 in sedentary individuals. This rate of change is associated with cardiac and skeletal muscle deterioration. The rate of decline, however, can be reduced with a regular exercise plan that includes aerobic exercise that generates a heart rate of approximately 70% of predicted maximum for 30 minutes and occurs at least three times per week.

Heart Rate

Fig. 5-9 shows the relationship between heart rate and cardiac output. As described earlier, cardiac output is directly related to the heart rate. An increasing or decreasing heart rate should result in an increase or decrease in cardiac output, respectively. A decreasing heart rate causes a proportionate decrease in cardiac output. However, increasing the rate generates a limited effect on cardiac output. This is because of the fact that the heart cannot pump more blood than is returned to it through the venous system.

The rate or rhythm, or **chronotropic state,** of the heart is established by the frequency of stimuli that are generated in the sinoatrial

(SA) node. SA node activity is, in turn, influenced by various extrinsic factors. Drugs or conditions that increase heart rate are known as positive chronotropic conditions and those that decrease rate are known as negative chronotropic conditions. The major factors are listed in Table 5-2.

Autonomic Nervous System Input

The SA node receives nerve impulses from both divisions of the autonomic nervous system. Impulses from branches of the sympathetic nervous system (fibers from sympathetic ganglionic chains that release **catecholamines**) cause an increase in SA node activity, which results in an increased heart rate. On the other hand, the parasympathetic nerve fibers (from the vagus nerve, which releases **acetylcholine**) carry impulses that inhibit SA node activity and cause a decrease in heart rate. Both divisions of the autonomic nervous system are active, but it is the most active division that influences SA node activity and heart rate the most. Sinus tachycardia is caused by a greater number of sympathetic impulses and fewer parasympathetic impulses, whereas a sinus bradycardia would be caused by just the opposite condition. Thus the auto-

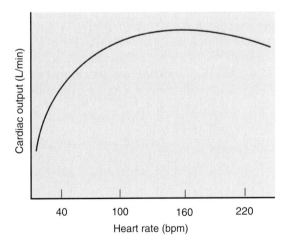

FIG. 5-9 Changes in cardiac output as heart rate is adjusted by electrical pacing. Cardiac output increases and then declines with increasing rate during conditions of constant venous return.

 Table 5-2 Factors that Influence Heart Rate

Factors	Effect on Heart Rate
Sympathetic nervous input	↑
Parasympathetic nervous input	↓
↑ Plasma catecholamines	↑
Parasympathetic blockade	↑
Ca^{++} channel blockade	↓
↓ Blood oxygen content	↑
↑ Core temperature	↑
↑ Plasma K^+ concentration	↓
↓ Plasma Ca^{++} concentration	↓

nomic nervous system influences heart rate through the balance of sympathetic and parasympathetic activity.

SA node activity is stimulated during physical and emotional stress. The sinus tachycardia associated with these conditions is produced by elevated levels of plasma catecholamines (e.g., **epinephrine** and **norepinephrine**). Catecholamines are released by the sympathetic nerve fibers and the adrenal gland during the response to stress (flight or fight response). After the stressful event, the catecholamines are rapidly metabolized or removed by the circulation.

The actions of the sympathetic nervous system can be inhibited by the use of a sympathetic receptor (β-adrenergic receptor) blocking drug (e.g., **propranolol**). A β-blocker inhibits the action of the catecholamines by preventing their binding to the myocardial cell receptor. This results in a reduction in heart rate or the inability to increase heart rate in response to stress. Another approach to reducing heart rate is through the use of Ca^{++} channel blocking drugs such as **verapamil.** Verapamil stops the opening of Ca^{++} channels, which reduces myocardial irritability, heart rate, and contractility.

Parasympathetic inhibition of the heart can be blocked by preventing the binding of acetylcholine to parasympathetic receptors in the SA node. **Atropine** is a parasympathetic blocker that prevents acetylcholine from binding to the receptors. Blockade of the parasympathetic system by the administration of atropine allows the sympathetic system to increase heart rate.

A variety of heart rate reflexes exist and utilize the autonomic nervous system pathways. For example, low blood pressure and hypoxia cause a reflex tachycardia. These and other reflexes are described in Chapter 8.

Metabolic Rate and Core Temperature

Increased metabolic rate causes increased heat production. The SA node is sensitive to local temperature and thus to the heat carried to it by blood from metabolically active tissues. Increased core temperatures cause the SA node to increase its frequency of discharge. Most individuals who are running fevers as the result of an infection have an associated tachycardia. Conversely, when core temperatures drop during conditions that produce hypothermia (core temperature less than 35° C), SA node activity decreases, resulting in bradycardia.

Cardiac rate changes approximately 20 bpm for each change of a degree in core temperature when using the Celsius scale. For example, if a patient's temperature climbs from 37° C to 39° C, their heart rate increases from a resting value of 70 to 110 bpm.

Electrolyte Balance

Blood electrolyte balance (see Chapter 3) is important for stable cardiac performance. Electrolyte imbalances are known to cause heart rhythm and rate disturbances (see Chapter 4). During conditions of **hyperkalemia** (increased plasma K^+ concentration greater than 5.0 mEq/L) the QRS and P-R intervals of the ECG are increased and, in severe conditions, heart block can occur. Generally, hyperkalemia causes bradycardia and, in severe cases, can induce ventricular fibrillation and asystole. Elevated concentrations of Na^+ **(hypernatremia)** above 155 mEq/L inhibit the inflow of Ca^{++}, which reduces cardiac rate. Alterations in plasma Ca^{++} concentration cause variations in cardiac rhythm and rate. Plasma Ca^{++} below 8 mEq/L **(hypocalcemia)** results in decreased sympathetic nervous impulse frequency, SA node activity, and myocardial responsiveness. This results in a bradycardia.

Age and Maximum Heart Rate

As an individual ages, the maximum heart rate achievable declines. This is the major factor that limits the ability to exercise and causes a gradual decline in exercise tolerance with age. Maximum heart rate can be estimated through the following relationship:

Maximum heart rate = 220 − Age

Most aerobic exercise training plans direct the subject to exercise to a point where the heart rate is at about 70% of their predicted maximum. Exercising at workloads that cause higher heart rates is excessively stressing and may cause the myocardium to work at metabolic rates that exceed the oxygen delivery capacity of the coronary circulation. This condition increases the risk of developing myocardial hypoxia and infarction.

Stroke Volume

The normal stroke volume for an adult is about 60 to 80 ml. The ventricles do not completely empty during the contraction and the delivery of the stroke volume. At the end of diastole each ventricle is filled with about 120 ml. This volume is known as the **end-diastolic volume (EDV).** The amount of blood remaining in the ventricle following systole is approximately 40 ml at rest and is referred to as the **end-systolic volume (ESV).** The ESV is a reserve volume of blood that can be used by the heart to increase stroke volume when the heart is stimulated to beat more forcefully. This commonly occurs in response to stress or during exercise. The relationship between these various volumes is shown in Fig. 5-10.

Determining the **ejection fraction (EF)** is a common method used to describe ventricular pump performance. The EF is that percent of the EDV that is pumped with each beat. It is calculated with the following relationship:

$$EF = \frac{SV}{EDV}$$

At rest, the normal ejection fraction is approximately 0.65, or 65%. In severe heart failure the EF can drop to values of 20% or less. In heart failure the EDV and ESV increase as the ejection fraction decreases and the heart swells with blood. The major factors that influence the amount of blood pumped with each beat are listed in Box 5-2. These factors can be organized into two general groups—*systemic* and *cardiac* factors. The amount of blood flowing back to the heart (e.g., venous return) constitutes the

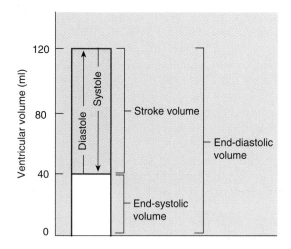

FIG. 5-10 Normal resting ventricular (left and right) volumes at various times in the cardiac cycle.

BOX 5-2

Factors that Influence Stroke Volume

FACTORS THAT INCREASE STROKE VOLUME
↑ Venous return
↑ Ventricular preload
↑ Ventricular contractility
↓ Ventricular afterload

FACTORS THAT DECREASE STROKE VOLUME
↓ Venous return
↓ Ventricular preload
↓ Ventricular compliance
↓ Ventricular contractility
↑ Ventricular afterload
↑ Heart rate

primary systemic factor. The ability of the heart to pump the blood it is presented with comprises the cardiac factors (e.g., filling, contractility, rates, and downstream resistance).

Venous Return and Preload

The amount of venous blood returning to the atria is commonly referred to as the **venous return.** Venous return is the most important factor that influences stroke volume and cardiac output. The other factors are important, but without an adequate supply of venous blood returning to the heart, the cardiac factors would be unimportant. Put simply, the heart cannot pump any more blood than the amount of venous return it receives. Similarly, under stable conditions, the venous return is equal to the cardiac output. Fig. 5-11 summarizes the major factors that govern venous return to the heart.

Venous return is propelled to the right atrium by the left ventricle and the elastic recoil force of the arterial and venous vessels. The left ventricle generates sufficient pressure during systole to propel blood into the arterial system. The distended arteries recoil and force blood through the arterioles and capillary bed and on to fill the veins. The veins distend and blood is forced on to the right atrium. A simi-

lar series of events occurs with the right side of the heart and the pulmonary circuit.

The recoil pressure of the circulatory system can be described through the concept of the **mean circulatory filling pressure.** This is the pressure generated by the vessels of a circuit when it is filled with the current blood volume. The mean circulatory filling pressure is difficult to measure in the human but can be measured in laboratory animals. In the laboratory setting it is measured just after stopping the heart and allowing aortic pressures to drop and vena cava pressures to climb. It is equal to the value of aortic pressure when it equilibrates with vena cava pressures. At this point the mean filling pressure reflects the force exerted on the blood volume by the elastic vessels. In humans the mean filling pressure in the systemic and pulmonary circuits is believed to be approximately 7 and 5 mm Hg, respectively. The mean filling pressure drops if blood volume is reduced or if vessel smooth muscle tone is reduced. Thus venous return is reduced during conditions of low blood volume and reduced vessel tone.

Venous Return Pumps

Venous return from the extremities would be very low or actually be reversed if it were only

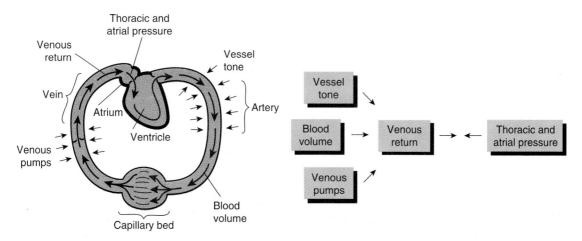

FIG. 5-11   Major factors that influence venous return to the ventricle.

driven by the arterial vessel recoil force. In fact, the venous return to the right atrium decreases approximately 20% when a person rapidly changes from a supine to a standing position. This drop is even greater if venous flow from the extremities was not retarded. To prevent blood from pooling in the veins of the extremities, these vessels are equipped with one-way venous valves. They direct blood flow back toward the heart. In addition, the veins are squeezed by the contracting skeletal muscles that lie along side them. During skeletal muscle contraction, the vessels of the extremities are squeezed. Blood within these vessels is forced through the valves and is prevented from flowing backward when the muscle relaxes (Fig. 5-12, *A*). This "venous pump" activity facilitates venous return and prevents blood from pooling in the extremities.

Venous return to the thorax is further aided by the rhythmic fluctuation of intrathoracic pressure generated by the diaphragm during the breathing cycle (Fig. 5-12, *B*). The intrathoracic cavity has a subatmospheric pressure that fluctuates between −2 and −7 mm Hg during the breathing cycle. During the inspiratory phase the diaphragm contracts, which enlarges the thorax. This causes intrathoracic pressure to become more negative and reaches a value of about −7 mm Hg. As intrathoracic pressure becomes more negative, venous blood flow into the thorax is enhanced. During the expiratory phase, intrathoracic pressure becomes more positive and returns to about −2 mm Hg. This slightly retards venous return into the thorax. This "respiratory pump" effect facilitates venous return to the thorax and heart. It is thought that cardiac output varies during the respiratory cycle by as much as ±25% and 7% for the right and left ventricles, respectively. The effects of the respiratory pump can be amplified when greater intrathoracic pressure changes occur during forceful breathing that accompanies exercise and cardiopulmonary disease.

Central Venous Pressure

Atrial pressure represents an important variable that affects venous return and, in turn, ventricular filling and output. In clinical prac-

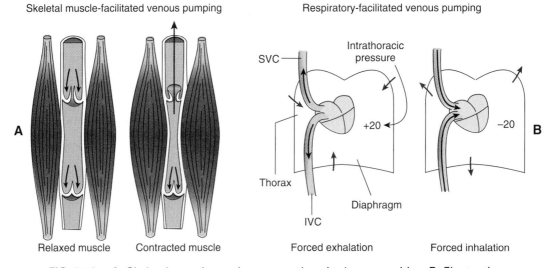

Skeletal muscle-facilitated venous pumping   Respiratory-facilitated venous pumping

A   Relaxed muscle   Contracted muscle   Forced exhalation   Forced inhalation   B

SVC   Intrathoracic pressure   +20   −20   Thorax   Diaphragm   IVC

FIG. 5-12   **A,** Skeletal muscles and venous valves in the extremities. **B,** Fluctuations in the intrathoracic pressure during breathing. Both act as venous return pumps to facilitate venous return to the right side of the heart. *SVC,* Superior vena cava; *IVC,* inferior vena cava.

tice, right atrial pressure is commonly called the **central venous pressure** (CVP).

Although the venous return rate is influenced by the cardiac output and recoil of the vessels at a given blood volume, it is apposed by the pressure within the thorax and atrium. Fig. 5-13 shows the relationship between right atrial pressure and venous return rate. Venous return declines as atrial pressure increases. This can be produced during elevated intrathoracic pressures (e.g., a Valsalva maneuver or positive pressure ventilation) or as a result of heart failure.

Preload Pressure and Ventricular Performance

Stroke volume and cardiac output are highly influenced by the EDV. The venous return rate is critical for proper diastolic filling. The degree of filling not only determines how much blood is available for pumping but also influences ventricular performance. This concept was introduced previously in the description of the Frank-Starling law of the heart, which basically states that ventricular strength

or the amount of force generated during systole increases with increasing filling or stretching during diastole. Greater stretching results in a greater force generation and an increased stroke volume. This relationship is an important intrinsic regulation property of the heart that enables it to adjust its pumping capacity as the amount of venous return varies.

The degree of ventricular stretch is commonly described as the **preload** for the ventricle. EDV would be an ideal choice for the evaluation of preload but it is not commonly measured. As an alternative, preload is most frequently determined by measuring the intraventricular pressure when the ventricle is filled with blood at end-diastole or by measuring atrial pressure. Fig. 5-14 illustrates the Frank-Starling law of the heart through the effect that preload pressure has on stroke volume and cardiac output. As preload pressure increases, ventricular filling and stretch increases and the heart responds with greater stroke work and volume. This improvement is limited, however. At higher preload levels the ventricle is over filled and the ability to

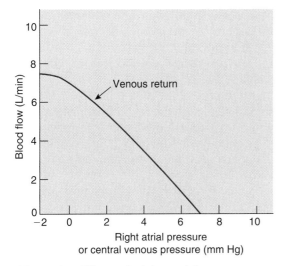

FIG. 5-13 Effect of right atrial pressure on venous return (blood flow) to the right ventricle. Increasing atrial pressure reduces venous return to the ventricle.

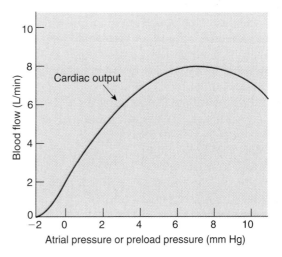

FIG. 5-14 Effect of atrial pressure or preload pressure on cardiac output. Increasing preload results in greater ventricular filling and output (Frank-Starling law of the heart).

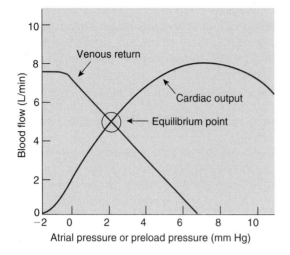

FIG. 5-15 Venous return and cardiac output curves are plotted together to show the equilibrium point where the two intersect. This point represents where the cardiovascular system normally operates with a normal blood volume and atrial pressure. Changes in the cardiovascular system (e.g., added blood volume or increased vessel tone) result in the establishment of a new equilibrium point and a new venous return and cardiac output.

work and generate a stroke volume actually decreases. This response is improved when the sympathetic nervous system stimulates the heart. In heart failure the ventricle responds to elevated levels of preload very poorly, which results in ventricular dilation.

Fig. 5-15 illustrates the critical link between venous return, CVP, and cardiac output. The point where venous return and cardiac output intersect is the equilibrium point at which the cardiovascular system is operating. Normal blood volume and vessel tone, coupled with a preload pressure of 2 mm Hg, results in a venous return rate and cardiac output that are both equal to 5 L/min. If the venous return curve was offset down by reduced blood volume or vessel tone, a new equilibrium point would be established at a lower cardiac output. Remember, the heart cannot pump more blood than is returned to it.

The relationship that preload pressure has on ventricular filling is highly influenced by ventricular compliance. Ventricular compliance, as described previously, is defined as the amount of blood volume change for a given amount of blood pressure change within the ventricle. This is a measure of the distensibility of the ventricle. With age or following myocardial injury, the ventricle becomes stiffer and compliance drops (less blood volume for the amount of pressure within). As compliance drops, the same preload pressure results in less ventricular filling and stretch. This, in turn, results in less myocardial force during systole. Stroke volume decreases at this preload pressure. Thus preload pressure is an unreliable indicator of EDV in conditions that cause decreased ventricular compliance.

Preload of the right side of the heart is measured with a CVP catheter whereas preload of the left side of the heart is determined by placing a special catheter in the left ventricle or by "wedging" a pulmonary artery catheter into one of the bifurcations of the pulmonary artery.

Contractility

The strength of ventricular contraction is influenced by numerous factors (Box 5-3). Those factors that increase contractility result in greater stroke volume and myocardial work.

An important intrinsic property of the ventricle, as stated in the Frank-Starling law, is the ability to increase the force of contraction as EDV or preload is increased. This relationship is illustrated in the ventricular function curve shown in Fig. 5-16.

A variety of extrinsic factors influence contractility. Extracellular concentrations of Ca^{++} and the cell membrane permeability for this ion influence the intracellular Ca^{++} concentration. Intracellular concentrations of Ca^{++} are critical for myocardial performance. Elevated intracellular levels of Ca^{++} enhance contractility, whereas reduced concentrations prevent actin and myosin binding and sliding.

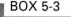

BOX 5-3

Factors that Influence Ventricular Contractility

FACTORS THAT INCREASE CONTRACTILITY
↑ End-diastolic volume
↑ Ca^{++} and adenosine triphosphate (ATP) concentrations
Exposure to catecholamines
Exposure to cardiac glycosides
Exposure to parasympathetic blockers

FACTORS THAT DECREASE CONTRACTILITY
↓ End-diastolic volume
↓ Ca^{++} and ATP concentrations
↑ Na^+ and K^+ concentrations
Exposure to acetylcholine
Exposure to Ca^{++} channel blockers
Exposure to β-receptor blockers
↓ Myocardial blood flow
↓ Blood oxygen content, pH, and temperature

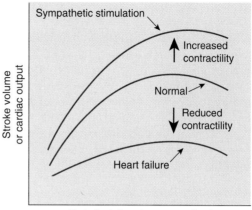

FIG. 5-16 Effect of adjusting contractility on ventricular function. Improved contractility through sympathetic stimulation results in greater stroke volume and cardiac output at all levels of preload. Reduced contractility, brought about by heart failure, produces reduced stroke volume and cardiac output despite elevated preload.

Myocardial hypoxia, malnutrition, or acid-base imbalance that is brought about by poor coronary circulation or respiratory or renal failure results in reduced contractility. Reduced levels of oxygen and nutrient (e.g., glucose or lactate) delivery to the myocardial cell result in reduced levels of ATP production. As ATP levels decline within the myocardial cells, the myosin cross bridges fail to bend and actin is not pulled along the myosin molecule. This results in failure of sarcomere shortening and reduced ability of the myocardial cell to contract. Alterations in acid-base balance (acidosis or alkalosis) cause enzymes and other proteins to malfunction, which leads to myocardial cell dysfunction.

Excitement, stress, exercise, and hypoxia activate the sympathetic nervous system, which releases catecholamines, which, in turn, bind to the β-receptors on the surface of the myocardial cells. β-receptor stimulation causes Ca^{++} channels to open, which results in an increase in intracellular Ca^{++} concentration,

leading to greater contractility. This response can be inhibited by the action of drugs that block β-receptors such as propranolol.

Patients with heart failure often have reduced contractility. The cardiac glycosides (e.g., digitalis or digoxin) are often used in the treatment of heart failure to increase cardiac output. They act by enhancing ventricular contractility and stroke volume. Their mechanism of action centers on inhibiting the Na-K ATPase pump, which causes an increase in intracellular Na^+ and Ca^{++} concentrations. These changes lead to more complete ventricular depolarization and contractility.

Parasympathetic release of acetylcholine results in a modest inhibition of contractility by binding to the muscarinic receptors of the myocardial cells. Activation of muscarinic receptors inhibits the opening of Na^+ and Ca^{++} channels in the cell membrane, leading to reduced contractility. The muscarinic receptors can be blocked with parasympathetic blocking drugs such as atropine. This leads to greater sympathetic action on the heart and increases contractility and heart rate.

The change in contractility that is brought about by various hormones or drugs is often referred to as a change in the heart's inotropic state. Those chemicals that cause decreased or increased contractility are said to have a negative or positive inotropic effect respectively. Dopamine and digitalis have positive inotropic effects on the heart, whereas propranolol has a negative effect.

Downstream Resistance

The ventricles must generate sufficient pressure to open the aortic or pulmonic semilunar valves and force blood into the vascular system. The ventricular pressure necessary to force blood through the valve must be greater than the diastolic pressure in the vessels. The right ventricle must generate more than 10 mm Hg, whereas the left ventricle must generate more than 80 mm Hg. The pressure needed to generate flow through the valve is referred to as the **afterload** of the ventricle.

Fig. 5-17 shows the effect high afterload levels have on stroke volume and cardiac output. A modest increase in afterload or diastolic pressure in the healthy heart causes an initial drop in stroke volume. This results in a greater EDV, which, in turn, causes increased contractility (the Frank-Starling law). The subsequent contractions are stronger and the ventricle generates the same stroke volume at the cost of greater ventricular work. With high levels of afterload, the heart is unable to compensate and stroke volume decreases. Individuals with severe heart failure generally cannot tolerate much of an increase in afterload. Their ventricles are typically unable to increase their contractility to compensate. As a result, they generate reduced stroke volumes and low cardiac output and their hearts swell as the EDV remains increased. Box 5-4 summarizes various conditions that increase or decrease ventricular afterload.

Another approach to the evaluation of afterload is the measurement of the resistance to blood flow or the **vascular resistance (VR).** VR is defined as the amount of pressure needed to propel blood at a certain flow rate through the vascular system. Systemic VR is normally about 10 times greater than pulmonary VR. A more complete description of the measurement of VR is found in Chapter 6.

VR is largely influenced by the smooth muscle tone in the walls of small arteries. Constriction of these vessels is brought about by

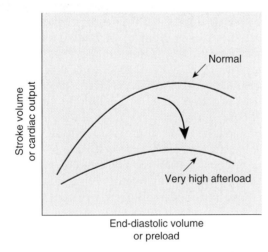

FIG. 5-17 High levels of afterload or downstream resistance result in reduced stroke volume and cardiac output.

> **BOX 5-4**
>
> ### Factors that Influence Ventricular Afterload
>
> **FACTORS THAT INCREASE AFTERLOAD**
> Aortic or pulmonic valve stenosis
> Aortic or pulmonary artery stenosis
> Vasoconstriction
> ↑Hematocrit
>
> **FACTORS THAT DECREASE AFTERLOAD**
> Vasodilation
> ↓Hematocrit

increased smooth muscle tone. Constriction of vessels results in a reduced internal diameter, which causes increased VR. When Hagen-Poiseuille's law (described in Chapter 1) is rearranged to solve for resistance, the impact that vessel size has on the resistance to flow is illustrated:

$$R = \frac{\Delta P}{Q_T} = \frac{8\eta l}{\pi r^4}$$

where η is the viscosity of the fluid, l is the length of the vessel, π is the constant (3.14), and r is the radius. This relationship shows that resistance to flow is inversely related to the radius of the vessel to the fourth power. Put another way, if the radius of the vessel decreases to half of its original size as a result of vasoconstriction, the resistance to flow increases 16 times. This means that the driving pressure the heart must generate to pump blood through the vasculature is directly related to vascular resistance—increasing vascular resistance requires increasing systolic pressure to maintain cardiac output.

CASE STUDY FOCUS

Heart Failure and Cardiac Transplantation

End-stage heart failure is characterized by chronically low cardiac output (<2.5 L/min), low systemic blood pressure, systemic venous and pulmonary circuit congestion, and cardiac dilation. The life expectancy of a person with this condition can be measured in months. Medical treatment in end-stage heart failure employs the use of various drugs to improve cardiac output, arterial vascular resistance, and urine output. Surgical treatment is focused on correcting the primary cause of heart failure, such as improving coronary blood flow or correcting a valve defect. In some cases the only treatment left is cardiac transplantation. The most common reason for heart transplantation is cardiac muscle failure (cardiomyopathy) that is caused by poor coronary circulation (ischemic cardiomyopathy) or that results from unknown causes (idiopathic cardiomyopathy). The 5-year survival after heart transplantation is about 65%.

A 55-year-old male has generalized and progressive coronary artery disease that is resulting in end-stage ischemic cardiomyopathy. He has had two coronary artery bypass graft surgeries in the past 8 years. He was found to be eligible for heart transplantation. He had blood and tissue typing and was placed on the waiting list. Six weeks later a donor heart became available from the victim of a car accident. The donor heart was harvested, preserved in iced cardioplegic solution, and transported to the hospital. The patient was anesthetized, underwent median sternotomy, and was placed on cardiopulmonary bypass. Blood was pumped from the vena cava to the gas exchange membrane, oxygenated, and pumped to the aorta to maintain a systemic blood pressure of 120/80. The patient's aorta and vena cava were clamped and cut, and the diseased heart was removed by cutting away the ventricles and leaving the upper portions of the atria. The donor heart was placed in the patient and attached by sewing the atrial tissues of the patient to the atrial tissues of the donor heart followed by attachment of the aorta and pulmonary artery. Care was taken to remove all air bubbles from the cardiac chambers and vessels. The aortic and pulmonary artery clamps were removed, and blood flowed through the donor heart muscle. The heart began to quiver (fibrillate) and was converted by electric shock to a steady sinus rhythm that resulted in a blood pressure of 110/70. The patient was transferred to the surgical intensive care unit and recovered. Immunosuppression was started and the patient recovered well without signs of tissue rejection and was discharged 7 days later with normal cardiac output and blood pressure.

Hagen-Poiseuille's law also shows that the viscosity of blood has a direct impact on the resistance to moving blood through vessels. The viscosity of blood is highly influenced by the number of erythrocytes and the amount of solute (primarily protein) that is dissolved in the plasma (Chapter 3). Generally, polycythemic conditions and the tendency of blood to form microscopic blood clots increase the viscosity of blood and afterload.

Individuals who are in chronic heart failure occasionally develop polycythemia as a compensatory mechanism to improve oxygen transport to their tissues. This, however, may increase myocardial work by increasing afterload. In some cases it may become necessary to reduce their hematocrits back toward normal by removing small amounts of blood. These patients are also put on anticoagulants such as **Coumadin** to prevent the formation of blood clots. The reduced blood flow that occurs in chronic heart failure increases the risk for the development of blood coagulation. Anticoagulants reduce this risk and further reduce the viscosity of blood by preventing the production of microscopic clots.

HOW HEART RATE AND STROKE VOLUME INTERACT TO AFFECT CARDIAC OUTPUT

Heart rate has a direct affect on cardiac output. That is, as the heart rate is increased, cardiac output increases. It turns out, though, that heart rate has a more complex influence on cardiac output. This is brought about by the effect heart rate has on stroke volume. Stroke volume is affected in two ways—alterations in filling time and contractility.

An increase or decrease in the heart rate changes the amount of diastolic time available for filling the ventricle. During low heart rates the amount of time available for filling is increased, which produces a greater EDV. With greater volume the heart contracts with more force. High heart rates, on the other hand, provide less filling time, which results

in less EDV and reduced contractility. The alteration of end-diastolic ventricular filling subsequently affects the stroke volume. Low heart rates (i.e., less than 40 bpm) provide more time for filling, but because 60% of the filling occurs in the first third of diastole, the stroke volume is not increased sufficiently to maintain cardiac output. At high heart rates (i.e., greater than 180 bpm) the ventricle has insufficient time to fill and stroke volume decreases. In this situation, although the heart rate may be high, the cardiac output actually falls. Fig. 5-9 shows these effects. This figure further supports the concept that the heart cannot pump any more blood than is provided to it in the form of venous return. To maximize cardiac output, the heart must be at its maximum rate, venous return must be maximal, contractility must be maximal, and the afterload must be minimal. Inability to bring any of these about decreases the maximal cardiac output that could be achieved.

METABOLIC REQUIREMENTS AND WORKLOAD OF THE HEART

Nutrient and Oxygen Requirements

The primary task of the myocardium is to contract rhythmically about 70 times per minute to pump blood. For this process to occur, the myocardial cells must be supplied with a steady flow of nutrients and oxygen to produce the necessary amounts of ATP needed for the sliding filament action of actin and myosin. At rest, approximately 60% of the ATP production is from the metabolism of free fatty acids and the remaining amount comes from the utilization of glucose, lactate, and amino acids (Fig. 5-18). The myocardium has the ability to shift the percentage of nutrients used according to what it is supplied with and the activity of the heart. These nutrients are used almost exclusively in aerobic metabolism, which requires a steady supply of oxygen for the phosphorylation of ADP to ATP.

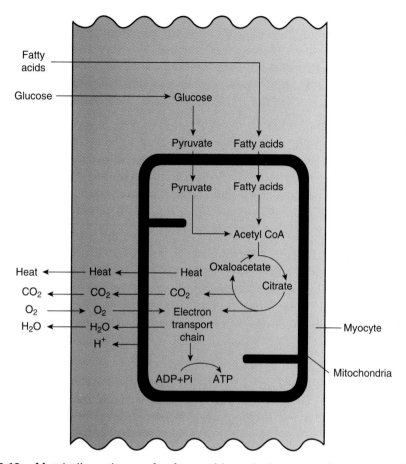

FIG. 5-18 Metabolic pathways for fatty acids and glucose in the myocyte. These nutrients and oxygen are utilized in the mitochondria for the production of adenosine triphosphate *(ATP)*. Primary waste products include carbon dioxide, water, and heat. *ADP,* Adenosine diphosphate.

Thus oxygen consumption is a good overall indicator of the metabolic rate of myocardial tissues.

Oxygen consumption by an organ is usually expressed as a volume of oxygen consumed per 100 g of tissue per minute. During resting conditions the oxygen consumption of the heart (M$\dot{V}O_2$) is about 8 ml of oxygen per 100 g/min. By comparison, this is two to three times greater than the values for brain and skeletal muscle tissues at rest. About 70% of the heart's metabolic rate is in the pumping of blood, whereas the rest supports basal tissue metabolism.

Myocardial Work

Mechanical work, as used in physics, is defined as the utilization of energy for the process of moving mass through a given distance. The heart performs mechanical work by pumping a mass of blood into the vascular system. To carry out this process, the heart converts metabolic energy into the generation of pressure and flow. The pumping of blood into the vascular system is termed *external work*. Mechanical work can be expressed as the number of grams × meters per beat or kilograms × meter per minute.

The normal amount of external work done by the heart per minute is about 5 kg × meters per minute. The measurement of cardiac work is further discussed in Chapter 6. The energy used to open and close valves and the amount dissipated as heat is termed *internal work*. Total cardiac work is the sum of all work done and is reflected by the metabolic rate of cardiac tissue. Oxygen consumption is used as the overall indicator of total cardiac work.

The primary factors that influence the amount of ventricular work done include the amount of tension developed, the velocity of the contraction, and the number of cardiac cycles completed each minute. Greater contractility (tension and velocity) and heart rate lead to greater myocardial work and metabolic rate.

Cardiac work can be further evaluated according to the major load placed on the heart. The heart works harder if greater pressure or flow is generated. For example, if the heart pumps a normal stroke volume against higher vascular resistance (afterload), a greater amount of work is performed to generate the higher pressure necessary to force the same blood flow against greater resistance. On the other hand, the heart also works more if a greater amount of blood is pumped per minute with the same systolic and diastolic pressures. It turns out that the $M\dot{V}O_2$ is greater with increased "pressure" work when compared to the same increase in "flow" work. Consequently, a subject with hypertension has greater demands for myocardial work and oxygen consumption than the exercising subject who has near normal blood pressure with an elevated cardiac output.

Myocardial Efficiency

The efficiency of a machine is defined by the ratio of the useful amount of work performed to the total amount of energy consumed. The useful amount of work performed by the heart is that amount of external work done to pump blood into the vascular system. The total amount of energy consumed is determined by measuring the $M\dot{V}O_2$. External work is determined by measuring the average amount of pressure generated for a given amount of blood volume pumped and converting it into work units of kilogram meters per minute. Total metabolic rate is determined by measuring $M\dot{V}O_2$ and converting it to mechanical work units by multiplying by the conversion factor 2 kg m/ml of oxygen consumed. Myocardial efficiency is determined through the following relationship:

% Efficiency =
$$\frac{\textbf{External work}}{M\dot{V}O_2 \times \textbf{2 kg m/ml oxygen}} \times \textbf{100\%}$$

Using normal resting values for external work and resting oxygen consumption, the efficiency of the heart is found to be about 10% at rest. The remaining 90% is lost in the form of dissipated heat. In patients with hypertensive heart failure the efficiency of the heart drops dramatically as a result of generating reduced stroke volume against high blood pressures. The exercising athlete has efficiencies that actually improve because they generate a high cardiac output against near normal blood pressures.

CHAPTER SELF-TEST QUESTIONS

1. Ventricular compliance is a measure of the ability of the ventricle to fill with blood. It is best defined by which one of the following relationships:
   a. end-diastolic volume divided by the distending pressure
   b. end-systolic pressure multiplied by the stroke volume
   c. end-diastolic pressure divided by the filling volume

d. end-systolic volume multiplied by the systolic pressure

2. Which one of the following factors influences ventricular filling the least?
   a. venous return
   b. ventricular compliance
   c. atrial contraction
   d. contractility

3. The Frank-Starling law of the heart basically states that the heart will
   a. generate less force at very high heart rates
   b. develop more force with increased ventricular filling
   c. beat more rapidly with reduced venous return
   d. pump a volume of blood equal to the venous return

4. Conditions or drugs that are described to have a negative inotropic property cause the heart to beat with
   a. less contractility
   b. greater diastolic filling
   c. less systolic volume
   d. a lower rate

5. The isovolumic contractile period is the phase of systole in which
   1. ventricular volume declines as blood flows out
   2. ventricular volume remains constant
   3. ventricular pressure builds rapidly
   4. ventricular pressure drops rapidly
      a. 1 and 3
      b. 2 and 4
      c. 1 and 4
      d. 2 and 3

6. Blood pressure within the left ventricle reaches _____ mm Hg during systole.
   a. 150
   b. 120
   c. 100
   d. 50
   e. 20

7. Cardiac murmurs are produced by all but which one of the following:

a. turbulent blood flow produced by partial obstructions
b. high flows within normal structures
c. swirling in dilated structures
d. normal closure of cardiac valves
e. regurgitation through leaky valves

8. Cardiac output is defined as the amount of blood pumped
   a. in one minute by one ventricle
   b. in one stroke from one ventricle
   c. by both ventricles over one minute
   d. through the systemic and pulmonary circuits per minute

9. Which one of the following would cause a positive chronotropic response by the heart?
   a. release of epinephrine
   b. administration of sympathetic receptor blockers
   d. release of acetylcholine
   e. administration of Ca^{++} channel blockers

10. Which of the following conditions would result in reduced stroke volume and cardiac output?
    1. reduced venous return
    2. reduced contractility
    3. increased vascular resistance
       a. 1 only
       b. 1 and 3
       c. 2 and 3
       d. 1 and 2
       e. 1, 2, and 3

For answers, see p. 475.

BIBLIOGRAPHY

1. Berne RM, Levy MN: *Cardiovascular physiology,* St Louis, 1992, Mosby.
2. Brandenburg RO et al: *Cardiology: fundamentals and practice,* Chicago, 1987, Year Book Medical.
3. Cohn PF: *Clinical cardiovascular physiology,* Philadelphia, 1985, WB Saunders.
4. Gray H: *Anatomy of the human body,* ed 30, Philadelphia, 1985, Lea & Febiger.

5. Hole JW: *Human anatomy and physiology,* ed 5, Dubuque, Iowa, 1993, Wm. C. Brown.

6. Langman J, Woerdeman MW: *Atlas of medical anatomy,* Philadelphia, 1978, WB Saunders.

7. Little RC: *Physiology of the heart and circulation,* ed 2, Chicago, 1981, Year Book Medical.

8. McMinn RMH, Hutchings RT: *Color atlas of human anatomy,* Chicago, 1977, Year Book Medical.

9. Netter FH: *The CIBA collection of medical illustrations,* vol 5, Summit, NJ, 1969, CIBA Pharmaceutical Products.

10. Rushmer RF: *Cardiovascular dynamics,* Philadelphia, 1978, WB Saunders.

11. Smith JJ, Kampine JP: *Circulatory physiology: the essentials,* ed 3, Baltimore, 1990, Williams & Wilkins.

12. Spence AP, Mason EG: *Human anatomy and physiology,* ed 4, St Paul, 1992, West.

13. Wilson DB, Wilson WJ: *Human anatomy,* New York, 1978, Oxford University Press.

CHAPTER 6

Hemodynamic Measurements

CHAPTER OBJECTIVES

Upon completing this chapter, you will be able to:
1 Define hemodynamics.
2 Describe the noninvasive and invasive methods of measuring blood pressure.
3 Define pulse pressure and mean pressure.
4 Describe the measurement of central venous pressure and the normal value.
5 Describe the Swan-Ganz catheter and how it is placed in the pulmonary artery.
6 Define normal, systemic, and pulmonary arteries and systolic, diastolic, and mean blood pressures.
7 Define hypertension and hypotension.
8 Describe how the pulmonary artery wedge pressure is measured, what a normal value is, and what it indicates.
9 Describe the various invasive and noninvasive methods of measuring cardiac output, cardiac index, stroke volume, and stroke volume index and their normal values.
10 Describe how systemic and pulmonary vascular resistance is determined and what the normal values are.
11 Define the double product and what the normal value is.
12 Describe the method used to determine stroke work index for the left and right ventricles and what the normal values are.
13 Describe the method used to determine cardiac work index for the left and right ventricles and what the normal values are.

The measurement of blood pressure, flow, vascular resistance, and cardiac work is used in the evaluation of the mechanical properties of the cardiovascular system. The term *hemodynamics* is a general reference to these mechanical properties. Hemodynamic measurements are frequently made in the critically ill patient who has unstable cardiovascular performance. The findings from these measurements are useful in diagnosing the type of cardiovascular dysfunction and in guiding the appropriate therapeutic interventions. This chapter surveys the various types of hemodynamic measurements.

◉ NORMAL BLOOD PRESSURES AND HOW THEY ARE MEASURED

Blood pressure is measured in a variety of vessels and cardiac chambers. Noninvasive methods are used to "spot" check systemic arterial pressure. The invasive method of placing a catheter in a vessel or cardiac chamber is used for more precise measurements and for continuous monitoring of the critically ill patient. Table 6-1 summarizes the normal adult blood pressure values in various locations.

Noninvasive Arterial Blood Pressure Measurement

The most common method used to measure arterial blood pressure is a noninvasive and indirect method that includes the use of a stethoscope and a **sphygmomanometer** (Fig. 6-1). These tools detect **Korotkoff's sounds,** which form at the systolic and diastolic pressures as blood flows through a partially occluded peripheral artery. A sphygmomanometer, or blood pressure cuff, is a tubular bladder of air that is inelastic in nature and equipped with a pressure gauge or mercury column and handbulb pump. The cuff is wrapped around the upper arm and inflated to a pressure above the systolic pressure (e.g., 250 mm Hg). This results in collapsing the brachial artery and stopping blood flow below the cuff. The stethoscope is placed over the brachial artery just below the cuff, and the pressure in the cuff is allowed to slowly drop by opening a small valve. As the pressure in the cuff drops, it falls to a value that is just equal to the systolic pressure and blood flows past the cuff and begins to cause a turbulent thumping or tapping sound under the stethoscope. This first sound heard is at the systolic pressure, which is noted by checking the pres-

◉ **Table 6-1** Normal Blood Pressure Values in Various Locations of the Cardiovascular System in a 25-Year-Old Supine Subject at Rest*

Location	Abbreviation	Systolic	Diastolic	Mean
Central venous pressure	CVP			−5-5
Right atrium	RAP	5	3	−2-5
Right ventricle	RVP	25	2	
Right ventricular end-diastolic	RVEDP			2-6
Pulmonary artery	PAP	25	10	10-20
Pulmonary artery wedge pressure	PAWP			5-13
Left atrium	LAP	12	4	1-12
Left ventricle	LVP	120	5	
Left ventricular end-diastolic	LVEDP			5-12
Systemic artery	SBP	120	80	80-100

*All pressures are in mm Hg.

sure on the pressure gauge or mercury column. The pressure in the cuff is allowed to continue to drop to the point where the thumping sound becomes muffled and disappears. This is at the point where cuff pressure is equal to the diastolic blood pressure and the gauge pressure should be noted and the value recorded.

To improve the accuracy of this noninvasive method, the following steps should be taken: (1) measurements should be made after the subject has been sitting quietly for at least 10 to 15 minutes, (2) the arm should be placed at the level of the subject's heart, (3) two measurements should be taken to confirm the values, and (4) the measurement should be carried out in both arms and the difference noted.

Normal adult systemic arterial blood pressure in the brachial artery is 120/80 mm Hg. Table 6-2 shows normal ranges and values that define **hypertension** (high blood pressure) and **hypotension** (low blood pressure). High cardiac output, hypervolemia, and systemic vascular resistance cause hypertension. Hypotension can be caused by reduced vascular

resistance, reduced blood volume, or reduced cardiac output secondary to failure of the left side of the heart.

The pressure difference between systolic and diastolic values is known as the *pulse pressure (PP)*. The normal value of arterial PP is 35 to 45 mm Hg. Elevated values indicate reduced arterial elasticity (normal with aging) or elevated levels of stroke volume.

The mean arterial blood pressure (MAP) is frequently evaluated and can be estimated by measuring the systolic blood pressure (SBP)

Table 6-2   Normal and Abnormal Systemic Arterial Blood Pressure Ranges*

	Systolic	Diastolic
Hypertension	>160	>95
Normal	140-100	90-60
Hypotension	<100	<60

*All pressures are in mm Hg.

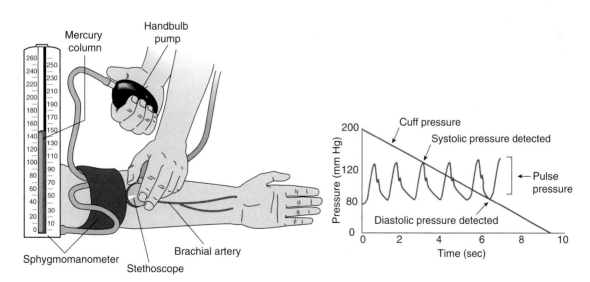

FIG. 6-1 Noninvasive measurement of blood pressure with a sphygmomanometer and stethoscope. Systolic pressure is detected when cuff pressure is dropped to point where the brachial artery opens and a tapping sound is heard. The diastolic pressure is detected when the tapping sound disappears as cuff pressure is allowed to drop further.

and diastolic blood pressure (DBP) and using the following relationship:

$$MAP = \frac{SBP + (2 \times DBP)}{3}$$

The following is an example of how to determine MAP:

$$SBP = 120 \text{ mm Hg}$$
$$DBP = 80 \text{ mm Hg}$$
$$MAP = \frac{SBP + (2 \times DBP)}{3}$$
$$= \frac{120 + (2 \times 80)}{3}$$
$$= \frac{280}{3}$$
$$= 93 \text{ mm Hg}$$

The normal MAP in the adult is 80 to 100 mm Hg. Mean SBP is an important hemo-dynamic variable. The MAP of the circulatory system is an important determinant of the amount of blood flow through an organ or tissue bed. For example, when MAP drops below 60 mm Hg, blood flow through the brain and kidney is reduced to the point of causing organ dysfunction after just a few minutes.

Invasive Arterial Blood Pressure Measurement

The surgical placement of catheters in vessels and cardiac chambers represents the major method of invasive measurement of hemodynamics. The first human cardiac catheterization was performed by Forssmann on *himself* in 1929. It was not until the 1950s that cardiac catheterization techniques were widely introduced to the hospital setting for the purpose of improving the diagnosis of various cardio-

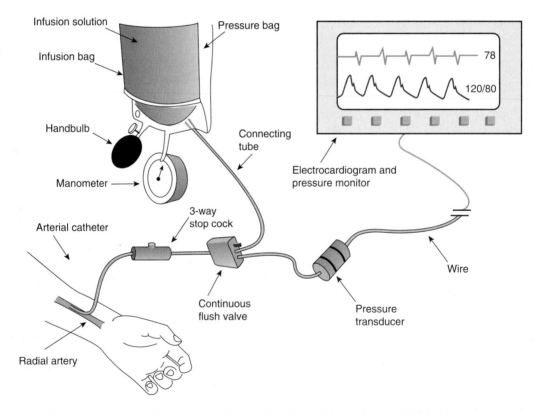

FIG. 6-2 Arterial catheter system for monitoring of systemic arterial blood pressure in the radial artery.

vascular disorders. Since that time, catheterization of the vessels and heart has become more common not only in the catheterization laboratory, but also in the emergency department, intensive care unit, and the operating room. It involves the use of intravascular catheters that are placed in various vessels and cardiac chambers for the measurement of blood pressure and blood flow (cardiac output) and for the injection of radiopaque material. Catheterization of the vessels and heart is undertaken if the noninvasive diagnostic techniques (e.g., echocardiography) indicate the need for more precise understanding.

Invasive measurement of blood pressure is carried out by placing plastic catheters directly into various vessels and cardiac chambers to "expose" the pressure changes to an electronic pressure transducer. Fig. 6-2 shows the arterial catheter setup used for measuring blood pressure in the radial artery. Catheters can also be placed in the temporal artery, brachial artery, dorsalis pedis artery, and umbilical artery for the monitoring of SBP. The transducer converts pressure changes into an electronic sig-

nal that can be processed and displayed as a numeric value or a pressure-vs.-time waveform (Fig. 6-3).

MAP is often measured by the invasive monitoring system by averaging the blood pressure over several seconds.

Measurements of left atrial and ventricular pressures or the injection of radiopaque material to study blood flow are carried out with special arterial catheters. Catheters placed in the left side of the heart are precisely bent and semirigid in nature. These catheters are inserted into the carotid, brachial, or femoral artery and are advanced upstream under fluoroscopy until they reach their desired destination. These catheters are used almost exclusively in the catheterization laboratory.

Central Venous Pressure

Right atrial pressure, or central venous pressure (CVP), is measured with catheters that are introduced into the internal jugular, brachial, subclavian, or femoral veins (Fig. 6-4). The catheter is advanced to the right atrium for the

---

DIAGNOSTIC FOCUS

Accuracy of Systemic Blood Pressure Measurements

Systemic blood pressure is the most frequently measured hemodynamic variable in acutely ill patients. Abnormally high or low values indicate altered perfusion that can threaten organ function and the need for fluids or medications. This demands an accurate measurement of blood pressure to avoid overlooking a problem or treating a nonexistent condition. Systemic blood pressure measured with a properly placed and calibrated arterial catheter system is more accurate than noninvasive cuff-measured pressure. In normal conditions, catheter-measured pressures are 2 to 8 mm Hg higher than cuff-measured pressures. In critically ill patients, catheter-measured pressures range from 10 to 50 mm Hg higher than cuff-measured pressures. Those situations in which significant differences are more likely to exist are conditions of significant vasoconstriction and low stroke volume. Patients who are most likely to produce these conditions are those who have lost significant quantities of blood and who are hypovolemic. Hypovolemia results in lower ventricular filling and compensatory neurogenic vasoconstriction. Postsurgical patients and trauma patients are at greatest risk for significant blood loss and the need for accurate blood pressure measurements.

measurement of CVP. The normal CVP in the adult is −5 to 5 mm Hg. A typical waveform is shown in Fig. 6-5.

Blood volume and venous return are indicated by the CVP value. CVP is frequently used to guide intravenous fluid administration and to monitor fluid volume in the circulatory system. Elevated CVP values greater than 10 mm Hg indicate that the subject has a relatively high blood volume, which is referred to as **hypervolemia.** CVP values that remain at or near 0 indicate that a subject has reduced blood volume or is in a state of **hypovolemia.**

Pulmonary Artery Pressure

Right atrial pressure, ventricular pressure, and pulmonary artery pressure (PAP) are most commonly measured with a pulmonary artery catheter that was developed in the late 1960s by Swan and Ganz (Fig. 6-6). The **Swan-Ganz**

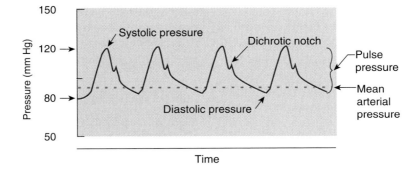

FIG. 6-3 Normal systemic artery blood pressure waveform.

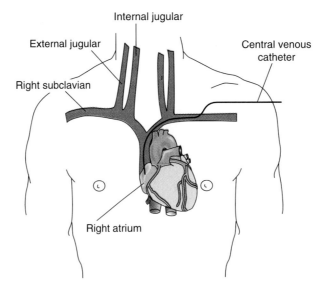

FIG. 6-4 Venous catheter placed in the left subclavian vein and advanced to the region of the right atrium for measurement of central venous pressure.

catheter is a balloon-tipped catheter that is introduced and advanced to the right atrium in the same manner as the CVP catheter. Once in the right atrium, the balloon is inflated with 1 ml of air and the catheter is advanced

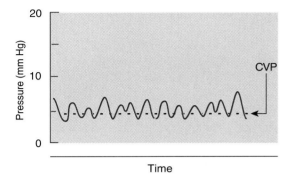

FIG. 6-5 Normal central venous pressure *(CVP)* waveform recorded from a catheter in the region of the right atrium.

blindly through the right side of the heart (Fig. 6-7). The inflated balloon permits the catheter to be directed by the blood flow through the right side of the heart and into one of the branches of the pulmonary artery without the need of fluoroscopy. The position of the catheter is determined by monitoring the blood pressure waveform in each vessel and chamber. Once the catheter is positioned in the pulmonary artery, the balloon is deflated and a chest x-ray is taken to confirm its location.

The catheter has two channels for the measurement of right atrial pressure and PAP. A proximal opening, or port, is placed 30 cm back from the tip of the catheter, and a distal port opens at the end of the catheter in the pulmonary artery. The proximal port allows measurement of the CVP. When the balloon is inflated the catheter wedges in a branch of the pulmonary artery. The pressure measured

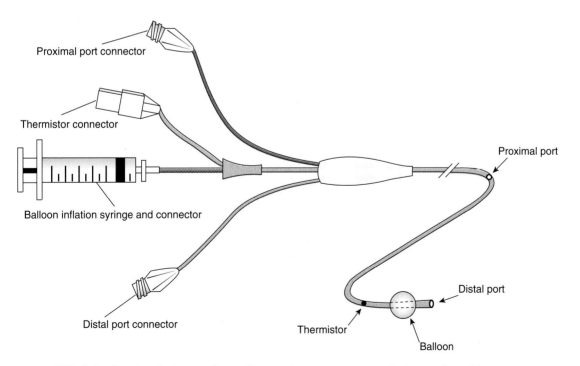

FIG. 6-6 Quadruple-lumen Swan-Ganz pulmonary artery catheter equipped to measure central venous pressure, pulmonary artery pressures (systolic, diastolic, mean, and wedge), and cardiac output by thermodilution.

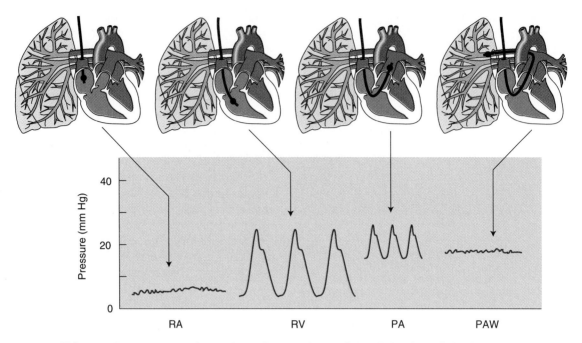

FIG. 6-7 Pressure waveforms in various regions of the right side of the heart and pulmonary circulation as the pulmonary artery catheter is advanced into the right pulmonary artery. *RA*, Right atrium; *RV*, right ventricle; *PA*, pulmonary artery; *PAW*, pulmonary artery wedge.

when the balloon wedges is termed the *pulmonary artery wedge pressure (PAWP)* or the *pulmonary capillary wedge pressure (PCWP).* The PAWP is an accurate reflection of PCWP and left atrial pressure (Fig. 6-8).

The Swan-Ganz catheter can measure CVP (preload for the right ventricle), PAP (afterload of the right ventricle), and PAWP (preload for the left ventricle). The normal PAP and PAWP in the adult are 25/10 and 10 mm Hg, respectively.

The PAP and PAWP are useful indicators of blood volume status and pump performance. If the patient is suffering from hypovolemia, the PAP and PAWP are often reduced. During conditions of failure of the right side of the heart, the PAP and PAWP are decreased. Vasoconstriction of the pulmonary vasculature and mitral valve stenosis causes the PAP and mean PAP to increase. In failure of the left side of the heart, PAP, mean PAP, and PAWP all increase.

Failure of the left side of the heart causes the increase in all the PAPs brought about by the ability of the right side of the heart to pump blood into the pulmonary circuit and the inability of the left side of the heart to pump the pulmonary blood that comes to it. As the pulmonary circuit blood volume increases, both the PAP and PAWP increase as a consequence. In severe cases of failure of the left side of the heart, PAP and PAWP can increase to levels that result in leakage of plasma into the interstitial and alveolar spaces of the lung, causing a condition known as **cardiogenic pulmonary edema,** which usually occurs when the diastolic PAP or PAWP exceeds 30 mm Hg.

PAWP is also useful in guiding fluid and diuretic drug administration. Because the PAWP reflects the preload pressure for the left ventricle, it can be monitored while fluids or diuretic drugs are given to a patient. Often a target PAWP is determined (e.g., 15 mm Hg)

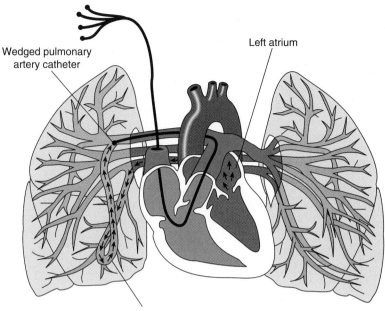

Wedged pulmonary
artery catheter

Left atrium

Pulmonary capillaries

FIG. 6-8 Inflation of the balloon on a pulmonary artery catheter allows the measurement of the "wedge" pressure. The wedged catheter is exposed to a nonflowing path of blood from the tip of the catheter to the left atrium. The wedge pressure is an accurate reflection of the pulmonary capillary and left atrial pressures.

for optimal stroke volume or cardiac output. Intravenous fluid administration (to increase fluid volume) or diuretic drug dosing (to decrease fluid volume by stimulating urine formation) is adjusted to reach and remain at this target pressure.

NORMAL VALUES FOR BLOOD FLOW AND HOW IT IS MEASURED

Cardiac output, cardiac index, stroke volume, and stroke index are common measurements of blood flow. The normal values for these hemodynamic variables in the adult are listed in Table 6-3.

Cardiac Output

The earliest method of blood flow measurement in the intact animal or human subject

 Table 6-3   Normal Blood Flow Values in a 25-Year-Old Supine Subject at Rest

Variable	Abbreviation	Normal Range
Cardiac output	CO	4.0-8.0 L/min
Cardiac index	CI	2.5-5.0 L/min/m²
Stroke volume	SV	60-100 ml/beat
Stroke index	SI	40-65 ml/beat/m²

was developed by Fick in 1870. Fick's principle describes the relationship between blood flow through tissue, the amount of a substance removed by the tissue, the concentration of the substance entering and leaving the tissue, and the principle of the conservation of matter. It can be used to determine the flow of blood through an organ or an entire organism.

Fick's method for measuring cardiac output (Fig. 6-9) uses the total oxygen consumption measured over several minutes and the oxygen content in mixed venous blood (from the pulmonary artery) and systemic arterial blood (from the radial artery). All of the measurements are done simultaneously. Cardiac output is determined by Fick's method with the following relationship:

$$\dot{Q}_T = CO = \frac{\dot{V}O_2}{CaO_2 - C_{\bar{v}}O_2}$$

where $\dot{Q}_T$ is the total blood flow, CO is the cardiac output, $\dot{V}O_2$ is the oxygen consumption per minute, and CaO_2 and $C\bar{v}O_2$ are the respective values of oxygen content in systemic arterial and mixed venous blood. The normal resting values in a subject are as follows:

$$\dot{V}O_2 = 300 \text{ ml of oxygen per minute}$$
$$CaO_2 = 200 \text{ ml of oxygen per liter of blood}$$
$$C\bar{v}O_2 = 150 \text{ ml of oxygen per liter of blood}$$

This yields a normal cardiac output:

$$CO = \frac{300 \text{ ml/min}}{200 \text{ ml/L} - 150 \text{ ml/L}}$$
$$= 6 \text{ L/min}$$

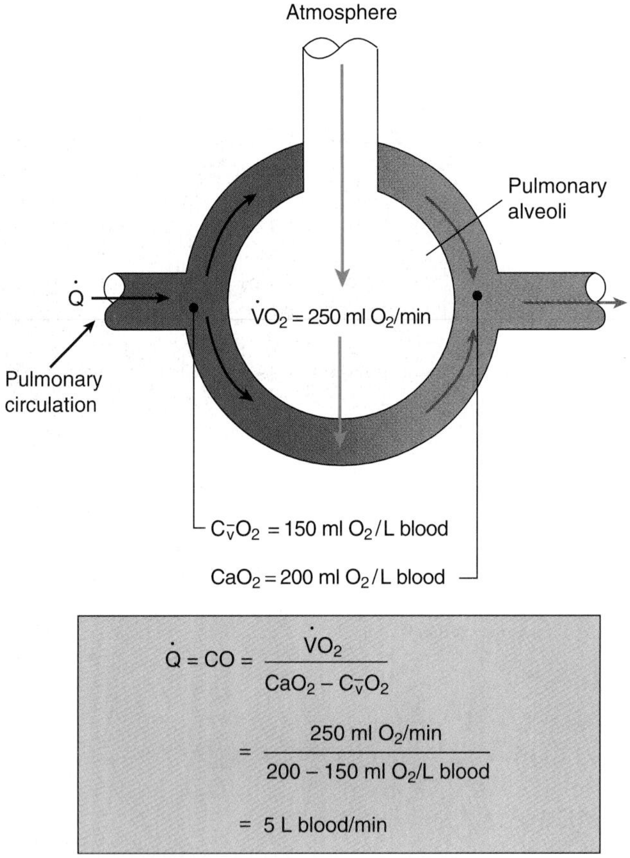

FIG. 6-9 Fick's method of measuring cardiac output *(CO)* by measuring the blood flow (Q̇) through the pulmonary circuit. Blood flow through the pulmonary circuit is determined by measuring the subject's oxygen consumption ($\dot{V}O_2$), mixed venous oxygen content ($C_{\bar{v}}O_2$) in the pulmonary artery, and arterial oxygen content (CaO_2) in the radial artery.

Fick's method is cumbersome, slow, and subject to error. Errors are produced when the subject is not quiet during the 3-minute determination of oxygen consumption, when there are intracardiac or intrapulmonary shunts that route blood around gas exchange sites, and when samples are contaminated or incorrectly measured. These reasons have driven the need for a method that is rapid and less technically demanding.

A more popular method is the indicator-dilution technique. This technique utilizes a dye (i.e., indocyanine green) that is injected into the right atrium where it mixes with blood. This is followed by the slow withdrawal of arterial blood from a catheter downstream and pulled through a dye detector (i.e., an optical densitometer). The concentration of the dye is recorded over time and a concentration-vs.-time curve is generated. Cardiac output is proportional to the amount of dye that is injected upstream divided by the average concentration of dye under the cardiac output curve measured downstream and the length of time the dye takes to pass the detector. This relationship is shown mathematically as follows:

$$\dot{Q}_T = \frac{I}{C \times T}$$

where I is the amount of dye injected, C is the average concentration of dye detected downstream, and T is the amount of time it takes for the dye to pass the detector. One of the primary limitations of this technique is the "recirculation" of the dye as it is pumped around the circulatory system. This prevents accurate determinations of cardiac output when more than three or four dye injections are used over short periods.

A variation of the indicator-dilution technique is the thermodilution technique, a method that utilizes ice-cold water as the "dye" and an electronic thermometer as the detector. Thermodilution is performed with a Swan-Ganz catheter that is equipped with a thermistor (Fig. 6-10). The cold water "dye" is a 10-ml volume of 5% dextrose in water (D_5W) that is cooled by an ice bath to about $2°\ C$ and injected into the right atrium through the proximal port of the Swan-Ganz catheter. The thermistor is placed downstream 4 to 6 cm back from the tip of the catheter to detect the cold solution as it is diluted with warm blood and moves past the catheter tip. A cardiac output curve (Fig. 6-11) is produced and analyzed in the same manner as in the indicator-dilution technique to determine the cardiac output. Thermodilution requires the placement of only one catheter and does not require blood sampling. Multiple injections of ice-cold D_5W can be given for multiple determinations of cardiac output without the problem of dye recirculation that is inherent in the dye-dilution technique. These features, coupled with a microprocessor for automated calculations, have made thermodilution the most popular invasive method for cardiac output determination in use today.

A variety of noninvasive methods have been developed over the past three decades for the measurement of cardiac output and stroke volume. The three most promising methods include thoracic bioimpedance, Doppler-enhanced echocardiography, and radionuclide ventriculography.

Thoracic bioimpedance was originally developed for monitoring U.S. astronauts in space, and since that time it has been improved. The technique utilizes four pairs of electrodes that are placed on the neck and lower thorax. Two pairs of electrodes inject a flow of safe, high-frequency (100 kHz), and low-magnitude alternating current while the other two pairs detect the impedance of current flow. Variations in impedance are caused by pulsatile blood flow, breathing, and movement. With the subject lying still and breathing quietly, the impedance changes correspond to the velocity and volume of blood being pumped into the aorta with each beat. This relationship, combined with heart rate detection, enables a microprocessor to calculate cardiac output and other blood flow parameters. The precision of this technique has improved but is not

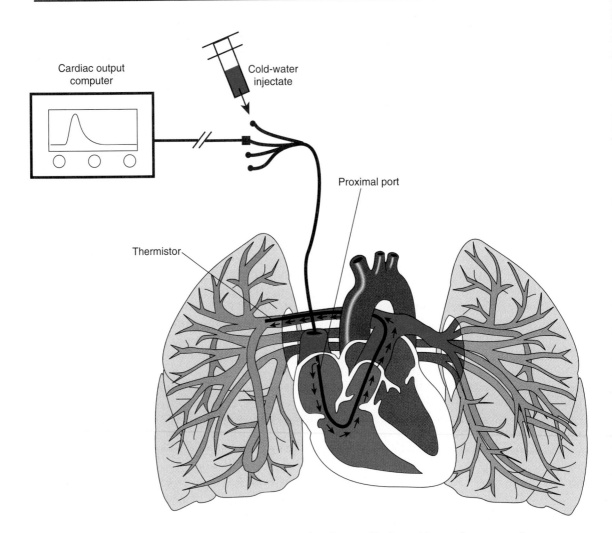

Cardiac output computer

Cold-water injectate

Proximal port

Thermistor

FIG. 6-10 Measurement of cardiac output by thermodilution with a pulmonary artery catheter. Cold water "dye" is rapidly injected into the right atrium by using the proximal port, and temperature change is detected downstream by the thermistor. The temperature change over time is analyzed by a computer and the cardiac output is determined.

as accurate as the indicator-dilution method. Although its absolute accuracy is low, it is a useful noninvasive technique for continuous trending of cardiac performance.

Echocardiography is an evolving technique that allows the imaging of cardiac structure through the use of high-frequency sound waves. The sound waves are directed into the chest by a transducer that is placed in contact with the chest. The sound waves are reflected back to the transducer by the structures within the thorax and displayed on a video screen. Recently, pulsed Doppler-enhanced echocardiography has become available. This technique detects the movement and direction of blood flow within vessels and cardiac chambers. With the transducer placed in the suprasternal notch or in the esophagus, the

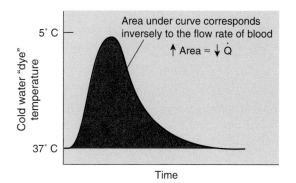

FIG. 6-11 Temperature change vs. time cardiac output curve produced by thermodilution.

dimensions of the aorta and the velocity of blood flow are detected. A microprocessor carries out the calculation of stroke volume and cardiac output. This technique is typically used to "spot check" cardiac structure and flow and has been shown to be a good indicator of cardiac performance.

Radionuclide ventriculography is a method of visualizing the cardiac chambers by detecting the gamma radiation emitted by radioactively tagged blood within the beating heart. A small amount of the patient's blood is tagged with the short lived technetium radioactive nuclide. The tagged blood is returned to the subject by injecting it into a peripheral vein. The labeled erythrocytes mix with the rest of the patient's blood volume to reach a stable concentration, and the image of the cardiac cycle is detected with an Anger scintillation camera and analyzed by a microprocessor. This allows the estimation of end-diastolic volume, stroke volume, end-systolic volume, and ejection fraction. This, coupled with heart rate, yields an estimation of cardiac output. This technique, like echocardiography, does not replace invasive catheterization techniques but is useful for "spot checking" cardiac performance.

The normal value for cardiac output in the resting adult is 4 to 8 L/min. Those factors that reduce cardiac output include reduced venous return, reduced blood volume, reduced contractility, faulty valvular action, and increased afterload. Reversing all of these factors improves cardiac output.

Stroke Volume

Stroke volume is frequently determined by measuring cardiac output and heart rate and using the following relationship:

$$SV = \frac{CO}{HR}$$

where SV is stroke volume, CO is cardiac output, and HR is heart rate. This method yields an average value for SV. The following is an example:

$$CO = 8.3 \text{ L/min}$$
$$HR = 125/\text{min}$$
$$SV = \frac{8.3 \text{ L/min}}{125/\text{min}}$$
$$= 0.066 \text{ L or } 66 \text{ ml}$$

Noninvasive measurements of stroke volume are carried out by thoracic bioimpedance, Doppler-enhanced echocardiography, and radionuclide ventriculography.

The normal stroke volume in the adult is 60 to 100 ml/beat. The factors listed previously that affect cardiac output basically affect stroke volume the same way.

Cardiac and Stroke Indexes

The effect of body size on resting values of cardiac pump performance has led to another approach in reporting stroke volume and cardiac output. **Stroke index (SI)** and **cardiac output index (CI)** are values of stroke volume and cardiac output that are adjusted for body size by dividing the respective values by the body surface area in square meters:

$$SI = \frac{SV}{BSA}$$

$$CI = \frac{CO}{BSA}$$

For a normal 70-kg adult with a body surface area of 1.63 m², the SI and CI are as follows:

SI = 75 ml/beat/1.63 m² = 46 ml/beat/m²
CI = 6.0 L/min/1.63 m² = 3.68 L/min/m²

The indexing of stroke volume and cardiac output allows the clinician to make easier comparisons between the actual and acceptable values for individuals of varying size.

The normal values of CI and SI in the resting adult are 2.5 to 5.0 L/min/m² and 40 to 65 ml/beat/m², respectively (see Table 6-3). **Shock** is a condition that typically presents with hypotension, a CI of less than 1 to 2 L/min/m², and an SI of less than 40 ml/beat/m². Shock can be caused by pump failure, hypovolemia, sepsis, and brain or spinal cord injuries. Hyperdynamic states are considered to be present when the CI is greater than 6 L/min/m². Stress, exercise, trauma, and early stages of sepsis often present with hyperdynamic conditions.

MEASURING VASCULAR RESISTANCE AND THE NORMAL VALUES IN EACH CIRCUIT

Measuring arterial blood pressure is one way of evaluating ventricular afterload. Higher than normal arterial blood pressure indicates elevated afterload for the ventricle to pump against. Another approach is the measurement of **vascular resistance.**

Vascular Resistance

Vascular resistance (VR) is defined as the amount of pressure needed to propel blood at a certain flow rate through the vascular system. It can be determined for each of the circuits with the following relationship:

$$VR = (\Delta P / \dot{Q}_T) \times 80$$

where VR is vascular resistance, ΔP is the pressure drop across the circuit, $\dot{Q}_T$ is the total blood flow, and 80 is a constant to convert the value into units of resistance (dyne $\times$ sec $\times$ cm^{-5}). Normal values of systemic and pulmonary vascular resistance are summarized in Table 6-4.

VR is an important hemodynamic measurement when vasoactive drugs and large amounts of intravenous fluids are being administered. Acute hypertension can be treated with a vasodilator such as **nitroprusside,** which causes vascular resistance to drop. Hypotension is treated with fluid administration and vasoconstrictive drugs such as **phenylephrine** or **dopamine,** which cause increased VR. These drugs can be more precisely administered by monitoring VR and other indicators of hemodynamic status.

Systemic Vascular Resistance

Systemic vascular resistance (SVR) can be determined by measuring the pressure drop across the systemic circuit (the difference between MAP and CVP), dividing by total blood flow or cardiac output, and multiplying by the constant 80. The SVR in a subject is determined in the following way:

$$SVR = \frac{MAP - CVP}{CO} \times 80$$

The following is an example:

Table 6-4   Normal Vascular Resistance Values in a 25-Year-Old Supine Subject

Variable	Abbreviation	Normal Range
Systemic vascular resistance	SVR	800-1500 dynes $\times$ sec $\times$ cm^{-5}
Pulmonary vascular resistance	PVR	50-100 dynes $\times$ sec $\times$ cm^{-5}

$$MAP = 90 \text{ mm Hg}$$
$$CVP = 2 \text{ mm Hg}$$
$$CO = 5 \text{ L/min}$$
$$SVR = \frac{90 \text{ mm Hg} - 2 \text{ mm Hg}}{5 \text{ L/min}} \times 80$$
$$= 1408 \text{ dyne} \times \text{sec} \times \text{cm}^{-5}$$

The normal range for SVR in the adult is 800 to 1500 dyne $\times$ sec $\times$ cm^{-5}. In cases of severe vasoconstriction the vascular resistance can climb to levels that reduce cardiac output as a result of excessive afterloads on the ventricle.

Pulmonary Vascular Resistance

Pulmonary vascular resistance (PVR) is determined in a similar manner by measuring the pressure drop across the pulmonary circuit (the difference between mean PAP]) and PAWP, dividing by pulmonary blood flow or cardiac output, and multiplying by 80. The PVR in a subject is determined with the following relationship:

$$PVR = \frac{\text{mean PAP} - \text{PAWP}}{CO} \times 80$$

For example:

$$\text{mean PAP} = 15 \text{ mm Hg}$$
$$PAWP = 8 \text{ mm Hg}$$
$$CO = 5 \text{ L/min}$$
$$PVR = \frac{15 \text{ mm Hg} - 8 \text{ mm Hg}}{5 \text{ L/min}} \times 80$$
$$= 112 \text{ dyne} \times \text{sec} \times \text{cm}^{-5}$$

The normal range for PVR is 50 to 150 dyne $\times$ sec $\times$ cm^{-5}. This is about one tenth of the resistance found in the systemic circuit.

PVR is normally decreased during exercise as the pulmonary circuit accepts greater cardiac outputs with little increase in pressures. Hypovolemic shock commonly causes the PVR to decrease. Conditions such as hypoxia, large pulmonary emboli, and lung injuries caused by infection or inhalation of toxic gases can cause PVR to dramatically increase. Conditions that cause elevated PVR can result in the right side of the heart having to work

harder and disruption of the distribution of pulmonary blood flow. Elevated PVR can be reduced by inhalation of elevated concentrations of oxygen or low concentrations (e.g., 20 parts per million) of gaseous nitric oxide, which reduces the workload of the right side of the heart and improves gas exchange within the lung.

● CARDIAC WORK AND ITS NORMAL VALUES

The amount of work done by the heart can be evaluated in a number of ways, all of which estimate the amount of mechanical work being done by the ventricle to pump blood into its vascular circuit. The various approaches and their normal values are summarized in Table 6-5.

Double Product

A simple approach to the estimation of left ventricular work is the calculation of the double product (DP). The DP is calculated from the noninvasive measurements of heart rate and SBP:

$$DP = \frac{HR \times SBP}{100}$$

Determine the following DP:

$$HR = 70/\text{min}$$
$$SBP = 120 \text{ mm Hg}$$
$$DP = \frac{70 \times 120}{100} = 84$$

The normal value for DP in the adult is less than 140 at rest and increases with increasing left ventricular work. Exercise (e.g., aerobics) in the normal subject typically causes the DP to increase to a range of 200 to 250, indicating elevated myocardial work.

Many subjects with significant coronary artery disease begin to complain of angina during exercise as their DP approaches twice their resting value. This signifies a limited

Table 6-5   Normal Cardiac Work Values in a 25-Year-Old Supine Subject

Variable	Abbreviation	Normal Range
Double-product	DP	<140
Left ventricular stroke work index	LVSWI	40-60 g × m/beat/m²
Right ventricular stroke work index	RVSWI	7-10 g × m/beat/m²
Left cardiac work index	LCWI	3.5-4.5 kg × m/min/m²
Right cardiac work index	RCWI	0.4-0.8 kg × m/min/m²

ability to increase myocardial work without having symptoms of insufficient blood flow in the coronary circulation. The development of angina and the evaluation of DP are a simple clinical indicator of the balance between the amount of work done by the heart and the blood flow in the coronary circulation.

Stroke Work

Another approach to determining the amount of mechanical work performed by the heart is through the analysis of a ventricular pressure-volume "loop." The loop is generated by simultaneous recordings of intraventricular pressure and volume changes during one cardiac cycle. The internal area of the loop, equivalent to the amount of mechanical work done during one stroke volume, is known as the *stroke work* of the ventricle.

Fig. 6-12 shows a normal pressure-volume loop generated by the left ventricle. The events of the cardiac cycle are indicated by the labeled points. *A* to *B* marks the start of systole with the isovolumic contraction period. The ejection phase occurs from *B* to *C*. The isovolumic relaxation period occurs from *C* to *D*, and the filling phase of diastole occurs from *D* to *A*. Then the cycle starts all over again. The internal area of the loop is equivalent to the amount of external work that is done by the ventricle, pushing blood into the respective vascular circuit.

The area of the loop can be measured by computer analysis or estimated by multiply-

ing mean intraventricular pressure times the stroke volume:

$$W_{ext} = \bar{P} \times SV$$

where W_{ext} is the external work done by the ventricle to pump blood into the major outflow vessel (e.g., aorta or pulmonary artery), $\bar{P}$ is the mean ventricular pressure, and SV is ventricular stroke volume.

Increasing stroke volume or pressure generation results in "opening" the loop and indicates greater stroke work. **Aortic valve stenosis** is a condition that results in narrowed valvular opening. The pressure-volume loop in this condition opens up considerably as the ventricle contracts with increasing force to pump blood through the narrowed valve.

Conditions leading to reduced stroke volume and systolic pressure cause the loop to "close down" and indicate reduced stroke work. Reduced coronary artery perfusion results in myocardial failure and typically produces smaller loops, which illustrates a reduced ability to perform work.

A simplified approach to determine stroke work is the calculation of **stroke work index (SWI)**. The SWI is calculated by using the measurement of mean blood pressure ($\bar{P}$), the stroke volume index (SI), and the constant 0.0136 to convert the volume × pressure units to g × m units of work, and the following relationship:

$$SW = SI \times \bar{P} \times 0.0136$$

The left ventricular stroke work index (LVSWI) and the right ventricular stroke work

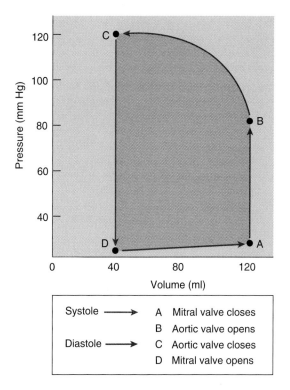

Systole ⟶	A Mitral valve closes
	B Aortic valve opens
Diastole ⟶	C Aortic valve closes
	D Mitral valve opens

FIG. 6-12 Normal left ventricular pressure-volume loop generated by simultaneous recording of pressure and volume changes. *A* to *B* to *C* is the systolic phase and *C* to *D* to *A* is the diastolic phase. The area within the loop is proportional to the amount of external work done to propel blood into the aorta.

index (RVSWI) are determined with the following relationships:

$$\text{LVSWI} = \text{SI} \times \text{MAP} \times 0.0136$$
$$\text{RVSWI} = \text{SI} \times \text{mean PAP} \times 0.0136$$

The normal values for LVSWI and RVSWI are 40 to 60 and 7 to 10 g × m/beat/m², respectively. This demonstrates that the left ventricle is doing about 6 times more work than the right ventricle even though they are both pumping the same amount of blood per minute.

This method is an estimate of stroke work because it does not use intraventricular pres-

sures. Instead, it uses downstream pressure measurements, which may not accurately reflect intraventricular pressure generation. Because of this, the SWI calculated with this method underestimates the amount of work in conditions with aortic or pulmonic valve stenosis. Intraventricular catheterization is necessary in these conditions.

Cardiac Work

The amount of mechanical work being done by the heart over time can also be estimated with the calculation of the **cardiac work index (CWI).** This method is similar to the calculation of SWI, but it uses the CI instead of the SI and thus indicates the amount of work being done per minute. The left ventricular CWI (LVCWI) and the right ventricular CWI (RVCWI) are calculated by using the following relationships:

$$\text{LCWI} = \text{CI} \times \text{MAP} \times 0.0136$$
$$\text{RCWI} = \text{CI} \times \text{mean PAP} \times 0.0136$$

where 0.0136 is the constant to convert to work units of kg × m/min/m².

The normal values for the left and right sides of the heart are 3.5 to 4.5 and 0.4 to 0.8 kg × m/min/m², respectively. The same limitations of accuracy apply in the calculation of CWI as they do in the calculation of SWI in patients with pulmonic or aortic valve stenosis.

CWI and SWI values correlate well with myocardial oxygen consumption. Conditions that increase myocardial contractility cause increased myocardial work and oxygen consumption. Those conditions that increase cardiac and stroke work include tachycardia, hypertension, increased cardiac output, and increased VR. The opposite conditions cause cardiac work to decline.

The patient experiencing heart failure often shows limited ability to increase their ventricular and cardiac work values during exercise. Those patients who have suffered a **myocardial infarction** in their left ventricle and develop

DIAGNOSTIC FOCUS

Cardiogenic Shock following a Myocardial Infarction

A 60-year-old woman was admitted to the emergency department for evaluation of chest pain, irregular pulse, sweating (diaphoresis), shortness of breath (dyspnea), and nausea. Vital signs were as follows:

Blood pressure	130/86
Heart rate	124
Respiration rate	27
Temperature	37° C

The electrocardiogram (ECG) shows S-T segment elevation, prominent Q waves in chest leads 3 and 4, and left bundle branch block. These are consistent with an anterior myocardial wall infarction. The patient was given oxygen via nasal cannula, sublingual nitroglycerin, aspirin, and intravenous morphine. She was then transferred to the coronary care unit.

Shortly after arrival in the unit, she became progressively dyspneic, her blood pressure dropped to 92/65, her heart rate increased to 132, and her ECG showed premature ventricular contractions and short runs of ventricular tachycardia. The patient was given lidocaine to reduce cardiac irritability and ventricular tachycardia. A portable chest x-ray showed pulmonary vessel engorgement and bilateral pulmonary edema. A radial artery and Swan-Ganz catheters were placed and the following data were gathered:

Cardiac output	2.1 L/min
Systemic blood pressure	86/43 mm Hg
Pulmonary artery blood pressure	48/31 mm Hg
Pulmonary arterial wedge pressure	30 mm Hg
Systemic vascular resistance	2095 dyne $\times$ sec $\times$ cm^{-5}
Pulmonary vascular resistance	228 dyne $\times$ sec $\times$ cm^{-5}
Left coronary work index	0.95 kg $\times$ m/min/m^2
Right coronary work index	0.60 kg $\times$ m/min/m^2

These data reveal severely reduced cardiac output, systemic hypotension, pulmonary artery hypertension, abnormally increased systemic and pulmonary vascular resistance, and abnormally reduced ventricular work. These findings are consistent with severe cardiogenic shock from a significant left ventricular myocardial infarction and failure. The goals of therapy to improve the circulation are to reduce the preload pulmonary artery wedge pressure and pulmonary hypertension, improve the contractility, and reduce the afterload resistance.

cardiogenic shock often show increased levels of work on the right side of the heart and reduced levels of work on the left side. This discrepancy in work performed is brought about by the fact that the right side of the heart has to pump blood to the failing left side of the heart. As the left side fails and is unable to pump blood effectively, pulmonary blood flow to the left atrium is impeded and pulmonary circuit pressures climb, causing increased work on the right side.

CHAPTER SELF-TEST QUESTIONS

1. Blood pressure is electronically converted from a pressure signal to an electrical signal by a/an
   a. transducer
   b. manometer
   c. arterial line
   d. regulator
2. Systemic hypertension is best defined as having

a. systolic pressure <120 and diastolic pressure >70 mm Hg
b. systolic pressure <130 and diastolic pressure >80 mm Hg
c. systolic pressure <140 and diastolic pressure >90 mm Hg
d. systolic pressure <150 and diastolic pressure >100 mm Hg

3. Central venous pressure is monitored by placing a catheter in the region of the
   a. inferior vena cava
   b. pulmonary vein
   c. left atrium
   d. right atrium

4. Inflation of the balloon on the Swan-Ganz catheter helps guide the catheter through the
   a. right ventricle and into the pulmonary artery
   b. carotid artery and into the left ventricle
   c. left atrium and into the pulmonary vein
   d. vena cava and into the left atrium

5. Pulmonary artery wedge pressure is a reflection of the pressures in the
   1. right atrium
   2. pulmonary capillaries
   3. left atrium
   a. 1 only
   b. 1 and 2
   c. 2 and 3
   d. 1 and 3
   e. 1, 2, and 3

6. Which one of the following is the best indicator of left ventricular preload?
   a. central venous pressure
   b. mean pulmonary artery pressure
   c. mean systemic artery pressure
   d. pulmonary artery wedge pressure

7. Which of the following are indicators of left ventricular afterload?
   1. systemic blood pressure
   2. systemic vascular resistance
   3. left ventricular stroke work index
   a. 2 only
   b. 1 and 2

c. 2 and 3
d. 1 and 3
e. 1, 2, and 3

8. The thermodilution method of measuring cardiac output utilizes
   1. injection of cold water "dye" into the right atrium
   2. a Swan-Ganz catheter equipped with a thermistor
   3. a densitometer to measure temperature in a systemic artery
   a. 2 only
   b. 1 and 2
   c. 1 and 3
   d. 2 and 3
   e. 1, 2, and 3

Use the following data to answer questions 9 and 10.

A 63-year-old female is recovering from open-heart surgery for placement of three coronary artery by-pass grafts to improve coronary artery blood flow. The following data are measured to monitor cardiovascular performance:

HR = 95 bpm   MAP = 102 mm Hg
CO = 6.8 L/min   CVP = 3 mm Hg
BSA = 1.55 m²   mean PAP = 18 mm Hg
PAWP = 10 mm Hg

Make a series of calculations to better characterize the hemodynamic status of the patient.

9. What is the patient's stroke volume index (ml/beat/m²)?
   a. 72
   b. 55
   c. 46
   d. 23

10. What are the patient's right and left ventricular stroke work indexes (g × m/beat/m²)?

	Right	Left
a.	64	11
b.	77	12
c.	93	16
d.	42	7

For answers, see p. 475.

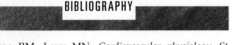
BIBLIOGRAPHY

1. Berne RM, Levy MN: *Cardiovascular physiology,* St Louis, 1992, Mosby.
2. Brandenburg RO et al: *Cardiology: fundamentals and practice,* Chicago, 1987, Year Book Medical.
3. Cohn PF: *Clinical cardiovascular physiology,* Philadelphia, 1985, WB Saunders.
4. Daily EK, Schroder JS: *Techniques in bedside hemodynamic monitoring,* ed 4, St Louis, 1989, Mosby.
5. Darovic GO: *Hemodynamic monitoring: invasive and noninvasive clinical application,* Philadelphia, 1987, WB Saunders.
6. Ganong WF: *Review of medical physiology,* ed 18, Stamford, Conn, 1997, Appleton & Lange.
7. Guyton AC: *Textbook of medical physiology,* Philadelphia, 1996, WB Saunders.
8. Martini FH: *Fundamentals of anatomy and physiology,* Upper Saddle River, NJ, 1998, Prentice Hall.
9. Shoemaker WC et al: *Textbook of critical care medicine,* ed 2, Philadelphia, 1989, WB Saunders.
10. Smith JJ, Kampine JP: *Circulatory physiology: the essentials,* ed 3, Baltimore, 1990, Williams & Wilkins.
11. Tilkian AG, Daily EK: *Cardiovascular procedures: diagnostic techniques and therapeutic procedures,* St Louis, 1986, Mosby.
12. Wilkins RL, Krider SJ, Sheldon RL: *Clinical assessment in respiratory care,* ed 3, St Louis, 1995, Mosby.

Circulation

The vessels of the systemic and pulmonary circuits form an endless loop through which blood is propelled by the heart. These circuits channel blood from region to region to sup-

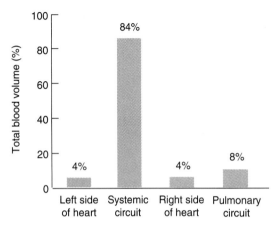

FIG. 7-1 Distribution of blood volume at rest.

port the exchange of various substances. In essence, the vascular system is an elaborate network of passages through the internal environment of the body. This chapter focuses on the organization and blood flow in various regions of the vascular system.

HOW THE CARDIOVASCULAR SYSTEM IS ORGANIZED

Fig. 7-1 shows the organization of the cardiovascular system and the volume of blood in each region. The systemic circuit contains 84% of total blood volume and disperses it to all the organs of the body to support their metabolism. The pulmonary circuit contains only 8% of the blood volume yet it receives the same cardiac output as the systemic circuit.

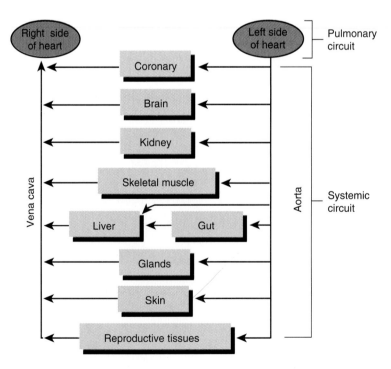

FIG. 7-2 Organization of the cardiovascular system.

HOW THE SYSTEMIC CIRCUIT IS ORGANIZED

The systemic circulation distributes blood to almost all cells of the body except for the gas exchange regions of the lung, which are supplied with blood from the pulmonary circuit. The systemic circuit, a parallel network of arteries that extends out from the aorta to the capillaries of various organs, drains blood through the veins back to the right side of the heart (Fig. 7-2).

Blood Volume, Pressure, and Flow Distribution

The distribution of blood volume and pressure within the cardiovascular system is summarized in Fig. 7-3. The arteries of the systemic circuit, which contain 16% of total blood volume, have a high mean blood pressure of about 90 mm Hg. Pressure drops rapidly and the pulse pressure disappears during transit through the arterioles. The capillaries, containing 4% of the blood volume, have a mean blood pressure of about 15 to 25 mm Hg. The veins contain 64% of the blood volume with a mean pressure of about 2 to 5 mm Hg. The much higher blood volume and very low pressure in the systemic veins reflect their greater distensibility.

The total blood flow from the left side of the heart is dispersed to the various organs at different flows to support the needs and functions of the various organs. Fig. 7-4 shows the distribution of systemic blood flow to the major organs in a subject at rest. This distribution remains stable while at rest and reflects

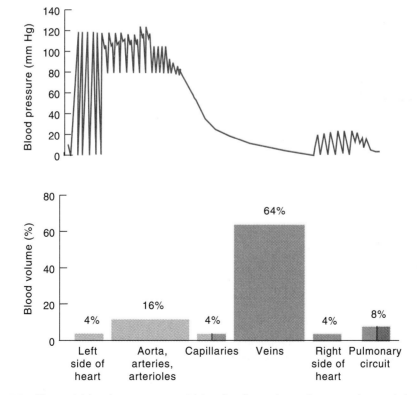

FIG. 7-3 Normal blood pressure and blood volume in various portions of the cardiovascular system at rest.

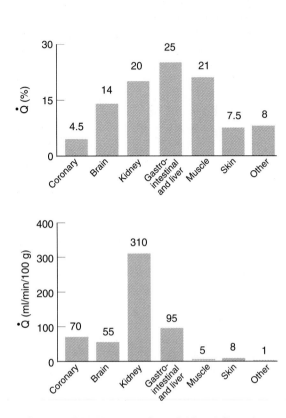

FIG. 7-4 Distribution of total blood flow (percent of cardiac output) and the average blood flow (ml min/100g of tissue) in various regions of the systemic circuit at rest.

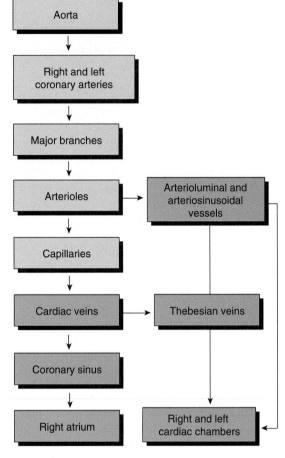

FIG. 7-5 Coronary circulation.

the regulation at work to maintain different organ perfusion rates.

Regional Circulations

Coronary Circulation

The general pathway of the coronary circulation is summarized in Fig. 7-5. Blood flows to the cardiac tissues from the right and left **coronary arteries.** Blood from these arteries perfuses the capillary network of the heart and drains into the coronary veins. About 65% to 75% of the coronary venous flow empties into the **coronary sinus** and on to the right atrium. The remaining amount of venous blood flows into the thebesian veins and other vessels that empty directly into the right and left cardiac chambers.

Fig. 7-6 shows a coronary angiogram, which is an x-ray picture of the coronary circulation produced by placement of a catheter in the base of the aortic arch and the injection of a radiopaque dye. The coronary angiogram enables the clinician to visualize the coronary

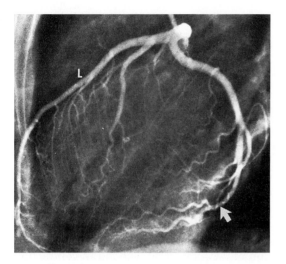

FIG. 7-6 Left lateral view of an angiogram of the left coronary artery system. *L,* Anterior descending branch of the left coronary artery; *arrow,* branches of the circumflex artery that provide blood flow to the inferior portions of the left ventricle. (From Braunwald E: *Heart disease: a textbook of cardiovascular medicine,* vol 1, ed 5, Philadelphia, 1997, WB Saunders.)

circulation and study it for abnormalities such as blockages or narrowing.

The normal adult heart at rest receives about 4% to 5% of the cardiac output or a flow of about 70 to 80 ml/min/100 g of cardiac mass. Coronary blood flow is influenced by four primary factors, which are summarized in Fig. 7-7.

The most important determinant of coronary blood flow is the **coronary perfusion pressure,** the pressure difference across the coronary circuit. It can be calculated by subtracting the central venous pressure from mean aortic blood pressure. The normal value is 75 to 95 mm Hg.

Coronary blood flow is relatively constant over a perfusion pressure range between 60 and 180 mm Hg. The heart accomplishes this stability through **autoregulation,** which is the ability to self-regulate blood flow through a tissue region. Autoregulation and coronary flow generally decrease when mean aortic pressure drops below 60 mm Hg.

The exact mechanism of autoregulation is not well understood. However, factors that

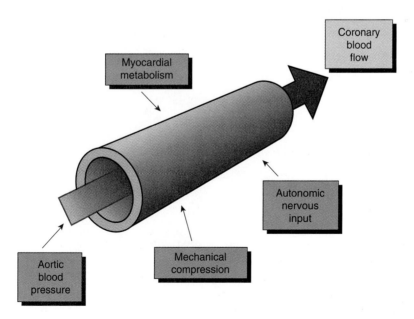

FIG. 7-7 Factors that affect coronary blood flow.

cause vasodilation and increased blood flow include local hypoxia and increased PCO_2, H^+, K^+, histamine, and a variety of different peptides and prostaglandins. Hypoxic vasodilation, the strongest stimulant, is triggered by the local production of **adenosine,** the product of adenosine triphosphate utilization.

Mechanical compression of the coronary vessels is responsible for about 25% of total coronary vascular resistance (VR) during a normal cardiac cycle and can increase during tachycardia when systole is a greater percentage of the total cycle. Flow through the left coronary artery is reduced to near-zero values during systole and is greater during diastole. Right coronary flow is not altered as dramatically. About 80% of total coronary blood flow occurs during diastole, making aortic diastolic pressure a major determinant of coronary perfusion.

Autonomic nervous system input also causes alteration in coronary perfusion. Activation of the sympathetic system generally results in increased coronary blood flow while parasympathetic stimulation results in reduced flow. In response to significant stress and sympathetic stimulation, coronary vasospasm can occur and result in reductions in coronary blood flow.

Flow through the coronary circulation can be further reduced by the development of coronary artery disease secondary to the development of **atherosclerosis.** This condition results in narrowing or blockage of the vessel. Significant reductions in myocardial contractility occur with a 10% to 20% reduction of coronary flow. The fall in contractility is proportional to the reduction in coronary flow. Ninety-five percent occlusion of coronary flow results in complete loss of contractility. Sudden occlusion of a coronary artery

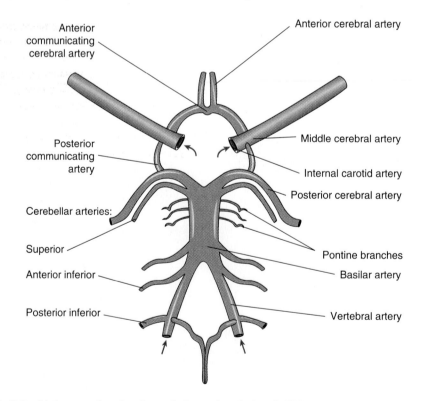

FIG. 7-8 Major arteries that branch from the circle of Willis and supply blood to the brain.

leads to dysfunction and necrosis of myocardial tissues. Death of myocardial tissue from coronary artery occlusion is known as a **myocardial infarction.** Coronary artery disease can be treated medically with vasodilators (e.g., **nitroglycerin** and **captopril**), surgically by balloon dilation called **angioplasty,** or by the removal of a portion of a vein from the leg (e.g., saphenous vein) and the placement of the vein around the coronary artery stenosis called a **coronary artery bypass graft.**

Cerebral Circulation

Systemic arterial blood is supplied to the brain by two **internal carotid arteries** and two verte-

bral arteries. The vertebral arteries fuse to form the basilar cerebral artery, which unites with the carotid arteries to form a network of vessels called the circle of Willis (Fig. 7-8). The primary arteries of cerebral circulation, which branch off from the circle of Willis, include the anterior, middle, and posterior cerebral arteries and the cerebellar arteries. The cerebral arteries supply different regions of the cerebrum as shown in Fig. 7-9. Venous blood drains back to the right heart through the **internal jugular veins.** The general pathway of the cerebral circulation is summarized in Fig. 7-10.

The capillaries of the central nervous system (CNS) prevent many chemicals from passing

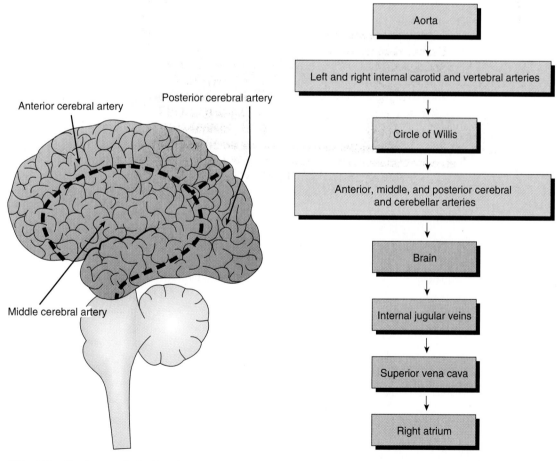

FIG. 7-9 Regions of the brain supplied with blood from the three cerebral arteries.

FIG. 7-10 Basic pathway of cerebral circulation.

through their walls. This selectivity is the product of a **blood-brain barrier** formed by tight junctions and glial cells that layer the surface of the capillary. The capillaries allow the passage of O_2, CO_2, glucose, small lipids, and various neurotransmitters. Large molecular weight compounds such as most proteins, ions, heavy metals, and numerous antibiotics pass through very poorly. The barrier effectively isolates the CNS from many neuroactive chemicals that would cause neural dysfunction.

The brain receives about 15% of cardiac output, which generates an average flow of 50 ml/min/100 g of brain at rest. Cerebral blood flow is influenced by cerebral perfusion pressure, **intracranial pressure,** local metabolism, and autonomic nervous input.

The skull protects the brain but also threatens cerebral perfusion. The CNS is surrounded by a colorless fluid called cerebral spinal fluid (CSF) that cushions and supports the brain and spinal cord. The CSF is formed by the choroid plexus within chambers of the brain at a rate of about 400 to 600 ml/day. It is absorbed at the same rate by the arachnoid villi of the dural sinuses on the superior surface of the brain (Fig. 7-11).

The pressure exerted by the CSF within the skull is termed the *intracranial pressure (ICP)*. The normal ICP is less than 10 mm Hg in the

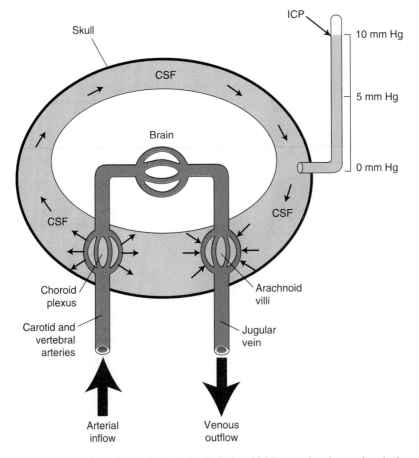

FIG. 7-11 Schematic of cerebral spinal fluid *(CSF)* production, circulation and absorption, and the intracranial pressure *(ICP)* it produces within the skull.

supine subject and can become negative when sitting upright. The volume of CSF, blood, and brain tissue determines the ICP. If the volume of any of these increases, the ICP increases rapidly within the rigid cranial vault. Intracranial hemorrhaging, brain swelling, CSF malabsorption, and tumor formations are all causes of increased ICP.

Normal brain function requires an adequate aortic pressure for sufficient blood flow. Total cerebral flow remains fairly constant over a mean aortic pressure of 60 to 130 mm Hg (Fig. 7-12, *A*). Loss of consciousness occurs if mean aortic pressure drops below 60 mm Hg or if cerebral blood flow is interrupted for as little as 5 to 10 seconds. Ischemia lasting more than a few minutes can lead to irreversible brain damage.

One of the most important determinants of normal perfusion is the cerebral perfusion pressure, the pressure difference between the mean aortic pressure (MAP) and ICP (Fig. 7-13). A normal MAP and ICP yields a normal cerebral perfusion pressure of about 80 to 100 mm Hg. Adequate blood flow and the ability to autoregulate flow are lost when the mean arterial blood pressure falls below 60 mm Hg or when the cerebral perfusion pressure drops below 50 mm Hg.

Increased ICP compresses the cerebral vessels and decreases cerebral perfusion pressure, leading to cerebral ischemia and dysfunction. The brain is capable of compensating for this by initiating a sympathetic induced increase in systemic blood pressure, which offsets the elevated ICP and maintains adequate perfusion pressure and cerebral blood flow. This reflex action is known as the cerebral ischemic reflex. During conditions of high ICP and low MAP, cerebral perfusion pressure and blood flow can decrease to a brain-damaging or lethal level.

Cerebral blood flow is autoregulated by the local metabolic rate of brain tissue in much the same way as the coronary circulation. Many of the same metabolic triggers (e.g., decreased

O_2 and increased CO_2) also cause cerebral vasodilation and increase cerebral blood flow (see Fig. 7-12, *B* and *C*). Moderate to severe hypoxia, a potent stimulant that causes an increase in cerebral perfusion, is thought to be mediated by the production of adenosine. Localized autoregulation occurs in the brain in

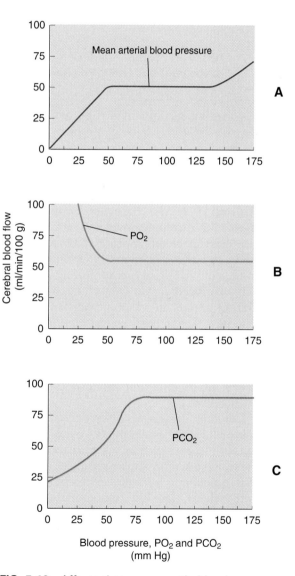

FIG. 7-12 Affects that mean aortic blood pressure, arterial PO_2, and arterial PCO_2 have on cerebral blood flow.

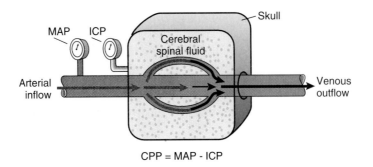

FIG. 7-13 Cerebral perfusion pressure *(CPP)* is the difference between mean arterial pressure *(MAP)* and the compressive force of the intracranial pressure *(ICP)*.

response to changes in mental activity. For example, reading, talking, problem solving, and manipulation of the hand cause increased metabolism in various regions of the brain, thereby increasing blood flow to those regions. Cerebral arteries are also sensitive to blood CO_2 and H^+ levels. **Hypoventilation** leads to elevated CO_2 (**hypercapnia**) and decreased pH (**acidosis**) in blood, causing cerebral vasodilation and increased blood flow. On the other hand, reduced CO_2 (**hypocapnia**) and increased pH (**alkalosis**) levels caused by **hyperventilation** results in vasoconstriction. Patients who have severe head injuries and are found to have elevated ICP from intracranial bleeding or swelling are frequently mechanically hyperventilated for short periods. The induced hypocapnia and alkalosis cause a reduction in ICP.

Cerebral vessels also react to autonomic nervous input. Sympathetic nerve activity causes vasoconstriction whereas parasympathetic nerve activity causes vasodilation. However, autonomic control over cerebral circulation is weak, leaving autoregulation as the most important control mechanism.

The cerebral blood flow can be disturbed by sudden occlusion of a major artery or by the rupture of an arterial aneurysm. These conditions are generally termed a **stroke**. Blood clot formation in a major cerebral artery is a form of occlusive stroke that leads to a set of neuro-

logic defects that correspond to the region of the brain that has lost its blood supply. A cerebral artery aneurysm forms by the weakening and ballooning of the vessel wall. A sudden hypertensive event can lead to the rupture of the aneurysm and the formation of a hemorrhagic stroke. Hemorrhagic strokes are rapidly lethal if they bleed excessively and increase the ICP causing a decrease in total cerebral perfusion.

Renal Circulation

The regulation of fluid and electrolyte balance, the major task of the kidney, is supported by a major portion of systemic blood flow. Blood is supplied to each kidney by a single renal artery. The renal artery divides into arcuate arteries and numerous **interlobular arteries** that supply blood to the functioning units of the kidney—the **nephron.** The one million nephrons in each kidney are the sites of plasma filtration and urine formation.

The interlobular vessels supply blood to each nephron from an afferent arteriole. Blood from the afferent arterioles passes through a capillary network called the glomerulus. The glomerular capillaries are the site of plasma filtration. Filtered fluid flows into the renal tubules. The amount of plasma filtered, known as the **glomerular filtration rate (GFR),** is normally about 125 ml/min or about 180 L/day. This means that the entire plasma volume is

DIAGNOSTIC FOCUS

Severe Headache and Loss of Consciousness

A 39-year-old woman was admitted to the emergency department with complaints of sudden left temporal headache, short-term loss of consciousness, nausea, photophobia, stiff neck, and mild disorientation. These findings suggested that she had had an intracranial hemorrhage. Her vital signs were as follows:

Blood pressure	150/81
Heart rate	108
Respiration rate	26
Temperature	37° C

A computed tomography scan of the head showed a small subarachnoid bleed in the base of the brain. The patient was moved to the critical care unit for monitoring and stabilization of her vital signs.

She is at increased risk for rebleeding and vasospasm. To prevent these problems, she was placed on "aneurysm precaution" protocol (i.e., kept quiet, supplemental oxygen therapy, and head of bed elevated 30 degrees). She was also given Amicar, which prevents the natural breakdown of clots to help prevent further bleeding, and nimodipine, a calcium channel blocker to prevent cerebral vasospasm, which can follow brain injuries.

Angiography of the cerebral circulation was performed and revealed a right vertebral artery aneurysm. Surgery was performed 24 hours later. A craniotomy was performed and a clip was placed on the aneurysm to prevent further bleeding or rupture. The patient did experience some vasospasm 36 hours postoperatively, which manifested itself with the sudden onset of a headache, disorientation, confusion, and weakness of the left hand. This was treated with a "hypervolemia/hyperperfusion" to increase cardiac output and blood pressure. This is done to improve cerebral blood flow and to minimize the effects of vasospasm. This process was continued for 5 days and the patient responded very well. She was discharged to the rehabilitation service in an alert and oriented state with some weakness in the left hand.

filtered about 60 times per day. The unfiltered glomerular blood leaves the glomerular capillary network through the efferent arterioles, which then branch into the **peritubular** capillaries. The peritubular capillaries surround the tubules of the nephron and are involved in the reabsorption of glomerular filtrate and the concentration of urine. Approximately 99% of the filtered plasma is reabsorbed into the peritubular capillaries. The remaining 1% of water and concentrated solutes are excreted in the form of urine. Blood from the peritubular capillary beds drains into **interlobular veins** and arcuate veins and out through a single renal vein to the inferior vena cava. This pathway is summarized in Fig. 7-14.

The kidneys receive about 20% of the cardiac output, producing a tissue perfusion rate of about 300 ml/min/100 g of renal tissue. This rate of blood flow, the highest of any major organ in the body, is necessary to support a high plasma filtration rate and the production of urine.

The main factors influencing renal blood flow include mean aortic pressure, autoregulation, autonomic nervous input, and hormones.

Renal blood flow is stable over a mean aortic pressure range from 75 to 160 mm Hg. The remarkable ability to maintain renal flow over such a wide range of aortic pressure is the result of a strong autoregulatory mechanism. Renal blood flow is strongly linked to a stable

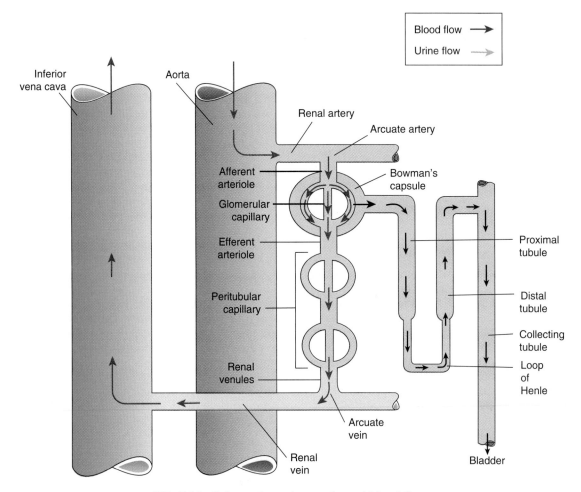

FIG. 7-14 Schematic pathway of renal blood flow.

GFR (Fig. 7-15). The primary benefit of stable blood flow is the ability to have a steady GFR and urine production rate. The kidney fails to form adequate amounts of urine when aortic pressure drops below 60 mm Hg.

A variety of regulatory mechanisms have been proposed to explain the linkage between renal blood flow and GFR, but the precise mechanism is not completely understood. The afferent arterioles vasoconstrict and vasodilate as aortic pressure increases and decreases, respectively, thereby maintaining stable glomerular blood flow. Another intrinsic regulatory mechanism is a negative feedback response

called the tubularglomerular feedback. This mechanism involves the sensation of tubular flow and electrolyte concentration in the distal tubule of the nephron, causing the production of a variety of vasoconstrictive substances. Increased tubular flow triggers efferent arteriole dilation, which reduces glomerular pressure, filtration, and urine production. During reduced tubular flow and electrolyte delivery to the tubule, the opposite actions occur. In addition, vasoconstrictors are produced, leading to efferent arteriole constriction and greater glomerular capillary pressure, GFR, and urine production. The balancing of these

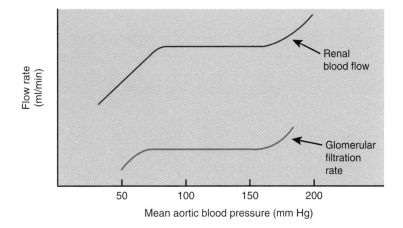

FIG. 7-15 Renal blood flow and glomerular filtration rate are stable over a wide range of mean aortic blood pressure, indicating considerable autoregulation.

autoregulatory features stabilizes renal blood flow, GFR, and urine production.

Neural control over renal blood flow is carried out by the action of the autonomic nervous system. Rage, anxiety, fear, and mild hypotension all activate the sympathetic system causing generalized renal vasoconstriction and reduced blood flow. Despite this general reduction in renal blood flow, GFR and urine formation are usually preserved as a result of autoregulation. Activation of the parasympathetic system appears to cause a generalized increase in blood flow and urine production.

Numerous hormones and humoral agents effect renal perfusion. **Histamine, dopamine, prostaglandins** A and E and **atrial natriuretic peptide** cause vasodilation and improve blood flow. **Epinephrine, antidiuretic hormone** (also known as **vasopressin**) and, **angiotensin II** cause renal vasoconstriction, but the elevated systemic pressures they produce actually can result in increased renal blood flow.

Splanchnic Circulation

The splanchnic circulation is a network of vessels that provides blood flow to the stomach, spleen, intestine, pancreas, and liver. The major arteries that supply blood to the splanchnic circulation include the celiac arteries and the **mesenteric arteries.** Blood drains from the stomach, intestine, spleen, and pancreas into the portal vein. The liver receives about 70% of its blood flow from the portal vein and the remaining 30% from the hepatic artery (a division of the celiac artery). Essentially all splanchnic flow is channeled through the liver and drained into the inferior vena cava by way of the **hepatic veins.** The splanchnic circulation is arranged into two large networks that are in series—blood flows first to the gastrointestinal (GI) system and then through the hepatic network (Fig. 7-16). This design allows absorption of nutrients by the GI circulation and then processing and detoxification by the liver.

At rest, the splanchnic circulation receives about 25% of the cardiac output and houses 25% of the total blood volume, the greatest amount when compared with any other major organ system. Regulation of flow is carried out by local, neural, and hormonal influences. Local flow is autoregulated by metabolism in much the same way as in the heart and brain and is further adjusted by digestive activity. Food ingestion generally increases splanchnic flow through the action of certain nutrients (e.g., glucose and fatty acids) and

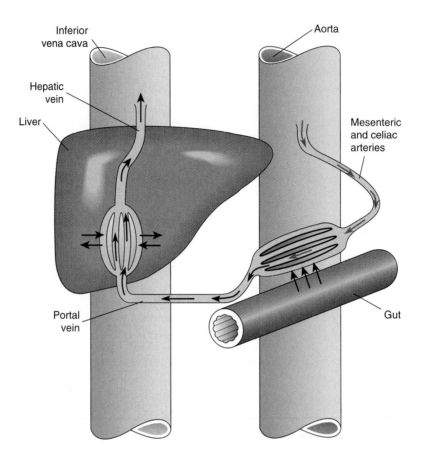

FIG. 7-16 Schematic pathway of splanchnic blood flow.

intestinal hormones such as gastrin and chole-cystokinin. This response enhances nutrient absorption.

Nervous influence on flow is mediated by the autonomic nervous system. Increased sympathetic activity causes generalized constriction of splanchnic vessels, which reduces blood flow and volume. This response shifts blood out of the splanchnic circulation and into other areas, which constitutes an important compensatory mechanism during times of stress. Parasympathetic stimulation results in vasodilation and improved blood flow.

Liver disease that leads to destruction of hepatic structure, such as cirrhosis secondary to chronic ethyl alcohol abuse, results in impaired hepatic blood flow. This causes portal venous hypertension, which can lead to fluid leakage and accumulation in the liver and the peritoneal cavity. This can result in distension of the abdomen commonly called **ascites.** Blood flow through the splanchnic circulation is forced through collateral routes, causing these vessels to distend. Distension of large vessels in the mucosa of the esophagus can lead to the formation of **esophageal varices.** These vessels can split open and result in hemorrhaging into the GI system, which can, along with the formation of GI ulcers and tumors, cause GI bleeds.

Skeletal Muscle Circulation

The circulation for skeletal muscle supports the metabolic needs of these tissues during both rest and exercise. This requires the circulatory supply to be robust in its ability to change as metabolic rate changes. At rest, skeletal muscles receive about 21% of the cardiac output or about 1200 ml/min. This flow can increase 10 to 20 times during exercise and represents about 90% of cardiac output.

Blood flow regulation in skeletal muscle can shift from neural to local autoregulatory control as the tissue moves from a resting to an exercising state. At rest, blood flow is largely regulated by sympathetic induced vasoconstriction. This keeps blood flow to a low perfusion rate of 5 ml/min/100 g of muscle. With exercise, muscle tissue heats up and the local chemical conditions change as metabolism increases (e.g., reduced O_2 and increased adenosine, CO_2, H^+, and K^+). Vessels dilate in response to the increased temperature and chemical changes. This overcomes the sympathetic induced vasoconstriction and blood flow increases.

Cutaneous Circulation

The skin normally receives about 7% to 8% of the cardiac output. The microcirculation of skin is organized in the familiar pattern of arterioles-capillaries-venules over most surfaces. The capillary densities are highest in the face and upper chest. In the palms, soles, lips, ears, and nose there are large arterioles that directly connect to venules and allow blood to bypass the capillary beds. These bypass vessels, known as arteriovenous anastomoses, function in the control of heat loss.

The skin has a relatively low perfusion rate of 8 ml/min/100 g. Regulated by a balance between autoregulation and autonomic nervous input, the skin is capable of tremendous blood flow changes in response to temperature changes. These flow changes are major factors in the release or retention of heat, which is important in thermoregulation.

Flow can increase 30 times with cutaneous heating to 50° C and decrease 10 times with cooling to 15° C. This response is mediated by the vasoactivity of the arterioles and the reflexes of the autonomic nervous system. Direct and indirect vasoconstriction occurs with cooling of the skin. The direct response is a localized vasoconstriction brought about by vessel cooling. The indirect response is a reflex triggered by thermoreceptors in the skin that results in sympathetic nervous induced vasoconstriction. Very low temperatures cause constriction of both arteries and veins and stop cutaneous blood flow. This condition can result in ischemia and can lead to the development of frostbite if allowed to last too long. Vasodilation is also stimulated by direct and indirect mechanisms. Heating the skin causes direct dilation of the arterioles and arteriovenous anastomoses. Indirect vasodilation occurs when cutaneous thermoreceptors are heated and a parasympathetic reflex causes vasodilation.

Mechanical irritation of skin produces red lines and weal formation. Red lines are formed by local vasodilation secondary to local irritation of the vessels. A weal, a round area of skin that is red and raised, is produced by the release of **histamine** and other inflammatory chemicals from secretory cells. Histamine causes the vessels to dilate and the capillaries to leak fluid, resulting in a localized **edema** formation.

Blushing of the face, neck, and upper chest with anger or embarrassment and blanching caused by fear is caused by CNS reflexes. These reactions are caused by inhibition and stimulation of sympathetic impulses to these regions, respectively.

Bronchial Circulation

The lung actually has two different blood supplies: (1) the pulmonary circuit, which supplies blood to the gas exchange regions, and (2) a small branch of the systemic circuit known as the bronchial circulation, which supplies blood to the other tissues of the lung. Minor branching from the aorta forms the bronchial arteries for each lung. The bronchial arteries supply blood to the tissues of the lung down to, but not including, the gas exchange tissues. About one half of the bronchial venous drainage passes into the pulmonary veins of the pulmonary circuit and the other half drains through azygos veins. The relationship between the bronchial and pulmonary circulation is summarized in Fig. 7-17.

The bronchial circulation, which receives less than 1% of the cardiac output, functions to support the metabolism of the airways, vessels, and connective tissue and normally participates little in gas exchange. The bronchial vessels enlarge and develop connections with the pulmonary circuit when the pulmonary blood flow is reduced (e.g., from a poorly developed pulmonary artery) over long periods. This form of compensation is helpful but does not entirely replace the gas exchange ability of the pulmonary circuit.

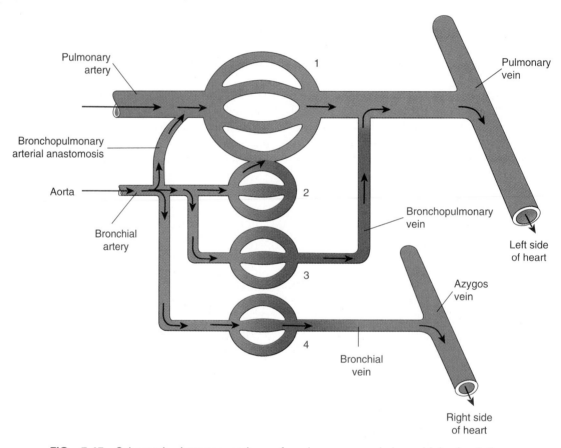

FIG. 7-17 Schematic interconnection of pulmonary and bronchial circulation. Bronchial blood flows to the pulmonary artery *(1)*, through the capillary bed of the large airways and into the pulmonary capillaries *(2)*, through the bronchopulmonary veins and into the pulmonary vein *(3)*, and through the bronchial vein and on to the azygos vein *(4)*. The route through the bronchopulmonary vein allows less oxygenated blood to mix with the better oxygenated blood, which returns to the left side of the heart.

PULMONARY CIRCUIT: FORM AND FUNCTION AND HOW IT IS REGULATED

The primary function of the lungs is the exchange of respiratory gases. This is carried out by "exposing" streams of gas and blood to one another. Ventilation of the lung provides a stream of gas from the atmosphere and the pulmonary circulation provides a stream of blood. These gas and blood streams come into close proximity in the gas exchange regions of the lung called the **respiratory zone.** The exposure of these two streams to one another results in gas exchange—O_2 moves into the blood stream and CO_2 moves into the gas stream.

The pulmonary and systemic circuits are organized so that blood flows from one circuit to the other. The blood flow is equal in both systems. The pulmonary circuit receives the entire output of the right side of the heart and carries out gas exchange with one-tenth the blood volume of the systemic circuit and at a significantly lower blood pressure. These and other distinctions make the structural and functional characteristics of the two systems different in many ways.

Anatomy

The right ventricle pumps blood through the pulmonic semilunar valve to the trunk of the pulmonary artery (Fig. 7-18). It bifurcates into the left and right pulmonary arteries, which leave the mediastinum, and enters a vertical slit called the **hilum** of each corresponding lung. The pulmonary vessels generally have thinner walls and are more distensible than the corresponding sized vessels in the systemic circuit. The arteries follow the airways into the lung and continue to bifurcate into numerous smaller arteries and arterioles that terminate in a dense capillary bed. The pulmonary capillary bed is organized in a different pattern than the typical systemic capillary network. The pulmonary capillaries, which wrap around the terminal air sacs of the

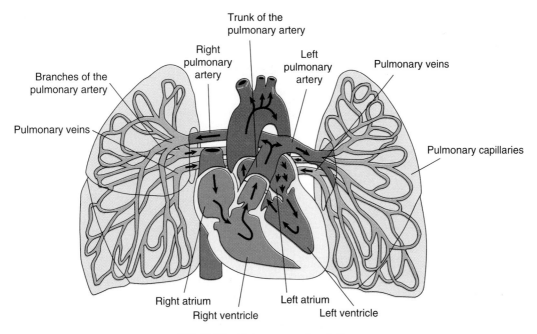

FIG. 7-18 Pulmonary circulation.

lung called **alveoli,** are arranged in a dense meshlike network (Fig. 7-19). The pulmonary microcirculation is sometimes described as being like a "sheet" of blood that has posts of tissue that hold the top and bottom of the sheet together. The capillaries are sandwiched between two gas-containing alveoli that permit gas exchange through both surfaces of the sheet. The oxygenated blood is collected by pulmonary veins and follows the airways back through the hilum to the left side of the heart. Four pulmonary veins (two from each lung) carry blood back to the left atrium.

Pulmonary Blood Volume

The pulmonary circuit contains about 8% of the total blood volume, or about 500 ml. With exercise, this volume can increase three to five times. Unlike the systemic circuit, where most of the blood is contained in the veins, more of the pulmonary blood volume is contained in the arterial and capillary portions of the circuit. The pulmonary capillaries contain about 75 ml of blood at rest. Despite this small vol-

ume, the capillary bed receives the entire cardiac output from the right side of the heart.

Pressures and Vascular Resistance

Pulmonary artery catheterization is frequently carried out with a balloon-tipped, flow-directed catheter for determining blood pressure and flow (see Chapter 6). The normal pulmonary artery pressure (PAP) is 25/10 mm Hg and the mean pressure is 15 mm Hg. These pressures are significantly lower than those found in the systemic circuit (see Fig. 7-3). The pressure in the pulmonary capillaries in the midlung region is about 10 mm Hg. Measurement of pulmonary capillary pressure is estimated by inflating the balloon on the pulmonary artery catheter to measure the wedge pressure or what is commonly referred to as the **pulmonary artery wedge pressure (PAWP)** or **pulmonary capillary wedge pressure (PCWP).** The capillary pressure is not uniform throughout the lung. Pressures are lower in the upper lung regions and greater in the lower lung regions. These differences are a result of the

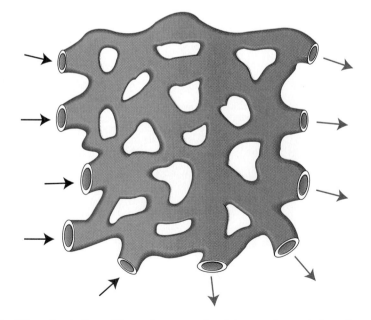

FIG. 7-19   Microcirculation of the pulmonary circuit is a perforated sheetlike structure.

effects of gravity. The pulmonary venous pressure is about 8 mm Hg. Unlike the systemic circuit where the bulk of the blood pressure drop occurs in the small muscular arteries and arterioles, there is a more uniform pressure drop across the entire pulmonary circuit. The normal pulmonary circuit pressures are summarized in Table 7-1.

The reason for having high systemic and low pulmonary circuit pressures is primarily because of their different functions. The systemic circuit provides blood flow to a variety of tissues at different flow rates. To provide these different flow rates, the systemic circuit is supplied with blood from a reservoir of high-pressure blood in the aorta. The pulmonary circuit, in contrast, does not require the ability to direct blood flow at different rates to different parts of the lungs. Low pulmonary blood pressure also minimizes fluid leakage in the lung. If the arterioles and capillaries of the pulmonary circuit were maintained at the same pressures as that found in the systemic circuit, excessive fluid would leak into the interstitial and air spaces and would increase the risk of a pulmonary hemorrhage.

The overall resistance to blood flow through the pulmonary circuit is referred to as the **pulmonary vascular resistance (PVR).** It is calculated by dividing the pulmonary perfusion pressure (mean PAP − PAWP) by the total pulmonary blood flow or cardiac output and multiplying by the constant 80 to produce units in dyne $\times$ s $\times$ cm^{-5} (see Chapter 6 for further discussion):

$$PVR = \left(\frac{MPAP - PAWP}{CO} \right) \times 80$$

The normal value for PVR when using this method ranges from 80 to 150 dyne $\times$ s $\times$ cm^{-5}. This is about one tenth of the value found in the systemic circuit. A variety of conditions can cause PVR to increase, including massive pulmonary embolization, positive pressure ventilation, and pulmonary vessel spasm triggered by sympathetic nervous stimulation, alveolar hypoxia, and vessel injury.

Blood Flow

Normally, the pulmonary circuit receives 100% of the output produced from the right side of the heart at a flow rate that can range from 5 L/min at rest to 20 or 30 L/min during maximum exercise. The marked increase in pulmonary blood flow brought on by exercise is accompanied by a modest increase in PAPs (Table 7-2). To accommodate a fivefold increase in blood flow with only a small

Table 7-1 Normal Pulmonary Circuit Pressures*

Site	Systolic	Diastolic	Mean
Right atrium			1-7
Right ventricle	25	0-7	
Pulmonary artery	25	10	15
Pulmonary capillaries			8-12
Pulmonary veins			6-12
Left atrium			6-12

*Pressures are in mm Hg.

Table 7-2 Pulmonary Hemodynamics During Rest and Maximal Exercise in a Healthy Subject

	Rest	Maximal Exercise
PRESSURES (mm Hg)		
Systolic/diastolic	25/10	40/12
Mean	15	25
Wedge	8	14
Right atrium	5	10
BLOOD FLOW (L/min)		
Cardiac output	6	25
PULMONARY VASCULAR RESISTANCE (dyne $\times$ sec $\times$ cm^{-5})		
	133	48

increase in blood pressure, the PVR must drop. The drop in resistance is produced by capillary recruitment (opening of a greater number of capillaries) and distension (expansion of those vessels already open) as depicted in Fig. 7-20. When cardiac output falls to resting levels, the vessels partially collapse in various regions of the lung.

Measurement of Pulmonary Blood Flow

Total pulmonary blood flow can be determined by the Fick method or, more commonly, by the thermodilution method, which utilizes a Swan-Ganz pulmonary artery catheter.

Regional blood flow in the lung can be determined by an **angiogram** or a perfusion scan.

Angiography typically involves the placement of a catheter in the pulmonary trunk and the injection of a radiopaque dye that casts a shadow in x-ray light and defines the location of blood flow. Fig. 7-21 shows a normal subtraction pulmonary angiogram. Pulmonary perfusion scanning utilizes the injection of albumin microspheres that have been tagged with the radioisotope technetium (^{99}Tc). The microspheres lodge in the pulmonary capillaries and the Anger scintillation camera detects and records the radioactivity. The albumin microspheres break down, clearing from the pulmonary circulation within 8 to 12 hours.

Fig. 7-22 summarizes the various factors that affect the distribution of pulmonary blood flow.

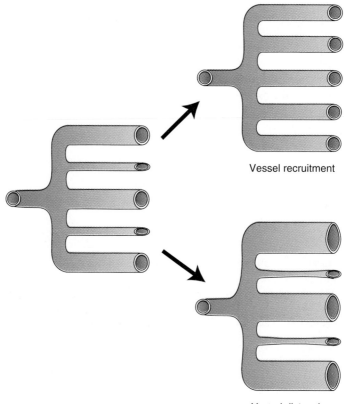

Vessel recruitment

Vessel distension

FIG. 7-20 Pulmonary circulation can accommodate additional flow through the recruitment and distension of vessels.

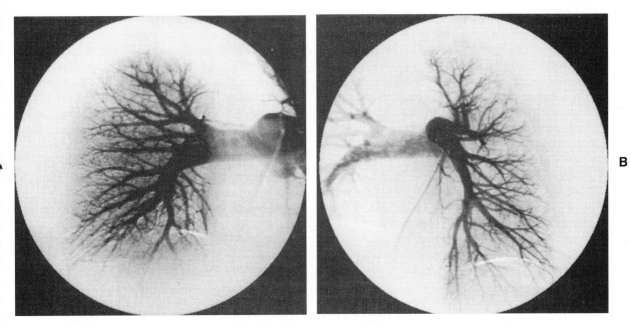

B

FIG. 7-21 Normal digital subtraction pulmonary angiogram. **A,** Right lung. **B,** Left lung. (From Wilkins RL, Pierson DJ: The heart and blood vessels. In Pierson DJ, Kacmarek RM, eds: *Foundations of respiratory care,* New York, 1992, Churchill-Livingstone.)

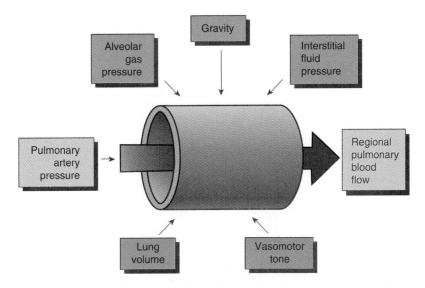

FIG. 7-22 Various factors that influence regional pulmonary blood flow.

Effects of Gravity and Pressure on Blood Flow

Regional pulmonary blood flow is highly influenced by the PAP, alveolar gas pressure and composition, interstitial fluid pressure, vasomotor tone, and gravity. The relatively low blood pressure, the distensible nature of the pulmonary vessels, and the effects of gravity cause local blood flow to be greatest in the base of the upright lung. The distribution of blood flow is shown in Fig. 7-23. This effect is produced by the earth's gravitation attraction for blood as it is pumped under low pressure into a vertical column within the upright lung. Blood pressure, flow, and volume are greater in the **dependent lung zone** (Fig. 7-24). Zero gravity conditions found during space flight produce a more even blood flow distribution.

The capillaries and vessels in the alveoli are thin-walled structures that can be collapsed or expanded by the surrounding alveolar gas and interstitial fluid pressures. Fig. 7-25 shows how positive and negative alveolar pressure disturbs the diameter of a vessel sandwiched between two alveoli. In addition, fluids can collect in the interstitial space around vessels and place pressure on these vessels. The pressure difference across the vessel wall (blood pressure—alveolar and interstitial pressure) is known as the **transmural pressure.** Positive

transmural pressures result in vessel distension whereas negative transmural pressures cause vessel collapse. Normally, alveolar pressure becomes negative during inspiration as the respiratory muscles contract and expand the lung. The combination of negative alveolar pressure and positive blood pressure results in a positive transmural pressure that causes the vessel wall to distend (Fig. 7-25, C). During exhalation, the respiratory muscles relax and the lung recoils back to its resting size, causing gas pressure to become positive. If alveolar pressure exceeds blood pressure, transmural pressures become negative, causing the vessel to collapse (Fig. 7-25, B). With the mouth and airways open and the respiratory muscles relaxed, alveolar pressure will equal atmospheric pressure. Atmospheric pressure is considered to be zero pressure and changes from this reference point are expressed as positive or negative values. When alveolar pressure is zero and there is sufficient blood pressure, the vessel remains open and permits blood flow (Fig. 7-25, A).

The interaction between low pulmonary blood pressure, gravity, and alveolar pressure produces three distinct flow patterns in the lung. These patterns have been described by West as a three-zone concept. Fig. 7-26 shows the three zones in an upright model lung. The model shows a normal mean PAP of 15 mm Hg upon entry into the lung. Arterial pressure varies from 25 mm Hg in the base to 2 mm Hg or less in the apex because of the gravitational pull on blood volume. Capillary pressures range from 20 to 0 mm Hg, and further downstream the venous pressures range from 15 to −5 mm Hg. The capillaries are exposed to alveolar pressures of 5 mm Hg throughout the lung. This is a typical alveolar pressure generated during the expiratory phase of ventilation.

The upper region of this model is classified as zone 1 because alveolar pressure (P_A) is greater than pressures in both the arterial (P_a) and venous (P_v) vessels. This results in a neg-

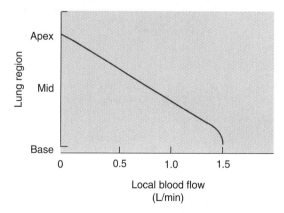

FIG. 7-23 Pulmonary blood flow in different regions of the upright lung.

ative transmural pressure and the vessels collapse, producing little or no blood flow through this zone. Ventilation of zone 1 is actually wasted ventilation because there is little blood flow with which to exchange respiratory gases. Normally, there is just sufficient PAP to perfuse the upper lung zones with a small amount of blood flow.

Zone 2 conditions occur in the midlung regions where Pa is greater than P_A and where P_A approaches or is greater than Pv. The arteriole end of the vessels in zone 2 is open by having a positive transmural pressure. The venous end of the vessel probably flutters open and closed as blood and alveolar pressures fluctuate at values that are about equal.

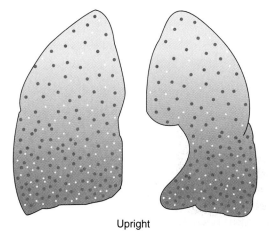

Upright

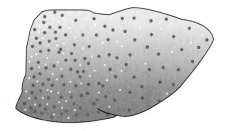

Supine

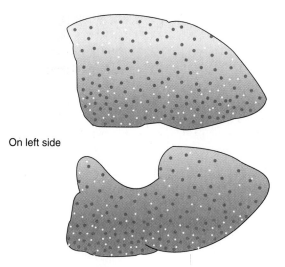

On left side

FIG. 7-24 Pulmonary blood flow (shaded region) is greater in the dependent regions of the lung in various positions.

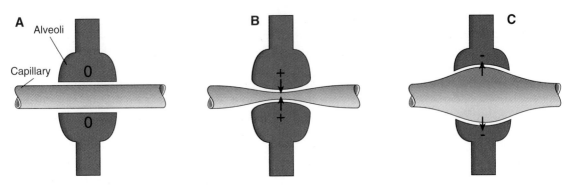

FIG. 7-25 Alveolar gas pressure affects capillary diameter. Alveoli at one atmosphere of pressure *(0)* allow greater flow, **(A)**. Positive pressure causes capillary collapse, **(B)**. Negative pressure causes capillaries to distend **(C)**.

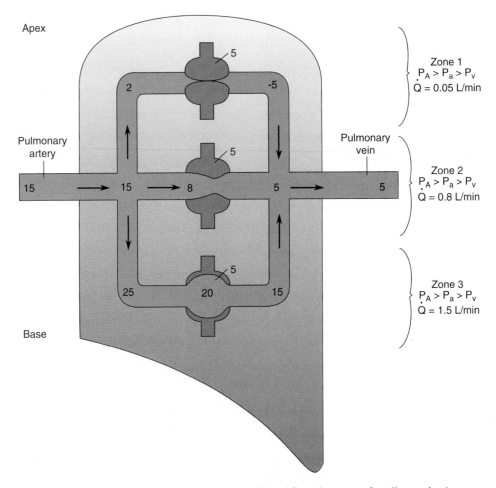

FIG. 7-26 Three zones of pulmonary blood flow (see text for discussion).

Blood flows through this region as long as the arterial pressure is higher than alveolar pressure. In the base of the model, P_a and P_v are significantly greater than P_A. This creates zone 3 conditions in which the transmural pressure along the entire length of the alveoli is positive with the vessels distending as a result. The higher blood pressures and distended vessels make zone 3 a region of high blood flow and volume.

Lung Volume and Blood Flow

Changes in lung volume can cause alterations in regional blood flow. Following a maximal inspiration and filling of the lung, the alveoli fill with air and their walls stretch. The mechanical stretching of the alveolar wall causes the compression of vessels. As a result, PVR increases with increased lung volume. During these conditions blood flow takes the path of least resistance and flows to the base of the lung where the vessels experience less collapse because of higher transmural pressures.

When a subject exhales completely, the alveoli deflate somewhat and their walls relax. This results in less compression of the vessels and allows vessel distension. PVR decreases and blood flow improves throughout the lung, resulting in a modest shift of flow from zone 3 to zones 1 and 2 of the lung.

Regulation of Pulmonary Blood Flow

The flow of blood through the pulmonary circuit is largely passive and is primarily influenced by the effects of PAP and gravity. It experiences little regulation during normal resting conditions. However, the pulmonary vessels are capable of autoregulating flow in response to a variety of stimuli.

The arteries and arterioles of the pulmonary circulation contain smooth muscle and respond to a variety of factors. The major factors that stimulate or inhibit contraction are summarized in Box 7-1.

The autonomic nervous signals influence the activity of pulmonary vessels. Sympathetic activity generally causes vasoconstriction, and parasympathetic activity produces vasodilation. Under normal resting conditions the autonomic nervous system is not very active, playing a minor role in the adjustment of blood flow through the lung. During times of stress, such as hypovolemia, the sympathetic system becomes active, causing vasoconstriction and an elevated PVR.

A variety of humoral substances cause pulmonary vasomotor adjustments. **Catecholamines,** such as epinephrine, **norepinephrine,** and dopamine, are released by the sympathetic nerve fibers and adrenal gland, circulating through the lung and generally causing vasoconstriction. Other vasoconstrictive substances released by various tissues include angiotensin II, prostaglandin $F_{2\alpha}$, vasopressin, and somatostatin. Vasodilation is stimulated by **acetylcholine, prostacyclin,** prostaglandin E, and histamine.

Unlike the systemic microcirculation, pulmonary vessels constrict in response to local

---

BOX 7-1	
Factors that Affect Pulmonary Vasomotor Tone	
VASOCONSTRICTION	**VASODILATION**
Chemical stimuli	
Hypoxia	Oxygen therapy
Acidosis	Alkalosis
Humoral agents	
Prostaglandin $F_{2\alpha}$	Prostaglandin E
Angiotensin II	Histamine
Vasopressin	Bradykinin
Somatostatin	Nitric oxide
Neurogenic stimuli	
Sympathetic activity	Parasympathetic activity
Norepinephrine	Acetylcholine
Epinephrine	
Pharmacologic agents	
Adrenalin	Nitroprusside
Levophed	Nitric oxide
Dopamine	Prostacyclin
Adenosine	

Persistent Pulmonary Hypertension in the Newborn

A full-term infant boy was born following an uncomplicated pregnancy. Significant bradycardia occurred following each uterine contraction during the later stages of delivery. These findings and the presence of meconium in the amniotic fluid and in the infant's mouth suggested some asphyxiation had occurred. Several minutes after delivery his heart rate was 167 bpm, his respiratory rate was 42/min, a loud S2 murmur was heard, and he continued to be cyanotic (gray-blue coloring of the skin) despite the administration of 50% supplemental oxygen via hood. Blood gas analysis revealed severe hypoxia (reduced oxygenation) and acidosis (blood pH of 7.15). He was intubated and his blood oxygenation improved with mechanical hyperventilation and 100% oxygen. The murmur, the response to hyperventilation with 100% oxygen, and echocardiography confirmed that the vessel between the trunk of the pulmonary artery and the aorta (ductus arteriosus) was open rather than closed. Normally, this vessel constricts shortly after birth as air breathing results in improved lung and blood oxygenation. In this situation the severe hypoxia and acidosis from the asphyxiation have resulted in a patent ductus arteriosus, increased pulmonary vascular resistance and pulmonary hypertension. This allows pulmonary artery blood to bypass the lungs and enter the aorta, which impairs the ability to oxygenate the blood fully. To improve oxygenation and pulmonary blood flow, 30 parts per million of nitric oxide (NO) was added to the inspired gas. Inhaled NO causes the pulmonary vascular dilation and improved oxygenation. The infant responded very well to this and the oxygen concentration and mechanical ventilation were weaned down over the next several days. Echocardiography confirmed closure of the ductus arteriosus and reduced pulmonary vascular engorgement. The infant was discharged from the hospital 12 days after birth without complication.

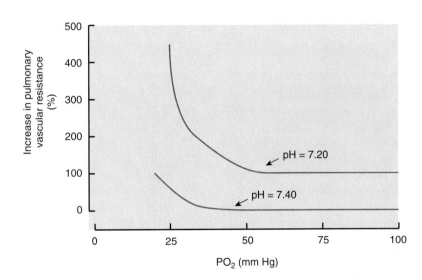

FIG. 7-27 Effects of PO_2 and pH on pulmonary vascular resistance. Hypoxia and acidosis cause a significant increase in pulmonary vascular resistance.

hypoxia. Reductions of both alveolar and arterial PO_2 cause vasoconstriction. In addition, decreased blood pH (increased H^+ concentration) causes pulmonary vasoconstriction. The changes in PVR in response to hypoxia and acidosis are illustrated in Fig. 7-27. These conditions can be generated in regions of the lung that are poorly ventilated. This localized reflex serves to shift blood flow from areas of poor ventilation toward those areas of better ventilation and with a higher alveolar PO_2. The hypoxic effect results in enhancing blood flow to those regions that are better ventilated.

Generalized hypoventilation of the lungs or breathing gas mixtures containing a low PO_2 both leads to pulmonary vasoconstriction and pulmonary hypertension. Chronic lung disease can lead to chronic alveolar hypoxia and chronic pulmonary hypertension. In these cases the right ventricle enlarges as it compensates for the added VR. This enlargement of the right side of the heart is called **cor pulmonale.**

Another situation that can cause chronic alveolar hypoxia is the breathing of air at high altitudes. The greater the elevation the lower the barometric pressure and PO_2 in the gas being breathed. Breathing air at very high altitudes (e.g., greater than 7000 m) can lead to pulmonary hypertension, pulmonary capillary fluid leakage, and pulmonary edema. High altitude pulmonary edema can be disabling and fatal. Breathing gas with supplementary oxygen (e.g., an FIO_2 of 100%) can elevate alveolar PO_2 which, in turn, produces vasodilation, decrease PAP, and decreased pulmonary fluid leakage.

Pulmonary vasodilation is caused by the local production of **nitric oxide (NO).** Nitric oxide, also known as **endothelial-derived relaxant factor (EDRF),** is thought to play an important role in maintaining a basal condition of vasodilation. Impaired NO production causes localized vasoconstriction, and pulmonary hypertension and enhances clot formation. Inhaling low concentrations of NO (e.g., 5 to 50 ppm) is becoming an important

tool in improving pulmonary blood flow and gas exchange.

Functions

The primary function of the pulmonary circuit is to supply a steady flow of blood to the alveolar capillaries for gas exchange. The functions of the pulmonary circuit, however, are not limited to gas exchange (Box 7-2). The pulmonary circuit receives the entire cardiac output, making it well suited to filter, eliminate, and secrete other substances from and into blood.

The metabolism of the lung is supported by both the bronchial circulation and the pulmonary circulation. The tissues that comprise the microscopic alveoli are metabolically active and are supplied with nutrients and cleared of waste by the pulmonary circulation. These tissues require adequate blood flow to support their metabolism and their various functions. Low pulmonary blood flow secondary to circulatory shock or the transport of

---

BOX 7-2

Functions of the Pulmonary Circuit

Respiratory gas exchange
Support of pulmonary tissue metabolism
Reservoir of blood for the left heart
Clot filtration
Quick source of neutrophils following traumatic stress
Clearance or inactivation of vasoactive substances
  Bradykinin is inactivated
  Angiotensin-converting enzyme is inactivated
  Serotonin is removed
  Norepinephrine partially removed
  Prostaglandins E and $F_{2\alpha}$ are removed
  Adenosine phosphate removed
Activation of vasoactive substances
  Angiotensin I converted to angiotensin II

toxins to the lung results in lung injury that causes the condition known as **adult respiratory distress syndrome (ARDS).** The alveolar tissues and microcirculation are injured in ARDS, which results in inflammation, alveolar collapse, and flooding. This leads to increased work of breathing and poor gas exchange.

The pulmonary circuit also acts as a reservoir of blood for the left side of the heart and systemic circuit. The pulmonary circulation can easily accommodate increased blood flow during exercise while continuing to supply oxygenated blood at a proper preload pressure to the left side of the heart. Hypovolemia following blood loss can cause sympathetic induced pulmonary vasoconstriction, which effectively shifts blood volume from the pulmonary circuit to the systemic circuit, helping improve blood pressure.

Blood clots can form in the sluggish blood flow in the systemic veins of the extremities. If these clots entered the arteries of the systemic circuit, occlusion of vessels in the brain, heart, and kidney could occur. This is prevented by the pulmonary circuit through its action as a filter. Small clots that are filtered are rapidly cleared from the pulmonary circuit by the fibrinolytic action of the enzyme **plasmin.** Large clots can move from the systemic veins to the pulmonary circuit, resulting in a **pulmonary embolism.** Large pulmonary embolisms or multiple emboli can cause poor gas exchange and reduce cardiac output. Ambulation and wearing elastic stockings or alternating pressure stockings by those patients at risk for developing clots is useful in promoting blood flow and preventing clot formation in the veins of the lower extremities. In some cases the patient is given anticoagulants to prevent clot formation. In severe cases of clot formation the patient can be treated with "clot-busting" drugs or, if necessary, surgical removal of the clot.

During times of sudden stress the lung can release large numbers of neutrophils, causing the leukocyte count to dramatically increase (**leukocytosis**). Release of neutrophils is a protective response that commonly occurs following trauma or extensive surgery.

A variety of vasoactive substances are cleared or inactivated with passage through the lung. The vasoconstrictor **serotonin** is almost completely absorbed and norepinephrine is absorbed to some degree. The vasodilators (adenosine triphosphate, **monophosphate,** and **bradykinin**) are almost completely cleared or inactivated. Prostaglandin E_2, a vasodilator, and prostaglandin F_{2a}, a vasoconstrictor, are also almost completely cleared. Clearance of these vasoactive molecules is necessary to avoid their continuous effects and to prevent their accumulation.

One vasoactive substance is formed by passage through the pulmonary circuit. Angiotensin I, formed by the action of the renal enzyme **renin** on the plasma protein angiotensinogen, is converted to angiotensin II in the pulmonary circulation. Angiotensin II, a potent vasoconstrictor, plays an important role in blood pressure regulation. The enzyme that carries out the conversion in the lung, called angiotensin-converting enzyme (ACE), is located on the surface of the endothelial cells of the pulmonary circuit.

FUNCTIONAL PROPERTIES OF MICROCIRCULATION

All living tissues require functioning capillaries to support their metabolism. The estimated 10 billion capillaries in the body are the centerpiece of circulatory function. Their walls are comprised of endothelial cells that are connected by junctions. Blood flows from an arteriole directly or from a smaller vessel called a **metarteriole** to the capillary (Fig. 7-28). Metarterioles primarily function to supply blood to capillaries, but in some disease states (e.g., septic shock) they can act as bypass channels that allow blood to flow from the arteriole directly to the venule. This bypass, or shunt-

Precapillary sphincters

Metarteriole

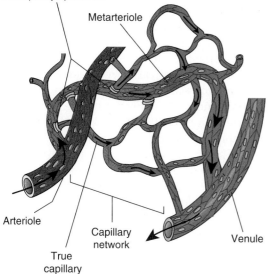

Arteriole

Capillary
network

True
capillary

Venule

FIG. 7-28 Microcirculation of the systemic circuit.

ing action, causes disturbances in cellular metabolism.

The microcirculation supports the exchange of water, respiratory gases, nutrients, hormones, and waste material between blood and tissue. The microcirculation disperses blood over a huge surface area that is estimated to be about 600 m² or about the area of four tennis courts. The extensive nature of the microcirculation enhances the exchange of material by permitting blood flow to slow down and come into close proximity to the cells.

Capillary Blood Pressure and Flow

Precise measurements of systemic capillary blood pressure have been made with different techniques. The systemic capillaries (at the level of the heart) have a pressure of about 35 mm Hg at the arterial end and about 10 mm Hg at the venous end. The mean pressure across the length of the systemic capillary ranges from about 15 to 25 mm Hg. This is

about two to three times that found in the pulmonary capillaries. Systemic capillary blood pressure varies widely from tissue to tissue. Capillaries that provide blood to the tissues in the upper portion of the body of a standing subject have the lowest pressures whereas the pressures in the capillaries of the lower extremities are much higher.

Blood flow through the capillaries is not continuous. It is intermittent, with the flow slowing to a stop every few seconds. The average velocity of blood through a capillary is about 1 mm/s. However, flow can range from 0 to 2 mm/s in some tissues and under various conditions.

The most important factors that influence the flow of blood through the capillaries are arterial blood pressure and microcirculatory vasomotor tone. Sufficient pressure is necessary to propel blood through a capillary and keep it open. If pressure is too low to move blood and distend the vessel, the capillary collapses. Capillary VR is adjusted in most capillaries by a thin band of smooth muscle that encircles the capillary at the point where they branch off from the arteriole or metarteriole. These "donuts" of smooth muscle are called **precapillary sphincters** (see Fig. 7-28). They control the flow of blood by constricting or relaxing. The degree of constriction generated by these muscles is referred to as *vascular tone*. The intermittent flow of blood within a capillary is brought about by a rhythmic dilation and constriction of the arteriole and precapillary sphincters known as vasomotion. Some capillaries also have smooth muscle sphincters at the outlet end of the capillary called postcapillary sphincters. Constriction of the postcapillary sphincters causes blood to collect in the capillary, increases capillary blood pressure, and enhances the leakage of material out of the capillary. The most important factor that influences capillary vascular tone and capillary blood flow is the local metabolic rate. Greater metabolism utilizes more O_2 and produces a variety of metabolic waste products that cause microcirculatory dilation and improved blood flow. Local control of blood flow is further described in Chapter 8.

Transport of Material across the Capillary Wall

The primary function of the capillary is the exchange of material between blood and the surrounding cells. The transport mechanisms utilized by the capillaries include pinocytosis, filtration, and diffusion (Fig. 7-29).

Capillary Pinocytosis

The endothelial cell moves material through the capillary wall by the formation of tiny

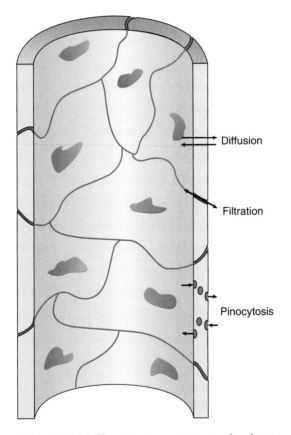

FIG. 7-29 Different transport mechanisms responsible for the movement of material through the capillary wall.

vesicles, a process called *pinocytosis.* Vesicles are produced by the pinching off of a portion of the cell membrane and the capture of a droplet of cytoplasm on the inside or a droplet of interstitial fluid from the outside of the capillary. Pinocytic vesicles move from one side of the capillary wall to the other side by Brownian movement. On contact with the cell membrane of the opposite side, the vesicle merges with the cell membrane and empties its contents. The small amount of material moved by this process appears to be responsible for the movement of large lipid-insoluble particles such as proteins.

Capillary Filtration

Substances can be forced through the capillary wall by a filtration mechanism. Substances move through openings between endothelial cells such as small gap junctions and large gaps or **intercellular clefts.** Continuous capillaries (Fig. 7-30), found in the nervous system, muscle, and lung, possess numerous small gap junctions and an outer basement membrane, which act together as a fine filter for material down to a diameter of about 4 nm. Discontinuous capillaries, or sinusoid capillaries (see Fig. 7-30), found in the liver, spleen, and bone marrow, have large intercellular openings between endothelial cells. These large gaps, which are not covered with a basement membrane, allow large particles, including cells, and large amounts of material to cross through the capillary wall. Substances can also move through openings in the endothelial cell called fenestrations. Fenestrated capillaries (see Fig. 7-30), found in the glomeruli of the kidney, small intestine wall, choroid plexus of the ventricles of the brain, and endocrine glands, have regions of numerous pores or fenestrations in the endothelial cell. The fenestrations can be as large as 100 nm in diameter. The openings in a fenestrated capillary enable it to be leaky.

The direction and amount of material filtered through the capillary wall is governed by the chemical nature of the material, the size of the particle, and the balance of forces on either side of the capillary wall. Water and inorganic ions such as Na^+, Cl^-, and K^+ can move relatively easily through the gap junctions of the continuous capillaries. Glucose moves through these junctions more slowly whereas proteins such as albumin are normally unable to pass through.

The primary forces that drive filtration and absorption of fluid through the capillary wall include the **hydrostatic fluid pressures** and protein-driven **colloid osmotic pressure (oncotic pressures)** found on either side of the capillary wall (Fig. 7-31). The most important factor behind the movement of fluid out of the capillary is the **transmural hydrostatic pressure** (difference between intracapillary

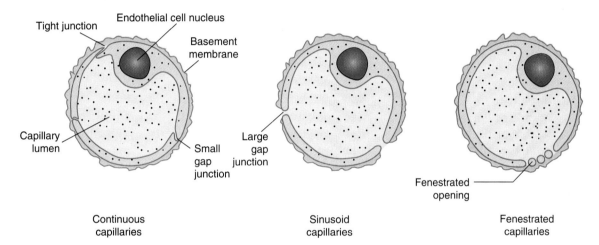

FIG. 7-30   Cross sections through different types of capillaries.

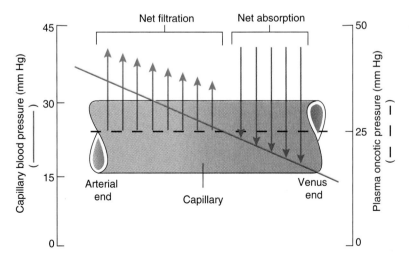

FIG. 7-31   Capillary blood and oncotic pressures along an ideal capillary result in regions of fluid filtration and absorption.

blood pressure and interstitial fluid pressure) across the capillary wall. The blood pressure within the systemic capillaries varies from region to region. The average pressure is about 35 mm Hg at the arterial end and 15 mm Hg at the venous end. These pressures can be increased by an increase in either arterial or venous pressures and decreased by a drop in either pressure. Pressures can also be increased by postcapillary sphincter (downstream) constriction or decreased by precapillary sphincter (upstream) constriction. When a subject is standing, capillary pressures are much greater in the legs and lower in the head as a result of the effects of gravity.

The capillary blood pressure generally forces fluid out through openings in the capillary wall. The interstitial fluid pressures on the outside of the capillary oppose filtration. However, the pressure in this region is known to be relatively negative with values in the −1- to −7-mm Hg range. This negative pressure is brought about by the constant drainage of fluid from this space into both the venous end of the capillary and the lymphatic capillaries.

The other major force effecting filtration and absorption is the water attracting osmotic forces generated by the proteins on either side of the capillary wall. Because of protein size, they are more important than the force generated by ions and other small solutes. Proteins, especially albumin, are normally too large to pass through the gap junctions in most capillary walls; this results in a much higher concentration of protein on the blood side of the capillary wall. Ions and smaller solutes can move through the capillary wall more easily which results in a more equal concentration of these solutes on either side of the capillary wall. The osmotic force generated by protein is referred to as a *colloid osmotic pressure* or *colloid oncotic pressure*. Plasma proteins actually exert more osmotic force than the simple number of molecules in solution can account for. The ability of proteins to cause more osmotic force is the result of their negative charges, which

attracts Na^+ and, in turn, attracts more water. This phenomenon is known as the Gibbs-Donnan effect. About 65% of plasma oncotic pressure is generated by albumin whereas the remaining amount is produced by the gamma globulins and fibrinogen. The plasma oncotic pressure is normally about 26 mm Hg. Normally, the small amount of protein found in the interstitial fluid exerts an oncotic pressure of about 1 mm Hg.

At the end of the late nineteenth century, Starling described the interaction between these various forces now known as Starling's law of the capillary. The following equation summarizes the modern version of Starling's law of the capillary:

$$F = k \times [(P_c - P_i) - (\pi_p - \pi_i)]$$

where F is the amount of fluid filtered, k is a filtration constant for a given type of capillary and fluid, P_c is the blood pressure in the capillary, P_i is the fluid pressure in the interstitial space, π_p is the plasma oncotic pressure, and π_i is the interstitial oncotic pressure. In essence, the equation describes the following relationship:

Filtration rate ≈
   Net transmural hydrostatic forces −
      Net oncotic forces

This means that the rate of fluid filtration across a capillary wall is a function of the balance between hydrostatic and oncotic pressure differences. If the blood pressure within the capillary is great enough to overcome the oncotic pressure exerted by the plasma proteins, fluid leaks out of the capillary. On the other hand, if the plasma oncotic pressure is greater than the blood pressure, fluid is absorbed. Fig. 7-32 shows the filtration forces across the arterial and venous ends of a model capillary. There is a net filtration of fluid out of the arterial end of the capillary and a net absorption of fluid at the venous end of the capillary. The balance of these two activities, which is not perfect, results in about 90% to

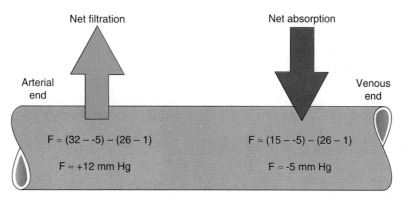

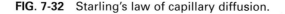

$$F \approx (P_c - P_i) - (\pi_p - \pi_i)$$

FIG. 7-32 Starling's law of capillary diffusion.

95% of the fluid being absorbed. This leaves about 5% to 10% of the fluid filtered into the interstitial space. In the average adult, the normal rate of net filtration overall is about 2 ml/min.

Most capillaries do not behave like this model. Some capillaries filter material along their entire length and others generally absorb material. Studies suggest that about 20 L of fluid are filtered out of capillaries daily and about 18 L of fluid is reabsorbed by capillaries. The 2-L difference is absorbed by the lymphatic system and returned to the circulatory system by way of the major lymph ducts that empty their fluid into the subclavian veins. Box 7-3 summarizes the factors that affect capillary filtration rate.

Diffusion across the Capillary Wall

Diffusion, the most important mechanism of capillary exchange, is responsible for the movement of respiratory gases, various small solutes (e.g., electrolytes, carbohydrates, fatty acids, and small proteins), and water. Small ions and molecules like water move about 5000 times better by diffusion than by filtration. The rate of diffusion through the capillary wall varies from substance to substance and from capillary to capillary. Lipid-soluble

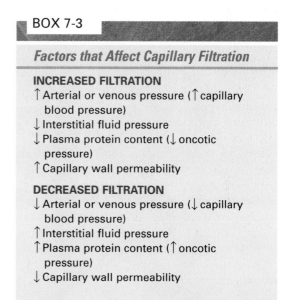

BOX 7-3

Factors that Affect Capillary Filtration

INCREASED FILTRATION
↑ Arterial or venous pressure (↑ capillary blood pressure)
↓ Interstitial fluid pressure
↓ Plasma protein content (↓ oncotic pressure)
↑ Capillary wall permeability

DECREASED FILTRATION
↓ Arterial or venous pressure (↓ capillary blood pressure)
↑ Interstitial fluid pressure
↑ Plasma protein content (↑ oncotic pressure)
↓ Capillary wall permeability

substances such as CO_2 move easily whereas water-soluble substances such as glucose diffuse more slowly. The diffusion of small substances through a capillary is described by a modification of Fick's law of diffusion:

$$J = P \times S \, (C_i - C_o)$$

where J is the amount of substance moved by diffusion per unit time, P is the permeability of a capillary wall for a substance, S is the surface area of the capillary wall, C_i is the concentration of the substance on the inside of the capillary, and C_o is the concentration of the substance on the outside of the capillary. Fick's law demonstrates that increases in capillary wall permeability, capillary bed size, and the concentration of the substance within the plasma increase the diffusion of the substance through the capillary wall and into the tissues.

Small molecules or ions and lipid-soluble molecules are very permeable when compared with large molecules. Small molecules such as water, respiratory gases, glucose, and inorganic ions move so easily through the capillary wall that their delivery to the tissues is said to be **perfusion limited.** Molecules with molecular weights of greater than 60,000 such as albumin and the globulin proteins, which are unable to diffuse across the capillary wall, are described as being **diffusion limited.**

FUNCTIONS OF THE LYMPHATIC SYSTEM

Water enters the interstitial space from both the capillaries and the tissues. Despite this

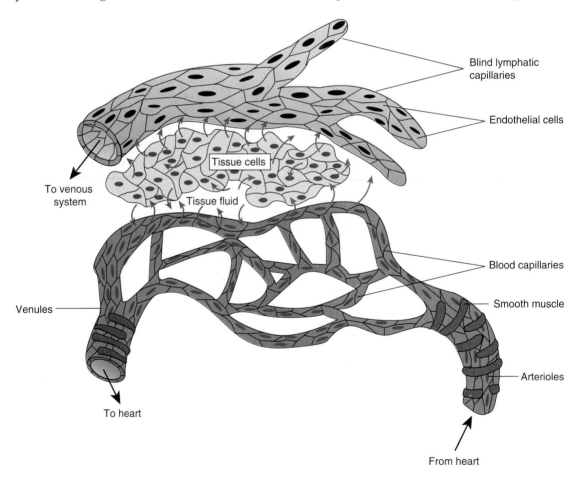

FIG. 7-33 Lymphatic capillaries lay in close proximity to the microcirculation and absorb excess fluid from the interstitial space.

continuous addition of more than 2 L of water per day, the interstitial space stays relatively dry, with a hydrostatic pressure that ranges from −1 to −7 mm Hg. The ability to move a relatively huge amount of water into the interstitial space and keep it relatively dry is one of the important functions of the lymphatic system.

The lymphatic system begins as a network of closed-ended capillaries held in position within the interstitial space by fine protein filaments (Fig. 7-33). Lymphatic capillaries have permeable walls that allow the absorption of water and particles as large as proteins. The balance between fluid and oncotic pressures drives fluid across the capillary wall and into the lymphatic system. Fig. 7-34 shows the various pressures in the various compartments and the gradient that drives fluid into the lymphatic system.

Fluid drains into larger lymph vessels that are equipped with one-way valves that direct lymph fluid flow through the vessels as fluid is collected and further propelled by the compression action of the nearby skeletal muscles of the extremities. Over 80% of lymph fluid flows through the thoracic duct. The remaining 20% or less is drained into the right lymph duct (Fig. 7-35). The thoracic duct drains into the left subclavian vein, and the right lymph duct drains into the right subclavian vein. Both of these veins ultimately drain lymph fluid back to the right side of the heart by way of the superior vena cava. The lymph fluid flow from these two ducts totals about 100 ml/hr in a normal adult.

In addition to draining water, the lymphatic system also drains proteins and fat from the interstitial space. The capillary walls in most tissues are impermeable to the movement of

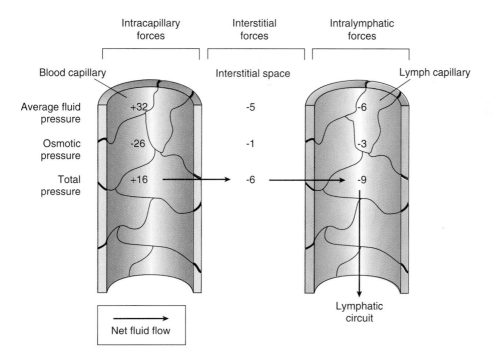

FIG. 7-34 Distribution of forces that affect fluid movement between the blood capillary, interstitial space, and lymphatic capillary that results in the production of lymphatic fluid.

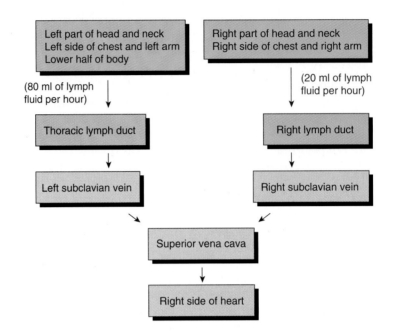

FIG. 7-35 Schematic pathway of lymphatic drainage from various regions of the body back to the right side of the heart.

protein, but some protein does leak into the interstitial space from cells and some highly permeable capillaries. The lymphatic system helps clear proteins from the interstitial space. If they were not cleared, they would act osmotically and attract more water into the interstitial space. Lymphatic capillaries in the wall of the intestine also play an important role in the absorption of lipids.

Lymphatic vessels pass their fluid through numerous lymph nodes, which house lymphocytes. This action is an important part of the host defense system. Fluid drained from the interstitial space may be contaminated with bacteria, viruses, or fungi. By presenting these foreign cells to the lymph nodes, phagocytic cells can remove the foreign cells and immune cells can start the production of antibodies. Unfortunately, the lymph vessels can also be used by microbe infections and cancer cells to spread to other regions of

the body when the immune system fails to stop them.

Edema Formation

Edema is the accumulation of excess fluid in the interstitial space. Edematous tissue appears to have a swollen or fluid expanded appearance as a result of fluid collection and the development of positive interstitial pressures. Edema occurs more commonly in dependent areas of the body as a result of the effects of gravity. The ankles, hands, and around the eyes are the most common sites of edema formation. The general mechanisms that produce edema are summarized in Fig. 7-36.

Increased capillary blood pressure can be caused by increased arterial or venous blood pressure. The more common cause of edema formation is venous hypertension. With normal venous pressures, the capillary is able to

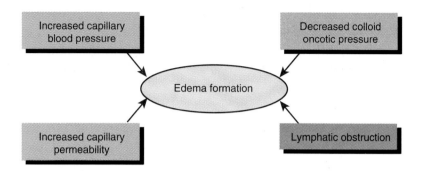

FIG. 7-36 Mechanisms responsible for edema formation.

absorb 90% to 95% of the water filtered. Increased blood pressure at the venous end of the capillary retards fluid absorption. Venous hypertension can be caused by venous obstruction, heart failure, and excessive blood volume.

Plasma protein concentration is normally about 10 g/dl. **Hypoproteinemia** (reduced plasma protein concentration) can be caused by inadequate protein in the diet, liver dysfunction, renal diseases, and hypermetabolic states such as the response to trauma. Reduced plasma protein concentration causes the colloid oncotic pressure to drop and reduces the ability to absorb fluid into the vascular space.

Increased capillary permeability results from enlargement of gap junctions between endothelial cells and injury to endothelial cells. This can occur as a result of vascular exposure to certain chemicals such as histamine, and proteolytic enzymes (released by leukocytes and injured tissues), and various cytokines, which are released during the inflammatory response to injury. Exposure to animal venoms, bacterial toxins, and certain viruses also causes hyperpermeability of the capillary. Enlargement of the gap junctions or the formation of openings in the endothelial cells allows the capillary to leak excessive amounts of fluid into the interstitial space and causes edema.

Drainage of fluid from the interstitial space can be impeded by failure of the lymphatic system to remove fluid. This can occur as a result of **lymphatic blockage** by tumor cells that are plugging a lymph vessel or tumor compression of a major lymphatic vessel. Venous hypertension, which also results in a form of lymphatic blockage, requires higher lymphatic pressures to drain at normal rates into the subclavian veins. Higher lymphatic pressure reduces the ability to drain the interstitial space and causes fluids to collect.

Pulmonary edema can result in the collection of fluid in the interstitial space and in the alveolar air space in severe cases. The causes are commonly classified as either **cardiogenic** or noncardiogenic pulmonary edema. Cardiogenic pulmonary edema, commonly caused by left ventricular failure or mitral valve stenosis, leads to excessive pulmonary capillary pressures. As the pressures exceed the colloid oncotic pressure, fluid is moved into the interstitial spaces of the lung at increasing rates. Pulmonary capillary pressures that exceed 25 mm Hg often result in fluid moving into both the interstitial and alveolar air spaces. This condition is further exacerbated by the development of systemic venous hypertension, which retards the ability of the pulmonary lymphatic system to drain the lung. Noncardiogenic pulmonary edema is caused by injury to the pulmonary capillaries, which results in their becoming hyperpermeable. Noncardiogenic pulmonary edema is often caused by aspiration of toxic liquids or gases, traumatic injury, and infection.

CHAPTER SELF-TEST QUESTIONS

Match the correct percentage of cardiac output that flows to each of the following portions of the systemic circuit (answers may be used more than once):

1. renal
2. cerebral
3. coronary
4. resting skeletal muscle

   a. 1% to 2%
   b. 5% to 7%
   c. 12% to 15%
   d. 20% to 25%

5. Which of the following factors influence coronary flow?
   1. mean arterial pressure
   2. mechanical compression of arteries
   3. myocardial metabolism
   4. autonomic nervous stimulation
     a. 2 and 4
     b. 1, 2, and 4
     c. 2, 3, and 4
     d. 1, 2, 3, and 4

6. The circle of Willis is supplied with systemic arterial blood from the
   1. internal carotid arteries
   2. subclavian arteries
   3. vertebral arteries
     a. 1 only
     b. 1 and 2
     c. 1 and 3
     d. 2 and 3
     e. 1, 2, and 3

7. Renal blood flow is about 300 ml/100 g of renal tissue. This very high blood flow is necessary to support
   a. the metabolic rate of the kidney
   b. tubular reabsorption
   c. venous return to the right side of the heart
   d. glomerular filtration rate

8. The splanchnic circulation is a network of vessels that provides blood flow to the
   1. stomach
   2. intestine
   3. pancreas
   4. liver
     a. 2 and 3
     b. 1, 3, and 4

     c. 1, 2, and 3
     d. 2, 3, and 4
     e. 1, 2, 3, and 4

9. The bronchial circulation arises from the aorta and supplies blood flow to the
   a. gas exchange region of the lung
   b. large airways and connective tissues of the lung
   c. pleural surface of the lung
   d. outer membranes of the lung and the thorax

10. Which of the following are true with regard to the normal resting hemodynamics of the pulmonary circulation?
   1. contains about 16% of total blood volume
   2. receives 5 to 6 L of blood per minute
   3. pulmonary artery pressure is about 25/10 mm Hg
     a. 3 only
     b. 1 and 3
     c. 2 and 3
     d. 1 and 2
     e. 1, 2, and 3

11. Which one of the following would *not* result in the formation of edema?
   a. decreased vessel permeability
   b. increased capillary blood pressure
   c. lymphatic blockage
   d. hypoproteinemia

For answers, see p. 475.

BIBLIOGRAPHY

1. Berne RM, Levy MN: *Principles of physiology*, St Louis, 1990, Mosby.
2. Berne RM, Levy MN: *Cardiovascular physiology*, St Louis, 1992, Mosby.
3. Brandenburg RO et al: *Cardiology: fundamentals and practice*, Chicago, 1987, Year Book Medical.
4. Cohn PF: *Clinical cardiovascular physiology*, Philadelphia, 1985, WB Saunders.
5. Ganong WF: *Review of medical physiology*, ed 18, Stamford, Conn, 1997, Appleton & Lange.
6. Gray H: *Anatomy of the human body*, ed 30, Philadelphia, 1985, Lea & Febiger.

7. Green JF: *Fundamental cardiovascular and pulmonary physiology,* ed 2, Philadelphia, 1987, Lea & Febiger.

8. Grover RF et al: Pulmonary circulation. In American Physiological Society: *Handbook of physiology,* vol 3, Bethesda, Md, 1984, American Physiological Society.

9. Guyton AC: *Textbook of medical physiology,* ed 8, Philadelphia, 1991, WB Saunders.

10. Langman J, Woerdeman MW: *Atlas of medical anatomy,* Philadelphia, 1978, WB Saunders.

11. Martini FH: *Fundamentals of anatomy and physiology,* Upper Saddle River, NJ, 1998, Prentice Hall.

12. Mathewson HS: Selective drug therapy for pulmonary hypertension, *Respir Care* 40:871, 1995.

13. Rushmer RF: *Cardiovascular dynamics,* Philadelphia, 1978, WB Saunders.

14. Slonim NB, Hamilton LH: *Respiratory physiology,* ed 5, St Louis, 1987, Mosby.

15. Smith JJ, Kampine JP: *Circulatory physiology: the essentials,* ed 3, Baltimore, 1990, Williams & Wilkins.

16. Spence AP, Mason EG: *Human anatomy and physiology,* ed 4, St Paul, 1992, West.

17. Staub NC: *Basic respiratory physiology,* New York, 1991, Churchill-Livingstone.

18. Tortora GJ, Grabowski SR: *Principles of anatomy and physiology,* ed 7, New York, 1993, Harper Collins College.

19. West JB: *Respiratory physiology: the essentials,* ed 4, Baltimore, 1990, Williams & Wilkins.

8

Cardiovascular Control

The average flow of blood through the tissues of a 75-kg subject with a normal cardiac output is about 8 ml/min/100 g of tissue. In reality, however, blood flow ranges from 0 to more than 300 ml/min/100 g of tissue. These differences are necessary to support the different functions and metabolic rates of specific tissues.

Fig. 8-1 shows the blood flow distribution in various regions in a subject at rest and after reaching stable conditions during moderate exercise. Total cardiac output increases 2½ times, the distribution of blood flow shifts from some organs to others, and the blood pressure changes very little. How is the cardiovascular system adjusted to deliver these different blood flows? This chapter answers this question by exploring the various mechanisms that maintain and adjust blood flow, pressure, and volume.

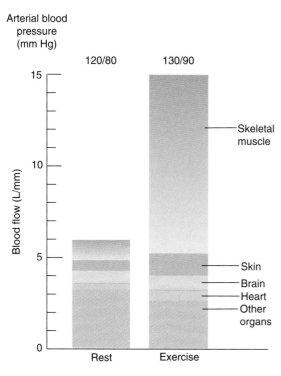

Arterial blood pressure (mm Hg)

FIG. 8-1 Total and regional blood flow in a subject at rest and during moderate exercise.

vascular resistance results in decreased blood flow.

The cardiovascular system utilizes this relationship to provide different flow rates of blood to different tissues. By maintaining a relatively high aortic blood pressure and adjusting the vascular resistance within each organ, blood flow can be delivered to different regions at different rates (Fig. 8-2). The high aortic pressure is maintained by the combined effects of ventricular pumping, vessel recoil, and vascular resistance. Different flow rates in each region are brought about by adjusting the local vascular resistance.

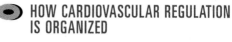

HOW CARDIOVASCULAR REGULATION IS ORGANIZED

The basic elements of cardiovascular regulation include the interplay between a control center, or **controller,** a set of **effectors** that influence blood flow and pressure, and an array of **sensors** that monitor blood flow and blood pressure. These elements are organized into a **feedback loop** (Fig. 8-3).

The controller, located in the central nervous system (CNS), sends signals to stimulate or inhibit various parts of the cardiovascular system. The effectors include the heart, smooth muscles of the vessels, kidney, and bone marrow. The products of effector activity are blood pressure, volume, and flow. An array of sensors is located in a number of major vessels and local tissues. Blood pressure and volume are monitored by stretch- or tension-sensitive cells called baroreceptors, which are located in various vessels and cardiac chambers. In addition, chemical-sensitive cells called *chemoreceptors* respond to a variety of metabolic products. These sensors generate and send information to both the controller and effectors. The anatomic components of the feedback loop are summarized in Fig. 8-4. The interaction between the elements of the control loop result in a stable and adequate flow of blood.

RELATIONSHIP BETWEEN BLOOD FLOW, BLOOD PRESSURE, AND VASCULAR RESISTANCE

Blood flow through a tissue region is generally the product of the perfusion pressure and the vascular resistance:

$$\dot{Q} = \frac{\Delta P}{R_{vas}}$$

where $\dot{Q}$ is the quantity of blood flow, ΔP is the perfusion pressure (arterial pressure − venous pressure), and R_{vas} is the vascular resistance. This equation, basically Ohm's law of electricity applied to fluid dynamics, tells us that blood flow is directly related to perfusion pressure. Increasing perfusion pressure causes an increase in blood flow whereas increased

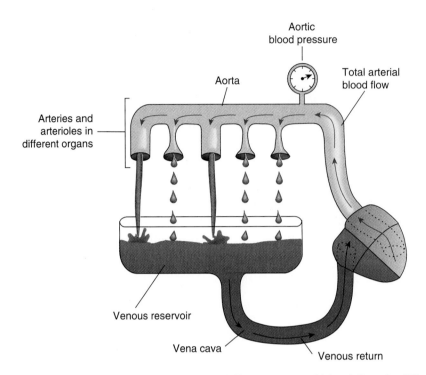

FIG. 8-2 Cardiovascular system produces different rates of blood flow in different regions by maintaining a high aortic pressure and variable vascular resistance in different regions.

Set Point Control

The activity of the sensors and controller directs the cardiovascular effectors to maintain a target, or **set point,** blood pressure. A variety of intrinsic and extrinsic regulatory mechanisms provide both short-term and long-term maintenance of a normal set point. The set point maintained by the effectors is a mean arterial blood pressure of 90 mm Hg (Fig. 8-5).

⬤ THE CARDIOVASCULAR CONTROLLER AND WHERE IT IS LOCATED

Cardiovascular Center

Various areas in the CNS are involved in cardiovascular control. Most of the control is exerted through the **cardiovascular center,** which is comprised of interconnected groups or "pools" of neurons located within the dorsal reticular region of the **medulla oblongata.** The neural pools of the cardiovascular region can be characterized according to their actions on the heart and blood vessels.

Cardiac Center

The pool of neurons in the medulla that cause a change in heart rate and strength of contraction is classified as the **cardiac center.** The region of the medulla oblongata that causes an increase in heart rate and contractility is called the cardiostimulatory center whereas the region that produces the opposite effect is called the cardioinhibitory center.

Signals from the cardiostimulatory center travel to the heart by way of sympathetic nerve fibers, causing increased heart rate (positive

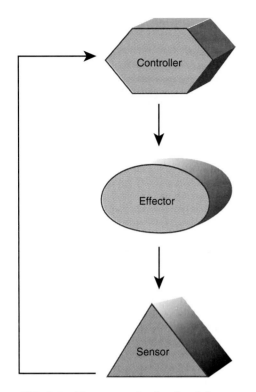

FIG. 8-3 Elements of a feedback loop.

chronotropism) and ventricular contractility (positive inotropism). The cardioinhibitory center sends signals to the heart through parasympathetic nerve fibers within the **vagus nerves** (the tenth cranial nerve). These parasympathetic signals cause a decrease in heart rate (negative chronotropism) and ventricular contractility (negative inotropism).

Vasomotor Center

The neuron pool in the cardiovascular center that causes changes in blood vessel tone is called the **vasomotor center.** Within the vasomotor center there is a vasoconstrictor area and a vasodilator area. Signals from the vasoconstrictor area are carried by sympathetic fibers to the blood vessels. Sympathetic signals cause smooth muscle contraction, which results in vasoconstriction. The vasodilator area sends signals to blood vessels by way of the parasympathetic fibers in the vagus nerve.

Parasympathetic signals cause smooth muscle relaxation leading to vasodilation.

Considerable interaction occurs between the various areas of the cardiovascular center. When one area is active the other area becomes less active. For example, when a stimulus triggers activity in the cardiostimulatory and vasoconstrictor areas, the output from these two areas not only stimulates the muscles of the heart and vessels but also inhibits the activity of the cardioinhibitory and vasodilator areas. This local inhibitory action helps ensure a rapid and powerful response.

Other Areas in the CNS that Influence Cardiovascular Function

A growing body of evidence now suggests that control of the cardiovascular system is not limited to an isolated cardiovascular center in the medulla oblongata. Although this region is the predominant area of control, interaction between different areas of the CNS provides a form of integrated control. Those areas outside the medulla that influence cardiovascular function include the cerebral cortex, thalamus, hypothalamus, cerebellum, and spinal cord.

Stimulation of the motor regions of the cerebral cortex and cerebellum cause elevation of blood pressure through selective vasoconstriction of splanchnic, renal, and cutaneous vessels. Simultaneously, the skeletal muscle vessels dilate, which enhances blood flow through this region. This response appears to be active during exercise and in response to pain and anxiety. The thalamus also appears active in causing elevation of heart rate and blood pressure during various emotional conditions such as anxiety, anger, and rage.

The hypothalamus plays a key role in thermoregulation as a controller of heat loss. Heat loss is primarily adjusted by regulating blood flow to the skin where heat can be radiated. Regions within the hypothalamus respond to core temperature as well as skin temperature, causing adjustment of vasomotor tone.

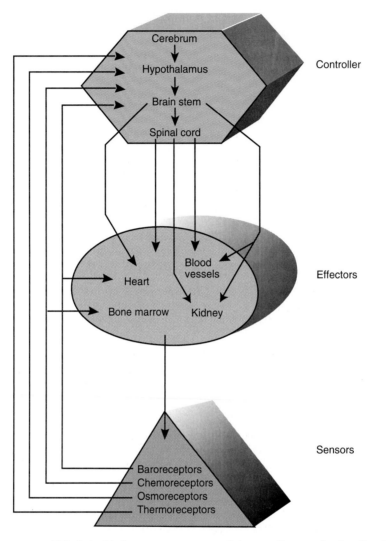

FIG. 8-4   Various components of the cardiovascular feedback loop.

The spinal cord is an important conduit for sympathetic signals traveling out from the medulla oblongata. Spinal cord injuries can produce hypotension through the loss of sympathetic stimulation of the heart and vessels. This condition is known as **spinal shock.** The spinal cord also participates in localized sympathetic vasomotor reflexes. Pain sensation from and cooling a particular region of skin causes reflex vasoconstriction in that area.

Conversely, warming a particular region of skin results in sympathetic suppression to that area and vasodilation.

In response to different stimuli, various areas of the CNS interact with each other and activate specific regions of the medulla oblongata to evoke a particular cardiovascular response. This more interactive concept of cardiovascular control is thought to be responsible for the range of reactions that the car-

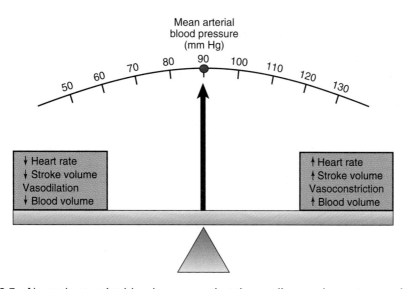

FIG. 8-5   Normal set point blood pressure that the cardiovascular system maintains is the result of balancing various activities.

diovascular system displays in response to various emotional and physical stimuli.

 HOW THE AUTONOMIC NERVOUS SYSTEM CAUSES CARDIOVASCULAR CHANGES

Autonomic Nervous System Signaling

The CNS distributes control signals to the heart and vessels through the peripheral nerves of the autonomic nervous system. The signals consist of a rapid series of action potentials, which, in turn, trigger the release of neurotransmitters. Action potentials generated in the sympathetic and parasympathetic fibers are virtually identical. The ability of these two systems to cause different cardiovascular effects lies in the different type of neurotransmitter released into the target tissue (Fig. 8-6).

Neural fibers of the sympathetic and parasympathetic systems are generally organized in the same way. A preganglionic fiber leaves the CNS and activates a postganglionic

fiber through the release of the neurotransmitter **acetylcholine.** Postganglionic fibers carry action potentials to the target tissue and release a neurotransmitter to either stimulate or inhibit the tissue.

Sympathetic preganglionic fibers leave the spinal cord along the thoracic and upper lumbar regions. These relatively short fibers stimulate longer postganglionic fibers in the paravertebral ganglions that lie on either side of the spinal cord. Postganglionic fibers of the sympathetic nervous system primarily release the neurotransmitter **norepinephrine,** which stimulates adrenergic receptors of the heart and vessels. Adrenergic receptors are classified according to the type of tissue and the type of response they evoke (Table 8-1). Alpha-adrenergic receptors are located on the smooth muscle of blood vessels. When these receptors are stimulated by norepinephrine, vasoconstriction results. Beta$_1$-adrenergic receptors are located on the sinoatrial (SA) node and ventricular myocytes. Stimulation of beta$_1$ receptors by norepinephrine causes an increase in heart rate and contractility. Beta$_2$-adrenergic

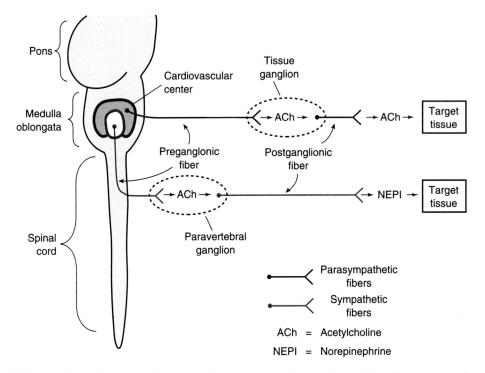

FIG. 8-6 Organization and types of neurotransmitters released by the autonomic nervous system.

Table 8-1   Types of Autonomic Receptors

Receptors type	Location	Action
SYMPATHETIC ADRENERGIC RECEPTORS		
Alpha	Vessels	Vasoconstriction
Beta$_1$	Myocardium	Increase rate and contractility
Beta$_2$	Vessels	Vasodilation
PARASYMPATHETIC CHOLINERGIC RECEPTORS		
Cholinergic	Vessels	Vasodilation
Cholinergic	Myocardium	Decrease rate and contractility

receptors are located on the smooth muscle of blood vessels and in other tissues such as the airways in the lungs, intestines, and uterus. Stimulation of beta$_2$ receptors by norepinephrine results in relaxation of vascular smooth muscle and subsequent vasodilation.

Parasympathetic preganglionic fibers exit the brain stem as part of the vagus nerve (see Fig. 8-6). Like the sympathetic fibers, the parasympathetic fibers have a ganglion where preganglionic fibers stimulate postganglionic fibers with acetylcholine. Unlike the sympa-

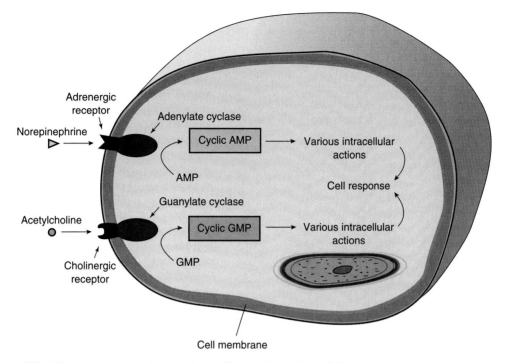

FIG. 8-7 Neurotransmitters released by the branches of the autonomic nervous system cause different cardiovascular cellular responses by the formation of different intracellular second messengers (cyclic AMP and cyclic GMP). *AMP,* Adenosine monophosphate; *GMP,* guanyl monophosphate.

thetic fibers, the parasympathetic preganglionic fibers are relatively long with the ganglions located in the target tissue. In addition, the relatively short postganglionic fibers release acetylcholine onto the target tissue. Acetylcholine stimulates cholinergic receptors in the heart and vessels. Cholinergic stimulation of the SA node and ventricular myocytes causes bradycardia and reduced ventricular contractility. Blood vessel response to cholinergic stimulation results in vasodilation.

Intracellular Second Messengers

Adrenergic and cholinergic receptors are located on the surface of the cell membrane of the target tissue. When activated by the appropriate neurotransmitter, these receptors cause

the production of a second messenger inside the cell (Fig. 8-7). Stimulation of adrenergic receptors causes the activation of the enzyme **adenylate cyclase.** Adenylate cyclase converts adenosine monophosphate (AMP) to the second messenger cyclic adenosine monophosphate (cyclic AMP). Parasympathetic stimulation of cholinergic receptors causes the production of a different second messenger. Cholinergic stimulation activates the enzyme guanylate cyclase, which converts guanyl monophosphate (GMP) to the second messenger cyclic guanyl monophosphate (cyclic GMP). Second messengers act within the cell to stimulate or suppress certain activities. For example, cyclic AMP's action in myocytes of the myocardium causes an increase of intracellular Ca^{++} whereas cyclic GMP's action causes the opposite effect. This results in either an increase or decrease in heart rate and contractility respectively.

⬤ WHERE CARDIOVASCULAR SENSORS ARE LOCATED AND TO WHAT THEY RESPOND

A variety of sensors are active in monitoring blood pressure, blood volume, chemicals, and the amount of solute dissolved in blood (Fig. 8-8). In addition, sensors for pain, temperature, and osmolarity also evoke cardiovascular responses.

Baroreceptors
Arterial Baroreceptors

High pressure-sensitive cells called *baroreceptors,* or pressoreceptors, are located in the walls of the carotid arteries and the aortic arch. When these cells are stretched by the force of blood pressure distending the walls of the vessel, they produce generator potentials, which are directed to the cardiovascular center. The baroreceptors of the carotid artery are localized in the carotid sinus where the internal and external carotid arteries branch from the common carotid artery (Fig. 8-9). The baroreceptors of the carotid sinus send signals

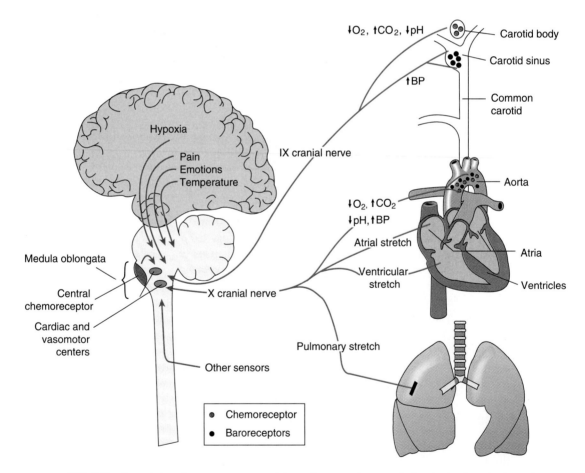

FIG. 8-8 A variety of sensors respond to numerous types of physical, chemical, and emotional stimuli and direct signals to the cardiovascular control center in the medulla oblongata. *O₂,* Oxygen; *CO₂,* carbon dioxide; *BP,* blood pressure.

via the **glossopharyngeal nerve** (ninth cranial nerve) to the cardiovascular center. Aortic baroreceptors, located on the anterior and posterior regions of the aortic arch (Fig. 8-10), produce signals that are sent to the cardiovascular center by way of the vagus nerves.

Increasing vessel pulsation brought on by greater blood pressure causes the number of signals per second generated and sent to the cardiovascular center to increase. With decreasing blood pressure, the number of signals sent decreases. The carotid sinus baroreceptors, which are more sensitive, cause greater cardiovascular center response than the aortic baroreceptors.

Cardiopulmonary Baroreceptors

Baroreceptors are also located in the walls of the vena cava, atria, ventricles, pulmonary vessels, and lung tissue. These stretch receptors, collectively referred to as cardiopulmonary

baroreceptors, send their signals to the cardiovascular center by way of the vagus nerve.

These receptors are more responsive to low-pressure changes caused by the effects of blood volume. When stimulated by chamber or vessel stretching brought on by increased blood volume, they generally cause inhibition of the cardiostimulatory center and vasoconstrictor area of the medulla. Stimulation of these receptors also suppresses the secretion of various hormones, which results in greater diureses (urine formation). These actions result in decreased blood volume and blood pressure.

Chemoreceptors

Chemoreceptors are located in a variety of areas and are stimulated by an assortment of chemicals. Upon stimulation they send signals to the CNS or they activate local vascular smooth muscle.

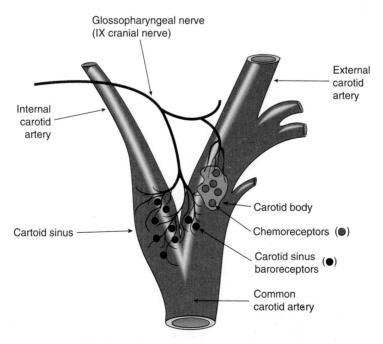

FIG. 8-9 Sensors of the carotid arteries.

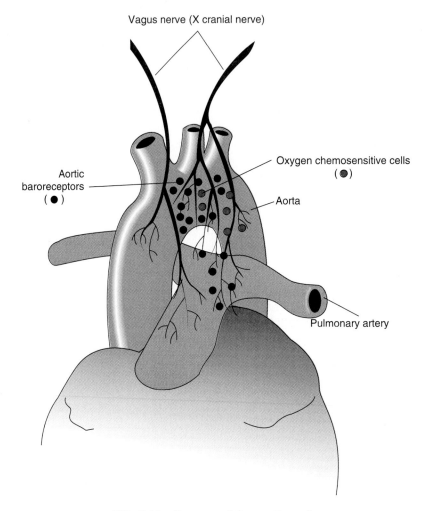

Vagus nerve (X cranial nerve)

Oxygen chemosensitive cells
(●)

Aortic
baroreceptors
(●)

Aorta

Pulmonary artery

FIG. 8-10 Sensors of the aortic arch.

Central Chemoreceptors

The anterior surface of the medulla oblongata has chemoreceptors sensitive to the H^+ concentration in the cerebral spinal fluid. Impulses from these sensors play an important role in the control of ventilation by the respiratory center, which is also located in the medulla oblongata. Impulses from these receptors also influence the cardiovascular center. Increased H^+ concentration (acidosis) generally results in activation of the vaso-

constrictor area of the cardiovascular center. Decreased H^+ concentration (alkalosis) causes reduced vasoconstrictor area activity and diminished sympathetic stimulation of the cardiovascular system.

Normal or elevated levels of oxygen have little or no effect on nervous system influence over cardiovascular function. The cerebrum and medulla oblongata do respond to hypoxia and cause vascular changes. Generally, reductions in O_2 content of the brain stimulate the vasomotor region of the cardiovascular center, causing sympathetic mediated vasoconstriction.

Arterial Chemoreceptors

Chemoreceptors, located in the carotid bodies and aortic arch, are called peripheral chemoreceptors. They are located near the sites of the arterial baroreceptors. These receptors respond to reductions in blood O_2 and less well to increases in blood CO_2 and H^+ concentration. Their primary role is to control ventilation, but some of their signals are sent to the cardiovascular center. When stimulated, the carotid and aortic bodies send signals to the cardiovascular center by way of the glossopharyngeal and vagus nerves, respectively. This causes stimulation of the vasopressor area and inhibition of the cardiostimulatory center. Hypoxia is the most powerful stimulant of the peripheral chemoreceptors. Acidosis and hypercapnia cause a more moderate response.

Cardiopulmonary Chemoreceptors

Chemical-sensitive nerve endings are also located in the chambers of the heart and pulmonary vessels with the greatest concentration found in the left ventricle. Those in the heart appear to respond to the local production of lactic acid, serotonin, prostaglandins, and bradykinin. These chemicals are produced by myocytes when stressed by hypoxic conditions that can be brought on by inadequate coronary blood flow. Stimulation of these receptors generally causes activation of sympathetic reflexes, which, in turn, causes increased heart rate, greater contractility, and vasoconstriction.

Local Chemoreceptors

The local vascular smooth muscle found in the walls of vessels of virtually all tissues is sensitive to a variety of chemicals, including O_2 (low levels), adenosine, H^+, K^+, histamine, bradykinin, prostaglandins, and other factors. The response to these chemicals plays a major role in the regulation of the microcirculation.

Other Receptors

Thermoreceptors, located in the skin, react to cooling and send signals to the spinal cord and hypothalamus, causing a reflex vasoconstriction of cutaneous and skeletal muscle vessels and reduction in heart rate. Cold-responsive thermoreceptors play an important role in the conservation of heat and trigger the **dive reflex.**

Within the hypothalamus are specialized cells that respond to the concentration of solutes dissolved in blood and interstitial fluid. The concentration of solutes in solution is referred to as the osmolarity of fluid. Decreased water intake or excessive water loss causes the osmolarity of blood and interstitial fluid to increase. Osmoreceptors in the hypothalamus respond to increasing osmolarity and trigger the release of antidiuretic hormone (ADH), which, in turn, causes vasoconstriction and water retention by the kidney.

TYPES OF SHORT-TERM REGULATORY MECHANISMS THAT INFLUENCE CARDIOVASCULAR ACTIVITY

The cardiovascular system utilizes a variety of short-term regulatory mechanisms to maintain a mean aortic pressure at the set point of 90 mm Hg. Input from various parts of the CNS and receptors is directed to the cardiovascular center. The cardiovascular center quickly reacts by sending signals to the heart and vessels by way of the autonomic nervous system.

Intrinsic Regulation

Regulatory reflexes that arise from the cardiovascular system are known as intrinsic regulation. These reflexes are the most important regulatory mechanisms for moment-to-moment control of cardiovascular function. The major intrinsic reflexes are summarized in Fig. 8-11.

Mechanical Circulatory Support Following Open Heart Surgery

A 71-year-old woman was experiencing unstable angina and was found to have complete blockage of several branches of her left coronary artery. She underwent emergent open-heart surgery for the placement of three coronary artery bypass grafts. After successful placement of the grafts, the heart-lung bypass pump, which was supporting her blood pressure during the open-heart procedure, was reduced to allow the patient's heart to assume the work of providing the cardiac output. When the pump's output was reduced to a minimum, it was discovered that the patient had a heart rate of 136, systemic blood pressure of 82/55, and a cardiac output of 2.9 L/min despite treatment with intravenous fluids and dobutamine. These findings are consistent with refractory failure of the left side of the heart and cardiogenic shock. To remove the patient from the heart-lung pump and to improve cardiac pump performance, the physician decided to employ temporary mechanical circulatory support with an intraaortic balloon pump (IABP).

The IABP technique involves the placement of a special intraaortic balloon catheter in the descending aorta just below the aortic arch. The catheter is equipped with a sausage-shaped balloon that extends down from the tip of the catheter. When the balloon in inflated, it is approximately 2 cm in diameter, 15 cm in length, and contains a volume of 40 ml. With the balloon deflated, the catheter is inserted percutaneously into the femoral artery and advanced up into the aorta. When in use, the balloon is rapidly inflated and deflated with helium or CO_2 gas. The inflation and deflation is synchronized to the cardiac cycle by sensing the R wave of the electrocardiogram. Balloon inflation during diastole improves coronary artery blood flow by increasing aortic arch blood pressure and helps propel blood out of the descending aorta toward the periphery. Deflation of the balloon produces a suction effect within the descending aorta, which reduces left ventricular afterload and enables the left ventricle to pump a larger stroke volume. Balloon pump inflation and deflation can be synchronized with every beat (1:1), with every second beat (1:2), or with every third beat (1:3).

The patient responded very well to the IABP technique and came off the heart-lung pump with an acceptable blood pressure and cardiac output. She was transferred to the intensive care unit where she remained sedated, supported by 1:1 synchronized IABP and mechanical ventilation. She was weaned from the IABP 4 hours later with a cardiac output of 4.7 L/min and a blood pressure of 110/75. The IABP catheter was removed without incident, mechanical ventilation was discontinued 12 hours later, and she recovered without incident.

Autoregulation of Cardiac Contractility

The heart self-regulates its contractility as the ventricle fills with different volumes of blood. This ability of the myocardium to increase contractility with increased ventricular filling is better known as **Frank-Starling's law of the heart.** This important compensatory mechanism allows the heart to autoregulate its strength of contraction as it distends with different volumes of blood.

Arterial Baroreceptor Reflex

The baroreceptor reflex is a negative feedback mechanism that is important in short-term regulation of arterial blood pressure (Fig. 8-12). As blood pressure drops below 80 mm Hg, the number of signals generated by the carotid and aortic baroreceptors decreases. This causes the cardiovascular center to increase sympathetic stimulation of the heart and vessels, resulting in increased blood pressure. With

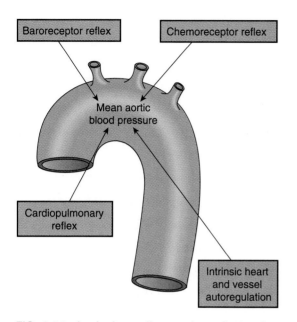

Baroreceptor reflex

Chemoreceptor reflex

Mean aortic blood pressure

Cardiopulmonary reflex

Intrinsic heart and vessel autoregulation

FIG. 8-11 Intrinsic cardiovascular reflexes that act to maintain arterial blood pressure at a set point.

increasing blood pressure, baroreceptor signaling to the cardiovascular center increases, causing suppression of sympathetic activity. Blood pressure drops until the cycle starts all over. The baroreceptor reflex acts quickly and oscillates to maintain mean blood pressure at the set point of about 90 mm Hg.

An example of the speed of the baroreceptor reflex is the response to body repositioning. Postural changes cause shifts of blood volume and threaten the maintenance of aortic blood pressure. When a subject moves from a reclining position to a standing position, about 10% to 15% of the blood volume moves into their lower limbs as a result of gravity. This results in brain and upper body hypotension if it were not for compensatory mechanisms. The baroreceptor reflex, an important compensatory response, causes vasoconstriction of the splanchnic circulation, which returns aortic blood pressure back to the set point in a matter of seconds. If a subject is unable to respond

and the carotid blood pressure falls, he or she experiences postural hypotension, which can lead to dizziness and syncope.

Manual pressure applied over the area of the carotid baroreceptors can elicit the baroreceptor reflex. Carotid massage with the fingertips is occasionally done to decrease the heart rate of a subject who is in an abnormal tachycardia. During vigorous application of the choke hold, where the neck of a subject is squeezed in a viselike arm grip, the baroreceptor reflex can be stimulated and may result in bradycardia, hypotension, cerebral hypoxia, unconsciousness, and even death.

Chemoreceptor Reflex

The chemoreceptors of the carotid and aortic bodies send increasing numbers of nerve signals to the cardiovascular center when the blood contains decreasing amounts of O_2 or increasing amounts of CO_2 and H^+. This is known as the chemoreceptor reflex. In response, the cardiovascular center sends increasing numbers of parasympathetic signals to the heart and increasing sympathetic signals to the peripheral vessels (Fig. 8-13), resulting in peripheral vasoconstriction and a moderate decrease in heart rate. The coronary and cerebral vessels are not constricted. The net effect is an increase in aortic blood pressure, decreased peripheral blood flow, and improved cerebral and coronary perfusion. With increasing O_2 and decreasing CO_2 and H^+, the reflex subsides.

The chemoreceptor reflex is important for the maintenance of proper respiratory gas transport to and from the CNS and cardiac tissues because conditions cause respiratory gas concentrations to change. Exposure to hypoxic environments, such as high altitude or a breath hold while diving, is a threat to cerebral and coronary function. The chemoreceptor reflex is a compensatory mechanism that results in enhanced blood flow to the brain and myocardium to better support their metabolism.

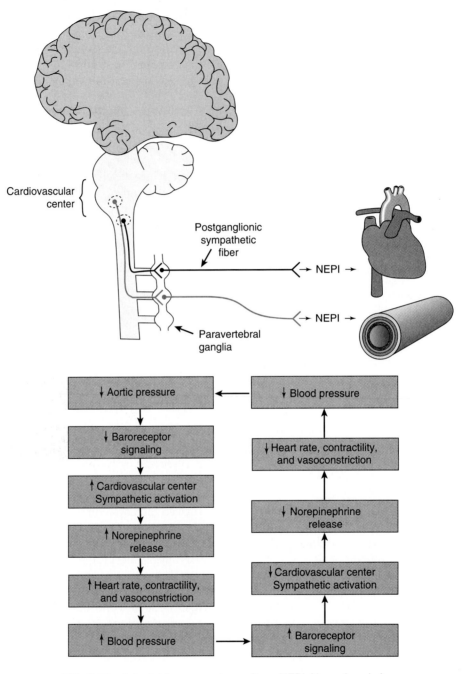

FIG. 8-12 Arterial baroreceptor reflex. *NEPI,* Norepinephrine.

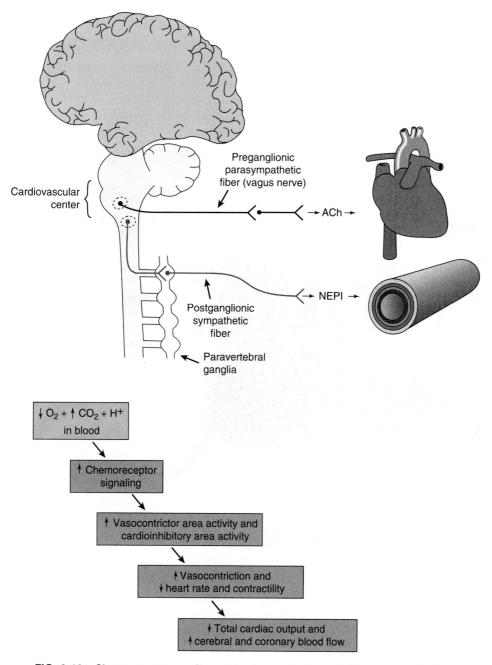

FIG. 8-13   Chemoreceptor reflex. *ACh,* Acetylcholine; *NEPI,* norepinephrine.

During sudden and severe hypoxic conditions, the chemoreceptor reflex can cause profound bradycardia and hypotension. When carotid chemoreceptors are exposed to blood that has a low O_2 content, the cardioinhibitory center activates and a reflex bradycardia occurs. This rather strong parasympathetic reflex is commonly referred to as a vagal reflex.

Cardiopulmonary Stretch Receptor Reflexes

The low-pressure receptors of the vena cava, atria, and ventricles are sensitive to blood volume and the stretching it causes in these regions. With increasing blood volume, these receptors send signals to the cardiovascular center, which causes inhibition of the cardiostimulatory center and vasoconstrictor area. This decreased sympathetic activity results in less cardiac and vessel stimulation. The effect of this reflex is to prevent excessive sympathetic activity during hypervolemia and hypertension.

Individuals who have chronic hypertension are thought to have a blunted ability to suppress sympathetic activity. Their treatment often includes the use of beta-adrenergic blockers to inhibit sympathetic activity and reduce blood pressure.

Hypovolemia and hypotension decreases cardiopulmonary baroreceptor stretching. Decreased cardiopulmonary baroreceptor signaling causes the inhibitory effects on the cardiovascular center to subside. This allows greater sympathetic activity to arise from the cardiostimulatory center and vasoconstrictor area, causing increased blood pressure. This reflex action, an important compensatory response, helps correct aortic blood pressure during states of low blood volume and when blood volume redistribution occurs during postural changes.

A localized effect of atrial distension, the Bainbridge reflex, occurs when the atria rapidly fill with fluid, causing distension and tachycardia. This appears to be a compensatory reflex for rapid filling of the atria.

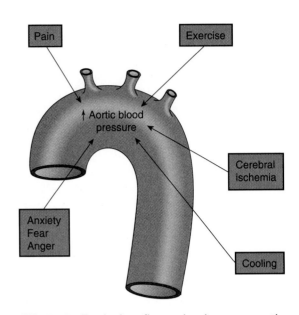

FIG. 8-14 Extrinsic reflexes that increase aortic blood pressure.

Extrinsic Regulation

A variety of extrinsic reflexes originate outside the cardiovascular system and influence its activity. The major extrinsic reflexes are summarized in Fig. 8-14. The combination of intrinsic and extrinsic reflex actions results in both stable cardiovascular performance and the ability to respond to a variety of conditions.

Pain

Pain can stimulate and inhibit cardiovascular activity. Pain generally causes a stress response that activates sympathetic stimulation of the heart and vessels, yielding an increase in heart rate and blood pressure. Extreme pain brought on by trauma or distension of the gall bladder, intestine, or ureter can produce a parasympathetic vagal reflex, which results in bradycardia and hypotension. The exact mechanisms that cause these different responses are not well understood.

Thermal Reflexes

Thermal receptors in skin respond to cooling and send signals to the spinal cord and hypothalamus. The hypothalamus sends signals, by way of sympathetic pathways, to cutaneous vessels and causes vasoconstriction and increased blood pressure. Intense cooling of an extremity triggers the cooling reflex and pain-induced vasoconstriction and hypertension.

A variation on the cutaneous cooling reflex, the dive reflex, enhances breath-holding time, produces a vagal nerve-mediated bradycardia, and causes extensive sympathetic peripheral vasoconstriction. Exposure of facial thermoreceptors to cold water and breath holding trigger the dive reflex. This response enables various animals to remain submerged for prolonged periods. In humans, heart rate drops about 25%, cutaneous blood flow drops about 75%, skeletal muscle blood flow drops 50%, and breath-holding time lengthens. Despite the drop in heart rate, the peripheral vasoconstriction actually causes an aortic hypertension of about 20% above normal. This effect, combined with a general lack of cerebral and coronary vasoconstriction, results in enhanced CNS and cardiac perfusion. As the dive proceeds and hypoxia and hypercapnia occur, the chemoreceptor reflex begins to maintain the peripheral vasoconstriction and bradycardia. Some young victims of accidental cold-water immersion have survived following more than 30 minutes of total immersion. Their survival is attributed to immersion in profoundly cold water, an intense dive reflex, reduced metabolism secondary to cooling, and their young age, which appears to enable them to better tolerate severe hypoxia.

Heating results in vasodilation and suppression of hypothalamic and spinal cord-triggered vasoconstriction. Excessive heating can result in widespread vasodilation, tachycardia, and fluid loss. The hypotension and fluid loss that result from hyperthermia can lead to reduced cerebral circulation and loss of consciousness. This condition is commonly called a heat stroke.

Exercise Pressor Response

Physical exercise appears to stimulate sensory nerve fibers in skeletal muscle, which, in turn, triggers a sympathetic-mediated vasoconstriction, tachycardia, and increased contractility. The pathways of this reflex are not well understood. Both **isotonic** (tension with muscle shortening) and isometric (tension without muscle shortening) exercises cause this response; the greater the amount of muscle mass exercising, the greater the response. The greatest response is brought on by isometric work of the arms. For example, sudden and sustained hand grip at about 30% of maximum or holding a 25-kg weight for 3 to 4 minutes elicits a powerful cardiovascular response that can result in a 25% to 35% increase in heart rate and blood pressure. This type of response can uncover "silent" coronary artery disease by inducing vessel spasm, which produces angina pectoralis and decreased ventricular wall motion—hence the admonition to individuals with coronary artery disease to refrain from lifting heavy objects.

CNS-Induced Changes

Activity in various parts of the brain can cause a number of extrinsic cardiovascular responses. Fear, anxiety, and anger cause activation of regions in the cerebrum, thalamus, and hypothalamus. This increases sympathetic activity and results in tachycardia and hypertension. This response is part of the protective fight-or-flight response, which enhances O_2 and nutrient transport to skeletal muscle. However, overpowering stimulation brought on by intense surprise or fear can activate regions of the hypothalamus, which causes sympathetic suppression and parasympathetic-induced bradycardia and hypotension. This offers a third option to an intense threat—syncope. This can also be viewed as a protective response known as the defense reaction. his reaction, which offers oblivion in the face of an overwhelming threat, is thought to be responsible for the act of playing dead that some animals use to reduce the chance of attack.

Abrupt and severe hypoxia of the brain brought on by sudden hypotension to levels of 40 to 50 mm Hg results in a powerful vasoconstrictive response. This action, known as the CNS ischemic response, is thought to be a "last ditch" attempt by the cardiovascular center to correct a life-threatening situation. However, this action is short lived as a result of general CNS dysfunction brought on by severe hypoxia. After prolonged ischemia or hypoxia, the cardiovascular center activates a vagal reflex, causing bradycardia and hypotension.

Other Extrinsic Reflexes

Rhythmic respiratory center activity coupled with incoming vagal signals that are produced by stretch receptors in the lung cause variations in sympathetic and parasympathetic stimulation of the heart and vessels. Vagal parasympathetic activity increases during inspiration and decreases during exhalation, resulting in a cyclic inhibition of heart rate that is synchronized with inflation of the lung. This reflex is not apparent in all subjects but can be conspicuous in some.

An interesting vagal reflex is triggered by manual massaging of the lateral walls of the eyeball. The oculocardiac reflex causes bradycardia and reduced blood pressure. It has been found useful, like the massaging of the carotid bodies in the neck, in reducing heart rate in those subjects who develop tachycardia secondary to an abnormal atrial pacemaker.

Hormonal Influences

The most important hormones released that influence cardiovascular function are the catecholamines **epinephrine** and norepinephrine. They are released from the adrenal gland and postganglionic sympathetic nerve endings following sympathetic stimulation. During exercise, hypovolemia, and emotional stress, the concentration of these hormones in blood plasma markedly increases and enhances sympathetic stimulation of the heart and vessels. Epinephrine has the ability to cause both alpha-adrenergic vasoconstriction and beta-adrenergic cardiac stimulation whereas norepinephrine is primarily an alpha-adrenergic vasoconstrictor. However, this route of catecholamine "delivery" to the cardiovascular tissues is less effective than through the sympathetic nervous system.

Numerous drugs have been developed to stimulate or block adrenergic and cholinergic receptors. Table 8-2 summarizes some of these drugs and their actions. Most are used to treat cardiovascular dysfunctions that cause abnormal blood pressure and flow.

Many other hormones and humoral agents are released into blood and influence blood pressure and blood flow. The atria produce the hormone **atrial natriuretic peptide (ANP),** which causes vasodilation and diuresis. ADH, also known as **vasopressin,** is secreted by the posterior pituitary gland and causes vasoconstriction and reduced urine

Table 8-2   Drugs that Act on Autonomic Receptors

Drug	Receptor Action	Use
Phenylephrine	Alpha stimulation	Vasoconstriction stimulation
Tolazoline	Alpha blockade	Vasodilation
Dopamine	Beta$_2$ stimulation	Cardiac stimulation
Propranolol	Beta blockade	Cardiac inhibition
Atropine	Cholinergic blockade	Cardiac stimulation

production. **Angiotensin II,** produced by the actions of the liver, kidney, and lung, is a powerful vasoconstrictor that plays an important role in long-term vasoconstriction and the regulation of urine formation. **Serotonin,** secreted by platelets and selective neurons, causes systemic vasoconstriction. Bradykinin is a potent vasodilator that is secreted by various exocrine glands. Many tissues produce and secrete prostaglandin E or prostaglandin F. Prostaglandin E has vasodilating properties whereas prostaglandin F has vasoconstricting properties. **Histamine,** another humoral factor that is secreted by a variety of cells in response to injury, causes local vasodilation and increases capillary permeability.

REGULATION OF LOCAL BLOOD FLOW

Autoregulation of Microcirculation

The autoregulation of local blood flow is another type of intrinsic regulation. The microcirculation relies on autoregulation to adjust blood flow locally to match nutrient and respiratory gas delivery with the local metabolic rate of the tissue. Virtually all tissues utilize local autoregulation to some degree. Those tissues with the least amount of autonomic nervous system control, such as the heart, brain, and kidney, show the greatest degree of autoregulation. The skin, which has well-developed autonomic control, has little autoregulation by comparison. A variety of physical conditions and chemical factors are known to be active in the autoregulation of blood flow (Fig. 8-15).

Physical Stimuli

Temperature changes and vessel stretching are important physical changes that cause blood flow fluctuations at the microcirculatory level. Increased tissue temperature causes the arterioles and precapillary sphincters to dilate,

allowing increased perfusion. Decreased temperature causes the opposite reaction. Arterioles also respond to mechanical stretching. This response is known as the **myogenic reaction.** Increased arteriole and capillary pressure and distension cause a reflex vasoconstriction. Decreased pressure results in vessel dilation. The myogenic reaction results in a relatively stable blood flow as blood pressure changes. The exact mechanisms behind the temperature response and myogenic reaction are not well understood.

Chemical Stimuli

A number of chemical factors produced locally influence blood flow (Box 8-1). These chemicals, produced in response to metabolic and physical changes, cause local adjustments of blood flow. Factors that cause dilation appear to be linked with metabolism. The waste products of metabolism such as adenosine, CO_2, H^+, and K^+ cause arteriole and precapillary sphincter vasodilation. This improves blood flow to better support metabolism. Vasoconstrictors such as serotonin, commonly produced following local tissue and vessel injury,

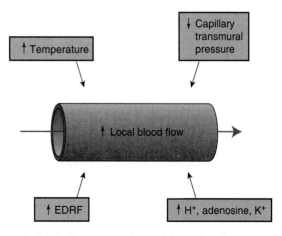

FIG. 8-15 Factors and conditions that influence capillary blood flow. *EDRF,* Endothelial-derived relaxing factor.

BOX 8-1

Locally Produced Vasoactive Chemicals that Affect Microcirculation

VASOCONSTRICTORS
Prostaglandin $F_{2\alpha}$
Thromboxane A_2
Superoxide-free radicals
Endothelial-derived constricting factor
  (endothelin)

VASODILATORS
Adenosine
H^+ and K^+
Lactic acid
Carbon dioxide
Prostaglandin E
Endothelial-derived relaxing factor (nitric
  oxide)
Histamine
Bradykinin

---

appear to act as part of a protective mechanism to help prevent blood loss.

Growing evidence demonstrates that the endothelium of microcirculation is not just a passive barrier that separates blood from the surrounding interstitial fluid, but it is also capable of producing and secreting a number of vasoactive chemicals that adjust blood flow locally. Vasodilation is caused by the local production of an **endothelial-derived relaxing factor (EDRF).** Stimulation of the endothelium by increased perfusion pressure and the presence of acetylcholine, bradykinin, and histamine cause the production and secretion of EDRF. **Nitric oxide (NO),** now known to be one of the forms of EDRF, causes vasodilation by activation of the enzyme **guanyl cyclase,** which causes the production of **cyclic GMP** and a decrease in the intracellular concentration of Ca^{++}. Reduced Ca^{++} concentration results in vasodilation. The production of NO and other forms of EDRF are thought to play an important role in maintaining local blood flow. The use of inhaled NO in low concentra-

tions (5 to 50 ppm) has been effective in improving pulmonary blood flow and gas exchange.

The endothelium also synthesizes and releases an endothelial-derived constricting factor (EDCF), which promotes vasoconstriction. One such factor is the small protein **endothelin,** a potent vasoconstrictor. Endothelin appears to play a role in the regulation of local and regional circulation. Its production is dramatically increased in those patients in renal failure, shock, and posttrauma. It may function in these circumstances to help compensate for low blood pressure through its potent vasoconstrictive action. The mechanisms that endothelin and other forms of EDCF utilize to stimulate vasoconstriction are not well understood.

Endothelial cell injury has been implicated in the microcirculatory abnormalities that commonly occur in patients who are in shock. The release of various vasoactive factors such as EDRF and EDCF following endothelial injury appears to be part of the cause of local overperfusion and underperfusion of the microcirculation. This contributes to the tissue dysfunction commonly seen in shock states.

MECHANISMS THAT ARE PART OF LONG-TERM CIRCULATION CONTROL

The concept of long-term control of blood flow and pressure, first proposed by Guyton in the 1960s, focuses on the maintenance of blood volume. The development of blood vessels can also be viewed as a form of long-term regulation.

Blood Volume Control

Water balance and erythrocyte production are the major influences on blood volume. Maintenance of fluid volume and solute concentration (osmolarity) is carried out by balancing the intake and output of water and solutes.

CASE STUDY FOCUS

Hypertensive Crisis

Sudden systemic hypertension (diastolic blood pressure >100 or a 30-mm Hg increase above baseline pressure) is a dangerous condition that should be confirmed by measuring the blood pressure in both arms and in one leg. It can be caused by emotional distress (e.g., pain, anxiety, and anger), intracerebral catastrophes (e.g., hemorrhages and strokes), encephalopathy (e.g., tumors), coronary surgery, acute myocardial infarction, renal insufficiency (those causing excessive renin secretion), pheochromocytomas of the adrenal gland (those causing excessive catecholamine secretion), toxemia of pregnancy, drug overdose (e.g., amphetamines and cocaine), and drug interactions (e.g., monoamine oxidase inhibitors and tyramine-rich foods). When blood pressure rapidly climbs to dangerous levels, there is greater risk of myocardial infarction, rupturing arteries in the brain, and dissection of the aorta. The treatment of hypertensive crisis is carried out in a controlled and progressive manner in such a way that the patient does not experience hypoperfusion of the brain, heart, or kidney. This is done by gradually reducing the mean arterial pressure about 20 to 30 mm Hg in the first hour and to 110 mm Hg in the first day. This is often carried out by placing the patient in a quiet environment and using vasodilators (e.g., nitroprusside), central sympathetic nervous blockers (e.g., clonidine), sympathetic receptor blockers (e.g., phentolamine and propranolol), calcium channel blockers (e.g., nifedipine), and diuretics (e.g., furosemide). These therapies are used with continuous monitoring of blood pressure to reach the appropriate target blood pressure in a gradual fashion to avoid hypoperfusion.

Renal function plays a dominant role in the regulation of fluid volume and solute concentration. The kidney also plays a role in the regulation of erythrocyte production by the bone marrow.

Generally, increased blood pressure normally triggers a series of actions that results in increased urine formation, decreased fluid volume, decreased cardiac output, and a return of blood pressure to the set point. Conversely, decreased blood pressure brought on by hemorrhaging or dehydration causes the opposite reaction, which results in retention of water, less urine production, greater cardiac function, and correction of blood pressure. These changes are triggered by a variety of neural and hormonal actions (Fig. 8-16).

Sympathetic Adjustment of Blood Volume

Hypotension brought on by hypovolemia causes the carotid, aortic, and cardiopulmonary baroreceptors to decrease their signaling of the cardiovascular center, resulting in vasoconstriction of the renal arterial network. Sympathetic vasoconstriction coupled with generalized reduction in arterial blood pressure causes reduced renal perfusion and subsequent reduction in glomerular filtration rate and urine formation. The resulting water retention helps compensate and improve cardiac output and blood pressure but requires time to be effective.

Hypervolemia and hypertension cause the opposite effect through suppression of sympathetic activity. The resulting renal vasodilation increases urine production and reduces plasma volume. In the normotensive subject, sympathetic activity suppresses renal blood flow sufficiently to help regulate urine formation.

Hormonal Adjustments of Blood Volume

Hormonal actions on the kidney and bone marrow are the most influential regulators of blood volume.

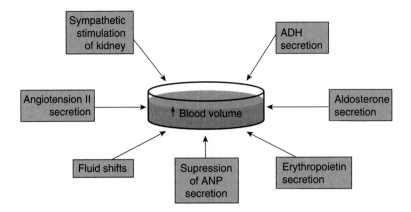

FIG. 8-16 Factors that cause an increase in blood volume. *ADH,* Antidiuretic hormone, *ANP,* atrial natriuretic peptide.

ADH, secreted by the posterior pituitary gland, is a potent vasoconstrictor and inhibitor of urine formation. Its release is triggered by hypovolemia and increased fluid osmolarity. Hypovolemia causes decreased carotid, aortic and atrial baroreceptors signal generation, which, in turn, causes an increase in sympathetic activity and ADH production. Decreased water intake or excessive water loss results in increased fluid osmolarity. This stimulates osmoreceptors in the hypothalamus, which triggers the release of ADH. ADH causes decreased urine formation by improving the water retention properties of the distal tubules of the renal nephrons. The combined effects of vasoconstriction and water retention brought on by ADH results in greater blood volume over time. Hypertension, hypervolemia, and hyposmolarity suppress ADH secretion and increase urine formation.

The renin-angiotensin-aldosterone system is another mechanism that is important in the control of blood volume. Decreased blood volume and pressure leads to reduced renal blood flow, glomerular filtration, and increased sympathetic activity. The combination of decreased fluid flow through the nephron tubules and

the increased sympathetic activity causes secretory cells in the juxtaglomerular apparatus of the renal nephron to secrete the enzyme renin. Renin acts to convert the plasma protein angiotensinogen (produced by the liver) to angiotensin I. Angiotensin I circulates through the lung where a second enzyme, angiotensin-converting enzyme, converts angiotensin I into angiotensin II. Angiotensin II is a potent vasoconstrictor and an important stimulant for the production of aldosterone. Aldosterone, a steroid hormone produced by the adrenal gland, causes the renal nephrons to retain Na^1, which, in turn, causes the retention of water. The collective actions of vasoconstriction by angiotensin II and Na^1 and water retention by aldosterone return blood volume and pressure back toward the normal set point. The production and secretion of angiotensin II and aldosterone are suppressed by a negative feedback mechanism induced by increases in hormone concentration and increased blood pressure and volume.

ANP, also known as atrial natriuretic factor, is another important hormone that influences blood volume regulation. It is a small peptide secreted by the atria of the heart in response to

Table 8-3   Hormones and Humoral Agents that Participate in the Long-Term Regulation of Blood Volume and Pressure

Hormone	Source	Target Tissue	Action
Antidiuretic hormone	Pituitary gland	Vessels	Vasoconstriction
		Renal tubules	Water retention
Angiotensin II	Lung	Vessels	Vasoconstriction
		Adrenal gland	Secretion of aldosterone
Aldosterone	Adrenal gland	Renal tubules	Na^+ and water retention
Atrial natriuretic peptide	Atrium	Vessels	Vasodilation
		Renal tubules	Na^+ and water excretion
Erythropoietin	Kidney	Bone marrow	Stimulates erythrocyte production

atrial distension and cardiopulmonary baroreceptor stimulation. The actions of ANP cause dilation of renal vessels, improved renal blood flow, increased glomerular filtration, and inhibition of Na^+ retention. This results in greater urine formation, greater Na^+ excretion (natriuresis), and reduced blood volume. These actions oppose the effects of ADH, angiotensin II, and aldosterone, suggesting that it helps retard the actions of these hormones. Reduced blood volume and venous return to the atria suppresses ANP production.

The hormones described previously are active in the regulation of plasma volume but have little influence over the number of erythrocytes in blood. Erythrocyte production is stimulated by the renal hormone **erythropoietin.** The production of this hormone is stimulated by reduced O_2 content in the blood delivered to the kidney. Individuals exposed to chronic hypoxia such as those living at high altitudes and who have chronic heart or lung failure compensate by increasing the production of erythrocytes. This is often shown by elevated hematocrit and erythrocyte counts. Increased blood O_2 content suppresses the production. More discussion about this hormone is found in Chapter 3.

The actions of these various hormones are summarized in Table 8-3.

Fluid Shifts

A decrease in arterial, capillary, and venous blood pressure results in a reduction of the hydrostatic pressure driving fluid out of the capillaries. The loss of pressure on the blood side of the capillary wall causes fluids to move from the interstitial space into the vascular space. The driving force behind this is the much higher colloid oncotic pressure of the plasma relative to the interstitial fluid. Following minor blood loss (i.e., the donation of a unit of blood), fluid shifts from the interstitial and intracellular compartments coupled with the other neural and hormonal changes provide an adequate response to normalize blood volume and blood pressure. The same responses occur following more severe blood loss (i.e., 40% to 50% of blood volume); however, the ability to normalize blood pressure is limited to only a few hours if fluid replacement is not started. Without adequate fluid replacement, wide spread metabolic dysfunction can occur leading back to hypotension and a lethal cycle that may not respond to therapy. This is better known as hypovolemic shock.

Hypervolemia and hypertension cause the opposite shifting of fluid. Increased blood pressure facilitates greater fluid filtration into the interstitial space, resulting in lower blood volume and blood pressure. In severe conditions, this can lead to the accumulation of excessive volumes of fluid in the interstitial space, which is called **edema.**

Numerous humoral and toxic agents influence fluid shifting. Histamine enhances fluid shifts through its actions on the microcirculation. Cortisol, a steroid hormone secreted by the adrenal gland, reduces fluid shifts. Some bacterial toxins can cause extensive fluid shifts out of the vascular compartment and vasodilation to the point of lethal hypotension—a condition known as septic shock.

Blood Vessel Development

The driving force behind local changes in blood flow is the local metabolic rate. The autoregulatory changes described previously are relatively short-term mechanisms. Other changes take more time during conditions of chronic hypoxia or low perfusion. Tissues exposed to a gradual decrease in blood flow begin to develop and dilate **collateral vessels** and capillary beds to improve blood flow. A good example of this is found in the myocardium following a nonlethal myocardial infarction. However, some tissues such as the brain and kidney do not have the ability to form collateral vessels. The ability to develop collateral vessels and extend capillaries (angiogenesis) is under the influence of a variety of growth hormones or angiogenic factors. Heparin, in addition to its ability to block blood clot formation, stimulates capillary formation. Angiogenic peptides and steroid hormones are known to stimulate and retard angiogenesis. The primary stimulus for angiogenesis appears to be chronic hypoxia.

1. The cardiovascular control center is located in the
   a. medulla oblongata
   b. cerebellum
   c. hypothalamus
   d. thalamus

2. Signals from the cardiostimulatory center result in positive chronotropism and inotropism through activation of
   a. parasympathetic nerve fibers
   b. motor nerve fibers
   c. sensory nerve fibers
   d. sympathetic nerve fibers

3. The vasodilator area of the vasomotor center is located in the
   a. cerebrum
   b. medulla oblongata
   c. cerebellum
   d. thalamus

4. Following stimulation, which one of the following adrenergic receptors generally results in vasoconstriction?
   a. alpha1
   b. beta$_2$
   c. alpha$_2$
   d. beta$_1$

5. The arterial baroreceptors are located in the walls of the
   1. carotid arteries
   2. cerebral arteries
   3. aorta
   a. 3 only
   b. 1 and 2
   c. 2 and 3
   d. 1 and 3
   e. 1, 2, and 3

6. Chemoreceptors that cause changes in cardiovascular function are located in
   1. aortic bodies
   2. carotid bodies

3. surface region of the medulla oblongata
   a. 1 only
   b. 1 and 2
   c. 2 and 3
   d. 1 and 3
   e. 1, 2, and 3

7. Frank-Starling's law of the heart is an example of
   a. extrinsic long-term regulation
   b. intrinsic short-term regulation
   c. extrinsic short-term regulation
   d. intrinsic long-term regulation

8. Pain generally causes
   1. tachycardia
   2. bradycardia
   3. hypertension
   4. hypotension
      a. 1 only
      b. 1 and 3
      c. 2 and 3
      d. 2 and 4
      e. 1 and 4

9. Which of the following causes the micro-circulation of the systemic circuit to dilate and to increase local blood flow?
   1. production of adenosine
   2. reduction of H^+ concentration
   3. production of endothelial-derived relaxing factor
      a. 3 only
      b. 1 and 3
      c. 2 and 3
      d. 1 and 2
      e. 1, 2, and 3

10. Which one of the following would result in greater fluid loss and cause blood volume to decrease?
    a. increased secretion of atrial natriuretic peptide
    b. sympathetic stimulation of the kidney
    c. increased secretion of antidiuretic hormone
    d. increased secretion of aldosterone
    e. increased secretion of erythropoietin

For answers, see p. 475.

BIBLIOGRAPHY

1. Athanassopoulos G, Cokkino DV: Atrial natriuretic factor, *Prog Cardiovasc Dis* 33:313, 1991.
2. Berne RM, Levy MN: *Cardiovascular physiology*, St Louis, 1992, Mosby.
3. Boldt J et al: Alterations in circulating vasoactive substances in the critically ill: a comparison between survivors and non-survivors, *Intensive Care Med* 21:218, 1995.
4. Brandenburg RO et al: *Cardiology: fundamentals and practice*, Chicago, 1987, Year Book Medical.
5. Cohn PF: *Clinical cardiovascular physiology*, Philadelphia, 1985, WB Saunders.
6. Ganong WF: *Review of medical physiology*, ed 18, Stamford, Conn, 1997, Appleton & Lange.
7. Guyton AC: *Textbook of medical physiology*, ed 8, Philadelphia, 1991, WB Saunders.
8. Little RC: *Physiology of the heart and circulation*, ed 2, Chicago, 1981, Year Book Medical.
9. Lüscher TF: Endothelin: systemic arterial and pulmonary effects of a new peptide with biologic properties, *Am Rev Respir Dis* 146:S56, 1992.
10. Martini FH: *Fundamentals of anatomy and physiology*, Upper Saddle River, NJ, 1998, Prentice Hall.
11. Perreaut T, Gutkowska J: Role of atrial natriuretic factor in lung physiology and pathology, *Am J Respir Crit Care Med* 151:226, 1995.
12. Rose BD: *Clinical physiology of acid-base and electrolyte balance*, New York, 1984, McGraw-Hill Book.
13. Smith JJ, Kampine JP: *Circulatory physiology: the essentials*, ed 3, Baltimore, 1990, Williams & Wilkins.
14. Spence AP, Mason EG: *Human anatomy and physiology*, ed 4, St Paul, 1992, West.
15. West JB: *Best and Taylor's physiological basis of medical practice*, ed 12, Baltimore, 1990, Williams & Wilkins.

Anatomy of the Pulmonary System

Upon completing this chapter, you will be able to:
1 Describe the four phases of lung development.
2 Describe the anatomy of the thorax.
3 Describe the structure, location, and function of the pleural membranes and fluid.
4 Define *conducting zone airway* and *respiratory zone airway.*
5 Describe the structures of the upper airway.
6 Describe the organization of the lobes and segments of the lungs.
7 Describe the structure and function of the trachea and bronchial tree.
8 Describe the structure and function of the various layers of the bronchial airway wall.
9 Describe airway mucus production and transport.
10 Define *alveolus, acinus,* and *primary lobule.*
11 Describe the structure of the alveolus and alveolar-capillary membrane.
12 Describe the types of nervous system inputs and outputs of the lung and what their general functions are.
13 Describe the nonspecific defenses of the lung.
14 Describe the specific defenses of the lung.

The respiratory tract brings air from the external environment into close contact with blood. Epithelial, connective, muscle, and nervous tissues are all found in the pulmonary system or support it. The system is organized around a complex arrangement of airways and blood vessels that terminate in delicate structures that carry out gas exchange. This chapter describes the anatomy of the pulmonary system and lays an important foundation for later discussions about the various functions of the pulmonary system.

HOW THE PULMONARY SYSTEM DEVELOPS

Organs of the pulmonary system begin forming 3½ weeks after conception and are complete at 8 or 10 years of age. This elaborate

| Table 9-1 | Major Events during Pulmonary System Development |

Developmental Phases	Structural Changes
Embryonic phase (fertilization to 5 weeks' gestation)	Lung bud formation Trachea and main stem bronchi form
Pseudoglandular phase (6 to 16 weeks' gestation)	Bronchial tree forms Mucus membrane forms Pulmonary arteries and veins form Lobes of lung form Diaphragm forms
Canalicular phase (17 to 25 weeks' gestation)	Respiratory bronchioles form Pulmonary capillary bed begins to form Surfactant begins to be synthesized
Terminal sac phase (26 weeks' gestation to 8 to 10 years)	Numerous saccules form Alveoli appear between 29 and 36 weeks' gestation Alveolar number increases to 50 million at birth Alveolar surface area is 3 to 4 m² at birth Pulmonary capillary bed continues to form Surfactant production increases
Postnatal phase (birth to 8 to 10 years)	Alveolar numbers increases to 300 to 350 million Alveolar surface area increases to 70 m²

process begins as a simple out-pouching of the primitive esophagus and culminates in the formation of an intricate network of airways that terminates in about 300 million microscopic air sacs called **alveoli.**

Developmental Phases of the Respiratory Tract

Development of the lung is a continuous process from start to finish. The major events of development are divided into four periods (Table 9-1). The exact length of time each period lasts in the human is still disputed largely because different methods and definitions have been used in the study of lung development.

Embryonic Period

During the embryonic period the pulmonary system begins to form 26 days after conception. The first structure to form is a pouch or

bud from the primitive esophagus (Fig. 9-1). Growth of the lung bud continues over the next several days and results in the first branching, or bifurcation. This division forms the left and right main stem bronchi. The main stem airways continue to grow and further divide into the airways that will form each lobe of the lung.

Pseudoglandular Period

The appearance of the pulmonary system during weeks 6 to 16 after conception is referred to as the pseudoglandular period. This name is given to this period because the developing lungs look like fluid-filled glands. In week 7 the airways have bifurcated to the point that 10 identifiable airways are present as branches from each main stem bronchus. The airways that form during this period constitute the basis of the familiar pattern of lobes and segments into which each lung will develop. At the end of this period the airways have branched approximately 20 times and have formed thousands of terminal bronchioles. Formation of the terminal bronchioles completes the development of the conducting airways. The conducting airways include all

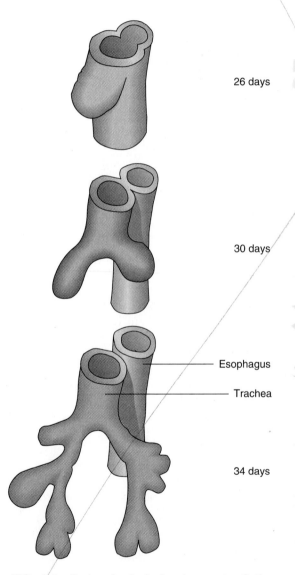

26 days

30 days

Esophagus

Trachea

34 days

FIG. 9-1 Embryological development of the respiratory tract at different points following conception.

the airways from the mouth and nose to the terminal bronchioles. These airways will supply gas to the airways that will participate in gas exchange. Few terminal bronchioles form following the pseudoglandular period. During this time the mucus membrane of the inner surface of the airways forms. Later in this period vessels grow and branch out in a pattern that parallels the airways. These vessels will eventually become pulmonary arteries and veins. During week 7 the diaphragm forms, and the first breathing motions of the fetus are detected during the twelfth week.

Canalicular Period

The canalicular period continues the refinement of the airways from 17 through 25 weeks' gestation and is named for the vascular changes that take place during this period. Airway and vessel branching continues, and numerous respiratory bronchioles form from the terminal bronchioles. Pulmonary capillary development begins during this period with the formation of vessel loops around the respiratory bronchioles.

At the end of this period the chemical **surfactant** begins to be formed by specialized secretory cells found in the walls of the respiratory bronchioles. Surfactant reduces surface tension that forms when the lungs fill with air. By reducing surface tension, surfactant plays an important role in helping prevent airway collapse when breathing air following birth.

The presence of respiratory bronchioles and pulmonary capillaries near the surface of the bronchioles and surfactant production around 24 weeks' gestation make air breathing gas exchange possible at the end of the canalicular period.

Terminal Sac Period

The last phase of pulmonary development is the terminal sac period, which extends from about the 26 weeks' gestation to 8 to 10 years after birth. Some researchers divide this period into saccular and alveolar stages, reflecting different changes that take place in the terminal airway. It is during this period that the respiratory airways are refined for better gas exchange. Early in this period the respiratory bronchioles branch out into multiple saccules with smooth walls of flattened epithelia and capillary beds that wrap around them. The saccules become subdivided by the development of cellular walls with capillary beds in them. These subdivisions are refined into numerous microscopic alveoli. True alveoli have been reported to form as early as 29 weeks' gestation by some researchers, and virtually all researchers report them by 36 weeks' gestation. The total number of alveoli at birth continues to be debated, but most agree that the number is approximately 50 million with a gas exchange surface area of about 3 to 4 m². This represents about 15% of the total number that form and about 5% of the surface area found in the adult lung.

Over the next 10 years following birth, alveolar number and size increase. The total number climbs and stabilizes at about 300 to 350 million. Most of the increase occurs in the first 2 years when the number increases about sixfold. By adulthood, lung volume, surface area, and weight increase approximately 20 times. The increase in lung size after 2 years of age is primarily caused by enlargement of alveoli.

● HOW THE THORACIC CAVITY IS ORGANIZED

The thoracic cavity is formed by the tissues of the chest, upper back, and diaphragm. It is a cone-shaped cavity that houses the lungs and the contents of the mediastinum (Figs. 9-2 and 9-3). It functions to protect the vital organs within and has the capability of changing shape to enable air to be moved into and out of the lungs. To carry out these actions, the thoracic cavity is arranged from epithelial, connective, and muscle tissues.

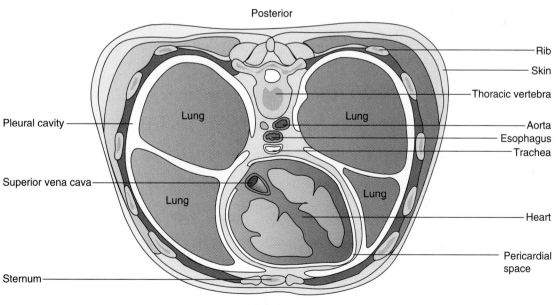

FIG. 9-2 Cross sectional view of the thorax showing its contents.

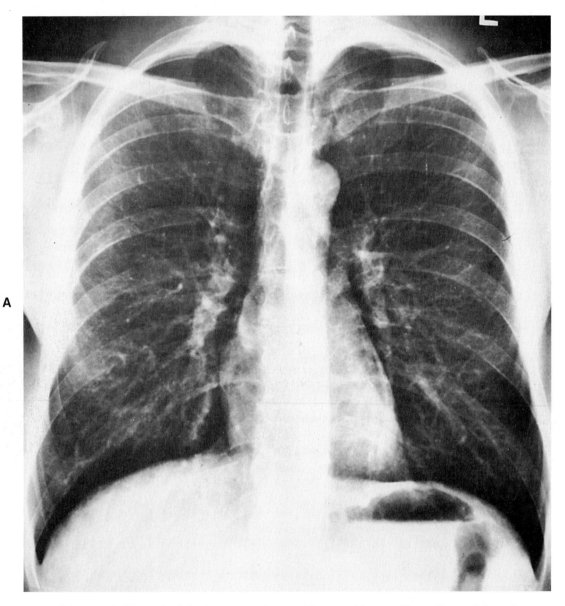

FIG. 9-3   A, Normal adult chest x-ray from a 28-year-old man. (From Fraser RS et al: *Synopsis of diseases of the chest,* ed 2, Philadelphia, 1994, WB Saunders.)

Components of the Thoracic Wall

The various parts of the thoracic wall are shown in Fig. 9-4. The outer covering of the thorax is formed by the integumentary system, which includes skin, hair, and subcutaneous fat. Skin is a composite of an outer epi-dermis and an inner connective tissue layer called the dermis. Below the dermis is a layer of subcutaneous fat. Skeletal muscle, encased in a layer of connective tissue called fascia, is found under the subcutaneous fat. Skeletal

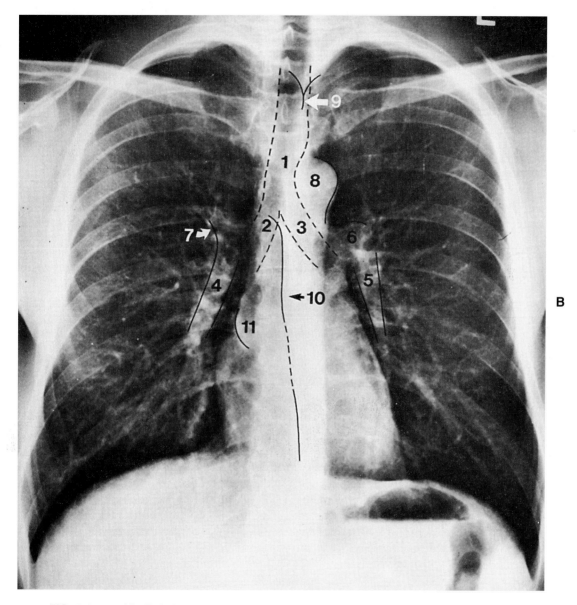

FIG. 9-3, cont'd   B, Labeled view showing *1,* trachea; *2,* main stem bronchus; *3,* left main stem bronchus; *4,* right interlobar artery; *6,* left main pulmonary artery; *7,* right superior pulmonary vein; *8,* aortic knob; *9,* posterior junction line; *10,* azygo-esophageal interface; and *11,* right pulmonary venous confluence.

muscle tissue forms the various muscles of the chest and back and lies over and between the ribs. The ribs of the rib cage lie in the inner portion of the thoracic wall. The inner layer of the thoracic wall is lined with a serous mem-brane called the **parietal pleura.** It is apposed by another serous membrane called the **visceral pleura** which covers the lung. A thin, fluid-filled pleural space forms between the parietal and visceral pleural membranes.

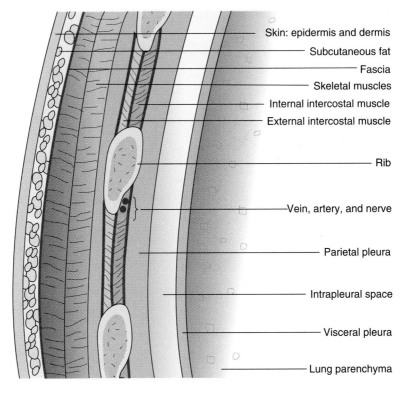

Skin: epidermis and dermis
Subcutaneous fat
Fascia
Skeletal muscles
Internal intercostal muscle
External intercostal muscle

Rib

Vein, artery, and nerve

Parietal pleura

Intrapleural space

Visceral pleura

Lung parenchyma

FIG. 9-4 Thoracic wall.

Skeletal Frame of the Thorax

The rigidity of the thorax is provided by the bone tissue of the rib cage (Fig. 9-5). This bony case includes the sternum, or breastbone, which is a long, vertical flat bone found on the anterior side. It is comprised of three bones: the manubrium, the body (or gladiolus), and the **xiphoid process.** The superior edge of the manubrium forms a shallow depression that is known as the jugular notch. The fused connection between the manubrium and the body is known as the sternal angle. On the lateral edges of the manubrium and body is a cartilaginous joint called the *costal cartilage* that forms the attachment between the ribs and sternum. This joint allows the rib cage to bend and permits the thorax to increase and decrease in size.

Twelve pairs of ribs form the rib cage. Rib pairs 1 through 7 are known as the true ribs because they are attached directly to the sternum. Ribs 8 through 12 are called *false ribs* because they are either indirectly attached to the sternum or not attached at all. The vertebrochondral ribs include rib pairs 8, 9, and 10, which are indirectly attached to the sternum through a common cartilaginous strap. Rib pairs 11 and 12 are called **floating ribs** because they are not attached to the sternum. Each rib has a sternal end, a long, curved, and relatively flat body, and a head that articulates with the vertebral bones. **Intercostal muscles** lie between the ribs and hold them together. Just bellow each rib is a thoracic artery, vein, and nerve that supplies blood flow and nerve communications to that region of the chest wall (see Fig. 9-4).

The 12 thoracic vertebrae constitute the bones of the thoracic vertebral column. These vertebrae form a somewhat flexible posterior

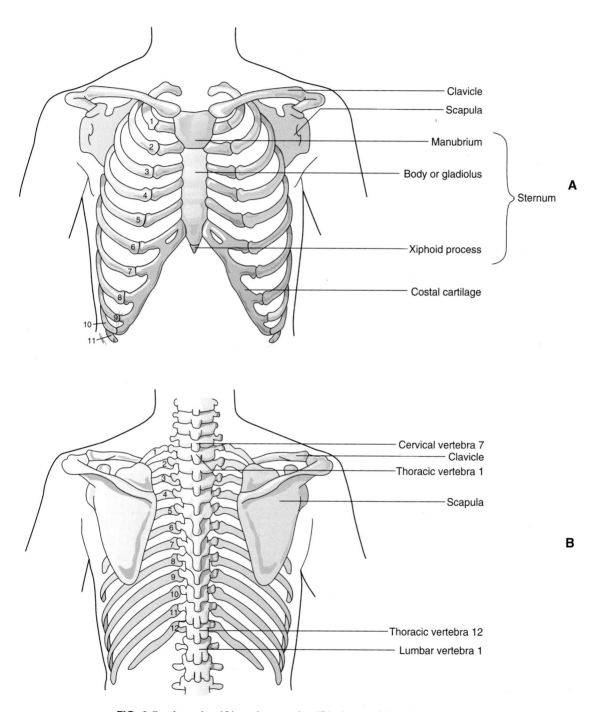

Clavicle
Scapula
Manubrium
Body or gladiolus
Sternum
Xiphoid process
Costal cartilage

A

Cervical vertebra 7
Clavicle
Thoracic vertebra 1
Scapula

B

Thoracic vertebra 12
Lumbar vertebra 1

FIG. 9-5 Anterior **(A)** and posterior **(B)** views of the rib cage.

support post for the rib cage to hang from and rotate against. The head end of the first nine pairs of ribs rotates against the bodies of two adjacent vertebrae and with the transverse process of the lower vertebrae. The tenth rib pair rotates against one vertebral body and transverse process. Rib pairs 11 and 12 rotate against only one vertebral body. The motion of the ribs against the vertebral column is commonly described as being like the motion of a bucket handle. This motion allows the thoracic cavity to increase and decrease in size as the ribs rotate upward and downward against the vertebral column. During a deep inspiration, the ribs move upward from a downward-projecting angle to a more horizontal position.

The upper and lateral regions of the thorax house the bones of the pectoral girdles. The pectoral girdle on each side is formed by the clavicle (collarbone) and scapula (shoulder blade). The scapula forms the socket for the shoulder joint and is stabilized or moved by skeletal muscles of the upper back. The clavicle supports and stabilizes the shoulder joint through a flexible attachment to the manubrium of the sternum.

Pleural Membranes and Space

The inner lining of the chest wall and the outer covering of the lungs are comprised of serous membranes called the *pleural membranes* (see Fig. 9-4). The membrane lining the chest wall is called the *parietal pleura*, and the membrane covering the lungs is called the *visceral pleura.* Both membranes are constructed from a thin layer of mesothelial cells, and below that is a layer of connective tissue that houses blood vessels, lymphatic vessels, and nerve fibers. The parietal pleura contains sensory fibers that are responsible for the painful sensation-associated inflammation of the pleura—a condition called **pleurisy.** The space between the membranes is called the *pleural space* and is filled with just a few milliliters of pleural fluid. This small volume of fluid is spread out over the entire surface of both lungs and functions as a lubricant to reduce friction as the lungs move within the thorax and as an airtight seal that adheres the two pleural membranes together.

Pleural fluid is secreted and reabsorbed by the two pleural membranes. Using the concepts described by Starling's law of the capillary (see Chapter 7), researchers conclude that most of the pleural fluid is produced by the parietal pleura and that most of the reabsorption is carried out by the visceral pleura. The systemic circulation supplies high-pressure blood to the parietal pleura, which causes fluid filtration into the pleural space. This process is estimated to produce about 5 to 10 ml of pleural fluid per day. The visceral pleura is supplied with blood from the low-pressure pulmonary circuit, which enables it to absorb the pleural fluid. The fluid absorbed by the visceral pleura is carried off by the pulmonary lymphatics and veins that eventually drain it back to the heart.

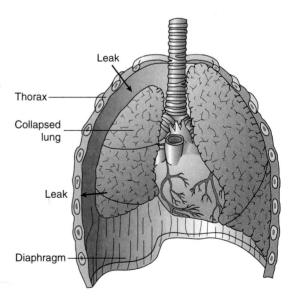

FIG. 9-6 Pneumothorax (see text for description).

Fluid and air can accumulate in the pleural space. Excess fluid filtration or lymphatic blockage can result in a pleural fluid accumulation called a **pleural effusion.** Blood vessels in the chest wall or lung can be injured, and blood can flow from them and accumulate in the pleural space. This is known as a **hemothorax.** Air can also move into the pleural space from open wounds through the chest wall, lung, or airways (Fig. 9-6). This condition is called a **pneumothorax.** When fluid or air moves into the pleural space, the lung is partially collapsed. Minor cases are allowed to reabsorb on their own. Situations that result in greater than 25% collapse usually require removal of the fluid or air.

HOW CONDUCTING ZONE AIRWAYS ARE ORGANIZED

Upper Airway

The upper airway is defined as those airways starting at the nose and mouth and that extend down to the trachea (Fig. 9-7). The upper airway is open to the outside environment through the external nares or nostrils of the nose and the mouth of the oral cavity. Most of the air moved through the respiratory tract during breathing at rest enters through the nares and nasal cavity. Mouth breathing is utilized during exercise to reduce the resistance to gas flow. The functions of the upper airway are summarized in Box 9-1.

Nasal and Oral Cavities

The left and right nasal cavities are formed by cartilage and numerous skull bones. The roof is formed by the nasal, frontal, sphenoid, and ethmoid bones. The septum separating the two cavities is formed by cartilage and the **ethmoid** and vomer bones. The lateral walls are created by the maxilla, concha, lacrimal, and palatine bones. The floor of the cavity, or palate, is primarily formed by the maxilla.

Three shelflike bones protrude into the cavity from the lateral walls. These bony shelves are called the superior, middle, and inferior conchae. The conchae are also known as the **turbinates.** The conchae function to increase the surface area and complexity of the nasal cavity. This enables the nasal cavity to work as a passageway, filter, humidifier, and heater of inhaled air. The posterior opening of the nasal cavity is called the internal nares and is, in part, formed by the flexible soft palate.

The surface of the nasal cavity is covered with epithelia. The anterior portion is covered with stratified squamous cells and possesses hair. This is the same type of tissue that forms the epidermis. The middle portion of the cavity is covered with a mucous membrane that is comprised of ciliated, pseudostratified epithelia and goblet cells. The mucous membrane functions to secrete mucus and to propel it toward the posterior portion of the nasal cavity and the mouth. Just below the mucus membrane is an extensive network of veins that forms a venous plexus. These vessels supply water and heat to the gas within the nasal cavity. Inflammation of this mucous membrane is brought on by irritation or infection. This is produced by vasodilation and increased vessel leakage. The consequence of nasal cavity inflammation is partial or complete blockage of the air passage. The vessels of the venous plexus can rupture as a result of breathing dry air or of passing foreign bodies

---

BOX 9-1

Functions of the Upper Airway

Passageway for gas flow
Filter
Heating
Humidification
Phonation
Protection of the lower airways

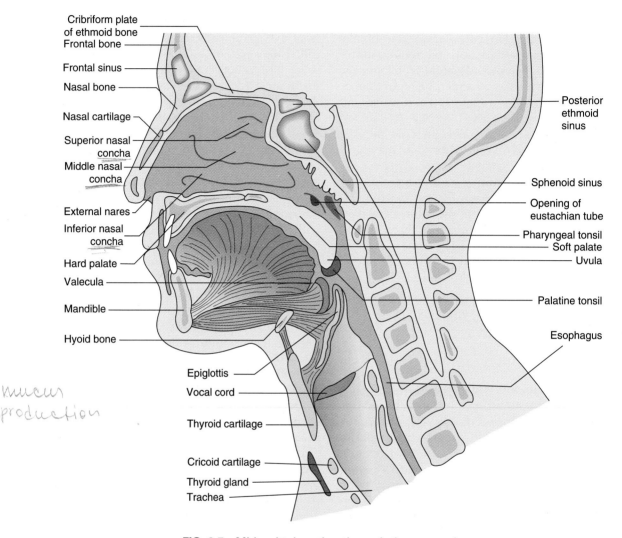

Cribriform plate of ethmoid bone
Frontal bone
Frontal sinus
Nasal bone
Nasal cartilage
Superior nasal concha
Middle nasal concha
External nares
Inferior nasal concha
Hard palate
Valecula
Mandible
Hyoid bone
Epiglottis
Vocal cord
Thyroid cartilage
Cricoid cartilage
Thyroid gland
Trachea

Posterior ethmoid sinus
Sphenoid sinus
Opening of eustachian tube
Pharyngeal tonsil
Soft palate
Uvula
Palatine tonsil
Esophagus

mucus production

FIG. 9-7 Midsagittal section through the upper airway.

through the nose. Rupture of these vessels can cause considerable nasal bleeding. The posterior portion of the nasal cavity is covered with stratified squamous just like the tissue covering the nearby oral cavity.

Within the skull bones and around the nasal cavity are the sinuses (Fig. 9-8). These hollow spaces are named for the bones in which they are found. The sinuses are lined with a mucous membrane and drain into the nasal cavity through numerous ducts. Sinus infections (sinusitis) are more common when these ducts become blocked or narrowed by inflammation commonly caused by repeat infections and allergies. Because of their proximity to both the upper respiratory tract and the surfaces of the brain and eye, the sinuses are an excellent route for infections to reach the meninges, brain, and eyes.

The nasal cavity functions to conduct air to and from the respiratory tract, to condition inhaled gas, to act as a region for sinus and eye

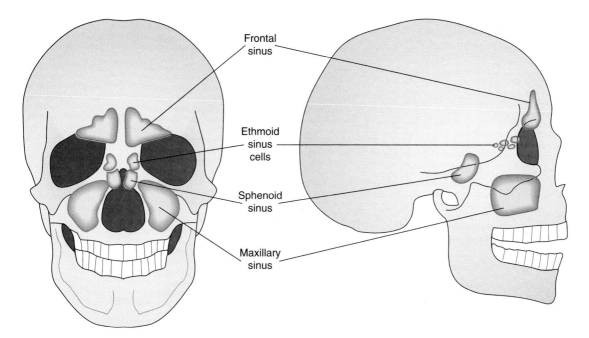

FIG. 9-8   Sinuses.

fluid to drain, and to contain olfactory sensors for the sensation of smell. Conditioning inhaled gas involves filtering, heating, and humidifying air. Filtration of inhaled air is carried out by the hair in the anterior portion of the cavity and by the sticky mucous membrane that covers the complex surface of the cavity. Almost all particles that are greater than 10 μm in diameter impact on the sticky surface of the membrane and are effectively filtered out. The mucous membrane of the cavity is also wet and warm and is able to heat and humidify the inhaled gases to 100% relative humidity and body temperature by the time it reaches the trachea. In addition, the mucous membrane in the superior portion of the cavity has chemoreceptors that send signals to the olfactory nerve for the sensation of smell.

Air can also enter and exit from the respiratory tract through the oral cavity (Fig. 9-9). The anterior roof of the oral cavity is called the *hard palate* and is formed by the maxillary bone. The posterior portion is known as the soft palate because of its soft-tissue composition and ability to move upward to seal off the nasal cavity when swallowing. The end of the soft palate hangs down into the posterior portion of the oral cavity. This part of the soft palate is called the *uvula*. The walls of the oral cavity are formed by the cheeks, and the floor is dominated by the tongue.

Pharynx

The posterior portion of the nasal cavity and the oral cavity opens into a region called the **pharynx.** The pharynx is subdivided into the nasopharynx, **oropharynx,** and **hypopharynx** (or **laryngopharynx**) (Fig. 9-10).

The nasopharynx lies at the posterior end of the nasal cavity and extends to the tip of the uvula. Gas flow undergoes a major change in direction as it travels into the nasopharynx. This causes a large number of foreign particles to impact on the surface of the nasopharynx. Exposure of the nasopharynx to such a large

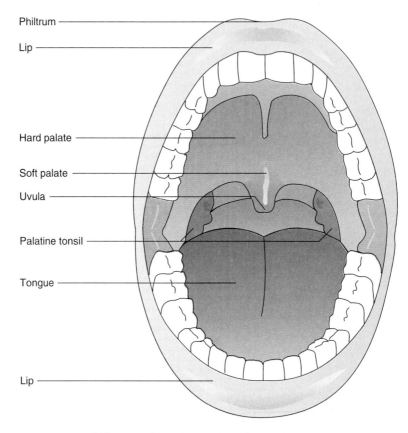

Philtrum

Lip

Hard palate

Soft palate

Uvula

Palatine tonsil

Tongue

Lip

FIG. 9-9 Frontal view into the oral cavity.

number of foreign particles makes it a logical place for the body to position lymphoid tissues to detect and interact with infectious microorganisms. The lymphoid tissues are housed in two pharyngeal tonsils (also called the adenoids) that are located on either side of the lateral and posterior walls of the pharynx. In the same region are two openings into the left and right eustachian tubes that link the upper airway with the middle ear (see Fig. 9-7). The eustachian tubes drain fluid out of the middle ear and allow gas to move in or out of the middle to equalize pressure on either side of the tympanic membrane.

The oropharynx is located in the posterior region of the oral cavity that spans the space between the uvula and the upper rim of the epiglottis. This region is also equipped with a pair of palatine tonsils that are located on the lateral walls of the oropharynx. These tonsils can become chronically swollen and cause partial airway obstruction. If the swelling is excessive and the individual has numerous repeat throat and ear infections, these tonsils can be removed by the surgical procedure known as a tonsillectomy.

The region below the oropharynx is known as the *hypopharynx*. It extends from the upper rim of the epiglottis to the opening between the vocal cords.

The tissues of the nasopharynx and hypopharynx can move and undergo shape changes during speech and swallowing. During unconsciousness, the muscles of the tongue and hypopharynx can relax and allow the tongue and other soft tissues to collapse and occlude the opening of the hypopharynx. This condition can result in partial to complete

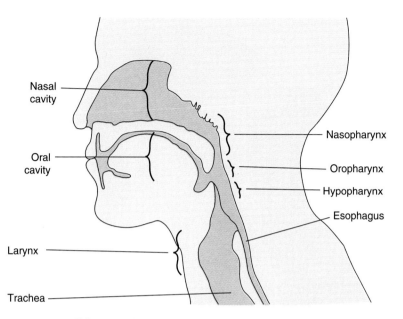

FIG. 9-10   Location and parts of the pharynx.

blockage of the upper airway and limit air movement to and from the respiratory tract. This is a primary cause of obstructive sleep apnea.

Larynx

The larynx lies below the hypopharynx and is formed by a complex arrangement of cartilages (Fig. 9-11). The thyroid cartilage forms most of the upper portion of the larynx and is generally referred to as the Adam's apple. This cartilage is named for the thyroid gland, which lies over its outer surface. Just below the thyroid cartilage is the **cricoid cartilage,** the only laryngeal structure that forms a complete ring of cartilage around the airway. A membrane of connective tissue called the *cricothyroid ligament* spans the space between the thyroid and cricoid cartilage. This membrane is occasionally used as the location for placement of an emergency prosthetic airway in those who have a life-threatening blockage of the upper airway.

The cartilaginous and leaf-shaped **epiglottis** lies within and is attached to the thyroid cartilage by a flexible joint. While air breathing, the thyroid cartilage slides down and remains apart from the epiglottis, allowing air to move in and out of the respiratory tract. The epiglottis functions to prevent liquids and food from entering the respiratory tract by forming a tight seal with the thyroid cartilage during swallowing. The act of swallowing is a complex series of muscular contractions that pulls the thyroid cartilage up and the epiglottis down to form a tight seal as food is propelled to the back of the mouth and toward the esophagus. Infection of the epiglottis can cause it to swell; this is known as **epiglottitis.** Epiglottitis can partially or totally block the airway and may necessitate the emergent placement of a prosthetic airway to maintain a patent air passage.

Within the thyroid cartilage and just above the cricoid cartilage are the arytenoid cartilages. They play an important role in the opening and closing of the vocal cords, which lie within the larynx (Fig. 9-12). The posterior portion of the vocal cords is formed by the arytenoid cartilages. When the two arytenoid cartilages rotate, they slide outward and the vocal cords are pulled open. The opening

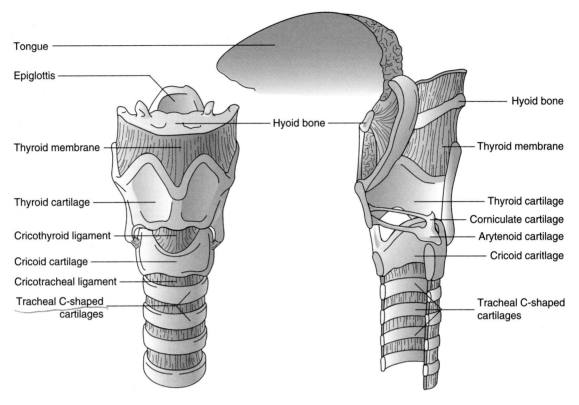

Tongue

Epiglottis

Thyroid membrane

Thyroid cartilage

Cricothyroid ligament

Cricoid cartilage

Cricotracheal ligament

Tracheal C-shaped cartilages

Hyoid bone

Hyoid bone

Thyroid membrane

Thyroid cartilage

Corniculate cartilage

Arytenoid cartilage

Cricoid caritilage

Tracheal C-shaped cartilages

FIG. 9-11 Anterior and lateral views of the larynx.

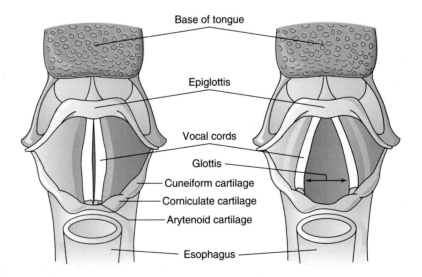

Base of tongue

Epiglottis

Vocal cords

Glottis

Cuneiform cartilage

Corniculate cartilage

Arytenoid cartilage

Esophagus

FIG. 9-12 Looking into the larynx from above and behind with the vocal cords closed and open.

formed between the vocal cords is called the *glottis*. Damage to the cricoarytenoid joint, which allows the arytenoid cartilages to rotate, could result in inability to open the vocal cords properly and cause difficulties with speaking and breathing. In the same region are the corniculate and cuneiform cartilages that function to support the soft tissue on either side of the vocal cords.

The vocal ligaments, or cords, span the opening in the larynx by attachments to the thyroid and movable arytenoid cartilages. The vocal cords function like a vibrating reed to form sound during phonation. They also help protect the lower airways by closing during the swallowing reflex.

The muscles of the larynx are innervated by the inferior laryngeal nerve, also called the *recurrent laryngeal nerve*. It is a motor nerve that branches off from the vagus nerve. Impulses carried by this nerve are important in phonation and swallowing. Injuries to this nerve can cause partial or complete paralysis of the vocal cords and inability to swallow correctly. This results in difficulty with phonation and can, in severe cases, cause airway obstruction as a result of vocal cord closure.

Tracheobronchial Tree and Lungs

The airways of the tracheobronchial tree extend from the larynx down to the airways that participate in gas exchange. The various types of airways and their dimensions are summarized in Table 9-2. Each branching of an airway produces subsequent generations

Table 9-2　Types of Airways Found in the Tracheobronchial Tree

Name	Generation	Diameter (cm)	Length (cm)	Number per Generation	Comments
Trachea	0	1.8	1.2	1	C-shaped cartilaginous rings
Primary bronchi	1	1.2	4.8	2	Complete cartilaginous rings
Lobar bronchi	2	0.8	0.9	5	Three on right, two on left
Segmental bronchi	3	0.6	0.8	20	10 in each lung
Subsegmental bronchi	4	0.5	1.3	20	
Small bronchi	5	0.4	1.1	40	Possesses cartilage and a mucous membrane
	10			1020	
Bronchioles	11	0.1	0.4	2050	No cartilage; lined with mucous membrane
	13	0.1	0.3	8190	
Terminal bronchioles	14	0.1	0.2	16,380	No goblet cells; layered with cuboidal cells, smooth muscle, and connective tissue
	15	0.1	0.2	32,270	
Respiratory bronchiole	16	0.1	0.2	65,540	No smooth muscle
	18	0.1	0.1	262,140	No cilia
Alveolar duct	19	0.05	0.1	524,290	Lined with alveoli
	23	0.04	0.05	8,390,000	
Alveolus	24	240	240	300,000,000	Dimensions in micrometers

Data from Weibel ER: *Morphometry of the human lung,* New York, 1973, Springer-Verlag.

of smaller airways. The first 15 generations are known as conducting airways because they function to convey gas from the upper airway to the airways that participate in gas exchange with blood. These airways are revealed in Fig. 9-13, which shows a special chest x-ray called a *bronchogram* that uses radiopaque fluid to coat the airways and to make them stand out. The microscopic airways beyond the conducting airways that carry out gas exchange with blood are classified as the *respiratory airways*.

Trachea and Bronchi

The trachea extends from its connection to the cricoid cartilage down through the neck and into the thorax (Fig. 9-14). The adult trachea is approximately 12 cm long and has an inner diameter of about 1.8 cm. Fig. 9-15 shows the different layers of tissue that form the trachea. The outermost layer is a thin connective tissue sheath. Below the sheath is a number of C-shaped cartilaginous rings that provide support and maintain the trachea as an open tube. The typical adult trachea has between 16 and 20 of these rings. The inner surface of the trachea is covered with a mucous membrane. In the posterior wall of the trachea, a thin band of tissue called the *trachealis muscle* supports the open ends of the tracheal rings. The esophagus lies just behind the trachea.

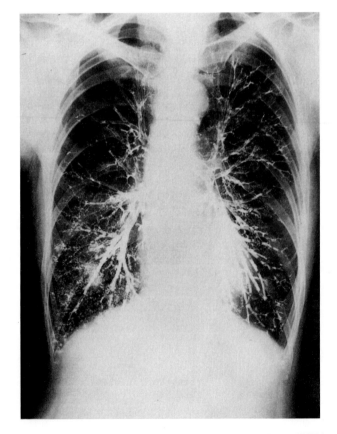

FIG. 9-13 Normal bronchogram (see text for description). (From Wilkins RL, Pierson DJ: The heart and blood vessels. In Pierson DJ, Kacmarek RM, eds: *Foundations of respiratory care,* New York, 1992, Churchill Livingstone.)

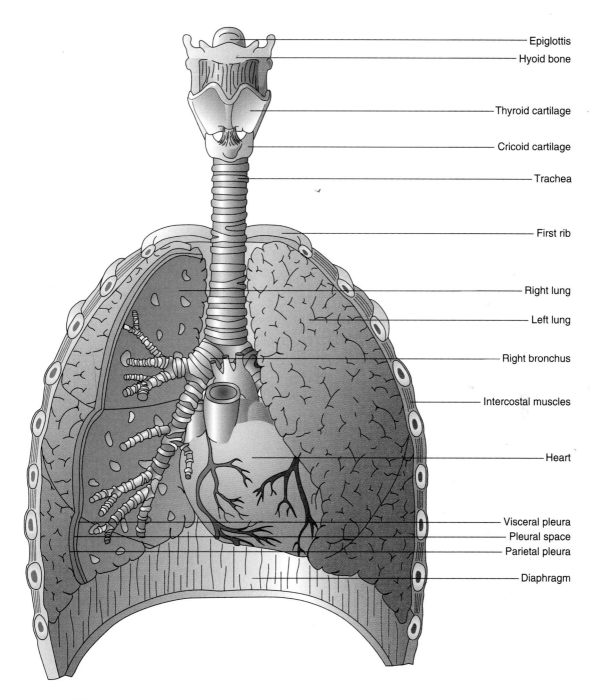

FIG. 9-14   Anatomical relationship of the larynx, trachea, lungs, heart, rib cage, and diaphragm.

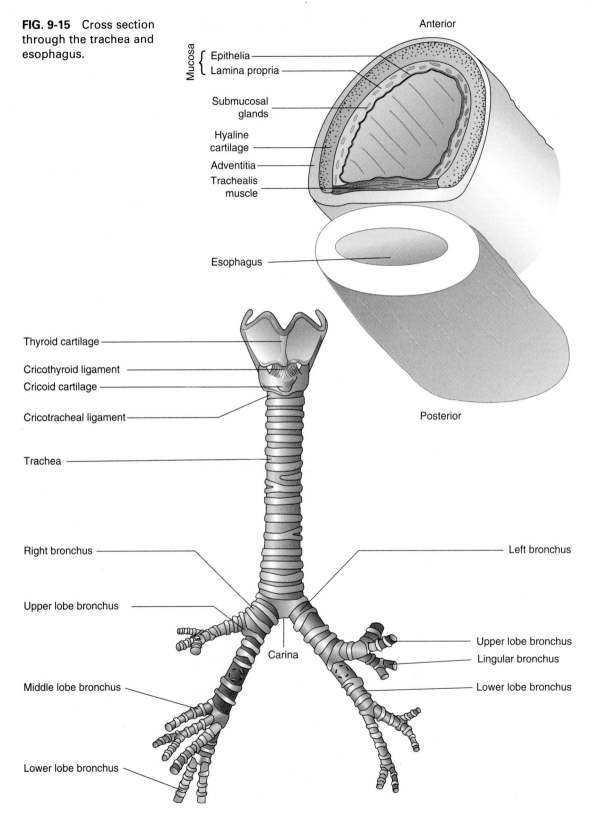

FIG. 9-15 Cross section through the trachea and esophagus.

Mucosa
{ Epithelia
Lamina propria

Submucosal glands

Hyaline cartilage

Adventitia

Trachealis muscle

Anterior

Esophagus

Posterior

Thyroid cartilage

Cricothyroid ligament

Cricoid cartilage

Cricotracheal ligament

Trachea

Right bronchus

Upper lobe bronchus

Middle lobe bronchus

Lower lobe bronchus

Carina

Left bronchus

Upper lobe bronchus

Lingular bronchus

Lower lobe bronchus

FIG. 9-16   Major airways of the tracheobronchial tree.

The trachea normally moves. The cartilaginous rings armor the trachea so that it does not collapse during exhalation. Some compression does occur when the pressure around the trachea becomes positive. During a strong cough, for example, the trachea is capable of some compression and even collapse. The negative pressure generated around the trachea during inhalation causes it to expand slightly.

The trachea branches into right and left main stem bronchi (Fig. 9-16). At the base of the trachea, the last cartilaginous ring that forms the bifurcation for the two bronchi is called the **carina.** The carina is an important landmark that is used to identify the level of the trachea from which the two main stem bronchi branch off. Normally this is just below the level of the aortic arch. The right bronchus branches off from the trachea at an angle of about 20 to 30 degrees, and the left bronchus branches off at an angle of about 45 to 55 degrees. The right bronchus's lower angle of branching results in a greater frequency of foreign body passage into the right lung because of the more direct pathway.

Each bronchus conveys gas to and from one lung. It enters the lung with the pulmonary vessels, lymph vessels, and nerves through a region on the medial surface called the **hilum.** The bronchus branches repeatedly within each lung to supply gas to separate regions of each lung.

The lungs have an apex and base and are subdivided by fissures into lobes (Figs. 9-17 and 18). The right lung is divided by horizontal and oblique fissures into upper, middle, and lower lobes. The left lung is divided by a single oblique fissure into an upper and lower lobe. Although the left lung lacks a middle

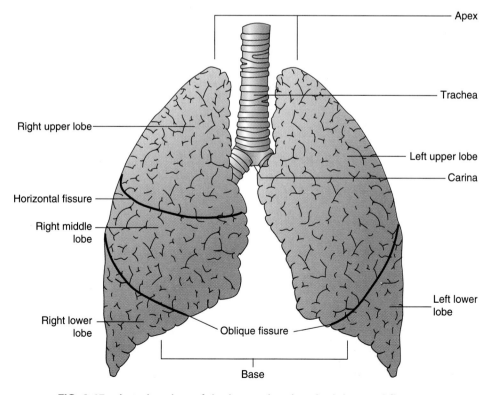

FIG. 9-17 Anterior view of the lungs showing the lobes and fissures.

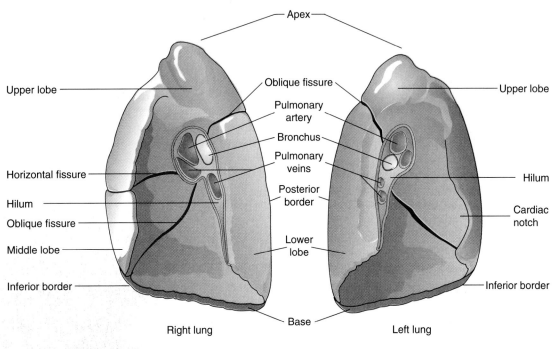

FIG. 9-18 Medial surface of each lung.

 Table 9-3 Bronchopulmonary Segments*

Right Lung		Left Lung	
Segment	**Location**	**Segment**	**Location**
RIGHT UPPER LOBE		**LEFT UPPER LOBE**	
Apical	1	Apical-posterior	1 and 2
Posterior	2	Anterior	3
Anterior	3		
RIGHT MIDDLE LOBE		**LINGULAR DIVISION**	
Lateral	4	Superior lingula	4
Medial	5	Inferior lingula	5
RIGHT LOWER LOBE		**LEFT LOWER LOBE**	
Superior	6	Superior	6
Medial basal	7	Anteromedial	7 and 8
Anterior basal	8	Lateral basal	9
Lateral basal	9	Posterior basal	10
Posterior basal	10		

*See Fig. 9-19 for anatomic location of each segment.

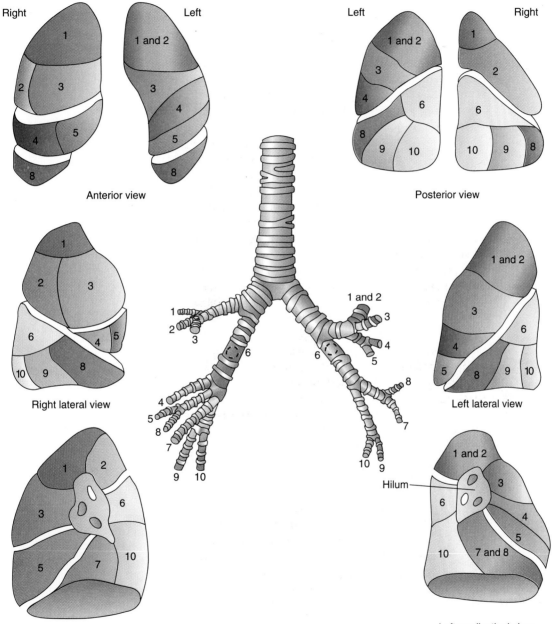

FIG. 9-19 Bronchopulmonary segmental divisions of the lungs. (See Table 9-3 for names of individual segments.)

lobe, it possesses a subdivision within the upper lobe called the **lingula** that corresponds developmentally to the right middle lobe. Each lobe receives air through one lobar bronchus. The right lung is approximately 15% larger than the left lung because of the position of the heart, which extends into the left hemithorax.

The lobes are subdivided further into bronchopulmonary segments (Fig. 9-19 and Table 9-3). Each segment is supplied with gas from a single segmental bronchus. Some con-

DIAGNOSTIC FOCUS

Bronchogenic Carcinoma

A 61-year-old business man was in good health until about 3 weeks ago, when he developed a productive cough of yellow-green sputum, some dyspnea, weight loss, and a general feeling of being ill (malaise). He is thin but well developed. His vital signs were as follows:

Heart rate	128/min
Blood pressure	146/88
Respiratory rate	31/min
Temperature	100° F

His breath sounds were diminished throughout the right lung.

He reported that he smoked one to two packs of cigarettes per day for the past 43 years and used alcohol moderately. A 12-lead electrocardiogram revealed a sinus tachycardia with occasional premature ventricular contractions and no signs of myocardial ischemia or infarction. A chest x-ray showed a 3-cm mass in the right hilar region with generalized loss of air volume and atelectasis throughout the right lung. The patient was given broad-spectrum antibiotics for what appeared to be pneumonia that was complicating the mass in the right lung. The patient underwent fiberoptic bronchoscopy to evaluate the mass.

Fiberoptic bronchoscopy is a diagnostic and therapeutic technique that entails the use of a flexible scope that is 5 mm in diameter, about 1 m long, and equipped with a viewing channel, a light channel, and suction/instrument channels. The viewing and light channels are comprised of bundles of fine glass fibers. The scope is capable of being bent by the operator so that it can be advanced into and around anatomic structures. It can be used to observe the airways, to collect specimens of fluid or tissue, and to clear mucous plugs from airways.

The patient was sedated and given supplemental oxygen and underwent bronchoscopy on an outpatient basis. His larynx, vocal cords, trachea, and carina all appeared normal. Upon advancing the scope into the right main stem bronchus, a tumor was observed to be encroaching into the airway and blocking about 80% of the lumen. A biopsy was taken from the tumor wall with a miniature forceps without excessive bleeding. The biopsy was sent to the laboratory and was found to be dominated by squamous cell carcinoma. The next day the patient was admitted to the hospital for surgical evaluation and treatment. A bone scan was performed and was found to be negative. A mediastinoscopy was done to collect mediastinal lymph nodes to determine if tumor cells had spread from the lung. The lymph nodes were negative for cancer cells. A right pneumonectomy was performed to remove the entire right lung along with the tumor. The patient then underwent radiation therapy to the mediastinum as a prophylactic measure to kill any cells that may have escaped the lung. The patient recovered from these procedures with some exercise limitations because of the loss of the right lung.

troversy exists over the exact number of segments. Some anatomists believe that each lung has 10 segments whereas others maintain that the right lung has 10 segments and the left lung has 8. Knowledge of segmental anatomy is important in the physical examination of a patient to identify the location of a defect such as an infection site or tumor mass in the lungs.

The airways continue to divide as they penetrate deeper into the lungs. The segmental bronchi bifurcate into about 40 subsegmental bronchi, and these divide into hundreds of smaller **b**ronchi. Thousands of bronchioles branch from the smaller bronchi. Bronchioles do not possess cartilage in their walls.

Tens of thousands of terminal bronchioles arise from the bronchioles. Terminal bronchioles are the smallest conducting airways and function to supply gas to the respiratory zone of the lung.

Layers of the Airway Wall

All of the conducting airways have walls that are constructed of three layers (Figs. 9-20 and 21): an inner layer that forms a mucous membrane called the **mucosa** and a submucosa comprised of connective tissue and bronchial glands, a middle layer containing smooth muscle fibers that wrap around the airway,

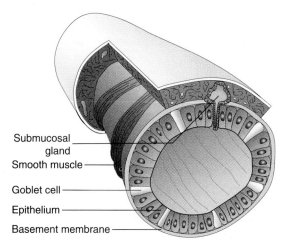

Submucosal gland

Smooth muscle

Goblet cell

Epithelium

Basement membrane

FIG. 9-20 Cross section of a bronchiole.

and an outer covering of connective tissue called the *adventitia*. The cartilaginous rings found in larger airways are located in the adventitia.

Mucous Membrane

The mucosa is comprised of different types of specialized epithelial cells that sit on top of a basement membrane. The most common type of epithelia is the numerous pseudostratified, ciliated, columnar epithelia. Below the pseudostratified cells is a layer of basal cells that mature into pseudostratified cells. Dispersed between the pseudostratified epithelia are mucus-producing goblet cells, serous cells, Clara cells, and the openings of submucosal bronchial glands. The bronchial glands are exocrine glands formed by secretory epithelial cells that sit on an invaginated portion of the basement membrane, which extends down into the lamina propria and into the submucosa. The bronchial glands are wrapped with smooth musclelike cells called *basket cells.* Basket cells contract and squeeze the bronchial gland when they receive signals from parasympathetic nerve fibers.

The secretory cells and bronchial glands produce about 100 ml of mucus per day. This amount can more than double with airway diseases such as chronic bronchitis. Mucus is spread over the surface of the mucus membrane to a depth of only 10 to 20 μm and is propelled by the ciliated epithelia toward the pharynx. The outer layer of mucus, called the *gel layer,* is more gelatinous. The inner layer is much more fluidlike and is referred to as the sol layer. Mucus produced by the respiratory tract is 95% water and 5% solute. The solutes include 3% protein (predominately glycoproteins), 1% lipids (primarily phospholipids), and 1% minerals (mainly inorganic electrolytes). The glycoprotein and water content of mucus gives it its viscoelastic gel nature. This refers to the ability of mucus to deform and spread when force is applied to it. It is also sticky and traps particles that make contact with it.

Mucus functions to protect the underlying tissue. It helps prevent excessive amounts of water from moving into and out of the epithelia. It shields the epithelia from direct contact with potentially toxic materials and microorganisms. It acts like sticky flypaper to trap particles that make contact with it. This makes mucus an important part of the pulmonary defenses. The regulation of mucus production and its composition is poorly understood.

The ciliated, pseudostratified epithelia play a crucial role in the defense of the respiratory tract by propelling mucus toward the pharynx. Ciliated cells are found in the nasal cavity as well as all the airways from the larynx to the terminal bronchioles. Each of the pseudostratified cells possesses about 200 cilia on its luminal surface. Under the electron microscope the surface of the mucus membrane looks like a "shag carpet" of cilia with about

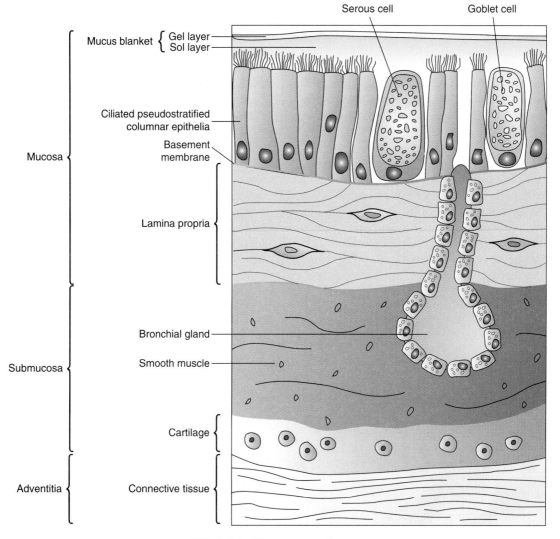

FIG. 9-21   Mucous membrane.

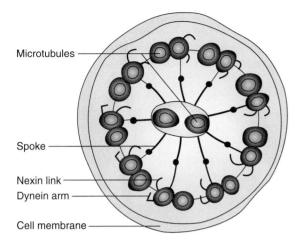

Microtubules

Spoke

Nexin link

Dynein arm

Cell membrane

FIG. 9-22 Cross section through a cilium showing one central and nine outer pairs of microtubules that interact to cause the whipping action of a cilium.

1 to 2 billion cilia per square centimeter. Each cilium is an extension of the cell with an average length of about 6 μm and a diameter of about 0.2 μm. A cross-sectional view through the cilium reveals it to be constructed of one inner pair and nine outer pairs of microtubules that are encased in the cell membrane (Fig. 9-22). The outer pairs are interlinked by a filamentous protein called *nexin*. From each of the outer pairs of microtubules, protein filaments (called *dynein*) extend toward the adjacent pair of microtubules. Each of the outer pairs also extends a protein spoke toward the central pair of microtubules. The presence of magnesium and adenosine triphosphate within the cilium causes the dynein arms and spokes to attach and slide along the outer and inner microtubules much like the action of

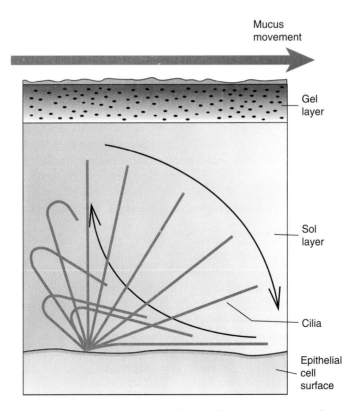

Mucus movement

Gel layer

Sol layer

Cilia

Epithelial cell surface

FIG. 9-23 Whipping action of a cilium within the sol layer of mucus.

actin and myosin. This action results in rapid bending of the cilium that resembles a whipping motion (Fig. 9-23). The cilia "stroke" at a rate of about 20 times per second. The stroking action of millions of cilia propels the surrounding mucus at a speed of about 2 cm/min. This action is commonly referred to as the *ciliary escalator.* It propels mucus and trapped particles over the surface of the airways toward the pharynx. The control and coordination of ciliary motion is not understood and is one of the many fascinating properties of pulmonary tissues.

The production of mucus and the rate of ciliary beating are sensitive to a variety of conditions and chemicals. Mucus production increases when the respiratory tract is irritated by particles and various chemicals and during increased parasympathetic nervous stimulation. Ciliary beating can be effectively slowed or even stopped if the viscosity of the sol layer is increased by exposure to dry gas. Ciliary motion is also stopped following exposure to smoke, high concentrations of inhaled oxygen, and drugs such as atropine.

● STRUCTURE AND ORGANIZATION OF RESPIRATORY ZONE AIRWAYS

Respiratory Zone

The airways beyond the terminal bronchioles are classified as respiratory zone airways (Fig. 9-24). These airways include the respiratory bronchioles, alveolar ducts, and **alveoli.** A single-terminal bronchiole supplies a cluster of respiratory airways. Collectively this unit is referred to as the acinus, or primary lobule. Each acinus is comprised of numerous respiratory bronchioles, alveolar ducts, and approximately 2000 alveoli (Fig. 9-25). The adult lung is thought to contain about 150,000 acini. Each acinus is supplied with pulmonary blood flow from a pulmonary arteriole, and blood is drained away from several acini to a pul-

monary venule. In addition, each acinus is equipped with a lymphatic drainage vessel and nervous fibers. These features make the acinus the functional unit of the lungs.

Respiratory bronchioles have walls that are formed from flattened squamous epithelia and a thin outer layer of connective tissue. They have some ciliated cells at the connection with the terminal bronchiole and generally lack mucus-producing cells and smooth muscle. In their walls are small outpouchings known as alveoli. The alveoli and their pulmonary capillary bed enable the respiratory bronchioles to carry out gas exchange.

Alveolar Ducts, Sacs, and Alveoli

Alveolar ducts branch from each respiratory bronchiole. Alveolar ducts are tiny airways only 1 to 0.5 mm long. Their walls are comprised entirely of alveoli. Each alveolar duct ends in a cluster of alveoli, which is frequently referred to as an *alveolar sac.* Each alveolar sac opens into about 10 to 16 alveoli.

The adult lungs contain about 300 million alveoli. Each alveolus is formed by walls or septa that are shared with surrounding alveoli (Fig. 9-26). The alveolar septa are covered with extremely flat squamous epithelia called *Type I alveolar cells.* These cells form a patchworklike surface. Although they represent only about 8% of all the cells found in the alveolar region, the Type I cells cover about 93% of the alveolar surface. The diameter of the average alveolus is about 250 μm.

Interspersed on the alveolar surface are cuboidal epithelia called *Type II alveolar cells* (Fig. 9-27). These cells are twice as numerous as the Type I cells, yet they occupy only 7% of the alveolar surface. Type II cells manufacture **surfactant,** store it in vesicles called *lamellated bodies,* and secrete it onto the alveolar surface. Surfactant is primarily comprised of phospholipids and functions to reduce the surface tension of the alveolus. Insufficient surfactant production leads to alveolar collapse.

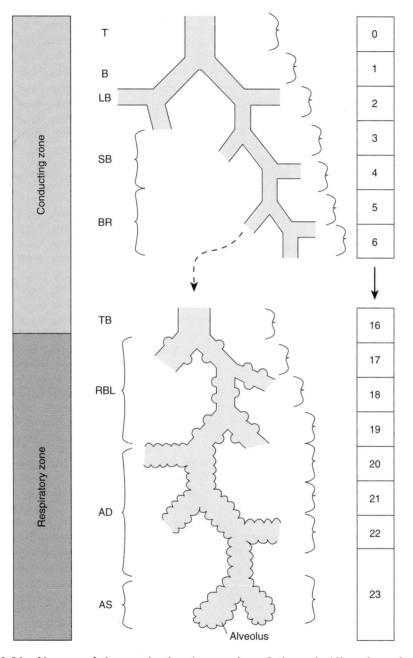

FIG. 9-24 Airways of the conducting (generations 0 through 16) and respiratory (generations 17 through 23) zones. *T,* Trachea; *B,* right and left bronchi; *LB,* lobar bronchi; *SB,* segmental and subsegmental bronchi; *BR,* bronchioles; *TB,* terminal bronchioles; *RBL,* respiratory bronchioles; *AD,* alveolar ducts; and *AS,* alveolar sacs.

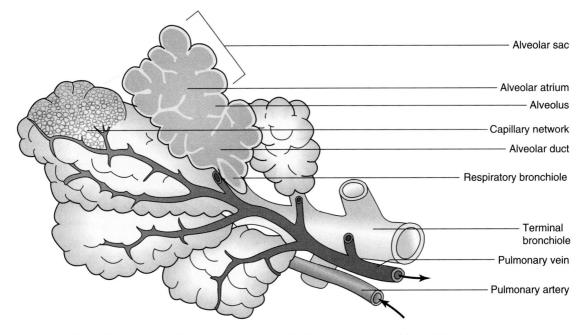

FIG. 9-25 Acinus of the lung is comprised of a single terminal bronchiole, numerous respiratory bronchioles, alveolar ducts, sacs of alveoli, and about 2000 alveoli. Pulmonary blood flow is delivered to it by a pulmonary arteriole and drained from it by a pulmonary venule.

Within the interalveolar septum is an interstitial space that contains the pulmonary capillaries. Also found in the interstitial space toward the opening of each alveolus is a collagen fiber ring that holds the "mouth" of the alveolus open. Small openings are located in the alveolar septa. Some of the openings allow gas to move from one alveolus to another. These are called the **pores of Kohn.** Other openings connect alveoli with second respiratory bronchioles. These passageways are called the **canals of Lambert.** All of the alveolar openings facilitate the movement of gas and help maintain alveolar volume.

Other cells are present in the alveolus. Alveolar macrophages wonder through this region and function as phagocytic cells that engulf particles, debris, and foreign cells. Different types of interstitial cells are found in the

septa of the alveoli. Some of these cells manufacture **collagen** and elastin protein fibers. These fibers form a septal fiber system within the interstitial space that supports alveolar structure.

Alveolar-Capillary Membrane

Gas exchange between alveolar gas and pulmonary blood takes place across the alveolar-capillary membrane (Fig. 9-28). This membrane is stretched over a surface area of more than 70 m² and is only 1 to 2 μm thick. This makes the membrane more than 40 times larger than the area covered by skin and 2000 times thinner.

The alveolar-capillary membrane is comprised of a number of different layers. The outermost layer is a thin film of fluid comprised primarily of surfactant. Below the

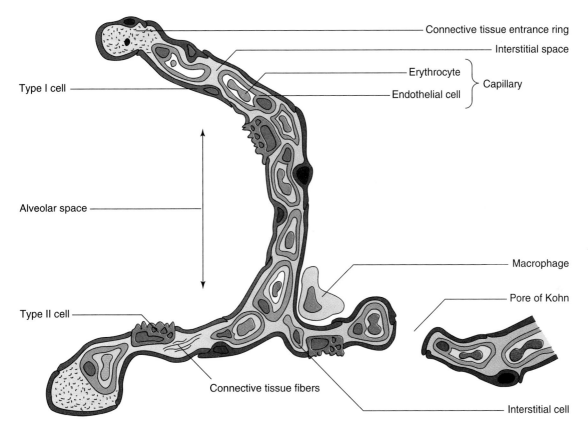

Connective tissue entrance ring

Interstitial space

Erythrocyte

Endothelial cell

Capillary

Type I cell

Alveolar space

Macrophage

Pore of Kohn

Type II cell

Connective tissue fibers

Interstitial cell

FIG. 9-26 Highly magnified view of a cross section through an alveolus (see text for description).

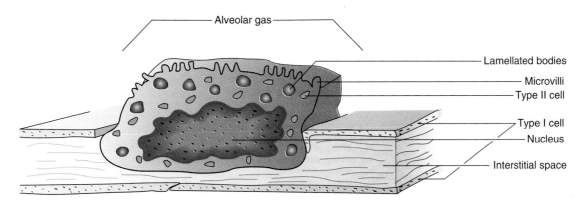

Alveolar gas

Lamellated bodies

Microvilli

Type II cell

Type I cell

Nucleus

Interstitial space

FIG. 9-27 Highly magnified view of Type II pneumocyte cells found in and around the alveolar-capillary membrane. They manufacture surfactant (primarily the phospholipid diphosphatidylcholine), store it in vesicles called *lamellated bodies,* and secrete it onto the alveolar surface. Surfactant functions to reduce the surface tension of the alveolus.

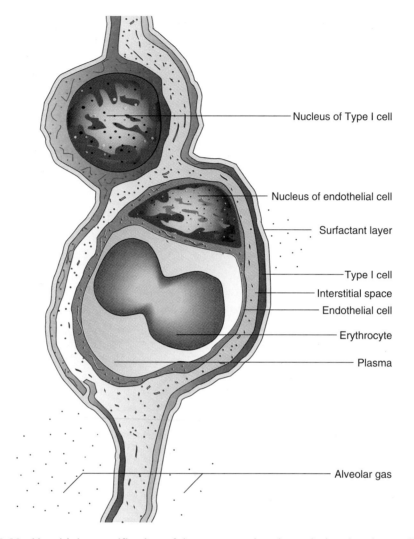

Nucleus of Type I cell

Nucleus of endothelial cell

Surfactant layer

Type I cell

Interstitial space

Endothelial cell

Erythrocyte

Plasma

Alveolar gas

FIG. 9-28 Very high magnification of the cross section through the alveolar-capillary membrane found in the septum between two alveoli.

fluid layer is the thinly stretched Type I cell. The delicate structure of the Type I cell makes them highly susceptible to injury from toxins carried to them by either airborne or bloodborne routes. These cells sit on an extremely thin basement membrane. The **interstitial space** and its contents lay below. This space is also very thin over most of the membrane. Regions of the interstitial space are thicker and contain connective tissue fibers and various types of cells. The capillary and its **endothelial cell** wall lie within the interstitial space. The endothelial cell is also a very thin cell and sits on a basement membrane like the Type I cell. Within the endothelial cell lies the **plasma** and finally the **erythrocyte.** Oxygen and carbon dioxide cross through the membrane during the transit to and from the hemoglobin and plasma of blood.

Gas exchange across the alveolar-capillary membrane can be disturbed by a number of different changes. The membrane can thicken as a result of fluid, fibers, cells, or debris depositing in the alveolus or the interstitial space. Surface area can decrease if alveoli lose their gas volume and collapse or if they rupture and decrease in number. The consequence of these changes is impaired gas exchange.

 HOW THE LUNG NERVOUS SYSTEM IS ORGANIZED

The lungs have a rich supply of sensors and motor nerve fibers that can be organized into efferent (incoming) and afferent (outgoing) fibers.

Efferent information is brought to various tissues in the lung by the sympathetic and parasympathetic fibers of the autonomic nervous system. These fibers travel into the mediastinum and penetrate the lung through the hilum. They branch out and follow the airway and blood vessels into the lung. Both branches supply nerve signals and release neurotransmitters onto the smooth muscles of the airways and blood vessels and onto the secretory cells of the mucus membrane.

Efferent sympathetic and parasympathetic nerve signals cause contrasting effects. Sympathetic stimulation causes the release of norepinephrine onto the smooth muscle of airways, vessels, and bronchial glands. This results in activation of beta-adrenergic receptors that cause bronchodilation. A weaker alpha-adrenergic vasoconstriction and inhibition of bronchial gland secretion also occurs. Parasympathetic activity results in the release of acetylcholine onto the various smooth muscles and activation of cholinergic receptors.

This causes bronchoconstriction, vasodilation, and mucus production. The opposing actions of the sympathetic and parasympathetic nervous systems bring about some level of control over air flow, blood flow, and mucus flow within the lung. Various conditions cause one system to dominate and thus influence lung function.

Afferent fibers carry information from sensors located on the surface and in the walls of the airways back to the central nervous system by way of the vagus nerve. **Irritant receptors** are found on the surface of the upper and first portion of the tracheobronchial tree. They respond to physical and chemical stimuli to elicit cough, gag, bronchoconstriction, and mucus production when irritated. **Stretch receptors** are located in the smooth muscle of the airway walls and generate signals when stretched by inflation. Injury to or fluid accumulation in the alveolar, airway, and blood vessel walls can cause C-fiber stimulation. Their signals cause the sensation of **dyspnea** (difficult breathing) and rapid breathing.

HOW THE RESPIRATORY TRACT IS DEFENDED

The delicate tissues of the conducting and respiratory airways are exposed to more than 10,000 L of air per day. This air may contain infectious microorganisms, toxic dust particles, or hazardous chemicals. Exposure to this foreign material can result in inflammation, necrosis, and cancerous pulmonary changes that can spread to systemic tissues. To prevent this from happening, the respiratory tract is equipped with a wide array of nonspecific and specific defenses to prevent and limit tissue injury, infection, and the spread of cancer cells (Box 9-2). These mechanisms are so effective that foreign microorganisms are not normally found below the larynx.

Traumatic Chest Injury

A 38-year-old woman was involved in a motor vehicle accident and received blunt-force injuries to the chest. She was extricated from the wreck, stabilized at the scene, and air evacuated to the nearest trauma center. On admission, she was found to be agitated and in obvious respiratory distress. Her right humerus was fractured, and her vital signs were as follows:

Heart rate	111/min
Blood pressure	92/60
Respiratory rate	38/min
Temperature	98° F

Her chest moved in a highly abnormal motion with the left side of the chest collapsing inward and the right side of the chest expanding outward during inspiration instead of in a unified manner. This paradoxical motion is known as a flail chest. A chest x-ray revealed that ribs 4 through 8 were fractured and that a hemopneumothorax was present in the left side of the chest.

The patient was sedated, her trachea was intubated with an endotracheal tube, and she was placed on mechanical ventilation. Two chest tubes were placed into the left pleural space and attached to suction to remove the air and blood that had collapsed the left lung.

Approximately 300 ml of air and 150 ml of blood was evacuated from the left pleural space. A repeat chest x-ray revealed that the left lung was about 80% reexpanded. It also showed that the left lung had patchy infiltrates, which are consistent with lung contusion. The blood pressure improved with the infusion of fluid and several units of blood. She was transferred to the intensive care unit (ICU) where she was further stabilized. Over the next 24 hours she developed adult respiratory distress syndrome (ARDS). This was managed with careful fluid administration, antibiotics, and ventilatory support. On the fourth day after the accident the physician decided to surgically "plate" the broken ribs with titanium straps that were attached to each rib to stabilize the fractures and aid their healing. The patient remained in the ICU for the next 2 weeks, and during this time she was supported with intravenous fluids, pain medications, intravenous feeding, and mechanical ventilation while the ARDS resolved and her injuries continued to heal. She eventually was weaned from ventilatory support, transferred to the surgical floor of the hospital, and discharged 27 days after admission. The titanium rods were eventually removed and she recovered.

Nonspecific Defenses

The respiratory tract possesses a large number of nonspecific defenses to protect itself. These mechanisms do not stop specific types of foreign particles. They function more generally against a wide array of chemicals, particles, and microorganisms.

Warming and Humidification

The delicate respiratory zone airways and tracheobronchial tree are sensitive to the temperature and humidity content of gases that enter them. The upper airway is capable of heating the gas to body temperature and humidifying it to 100% relative humidity before it reaches the carina. Mouth breathing cold air results in cooler gas reaching further into the tracheobronchial tree. In some people, mouth breathing cold air can trigger bronchospasm. Gas that is not humidified completely can cause the mucus blanket to thicken and become more difficult to move. As a consequence,

BOX 9-2

Pulmonary Defenses

NONSPECIFIC DEFENSES
Warming and humidification
Filtration and clearance
Reflex actions
Secretions
Inflammation
Cellular defense

SPECIFIC DEFENSES
Antibody-mediated immunity
Cell-mediated immunity

mucus collects and blocks small airways, causing reduced ventilation in those regions beyond the blockage.

Filtration and Clearance

The term **aerosol** refers to liquid or solid particles that are suspended in air. Aerosols that are less than 10 μm in diameter pose the greatest threat to the respiratory tract because they can penetrate furthest into the lung. Aerosol deposition in the delicate respiratory zone of the lung is prevented by the filtering mechanism of the upper airway and tracheobronchial tree.

The nasal cavity acts as a first-stage filter by removing essentially all of the particles larger than 10 μm in diameter. Particles in the gas stream of the upper airway are forced to rapidly change their direction of movement as they travel through the airway. Particles also possess mass and, when in motion, they generate inertia. Inertia keeps particles moving in a straight line as they travel through the bends in the airway. Large aerosols are unable to complete all the turns and subsequently deposit on the airway wall. This is termed *inertial impaction* and is the primary factor behind filtration of particles in the upper airway.

Aerosols are also subject to the effects of gravity and settle out of the gas with time. This process, known as sedimentation, occurs more rapidly with more dense particles and in relatively still air. Sedimentation is most influential with particles between 0.2 and 5 μm in diameter and is the principal cause of particle deposition in the small airways of the tracheobronchial tree.

The upper airway and tracheobronchial tree protect the respiratory airways by filtering out most of the particles that are larger than 5 μm. Smaller particles can penetrate to the alveoli region and deposit there. Aerosol particles are continuously bombarded by the surrounding gas molecules. This causes small particles to move randomly in the air with a movement known as Brownian motion. This motion occurs with particles smaller than 1 μm in diameter. Brownian motion causes these small particles to make contact with the walls of the smallest airways. This process of diffusive impaction is an important cause of particle deposition in the respiratory zone airways. Particles in the 2- to 0.5-μm size have the greatest likelihood of reaching and depositing in the alveoli. Aerosols that are smaller than 0.1 μm in diameter have a greater probability of entering and exiting the respiratory tract without depositing on the walls of any airways.

Deposition of particles in the nasal cavity, tracheobronchial tree, and alveoli are cleared by two different mechanisms. The mucus layer over the airways of the nasal cavity and tracheobronchial tree protects the underlying tissue and traps particles that are deposited there. The ciliary action propels the mucus coating toward the pharynx where it is swallowed or expectorated. Clearance rates of particles that deposit in the tracheobronchial tree average about 500 minutes but vary widely from subject to subject. Those individuals with a history of chronic cigarette smoking have fewer ciliated cells and have impaired ciliary function. This causes poor clearance of particles and partially explains why these individuals have a higher frequency of respiratory tract infections when compared with nonsmokers.

Ciliated cells are not found along the respiratory zone airways. Particles that deposit in this region are cleared by phagocytic macrophages. Macrophages either digest the particles on the spot or carry them to terminal bronchioles where the ciliary escalator sweeps them to the pharynx for removal. Some particles are carried away through the lymphatic vessels by macrophages or as naked particles. Other particles that deposit in the alveolar region never leave the lung. Large and irregularly shaped particles, such as asbestos and fiberglass fibers, can be trapped in the interstitial spaces or lymphatic channels where they can remain for many years.

Reflex Actions

Irritation of the respiratory tract can elicit a number of different muscular reflexes. These reflexes are designed to prevent entry or to expel irritating foreign material. Virtually all of the respiratory reflexes are caused by either mechanical or chemical stimulation of irritant receptors that lie in the mucosa.

The sneeze is a sudden expulsion of air through the nasal cavity following stimulation of irritant receptors in the nasal cavity. Coughing occurs when irritant receptors in the pharynx, trachea (especial around the carina), and large bronchi are excited by mechanical and chemical stimuli. Irritant receptors cause nerve impulses to be transmitted to the medulla oblongata through the laryngeal and vagus nerves. The cough is comprised of a series of events: (1) deep inspiration, (2) closure of the glottis, (3) muscular constriction of the thoracic cavity, (4) elevation of intralung pressure, and (5) rapid opening of the glottis. This results in sudden high-velocity gas flow through the airways that is capable of shearing mucus from the airway wall and expelling it into the pharynx and mouth. The ability to

deep breath and cough is essential for pulmonary health. Without this ability, mortality is not far off.

Mechanical irritation to the base of the tongue, hypopharynx, and larynx triggers a gag reflex. This is also a vagal nerve- and medulla oblongata-mediated reflex that causes the muscles of the larynx to constrict and close the glottis and prevents foreign bodies from entering the lower airway.

Gag and cough reflexes are depressed when the nervous system is depressed by narcotics, anesthetics, and alcohol or following a stroke or head injury. Depression of the gag reflex leads to an increased risk of aspirating foreign material that can block or irritate the airways or cause an infection.

Like the cough and gag reflexes, a vagal nerve reflex can cause **bronchoconstriction** as a result of irritant receptor stimulation. Sensitive secretory cells known as **mast cells,** located in the mucosa of the airway, can trigger bronchoconstriction when they are exposed to certain irritants. They trigger this reaction by release of various chemicals (e.g., histamine and leukotrienes).

Bronchoconstriction helps prevent irritating material from penetrating further into the lung. Partial closure of the airway actually results in greater air flow and enhances mucus movement during exhalation. Although the process of irritant-stimulated bronchoconstriction is normal, severe reactions result in the symptoms commonly known as **asthma.**

Secretions

The surfaces of the airways and alveoli are not covered with the same fluids. Mucus, which lines the nasal cavity and tracheobronchial tree, acts as a moving mechanical barrier that eliminates trapped particles and helps prevent toxic materials from reaching the delicate epithelia below. Its secretion is increased in response to irritant receptor. Irritation of the digestive tract by spicy foods and milk products also triggers mucus production through a vagal nerve reflex.

The alveolar surface is coated with an extremely thin film of surfactant. This material reduces surface tension and helps repel water from the alveoli. In addition, it is known to enhance the phagocytic activity of macrophages.

Several antimicrobial chemicals are secreted by the respiratory tract. Digestive enzymes, such as lysozyme, are secreted by a number of cells. They are capable of breaking down the cell wall of bacteria. Several types of **interferon** are secreted by cells in the respiratory tract. These glycoproteins cause antiviral activity in the cells of the respiratory tract.

Like other tissues, pulmonary tissue is capable of inflammation when it is injured. Lung injury causes local blood vessels to dilate, capillaries to become leaky, and airway smooth muscle to constrict. As this occurs, fluid, proteins, and phagocytic cells move into the injured region. Initially blood flow is high and then almost stops as a result of increased blood viscosity because of water loss and the formation of blood clots in the microcirculation. These actions effectively dilute and minimize the spread of toxins, facilitate the clearance of cellular debris, and set the stage for tissue healing. The consequence of pulmonary inflammation is a swollen region of lung that has poor gas exchange capability.

A variety of chemical mediators are produced by injured lung tissue, mast cells, and leukocytes to cause the inflammatory response. **Histamine** is released by mast cells, basophils, and platelets. It causes vasodilation and increased vessel permeability. The kinins (e.g., bradykinin) are a group of small proteins that causes vascular changes and chemoattraction of leukocytes. **Complement** proteins are found in plasma and some are known to cross the capillary wall and enter the interstitial space and airway surface of the lung. Complement proteins stimulate vascular changes, promote cell lysis, cause the

release of lysozyme, enhance phagocytosis, and stimulate mast cell release of other mediators of inflammation. **Prostaglandins** (e.g., **prostaglandin E**) are fatty acids that play a role in the inflammatory process by causing vascular changes and prompt phagocytic migration and act as pyrogens by triggering fever. Leukotrienes are released by leukocytes in response to lung injury. These fatty acids are chemically similar to the prostaglandins and cause vascular changes, attract leukocytes, and stimulate bronchoconstriction and mucus production. The leukotrienes play an important role in the cause of asthma.

The lung also has the capacity to produce chemicals that protect it from the potentially damaging effects of phagocytic cells that invade the lung during inflammation. These cells utilize powerful proteolytic enzymes and oxidants to digest microorganisms and particles they have consumed. Damaged and dying phagocytes can leak these digestive chemicals into the lung and cause greater lung injury. Pulmonary diseases such as **emphysema** and **adult respiratory distress syndrome** have been linked to this mechanism of lung injury. Antiproteolytics and antioxidants help prevent these disorders. They are normally brought to the region of inflammation by the pulmonary blood supply and are secreted by local cells.

Excessive proteolytic enzyme release by the phagocytes can result in the breakdown of the proteins elastin and **collagen** that form the support fibers in the alveolar walls. Loss of these fibers results in alveolar expansion and rupture and the development of emphysema. The action of the proteolytic enzymes is normally inhibited by an antiproteolytic enzyme called **alpha-1-antitrypsin.** In some unfortunate individuals, a genetic defect is known to result in an alpha-1-antitrypsin deficiency. As a consequence, frequent lung infections stimulate frequent phagocytic invasions and the release of proteolytic enzymes that go uninhibited and thus damage elastin and collagen fibers. This defect is thought to be responsible for about 10% of emphysema cases. Recently, genetic engineering has brought about the availability of human alpha-1-antitrypsin. This can be given intravenously as a replacement and should slow the destructive effects of the genetic deficiency.

The lung is also exposed to powerful oxidants like hydrogen peroxide, oxygen radicals, and hydroxyl radicals. These toxic chemicals are produced within the phagocytes and can leak into the lung. In addition, the lung is exposed to oxygen radicals that form in the air in low concentrations. Oxidants are chemically reactive and are toxic to all the cells of the lung. They are implicated in the cause of a form of pulmonary edema known as *adult respiratory distress syndrome*. To help prevent oxidant injury, the lung produces or has a number of antioxidants available. These include superoxide dysmutase, catalase, alpha-tocopherol, ascorbic acid, reduced nicotinamide adenine dinucleotide phosphate, and others. However, the antioxidant system of the lung can be overwhelmed when exposed to excessive amounts of toxins such as breathing higher concentrations of oxygen (e.g., more than 70% at 1 atm of pressure) for several days. The lung injury associated with breathing high concentrations of oxygen is known as **pulmonary oxygen toxicity.**

Cellular Defense

Several types of cells contribute to the defense of the lungs. Infectious microorganisms and toxic particles are inhibited from entering the pulmonary circulation and lymphatics by the epithelia that cover all of the interior surfaces of the lungs. Injuries that result in loss of the epithelia barrier increase the risk of pulmonary infection and dissemination of the infection to the systemic tissues. Phagocytic **neutrophils** and **monocytes** circulate through the lungs and are known to move into lung tissue when the lungs are injured. They are drawn into the lung by the presence of various chemoattractant substances that are released by injured tissue.

The other major phagocyte that is responsible for removal of foreign particles and microorganisms is the alveolar **macrophage,** which patrols the interstitial spaces and airway, surfaces. Normally, they are found in higher numbers on the alveolar surfaces and are considered to be the primary phagocyte in the respiratory zone airways. Macrophages also secrete a large variety of chemical factors that promote the inflammatory process, leukocyte invasion, antibody production, and other defensive reactions. Reduced macrophage number and activity can occur as a result of emotional and physical stress. This reaction sets the stage for infection.

Specific Defenses

The immune response of eliminating a particular type of substance, cancer cell, or microorganism is the basis of the specific defense response. The immune system utilizes a highly complex set of reactions and cellular interactions that result in recognition and destruction of foreign substances. A foreign substance that triggers an immune response is called an *antigen.* Antigens typically have molecular weights greater than 8000 making many proteins, nucleic acids, and polysaccharides capable of eliciting an immune response. Groups of protein antigens, called *histocompatibility complexes,* are found on the surface of cells and are used by the immune system to differentiate between normal cells of the individual and foreign cells such as tumor cells or cells transplanted from another individual. Antibodies are specialized proteins formed by the immune system in response to exposure to an antigen. These proteins have the capability of binding to a specific antigen. Once bound in an antibody-antigen complex, the antigen is eliminated through a variety of different mechanisms.

Lymphocytes are the principal cells of the immune system. They respond in two general ways. One response is known as antibody-mediated immunity, or humoral immunity, where B lymphocytes secrete antibodies into body fluid. The other response is known as cell-mediated immunity, which involves a T-lymphocyte reaction. The immune system responds to an antigen by activating both of these responses and by developing memory cells to eliminate antigens encountered in the future. The response by these cells usually takes several days and during this time the toxic substance or foreign cells are battled by the nonspecific defenses.

Lymphocytes are found throughout the lungs in the pulmonary circulation, mucosa, lymphoid nodules in the airway walls, and in lymph nodes. Fluid, cells, and particles are carried out of the interstitial spaces of the lungs by lymphatic vessels. These vessels drain the fluid and other substances through numerous lymph nodes. Lymph nodes are found within and outside the lungs. Lymphatic drainage from the lungs is channeled through a maze of interconnected mediastinal and peritracheal nodes (Fig. 9-29) to the jugular and subclavian veins. Positioning lymphocytes in these different areas enables them to mount a specific immune reaction to foreign particles and cells that enter the lungs.

Antibody-Mediated Immunity

When antigens enter the body, they interact with B lymphocytes and macrophages to start antibody-mediated immunity. B lymphocytes bind to and engulf the invading antigen. At the same time, macrophages phagocytize the antigen and present a portion of the antigen to a particular T lymphocyte called a *T helper lymphocyte.* The T helper cell reacts by producing interleukins, also known as lymphokines, that stimulate the B lymphocyte to differentiate into plasma cells. Plasma cells secrete antibodies into lymph fluid and blood plasma. The antibodies drift throughout the body in blood plasma and lymph fluid and when they encounter the specific antigen, they bind to it and start its destruction.

The antibodies produced by this process are called the plasma **immunoglobulins (Ig).** They are classified into five types: IgA, IgD,

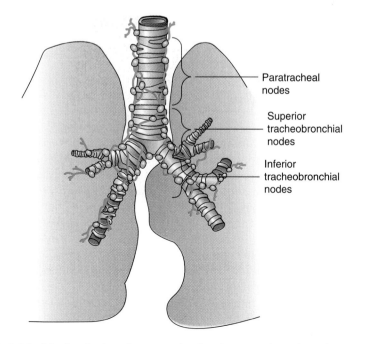

Paratracheal
nodes

Superior
tracheobronchial
nodes

Inferior
tracheobronchial
nodes

FIG. 9-29 Mediastinal and paratracheal pulmonary lymph nodes.

IgE, IgG, and IgM. Class IgA antibodies are the predominant antibodies found in fluids of the upper respiratory tract whereas IgG antibodies are found in greater concentration in the tracheobronchial and respiratory zone airways. The IgA and IgG antibodies function to neutralize viruses, bind to bacteria and reduce their attachment to epithelia, and neutralize toxins. Class IgE antibodies are highly involved with triggering asthmatic bronchoconstriction and mucus production. They are found on the surface of mast cells and function to sensitize these cells to specific antigens. When the specific antigens are encountered, the mast cells secrete a wide variety of inflammatory mediators that cause airway wall edema, bronchoconstriction, and mucus production. Class IgA and IgM antibodies are also found in respiratory tract fluid and are linked to antibacterial and antiviral activity.

Cell-Mediated Immunity

Viral- and bacterial-infected host cells, fungi, protozoa, cancer cells, and solid-tissue transplant cells can be recognized and destroyed by specialized T lymphocytes. This response is known as cell-mediated immunity and involves the interaction of killer T lymphocytes, helper T cells, and mast cells.

Cell-mediated immunity starts with exposure to an antigen found on the surface of a virus, bacteria, cancer cell, or foreign cell. The antigen is ingested by a macrophage and presented to a killer T lymphocyte that becomes active. The active killer T lymphocytes increase in number after exposure to an interleukin produced by a helper T lymphocyte. The growing number of active killer T lymphocytes that carry the specific antibody for the antigen are circulated throughout the body in blood and lymph fluid. When they make contact with a cell that has the antigen on its surface, they bind to the infected or foreign cell and inject it with highly toxic chemicals that cause the cell to lyse and die.

Solid-tissue transplants are recognized and evoke a cell-mediated immune response. The foreign proteins (histocompatibility complexes) on the surface of the transplant tissue cause the activation and proliferation of killer T lymphocytes. This results in attack and rejection of the transplant. Rejection can be minimized by selecting tissue from a donor that has a closer match to the type of histocompatibility complexes found on the surface of the recipient tissues. The second step in minimizing rejection is to suppress the recipient's immune response by giving them immunosuppressant drugs such as cyclosporine. However, the consequence of taking immunosuppressant drugs is the suppression of both nonspecific and specific defenses.

Immune Memory and Suppression

Both of the immune responses described previously develop the ability to quickly recognize and respond to subsequent encounters with specific antigens. This ability to "remember" the antigen and neutralize it quickly before toxic manifestations occur is one of the beauties of the immune system. When B and T lymphocytes are activated by exposure to a new antigen, some of them become memory cells. The memory cells are lymphocytes that contain regions of deoxyribonucleic acid that has been slightly altered. The instructions for unique antibody structure is recorded in these altered regions. Memory cells replicate themselves over time, pass the genetic information to their daughter cells, and continue the recognition and reactivity to future antigen exposure. After very long periods the memory cell line can die off, and the individual loses the immunity to a specific antigen.

Internal and external factors can suppress the immune response. The body can secrete a variety of chemicals that suppress immune cell function. These include the stress hormone cortisol. Cortisol is a steroid hormone secreted by the adrenal gland in response to stress. Leukocyte and macrophage activity is suppressed by this hormone. Some lymphocytes function to limit the immune response. Suppressor T lymphocytes secrete factors that inhibit B, killer T, and helper T lymphocytes. This effectively limits or shuts off the immune response. Drugs such as cyclosporine and methotrexate are used to suppress the immune response in several different situations. Organ transplants and the treatment of autoimmune disorders frequently employ these kinds of agents. However, the risk of infection increases when steroid hormones and immunosuppressant drugs are used. Infection with the human immunodeficiency virus causes immune suppression through the destruction of T helper lymphocytes. This results in a variety of different collections of opportunistic infections and cancers that is collectively referred to as acquired immunodeficiency syndrome. Aging also causes immune suppression as lymphocytic activity and numbers of specific types decline.

CHAPTER SELF-TEST QUESTIONS

1. The first evidence of pulmonary development can be seen as an outpouching of a primitive lung bud on
   a. day 21 of gestation
   b. day 26 of gestation
   c. day 16 of gestation
   d. day 35 of gestation
2. About 300 million alveoli are present in the lungs
   a. by 10 years of age
   b. at birth
   c. at the end of the canalicular phase
   d. at the beginning of the terminal sac period
3. Which portion of the sternum lies over the liver?
   a. xiphoid process
   b. body
   c. manubrium

4. What structures within the nasal cavity increase the surface area of this region and are covered with a mucous membrane?
   a. palatine tonsil
   b. pharyngeal tonsil
   c. uvula
   d. concha
5. Which of the following are functions of the upper airway?
   1. filtration
   2. humidification
   3. gas exchange with blood
   a. 1 only
   b. 2 and 3
   c. 1 and 3
   d. 1 and 2
   e. 1, 2, and 3
6. Which of the following are true regarding the adult trachea?
   1. approximately 12 cm long
   2. comprised of about 18 C-shaped cartilaginous rings
   3. has an inner diameter of about 1 cm
   a. 2 only
   b. 1 and 2
   c. 2 and 3
   d. 1 and 3
   e. 1, 2, and 3
7. How many lobes and segments are found in the left lung?

	Lobes	Segments
a.	2	12
b.	3	10
c.	2	10
d.	3	12

8. About 93% of the alveolar surface is covered with
   a. type II cells
   b. Clara cells
   c. type I cells
   d. endothelial cells
9. Nerve signals traveling to the lung (efferent impulses) are
   a. airway stretch receptor signals that stimulate rapid breathing

b. irritant receptor signals that will stimulate a cough

c. autonomic signals for the airways, vessels, and mucus glands

d. motor signals to stimulate the intercostal muscle

10. The upper airway clears aerosol particles that are _____ in diameter from air inhaled.
    a. smaller than 0.1 μm
    b. 0.5 to 2 μm
    c. 2 to 8 μm
    d. larger than 10 μm

For answers, see p. 475.

BIBLIOGRAPHY

1. Barnhart SL, Czervinske MP: *Perinatal and pediatric respiratory care,* Philadelphia, 1995, WB Saunders.
2. Gail DB, Lenfant CJM: Cells of the lung: biology and clinical implications, *Am Rev Respir Dis* 127:366, 1983.
3. Gray H: *Anatomy of the human body,* ed 30, Philadelphia, 1985, Lea & Febiger.
4. Guyton AC: *Textbook of medical physiology,* Philadelphia, 1996, WB Saunders.
5. Martin DE, Youtsey JW: *Respiratory anatomy and physiology,* St Louis, 1988, Mosby.
6. Martini FH: *Fundamentals of anatomy and physiology,* Upper Saddle River, NJ, 1998, Prentice Hall.
7. Murray JF: *The normal lung: the basis for diagnosis and treatment of pulmonary disease,* ed 2, Philadelphia, 1986, WB Saunders.
8. Proctor DF: The upper airways. I. Nasal physiology and defense of the lungs, *Am Rev Respir Dis* 115:97, 1977.
9. Proctor DF: The upper airways. II. The larynx and trachea, *Am Rev Respir Dis* 115:315, 1977.
10. Staub NC: *Basic respiratory physiology,* New York, 1991, Churchill Livingstone.
11. Thurlbeck WM: Postnatal growth and development of the lung, *Am Rev Respir Dis* 111:803, 1975.
12. Weibel ER: Morphological basis of alveolar-capillary gas exchange, *Physiol Rev* 53:419, 1973.
13. West JB: *Bioengineering aspects of the lung,* New York, 1977, Marcel Dekker.
14. West JB: *Respiratory physiology: the essentials,* ed 4, Baltimore, 1990, Williams & Wilkins.
15. Wilkins RL, Pierson DJ: The heart and blood vessels. In Pierson DJ, Kacmarek RM, eds: *Foundations of respiratory care,* New York, 1992, Churchill Livingstone.

CHAPTER 10

Pulmonary Mechanics

CHAPTER OBJECTIVES

Upon completing this chapter, you will be able to:

1 List the phases of thoracic cavity motion during the ventilatory cycle.

2 Describe the three types of rib motion that enlarge the thoracic cavity during inhalation.

3 Describe the origin, insertion, action, and innervation of the diaphragm.

4 Describe the origin, insertion, action, and innervation of the accessory muscles of breathing.

5 List the different locations of pressure changes that are important in gas movement.

6 List the important pressure gradients that exist across different regions of the respiratory system.

7 Define the phases of the ventilatory cycle by describing the changes in pressure, volume, and flow.

8 Describe the forces that move gas into and out of the lungs during resting breathing.

9 Describe why the lungs do not completely collapse within the thoracic cavity.

10 Name the volume of gas within the lungs when the respiratory muscles are relaxed.

11 Define *elastance, compliance, specific compliance,* and *dynamic compliance.*

12 Describe what *static compliance* of the lung, thorax, and total respiratory system is, the normal adult values for each, and how each is determined.

13 Describe the source and effect that surfactant has in the lung.

14 Describe the factors that influence lung and thorax compliance.

15 Define *tissue resistance, airway resistance,* and *airway conductance.*

16 Describe the factors that influence airway resistance.

17 Describe the nervous control of airway smooth muscle and submucosal glands.

18 Describe the normal values of adult airway resistance, airway conductance, specific resistance, and specific conductance and how they are determined.

19 Define *closing volume* and *time constant.*

20 Define the work of breathing in terms of its clinical appearance, mechanical properties, and metabolic cost and describe the most efficient breathing pattern.

21 Define *respiratory muscle strength* and describe how it is determined.

The term *pulmonary mechanics* describes those factors that influence the motion of the chest wall and lungs. Understanding pulmonary mechanics is central to understanding normal and abnormal conditions that influence lung volume and gas flow. This chapter describes the respiratory muscles, the mechanical factors that influence gas volume and flow, and the work done by the respiratory muscles.

MUSCLES THAT MOVE GAS INTO AND OUT OF THE LUNGS

Thoracic Cavity Motion during Breathing

Three distinct changes take place during inhalation. The first change is abdominal protrusion. Next, the lower and lateral chest expands outward. Last, the anterior chest expands outward. These changes are brought about by the coordinated actions of the diaphragm and other respiratory muscles. At end-inhalation the respiratory muscles relax and the elastic properties of the lungs and chest wall cause the thoracic cavity to return to its original position.

Rib movement occurs in three different ways: (1) pump handle motion, (2) bucket handle motion, and (3) caliper motion. The first six pairs of ribs move with a pump handle motion, rotating at their point of attachment with the vertebral bones in a forward and upward motion. Rib pairs 7 through 10 move with a bucket handle motion that causes the lower thorax to move upward and laterally. Rib pairs 11 and 12 rotate backward and laterally, causing lateral expansion of the lower thorax in a caliper motion. As a result of these different motions, anteroposterior enlargement

Table 10-1 Respiratory Muscles that Enlarge the Thorax during the Inspiratory Phase

Muscle	Origin	Insertion	Innervation	Action
Diaphragm	Inner surface of lumbar vertebra, abdominal wall and lumbar vertebra	Central tendon of dome	Phrenic nerves (C3-C5)	Diaphragm moves downward forced outward
External intercostals	Upper ribs	Lower ribs	Intercostal nerves	Lifts ribs upward (T1-T12)
Scalene	Lower 5 cervical vertebrae	First and second ribs	Cervical nerves (C3-C8)	Lifts first and second ribs
Sternocleidomastoids	Manubrium and clavicle	Mastoid process of occipital bone	Cranial nerve XI and cervical nerves (C1 and C2)	Lifts sternum
Trapezius	Occipital, seventh cervical, and all thoracic vertebrae	Scapula and clavicle	Cranial nerve XI	Stabilizes head
Pectoralis minor	Anterior region of ribs 3 to 5	Scapula	Pectoral nerves (C6-C8)	Lifts upper ribs
Pectoralis major	Clavicle and sternum	Humerus	Pectoral nerves (C5 to C8)	Lifts sternum

is most noticeable in the upper thorax while the lower thorax enlarges laterally.

Muscles of Breathing

The changes of thoracic cavity shape during breathing are the product of changes in respiratory muscle tension. These muscles include the diaphragm and the muscles of the neck, intercostal spaces, chest, and back (Tables 10-1 and 10-2). Different muscles are active at different times with different intensities as respiratory effort changes.

Diaphragm

The diaphragm is a thin, musculotendinous, dome-shaped structure that separates the thoracic and abdominal cavities (Fig. 10-1). It originates from the chest and abdominal wall and converges in a central tendon at the top of its dome. The posterior portion arises from the first three lumbar vertebrae. The lateral costal

Table 10-2 Respiratory Muscles that Compress the Thorax during the Expiratory Phase

Muscle	Origin	Insertion	Innervation	Action
Internal intercostals	Lower ribs	Upper ribs	Intercostal nerves	Pulls ribs down (T1 to T12)
External oblique	Anterior lower eight ribs	Linea alba and iliac crest	Lower intercostal and iliohypogastric nerves (T7 to T12)	Pulls abdominal wall inward
Internal oblique	Lumbar vertebrae, iliac crest, and inguinal ligaments	Costal region of ribs and pubis	Lower intercostal and iliohypogastric nerves (T10 to 12 and L1)	Pulls abdominal wall inward
Transverse abdominis	Costal region of lower ribs, iliac crest, and inguinal crest	Linea alba	Lower intercostal and iliohypogastric nerves (T7 to L1)	Pulls abdominal wall inward
Rectus abdominis	Costal region ribs 5 to 7	Pubis	Lower intercostal and iliohypogastric nerves (T7 to T12)	Pulls abdominal wall inward
Serratus anterior	Costal region of upper eight ribs	Scapula	Long thoracic nerves (T5 to T7)	Compresses thorax when arm is stabilized
Serratus, posterior superior	Lower cervical and upper thoracic vertebrae	Posterior ribs 2 to 5	Thoracic nerves	Pulls ribs downward
Serratus, posterior inferior	Lower thoracic and upper lumbar vertebrae	Posterior ribs 9 to 12	Thoracic nerves	Pulls ribs downward
Latissimus dorsi	Lower thoracic, lumbar, and sacral vertebrae, ilium, and lower ribs	Humerus	Thoracodorsal nerves (C6 to C8)	Compresses thorax when arm is stabilized

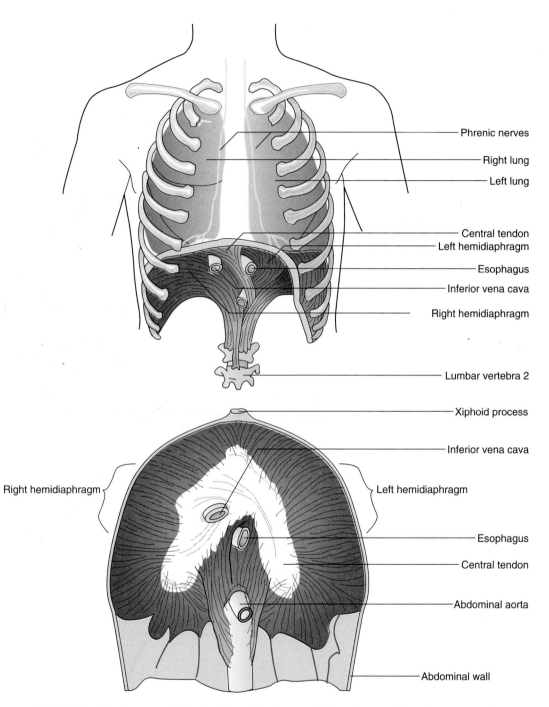

FIG. 10-1 Diaphragm originates from lumbar vertebra, lower ribs, sternum, and abdominal wall and converges in a central tendon. It enlarges the thoracic cavity and compresses the abdominal cavity when stimulated by the phrenic nerves.

portions arise from the inner surface of ribs 7 through 12 and transverse abdominal muscles on each side. The anterior portion arises from the inner surface of the xiphoid process of the sternum.

In an upright position and with the diaphragm relaxed, the dome of the diaphragm rests at the level of the eighth thoracic vertebrae. When lying down in a supine position, the weight of the abdominal contents forces the diaphragm further up into the thoracic cavity. During quiet breathing, muscle fibers of the diaphragm contract, causing the dome of the diaphragm to be pulled down 1 to 2 cm. This results in enlargement of the thoracic cavity and compression of the abdominal contents. During maximal inspiration, the diaphragm can be pulled down approximately 10 cm. Exhalation results when diaphragmatic tension decreases and the diaphragm returns to its relaxed position.

Large lung volumes cause the diaphragm to flatten out. Contraction of a flattened diaphragm can result in tension on the lower ribs that causes the ribs to be pulled inward, resulting in compression of the thoracic cavity. This condition can occur in individuals with severe cases of **emphysema** or **asthma.** To compensate, these individuals must recruit other muscles to enlarge the thorax. This results in less efficient breathing and excessive muscle work.

Functionally, the diaphragm is divided into a right and left **hemidiaphragm.** Each hemidiaphragm is innervated by a **phrenic nerve** that arises from branches of spinal nerves C3, C4, and C5. Spinal cord injuries at or above the level of the third cervical vertebrae result in diaphragmatic paralysis. In this situation the individual, having lost *all* nervous control of their respiratory muscles, is unable to breathe.

Accessory Muscles of Breathing

During quiet breathing, the diaphragm does the majority of the work. Other muscles that are slightly active during quiet breathing become more active with forceful breathing. These other muscles are generally known as the accessory muscles of breathing.

The accessory muscles of inspiration include a variety of muscles in the neck, chest, and upper back. Eleven pairs of intercostal muscles are found between the ribs. The external intercostal muscles (Fig. 10-2) originate on the upper ribs and attach to the lower ribs. The fibers of these muscles run at an oblique angle between the ribs. When they generate tension, they lift the ribs upward, causing the thoracic cavity to enlarge. The fibers receive nerve signals from the intercostal nerves that arise from thoracic spinal nerves. They are more active during the inspiratory phase of forceful breathing.

Three pairs of scalene muscles (scalenus anterior, scalenus medius, and scalenus posterior) arise from the lower five or six cervical vertebrae and insert on the clavicle and first two ribs (Fig. 10-3). The upper chest is lifted when the scalene muscles are active. The scalene muscles, slightly active during resting inhalation, become more active with forceful inspiration.

Sternocleidomastoid muscles (Fig. 10-4) originate from the manubrium and clavicle and insert on the mastoid process of the temporal bone. When the head is held in an upright position by tensing the trapezius muscle of the upper back and neck, the sternocleidomastoid muscles lift the upper chest. These muscles, active during forceful inspiration, become visible thick bands on either side of the neck during the inspiratory phase of an individual in respiratory distress. They receive nerve impulses from branches of the eleventh cranial nerve and cervical nerves C1 and C2.

The major and minor pectoralis muscles are broad, fan-shaped muscles of the upper anterior chest (Fig. 10-5). The pectoralis major originates on the clavicle and sternum and inserts onto the humerus. The pectoralis minor originates on the anterior portion of

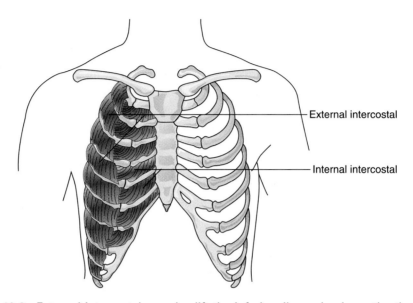

FIG. 10-2 External intercostal muscles lift the inferior ribs and enlarge the thoracic cavity. Internal intercostal muscles compress the thoracic cavity by pulling the ribs together.

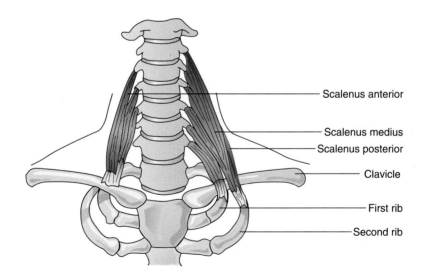

FIG. 10-3 Scalene muscles originate from the lower cervical vertebrae and lift the clavicle and first two ribs.

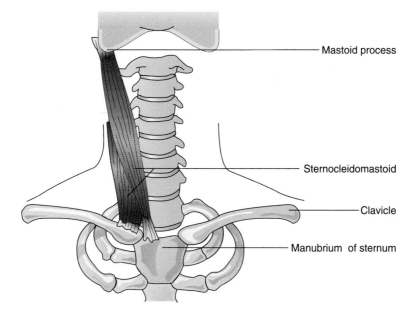

FIG. 10-4 Sternocleidomastoid muscles originate from the manubrium and clavicle and insert on the mastoid process of the temporal bone. They lift the upper thorax when the trapezius stabilizes the head.

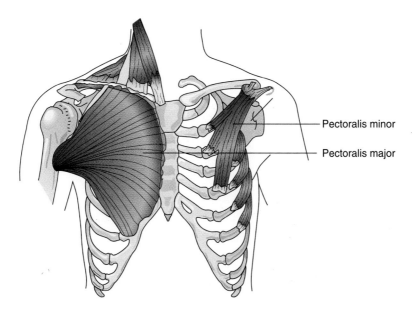

FIG. 10-5 Pectoralis major and minor can lift and enlarge the thorax when the arms are braced by leaning forward on the elbows.

ribs 3 through 5 and inserts onto the scapula. When these muscles receive impulses from the pectoral nerves, they normally function to adduct the arms in a hugging motion. They are also capable of generating some anterior thoracic lift when the arms are braced on a surface in front of a subject. Those individuals who suffer with chronic shortness of breath often use the pectoralis muscles by sitting in a "tripod" position. This is performed by sitting upright and leaning forward with both arms braced on a table.

The trapezius muscles are flat, triangular muscles located on the upper back and neck (Fig. 10-6). They arise from the occipital bone, seventh cervical vertebrae, and all of the thoracic vertebrae. They insert onto the scapula and lateral third of the clavicle. Their action is to rotate the scapula, lift the shoulders, and extend the head up and back. They become active during forceful inspiration by helping brace the head and allowing the sternocleidomastoid muscle to lift the thorax.

The accessory muscles of exhalation become active during forceful breathing. Generally, these muscles act to compress the thoracic cavity and to facilitate exhalation (see Table 10-2).

The internal intercostal muscles (see Fig. 10-2) lie between the ribs and just behind the external intercostal muscles. They originate along the inferior border of the upper ribs and insert into the superior border of the lower ribs. The muscle fibers of the internal intercostal muscles run downward and less obliquely than the external intercostal muscle fibers. This orientation causes these muscles to pull the ribs together, which results in compression of the thoracic cavity. The internal intercostal muscles are stimulated by branches of the intercostal nerves and are most active during forceful exhalation. They also become

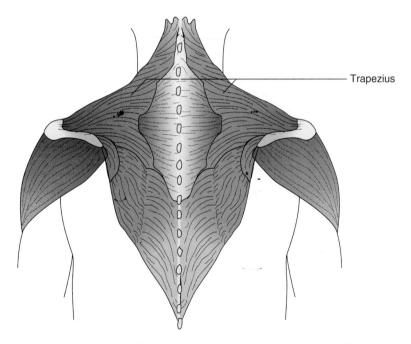

Trapezius

FIG. 10-6 Trapezius assists forceful inspiration primarily by stabilizing the head, which allows the sternocleidomastoid muscle to lift the anterior thorax.

active toward the end of deep inhalation, acting to antagonize the lifting effect of the external intercostal muscles.

When the abdominal wall muscles contract, they compress the abdominal cavity. This forces the diaphragm upward and compresses the thoracic cavity. The abdominal muscles include pairs of external oblique, internal oblique, transverse abdominis, and rectus abdominis muscles (Fig. 10-7). The external oblique muscles, the outermost layer of

abdominal wall muscle, lie over the lateral aspects of the abdominal cavity. They originate on the anterior surface of the lower eight ribs and abdominal aponeurosis and insert into the linea alba (a connective tissue band on the mid-anterior surface of the abdomen), iliac crest, and inguinal ligament. The internal oblique muscles lie just underneath the external oblique muscles. They originate on the lumbar vertebrae, iliac crest, and inguinal ligaments and insert into the pubis and costal

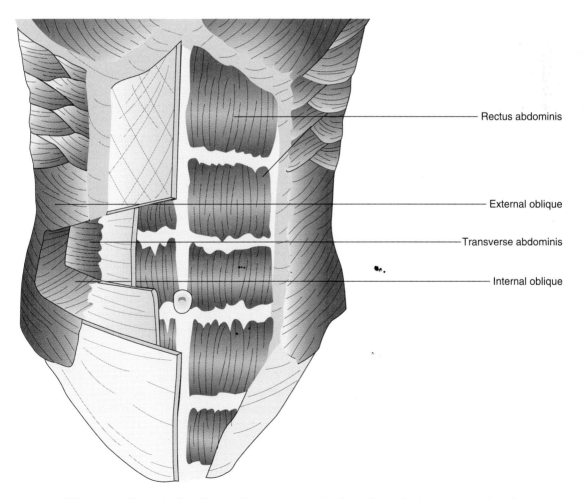

FIG. 10-7 Abdominal wall muscles compress the thoracic cavity by compressing the abdominal wall and forcing the diaphragm upward.

region of the lower ribs, resulting in a fiber orientation that is at right angles to those in the external oblique muscles. The transverse abdominis muscles lie below the internal oblique muscles. Muscle fibers of the transverse abdominis run around the lateral wall of abdomen by originating on the lower six ribs, the iliac crest, and the inguinal ligaments and by inserting into the linea alba. The rectus abdominis muscles are a pair of muscular bands that run vertically on the anterior surface of the abdomen. These muscular bands arise from the costal region of ribs 5 through 7 and the xiphoid process of the sternum, travel upward over the abdominal cavity, and insert into the pubis. The abdominal wall muscles, which receive nerve impulses from branches of the lower intercostal and iliohypogastric nerves, are most active during forceful exhalation, coughing, and loud talking.

● CHANGES THAT TAKE PLACE DURING THE VENTILATORY CYCLE

Pulmonary System Pressures

To move air, the pulmonary system generates pressure changes through the actions of the respiratory muscles on the thorax and lungs. Important factors in breathing include **barometric pressure (P_B)**, airway opening pressure (P_{ao}), **alveolar pressure (P_A), pleural space pressure (P_{pl}),** and abdominal cavity pressure (P_{abd}) (Fig. 10-8). The pressures are measured in centimeters of water (cm H_2O) or kilopascals (kPa) and are expressed in values that are relative (positive or negative) to atmospheric pressure.

The pressure differences between separate regions of an organ are referred to as pressure gradients, or transorgan pressures. Four pressure gradients are important in the study of ventilation and pulmonary mechanics (see Fig. 10-8). They are determined by subtracting the outermost pressure from the innermost pressure. These gradients quantify the amount

of force being applied to a particular region of the respiratory system.

The pressure gradient that is exerted across the chest wall is known as the **transthoracic pressure (P_w)**. It is the difference between atmospheric or body surface pressure and pleural space pressure:

$$P_w = P_{pl} - P_B$$

Transthoracic pressure indicates the amount of force that is being applied to the chest wall.

The pressure that expands the lung is the **transpulmonary pressure** (P_L). It is the difference between alveolar and pleural pressures:

$$P_L = P_A - P_{pl}$$

Negative pleural pressure creates a positive transpulmonary pressure that inflates the lung with a volume of gas.

The pressure difference between the airway opening and the alveoli is known as **transairway,** or transrespiratory, **pressure (P_{rs}):**

$$P_{rs} = P_A - P_B$$

Transrespiratory pressure produces air flow through the airways. Negative transairway pressure results in gas flow toward the alveoli, and positive transairway pressure causes flow out of the lungs.

The pressure differences that occur across the airway wall is known as the **transmural pressure (P_{tm}),** which is calculated by subtracting the pressure on the outside of the airway (P_{oAW}) from intraairway pressure (P_{iAW}):

$$P_{tm} = P_{iAW} - P_{oAW}$$

Pressure that is greater within the airway than that outside the airway produces positive transmural pressure, which tends to result in airway dilation. Pressure that is greater on the outside of the airway produces negative transmural pressure. A negative transmural pressure causes the airway to collapse.

When the diaphragm contracts, it develops enough tension to expand the thoracic cavity and to compress the abdominal cavity. The amount of tension produced during this event

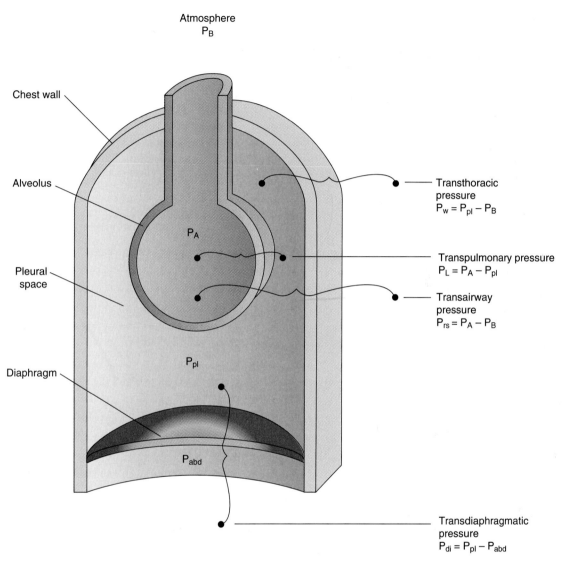

Atmosphere
P_B

Chest wall

Alveolus

Pleural space

Diaphragm

P_A

P_{pl}

P_{abd}

Transthoracic pressure
$P_w = P_{pl} - P_B$

Transpulmonary pressure
$P_L = P_A - P_{pl}$

Transairway pressure
$P_{rs} = P_A - P_B$

Transdiaphragmatic pressure
$P_{di} = P_{pl} - P_{abd}$

FIG. 10-8   Important regional pressures and pressure differences of the respiratory system.

is reflected by the transdiaphragmatic pressure (P_{di}), the difference between pleural and abdominal cavity pressures:

$$P_{di} = P_{pl} - P_{abd}$$

This pressure becomes negative during the inflation of the lungs and returns to 0 at end-exhalation.

Ventilatory Cycle

Like the cardiac cycle, breathing is also a sequence of events that repeats. This sequence, known as the **ventilatory cycle,** is comprised of an inhalation and an exhalation phase. The changes in pressure, volume, and flow that take place during each phase are shown in Fig. 10-9. Transorgan pressure changes that

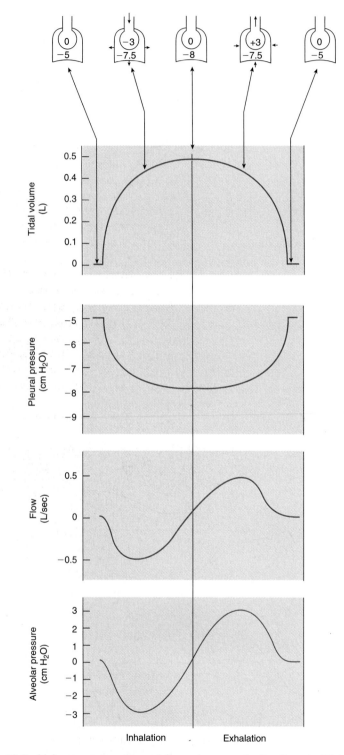

FIG. 10-9 Volume, pressure, and flow changes during the ventilatory cycle.

occur during the cycle are summarized in Table 10-3. The volume of gas moved in or out during the ventilatory cycle is termed the **tidal volume (V_T).**

At the beginning of the cycle the respiratory muscles are relaxed, the upper airway is open, and alveolar pressure is equal to atmospheric pressure. The average pleural pressure is -5 cm H_2O. The negative pleural pressure is the product of two apposing forces: (1) the tendency of the lungs to collapse and (2) the tendency of the chest wall to spring outward.

Inhalation begins as the respiratory muscles contract and enlarge the thoracic cavity. With thoracic cavity enlargement, pleural pressure becomes more negative, transpulmonary pressure becomes greater, and the lungs become enlarged. This causes alveolar pressure to become negative (Boyle's law of an inverse relationship between volume and pressure). When alveolar pressure becomes negative, transairway pressure becomes negative. During normal inflation, gas flows from the atmosphere to the alveoli at a rate of 0.5 L/sec. At end-inhalation, pleural pressure stabilizes at about -8 cm H_2O, creating a transpulmonary pressure that distends the lung with a tidal volume of 0.5 L. Without generating more respiratory muscle force, alveolar pressure equalizes with atmospheric pressure, transairway pressure returns to 0 cm H_2O, and gas flow drops to 0 L/sec.

Exhalation begins as the respiratory muscles relax their tension and the lungs recoil back toward their original position. Pleural pressures become less negative, causing transthoracic and transpulmonary pressure to return toward relaxation pressure levels. The lungs recoil and alveolar gas compresses. Transairway pressure now becomes positive and gas flows out of the lungs to the atmosphere at a flow of 0.5 L/sec. The lungs exhale a tidal volume of 0.5 L. This process ends at end-exhalation when the outward spring action of the thorax counterbalances the collapsing forces of the lung. At this point, pleural pressure returns to -5 cm H_2O and the lungs return to their preinhalation resting volume. Without further compression, alveolar pressure equilibrates with atmospheric pressure, transairway pressure drops to 0, and gas flow drops to 0. After a pause of 2 or 3 seconds, the cycle starts over.

FACTORS THAT INFLUENCE THE GAS VOLUME IN THE LUNGS

Static Properties of the Lungs

The lungs are flexible structures that change size and shape when force is applied to them. The flexibility of the lungs can be determined by inflating them with a known volume and measuring the pressure generated within them when they are allowed to recoil. This describes the static properties of the lungs. Understanding these static properties is important in

---

Table 10-3 Transorgan Pressure Gradients and their Values during the Ventilatory Cycle*

Pressure Gradient	Relaxed Respiratory Muscles	Inspiratory Phase	Expiratory Phase
Transthoracic pressure ($P_{pl} - P_B$)	-5	$-5 \rightarrow -8$	$-8 \rightarrow -5$
Transpulmonary pressure ($P_A - P_{pl}$)	$+5$	$+5 \rightarrow +8$	$+8 \rightarrow +5$
Transairway pressure ($P_A - P_B$)	0	$0 \rightarrow -3 \rightarrow 0$	$0 \rightarrow +3 \rightarrow 0$
Transdiaphragmatic pressure ($P_{pl} - P_{abd}$)	0	$0 \rightarrow +5$	$+5 \rightarrow 0$

*Pressures in cm H_2O.

understanding how various factors and diseases influence lung volume and the work necessary to move gas into and out of the lungs.

Elastic Properties of the Lungs

Elasticity is a property of matter that causes the lungs to return to their original size and shape after being stretched or compressed. This elastic property gives matter the ability to withstand external forces until it distorts or shears apart.

Fig. 10-10 illustrates this concept by showing a spring being stretched by the force of weights and a balloon being inflated with pressurized gas. The spring and balloon both stretch as more force is applied. At a certain point they no longer stretch despite the addition of more force. This point is known as the elastic limit. As more force is applied beyond the elastic limit, the spring and the balloon

reach a critical breaking point where the material that comprises them shears.

The relationship between stretch and force was first described by Hooke. Hooke's law of elasticity states that the stretch of an object is proportional to the amount of force applied to it. This can been seen in Fig. 10-10 where increasing stretch occurs with increasing force. Hooke's law states that the elastance (E) of an object equals the amount of force necessary to stretch it a given distance:

$$E = \frac{Force}{Stretch}$$

An object with high elastance requires a greater amount of force to stretch it a certain distance.

The elastic qualities of the lungs can be described by measuring the amount of pressure required to distend the lung with a cer-

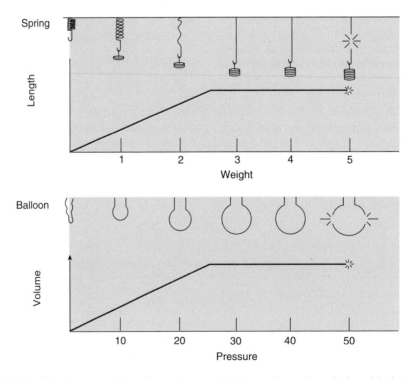

FIG. 10-10 Elastic properties of a spring and balloon show the relationship between force (weight and pressure) and stretch (length and volume).

tain volume. When inflated, the lung develops a greater tendency to collapse. The collapsing force, commonly described as the recoil pressure, is measured at the airway opening after the lungs are inflated and allowed to recoil against a blocked airway. By inflating the lung to its maximum capacity and measuring the recoil pressure at various volumes as the lung is deflated, an elastic profile of the lung can be created and analyzed. Fig. 10-11 shows this as a normal pressure-volume deflation curve for the lungs as they would behave if they were outside the body. Note that the curve is nonlinear. The region of lowest elastance (least pressure change for a given volume change) is at about 50% inflation where the curve is the steepest. The greatest region of elasticity (most pressure change for little volume change) occurs at about 100% inflation where the curve flattens out.

Lung Compliance

The elastic properties of the lungs are more commonly expressed in units of **compliance (C).** Compliance is the reciprocal of elasticity:

$$C = \frac{\text{Stretch}}{\text{Force}}$$

Lung stretch equals the change in lung volume (ΔV), and the force causing it is the change in transpulmonary pressure (ΔP). Using this approach, the equation for compliance can be written in the following form:

$$C = \frac{\Delta V}{\Delta P}$$

This indicates that a given amount of lung distension is generated for a given amount of inflating pressure. The units of compliance are liters or milliliters per centimeter of water.

The static compliance of the lung (C_{stL}) can be determined by examining a portion of the pressure-volume curve shown in Fig. 10-11. Deflation from point A to point B results in a decrease in volume and pressure. A straight line can be drawn from point A to point B and the slope of the line can be determined (rise divided by run). The slope of this line equals the static lung compliance:

$$C_{stL} = \frac{\text{Rise}}{\text{Run}} = \frac{\Delta V}{\Delta P}$$

Using this method, static compliance of the lung is found to be about 0.2 L/cm H_2O or 200 ml/cm H_2O at midinflation:

$$
\begin{aligned}
C_{stL} &= \frac{\Delta V}{\Delta P} \\
&= \frac{1.2 \text{ L}}{6 \text{ cm } H_2O} \\
&= \frac{0.2 \text{ L}}{\text{cm } H_2O}
\end{aligned}
$$

Note that different regions of the curve have different slopes. Those regions of the curve that are steeper represent greater lung compliance. This occurs toward the center of the curve. Regions where the curve flattens indicate reduced compliance. High lung inflation results in a nearly flat line, indicating low lung compliance as the lungs reach their elastic limits.

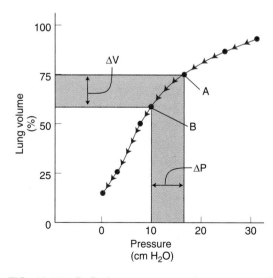

FIG. 10-11 Deflation pressure-volume curve of the lung (see text for description).

Specific Compliance

Compliance is highly influenced by lung size. Total lung compliance in an individual who has had one lung surgically removed **(pneumonectomy)** is half the normal value. This is the result of having half of the elastic tissue available for inflation. A similar situation exists when comparing adult and pediatric compliance. A child with a maximal lung volume that is half that of an adult has a compliance that is half the adult value. An alternative approach is to determine compliance with the fractional change in lung volume rather than the actual volume change. This can be done be dividing the volume change (ΔV) by the volume of gas in the lung before the change (V_L). This approach produces a value known as the specific lung compliance (SpC_L):

$$ SpC_L = \frac{\dfrac{\Delta V}{V_L}}{\Delta P} $$

Using this approach, pediatric and adult lungs are found to have about the same compliance. This indicates that the elastic properties of pediatric and adult lung tissue are similar and that the major differences are a result of lung size.

Elastic Tissues of the Lung

A significant portion of the elastic properties of the lung is produced by the elastic components of lung tissue. Lung tissue is largely comprised of epithelial cells that are found on the surfaces of the entire lung. Epithelia are supported and held in position by connective tissue fibers that are oriented in different ways and in different regions. Peripheral connective tissue of the lungs is located on the pleural surfaces that cover the lungs. Axial connective tissue arises from the hilum and extends into the lungs within the walls of the major airways and vessels. The parenchymal connective tissue, which is found in the interstitial space of the alveolar walls, effectively connects the peripheral and axial connective tissues.

The connective tissue network of the lungs is comprised primarily of **collagen** and elastin protein fibers that are deposited in the interstitial spaces by fibroblasts. Collagen fibers stretch poorly (high elastance) whereas elastin fibers stretch more freely (more compliant). In normal lungs there is an equal mix of these fibers. Lungs that are injured by exposure to toxins often heal with a greater deposition of collagen. Extensive injury and collagen fiber deposition can result in a condition known as **pulmonary fibrosis.** Increasing deposition of collagen fibers causes the lung compliance and gas diffusion properties of the lungs to decline.

Surface Tension Properties of the Lungs

The 300 million alveoli of the lungs are microscopic structures with wet surfaces. This creates a liquid-gas interface that possesses surface forces known as **surface tension** (see Chapter 1). In addition to the connective tissue fibers, surface tension causes alveoli to collapse.

Surface tension is produced by uneven forces that are exerted on molecules at the surface of a liquid-gas interface. Water molecules are attracted to one another by cohesive forces. Below the surface the cohesive forces between water molecules occur on all sides by the surrounding molecules (Fig. 10-12, *A*). The water molecules at the surface have unequal attractive forces applied to them (Fig. 10-12, *B*). They are attracted by water molecules around and below them with much more force than the more widely spread out gas molecules. This results in surface tension.

Surface tension is expressed as the amount of force necessary to break the surface cohesion exerted across a given distance in dynes per centimeter. For example, water has a surface tension of 70 dynes/cm, meaning that it requires a force of 70 dynes to open a 1-cm slit between the water molecules at the surface of the air-liquid interface.

Surface tension can be reduced by the addition of **surfactant** molecules to the surface of the liquid. Water molecules have little or no

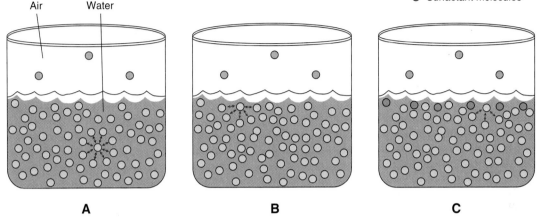

FIG. 10-12 **A,** Intermolecular cohesive attraction occurs equally below the surface. **B,** Unequal attraction at the surface produces surface tension. **C,** Surfactant molecules reduce cohesive attraction and surface tension.

attraction for surfactant molecules. The presence of surfactant results in a reduction in surface cohesive forces between surface molecules (Fig. 10-12, C). Soaps act as a surfactant, reducing surface tension sufficiently to allow the formation of bubbles. Without soap, bubbles that do form collapse or rupture quickly as a result of much higher surface tension.

The interrelationship between surface tension, bubble size, and distending pressure is described by **Laplace's law** (Fig. 10-13). Spherical structures like soap bubbles and alveoli have an inner and outer wet surface that develops surface tension. Laplace's law for this type of structure is as follows:

$$P = \frac{4T}{r}$$

where P is the distending pressure, T is surface tension, and r is the radius of the sphere. This relationship shows that the distending pressure necessary to inflate a spherical structure increases with increasing surface tension

or decreasing size. Laplace's law has practical implications for the size and volume of alveoli and the lung. Alveoli with increased surface tension have a greater tendency to collapse and require greater distending pressure to maintain their volume. If the distending pressure is low, alveoli collapse and lung volume decreases. Decreasing alveolar size increases the tendency of alveoli to collapse. Laplace's law states that the distending pressure necessary to inflate a sphere increases as the radius of the sphere decreases. Alveolar collapse can be triggered by increased surface tension and decreased alveolar size.

Laplace's law also helps explain why alveolar instability occurs when alveolar volume is low. An alveolus that is completely deflated requires sufficient distending pressure to snap it open. The amount of pressure necessary to overcome the cohesive forces that hold the walls together is known as the critical opening pressure. When a newborn infant takes his or her first breaths, pleural pressures of −40 to

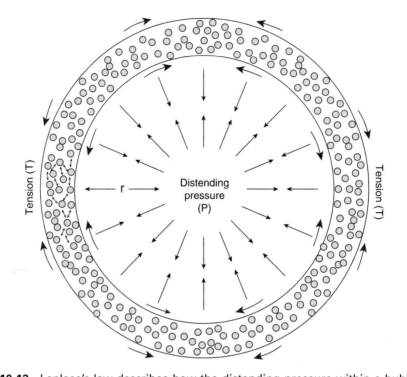

FIG. 10-13 Laplace's law describes how the distending pressure within a bubble is produced by surface tension and increases as the size of a bubble decreases.

−60 cm H_2O are generated to exceed the critical opening pressure of collapsed alveoli and to fill the alveoli with air. The reverse situation occurs when alveolar volume drops to a critical minimum and surface tension drives the remaining volume of gas out of the alveoli as they collapse. This minimum volume is known as the **closing volume.** According to Laplace's law, as the size of the alveolus decreases, the distending pressure, known as the **critical closing pressure,** needed to keep it inflated reaches a maximal value. It is mathematically equal to the same value as the critical opening pressure. Basically these are the same critical points that are arrived at from two different directions—inflation and deflation.

The effect of surface tension on the elastic properties of the lungs is substantial. This is shown in Fig. 10-14 where inflation and defla-tion pressure-volume curves are compared for lungs inflated with air and saline. The air-filled lungs generate greater recoil pressures during inflation and deflation than the saline-filled lungs at any lung volume. The saline-filled lungs do not possess an air-liquid inter-phase and thus have no surface tension properties. The recoil pressure generated solely results from the elastic behavior of the tissues. The air-filled lungs produce greater recoil pressure as a result of both the elastic nature of tissue and surface tension forces.

Because of the substantial effect that surface tension has on the amount of force that is necessary to inflate the lungs and keep them inflated, there is considerable interest in the use of liquids as a breathing medium. Fluoro-carbon liquids have been selected because of their fairly high O_2 and CO_2 solubilities. This type of liquid can support gas exchange and

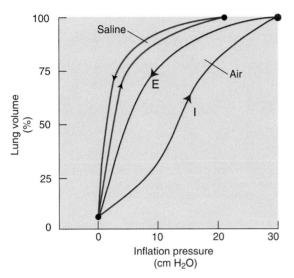

FIG. 10-14 Inflation and deflation pressure-volume curves of the lung filled with air and saline. The separation (hysteresis) between the inflation and deflation curves indicates different conditions exist during the two phases. *I,* Inflation; *E,* exhalation.

inflate the lungs more evenly with much lower distending pressure. It produces lower distending pressure because a liquid-filled lung lacks an air-liquid surface and thus the lung has no surface tension. Some alveoli in an air-filled lung may have higher surface tensions and are more difficult to inflate. The use of a liquid to inflate the lungs requires much less pressure and produces more uniform inflation of all lung regions.

Fig. 10-14 also demonstrates that the air-filled lungs develop marked separation between the inflation and deflation limbs of the pressure-volume curve. The inflation curve is displaced to the right and the deflation curve is displaced to the left. At any given volume, the lungs generate greater recoil pressure during inflation when compared with deflation. This separation, known as **hysteresis,** demonstrates that different conditions exist during

the two phases. During the inflation phase, the lung starts with a lower lung volume that is more difficult to inflate. During the deflation phase, lung volume starts out at a greater volume, and, with each step of deflation, the recoil pressure decreases. These different responses are partly described by Laplace's law. Low-volume alveoli require greater distending pressure to inflate them because of their smaller starting size. Higher volume alveoli require less pressure when deflated to a lower volume. Most of the difference is a result of changes in the surface tension acting across the surface of the alveoli as their size changes. Increasing lung volume causes the surface area and thus the surface tension of the alveoli to increase. Decreasing lung volume results in reducing surface area and surface tension. The saline-filled lungs lack these changes in surface tension and show little hysteresis between the inflation and deflation limbs.

Lung Surfactant and Surface Tension

The lungs produce a chemical solution called *surfactant* to reduce the surface tension properties of alveoli. Lung surfactant is produced by the type II alveolar epithelia and is secreted onto the surface of the alveoli. It is a complex mixture that is largely comprised of lipids (Table 10-4). The principal surface tension-lowering chemicals in surfactant are the phospholipids. The most important one is **dipalmitoyl phosphatidylcholine (DPPC)** (Fig. 10-15).

Surfactant is produced and stored within the type II cells in special organelles called *lamellar bodies.* The lamellar bodies merge with the cell membrane and release their contents onto the surface of the alveoli. Upon release, surfactant forms a latticelike network as a result of interconnection with different molecules. It then unravels and spreads out over the surface of the alveoli to a depth of one or two molecules. The DPPC molecules have hydrophobic and hydrophilic regions. The hydrophilic regions are oriented into the

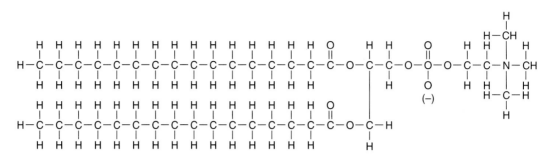

FIG. 10-15 Dipalmitoyl phosphatidylcholine is an important component of surfactant and functions by having lipid-soluble and water-soluble ends.

Table 10-4 Composition of Human Surfactant

Component	Percentage
Dipalmitoyl phosphatidylcholine	41.0%
Monoenoic phosphatidylcholine	25.0%
Phosphatidyl glycerol	9.0%
Protein	9.0%
Cholesterol	7.3%
Glycerides and glycolipids	3.2%
Serine and inositol	2.0%
Lysolecithin	1.5%
Sphingomyelin	1.0%
Free fatty acids	1.0%

liquid phase whereas the hydrophobic regions are oriented toward the air surface. This effectively reduces the contact of water molecules with the air surface and results in reduced surface tension.

The ratio of surfactant molecules to the surface area of the alveolus influences the alveolar surface tension. Increased surfactant to surface area ratio results in lower surface tension whereas a decrease in the ratio causes surface tension to increase. Changes of lung volume cause variations in this ratio and surface tension. With reduced lung volume, alveolar size and surface area are reduced. This results in an increased ratio of surfactant molecules to surface area and, as a result, surface tension is lowered. A low lung volume surface tension is about 10 to 15 dynes/cm. With increasing lung volume, the ratio of surfactant molecules to surface area decreases and surface tension increases. At maximum inflation, surface tension climbs to about 50 dynes/cm. The increased surface tension at high lung volume is an important cause of reduced lung compliance and a reduced ability to further inflate the lungs.

Interestingly, at high lung volume, more surfactant molecules move to the air surface (a suggested reason for sighing). When the lung deflates, a greater amount of surfactant is now at the surface and the ratio of surfactant molecules to surface area increases. This further reduces surface tension and this, coupled with reduced stretching of elastic fibers, generates a lower recoil pressure during lung deflation. These changes help produce the hysteresis effect. Surface tension changes do occur during resting tidal breathing. However, because the volume changes are small, surface tension does not fluctuate as much as that seen when comparing complete inflation and deflation. The small changes that do occur during resting ventilation oscillate around at an average surface tension of about 28 dynes/cm.

Surfactant functions in the lungs in a variety of ways (Box 10-1). Reducing surface tension helps prevent alveolar collapse and eases lung inflation by improving lung compliance.

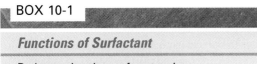

Functions of Surfactant

Reduces alveolar surface tension
Stabilizes alveolar size and shape
Improves lung volume and compliance
Reduces respiratory muscle work
Sheds water from the alveolus
Protects alveolar epithelial cells

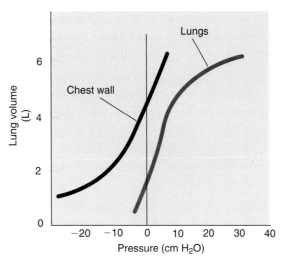

FIG. 10-16 Pressure-volume curves of the chest wall and lungs (see text for description).

This allows the outward spring effect of the chest wall to inflate the lungs with a resting volume of about 2.5 L. Surfactant reduces the respiratory muscle effort needed to inflate the lungs. This effectively reduces the work of breathing. Another general function of surfactant is its ability to help keep water out of the alveoli. The hydrophobic properties of surfactant help shed water from alveolar spaces toward the larger airways and the pulmonary circulation where it is carried away. Surfactant also provides protection for the delicate epithelial surface of the alveoli. The lipid and protein solution that surfactant is comprised of acts as a barrier and helps neutralize toxic chemicals that reach the alveolar surface.

Reduced surfactant synthesis results in the opposite effects. Alveolar surface tension increases and thus increases the tendency of alveolar collapse and reduced lung volume at end-exhalation. Increased surface tension causes reduced lung compliance and increases the work of breathing. Reduced surfactant also increases the risk of fluid collection and alveolar injury. The most common situation in which surfactant synthesis is reduced is in the premature infant. Surfactant production starts at about 24 weeks of gestation and gradually increases. Premature infants have lungs that have fewer alveoli and produce less surfactant. This sets the stage for the development of **neonatal respiratory distress syndrome (NRDS),** a condition of poor gas exchange and increased work of breathing.

Normally, surfactant is continually secreted and reabsorbed. The amount of time it takes to completely replace old surfactant with new surfactant (turnover time) is about 10 hours. Its concentration within the alveolus is dependent on the maturity and health of the type II cells. Surfactant synthesis is stimulated by a variety of humoral factors including glucocorticoids, thyroid hormone, epinephrine, and prostaglandins.

Static Properties of the Thorax

The chest wall is also an elastic structure. Its elastic properties can be studied in a similar manner as the method used to evaluate the properties of the lungs. The recoil pressure generated as the chest wall expands or contracts is shown as a pressure-volume curve in Fig. 10-16. When intrathoracic pressure equals atmospheric pressure (transthoracic pressure = 0), the chest wall springs outward with a volume of 4.5 L. Inflation of the thorax beyond this point requires positive transthoracic pressure whereas deflation requires negative transthoracic pressure.

The chest wall pressure-volume curve is shifted to the left of the lung's curve, indicating that inflation of the chest wall requires less pressure than that needed by the lungs. At a midinflation volume of 3 L, the chest wall has to be pulled inward with a force of -5 cm H_2O whereas the lungs require a distending pressure of 5 cm H_2O.

The chest wall pressure-volume curve is also parallel to the curve generated by the lung at midinflation. This means that chest wall compliance (C_W) is equal to the compliance of the lung in this region of the pressure-volume relationship. The compliance of the chest wall is computed in the same manner.

$$C_W = \frac{\Delta V}{\Delta P_W}$$

Chest wall compliance is found to have the same value of 0.2 L/cm H_2O or 200 ml/cm H_2O. With increasing volume, the slope of the lung's pressure-volume curve flattens out whereas the slope of the chest wall curve remains steeper. With inflation, the lung becomes much less compliant whereas the compliance of the chest wall remains relatively constant. Most of the elastic limitation that occurs at high inflation volume is caused by the lung reaching its elastic limit and having reduced compliance. The opposite conditions occur with deflation. Here, the lung has relatively well preserved compliance whereas the chest wall requires increasing force to collapse it. At low volume, the outward spring action of the chest wall increases and its compliance decreases.

Static Properties of the Total Respiratory System

The intact lungs and chest wall move together as a unit as gas inflates or deflates the system. The elastic properties of the intact system are influenced by the interaction of the chest wall and lungs.

At low volume the dominant force is the chest wall's tendency to spring outward. The respiratory muscles are incapable of overcoming the outward spring action of the chest wall to completely empty the lungs. As a result, a subject is incapable of exhaling all the gas from his or her lungs.

With inflation, it is the lung's elastic forces that dominate. With increasing volume, alveolar surface tension and the elastic recoil of tissue increase. Maximum inflation volume is reached when the respiratory muscles are unable to enlarge the lungs and thorax further.

The elastic properties of the intact system can be studied in the same manner as the elastic properties of the lungs and chest wall. The recoil force exerted by intact lungs and the chest wall results from their combined effects. The transrespiratory pressure (P_{rs}) reflects the overall recoil force generated by the respiratory system during relaxed breath holding. Fig. 10-17 shows the deflation pressure-volume relationship of the intact respiratory system and how it compares with the lungs and chest wall curves. With complete exhalation and holding the glottis closed (Fig. 10-17, A), the spring action of the chest wall creates negative pressure within the alveoli and pleural space. With the glottis open and the respiratory muscles relaxed, the chest wall pulls the lungs outward and inflates the lungs to an equilibrium point where transrespiratory pressure is 0 (Fig. 10-17, B). At this point the lung is inflated with a volume of 2.5 L by the springlike action of the thorax that creates a pleural pressure of -5 cm H_2O. This volume of gas within the lung at this resting equilibrium point is known as the **functional residual capacity (FRC).** With inflation and breath holding above the FRC volume (Fig. 10-17, C and D), alveolar and pleural pressures become progressively more positive as the recoil forces of the lungs and chest wall increase.

The slope of the respiratory system pressure-volume curve at midinflation is not as

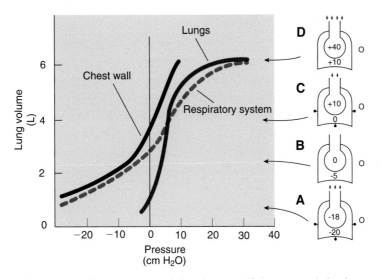

FIG. 10-17   Pressure-volume curves of the chest wall, lungs, and the intact respiratory system (see text for description).

steep as the chest wall or lung curves at this volume. This means that respiratory system compliance is lower than the compliance of the lungs and chest wall. The slope of the respiratory system curve compliance (C_{rs}) is determined with the following relationship:

$$C_{rs} = \frac{\Delta V_L}{\Delta P_{rs}}$$

where ΔV_{rs} is the change in volume within the lungs and ΔP_{rs} is the change of the transrespiratory pressure. Using this relationship during normal tidal volume and pressure changes, the normal respiratory system static compliance is found to be as follows:

$$C_{rs} = \frac{0.5\ L}{5\ cm\ H_2O}$$
$$= 0.1\ L/cm\ H_2O\ or\ 100\ ml/cm\ H_2O$$

This is half the value of lung or chest wall compliance.

When the respiratory system is inflated and stretched, both the lungs and chest wall stretch simultaneously. The total compliance for this parallel system is equal to the sum of the reciprocals of lung and chest wall compliance:

$$\frac{1}{C_{rs}} = \frac{1}{C_L} + \frac{1}{C_w}$$
$$= \frac{1}{200\ ml/cm\ H_2O} + \frac{1}{200\ ml/cm\ H_2O}$$
$$= \frac{2}{200\ ml/cm\ H_2O}$$
$$= \frac{1}{100\ ml/cm\ H_2O}$$
$$C_{rs} = 100\ ml/cm\ H_2O$$

This mathematical approach is necessary because of the parallel nature of these elastic components.

Factors that Influence Respiratory System Compliance

The static compliance of the respiratory system can be influenced by changes in the lung as well as the chest wall (Box 10-2). Changes in surfactant synthesis, amount of lung connective tissue, lung volume, and chest wall shape and flexibility, and abdominal cavity pressure

Factors that Influence Respiratory System Static Compliance

INCREASED STATIC COMPLIANCE
Decreased connective tissue fibers
Decreased surface tension
Increased surfactant production
Increased lung size
Decreased alveolar number
Increased rib flexibility and mobility

DECREASED STATIC COMPLIANCE
Increased connective tissue fibers
Increased surface tension
Decreased surfactant production
Decreased lung size
Thoracic wall distortion
Decreased rib flexibility and mobility
Excessive abdominal weight or cavity
   pressure

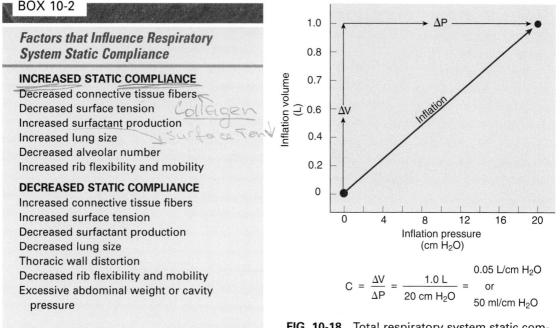

$$C = \frac{\Delta V}{\Delta P} = \frac{1.0\ L}{20\ cm\ H_2O} = \begin{matrix} 0.05\ L/cm\ H_2O \\ or \\ 50\ ml/cm\ H_2O \end{matrix}$$

FIG. 10-18 Total respiratory system static compliance during positive pressure ventilation can be determined by measuring the pressure that distends the lung with a measured volume.

all cause changes in total compliance. Various diseases cause changes in compliance by altering one or more of these factors.

Measuring Static Compliance

The measurement of static lung compliance can be done in a subject who is spontaneously breathing. Volume changes in the lungs can be determined by having a subject breath in and out of a spirometer. Simultaneously, pleural pressure changes are estimated by measuring esophageal pressure with a balloon-tipped catheter placed at midchest level. Following deep inflation, a series of pressure and volume changes is recorded as the subject exhales. This method produces a deflation pressure-volume curve (see Fig. 10-11). Lung compliance can be determined by measuring the slope of this pressure-volume curve.

Total respiratory system static compliance can be determined by having a subject fill his or her lungs and instructing them to relax as

the open airway is blocked by a valve. With the mouth and glottis open and the respiratory muscle relaxed, the pressure generated at the airway opening is equal to transrespiratory pressure, which, in turn, is equal to the recoil pressure of the lungs and chest wall. The subject then exhales some air through a series of exhalations. By measuring the total recoil pressure and changes in volume at each step, a deflation pressure-volume curve is generated. The slope of the curve equals the total respiratory system static compliance.

In mechanically ventilated patients, total respiratory system static compliance can be determined by inflating the lungs with a known volume and measuring the recoil pressure generated during a breath hold (Fig. 10-18). In this example, a 1.0-L breath is delivered, and airway pressure climbs as the system is

DIAGNOSTIC FOCUS

Pulmonary Edema Following Overhydration

A 61-year-old man with a history of heart disease had hip replacement surgery. During the procedure, he lost a significant amount of blood and received approximately 1500 ml of blood and intravenous solutions. He was transferred to the intensive care unit because his blood pressure was unstable and he was having dysrhythmias. Shortly after arrival he became increasingly dyspneic, he developed bilateral crackling and bubbling breath sounds, he lost consciousness, his heart rate increased to 137/min, and his blood pressure dropped to 91/60. Arterial blood oxygen levels were reduced despite breathing supplemental oxygen. His trachea was intubated, and he was put on mechanical ventilation. Within 5 minutes of starting mechanical ventilation, foamy, pink-tinged secretions flowed out of his lungs and into the endotracheal tube. The pressure needed to inflate his lungs with 700 ml of gas from the ventilator was 36 cm H_2O. His static respiratory system compliance was 19 ml/cm H_2O, which is markedly low when compared with a normal value of 70 to 100 ml/cm H_2O. An immediate x-ray revealed bilateral pulmonary edema and an enlarged heart.

Apparently the stress of the surgery and the large amount of fluid he was given caused his left ventricle to fail and his pulmonary artery pressure to climb. This resulted in excessive fluid movement into the lung tissue and alveolar spaces and disturbed the surfactant layer of the alveoli. The foamy secretion that came from the lung was surfactant-stabilized fluid coming from the alveoli. The excess fluid and loss of surfactant caused his work of breathing to increase, decreased his respiratory system compliance, appeared as a patchy infiltrate in both lungs on the x-ray, and caused his blood oxygen to decline.

The patient was given the diuretic Lasix to promote the renal release of water and dopamine to improve his systemic blood pressure. His ventilation was modified with the addition of 10 cm H_2O of positive end-expiratory pressure (PEEP). The addition of PEEP is intended to keep the lungs inflated and to prevent their collapse during exhalation. After 4 hours the pressure needed to inflate the patient's lungs with 700 ml of gas dropped to 21 cm H_2O, and the static respiratory system compliance increased to 33 ml/cm H_2O. The most recent chest x-ray showed some clearing of the pulmonary edema and reduction in heart size. This progress continued. The patient regained consciousness and hemodynamic stability, was weaned from ventilatory support 12 hours later, and was discharged to the rehabilitation service 7 days later.

inflated. At end-inflation the breath is held and the total recoil pressure is found to be 20 cm H_2O. Using the standard relationship, respiratory system static compliance can be determined:

$$C_{rs} = \frac{\Delta V_{rs}}{\Delta P_{rs}}$$
$$= \frac{1.0 \text{ L}}{20 \text{ cm } H_2O}$$
$$= 0.05 \text{ L/cm } H_2O$$
$$= 50 \text{ ml/cm } H_2O$$

The normal value for respiratory system static compliance in the mechanically ventilated patient ranges from 70 to 100 ml/cm H_2O.

Chest wall compliance in the spontaneously breathing subject is difficult to determine directly. It can be estimated by subtracting lung compliance from total respiratory system compliance with the following relationship:

$$\frac{1}{C_W} = \frac{1}{C_{rs}} - \frac{1}{C_L}$$

FACTORS THAT INFLUENCE GAS FLOW THROUGH THE AIRWAYS

Dynamic Properties of the Pulmonary System

Active inflation and deflation of the lungs and chest wall must overcome static as well as dynamic properties of the system. The static properties were described in terms of elastance and compliance of the system during breath-holding maneuvers. When gas and tissue are put into motion, a variety of additional properties must be overcome—inertia and friction. Inertial resistance is generated when an object with a given mass is accelerated into motion. The inertial resistance generated by the gas, lungs, and chest wall when they start into motion is small and can be ignored during resting tidal ventilation. Frictional resistance generated in the lungs is much more influential and is responsible for a significant portion of the total work done by the respiratory muscles.

Frictional Resistance

Gas flow through the airways is retarded by frictional resistance. Frictional resistance is produced in the gas stream by collisions between individual gas molecules and the molecules that contact the walls of the airway. Frictional resistance also occurs within the tissues of the lungs and chest wall as these tissues move, stretch, and slide past one another. The majority of frictional resistance produced during tidal ventilation is resistance caused by gas flow.

The amount of resistance resulting from friction can be determined in the same manner as vascular resistance. The general relationship used to determine respiratory system resistance is as follows:

$$\text{Resistance} = \frac{\Delta P}{\dot{V}}$$

where ΔP is the pressure difference ($P_1 - P_2$) that drives gas flow from a region of greater pressure to a region of lower pressure and $\dot{V}$ is the flow rate of the gas. Using this relationship and measuring different pressure gradients and flow permits the determination of resistance in different parts of the respiratory system, including **airway resistance, pulmonary tissue resistance,** and **chest wall tissue resistance.**

Pulmonary and Chest Wall Tissue Resistance

Expansion and contraction of the lungs and chest wall causes these tissues to move and stretch. Frictional resistance to this movement develops as these tissues slide over and past one another. This form of resistance is known as **tissue resistance.** Normally it represents about 15% to 20% of total frictional resistance during quiet breathing. It is determined by subtracting gas flow resistance from total resistance.

Airway Resistance

Airway resistance (R_{AW}), the gas flow resistance caused by friction between gas molecules and the airway wall, is generated along the entire length of airway from the airway opening to the alveolus. It represents about 80% of total frictional resistance produced during resting tidal breathing.

Poiseuille's law (see Chapter 1) reveals the major factors that influence gas flow (Fig. 10-19). This relationship shows that the amount of flow through an airway is directly related to the transrespiratory pressure that is exerted across the airway ($P_1 - P_2$) and the size of the airway as expressed by the radius (r) of the airway to the fourth power. It also shows that flow is inversely related to the length of the airway (L) and the viscosity of the gas (n). The constants 8 and π improve the accuracy of the equation.

Poiseuille's law can be rearranged to show how these major factors influence airway resistance:

$$R = \frac{P_1 - P_2}{\dot{V}} = \frac{8nl}{\pi r^4}$$

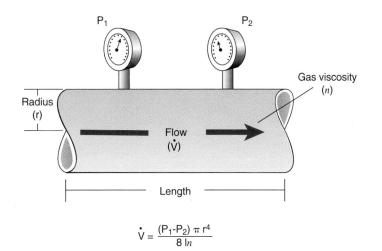

$$\dot{V} = \frac{(P_1-P_2)\ \pi\ r^4}{8\ ln}$$

FIG. 10-19 Poiseuille's law reveals that gas flow ($\dot{V}$) through a tube is increased when driving pressure (P_1-P_2) increases, tube size (radius [r^4]) increases, length of the airway (*l*) decreases, and viscosity of the gas (*n*) decreases (8 and π are constants).

This relationship demonstrates that airway resistance increases with greater gas viscosity and airway length. Normally, gas viscosity does not change while breathing air. In unusual situations the viscosity of the breathing medium can be significantly greater than that of air. This occurs when a patient is ventilated with fluorocarbon liquids.

Airway diameter is a much more influential factor of airway resistance. In Poiseuille's law the radius of the airway is a multiple to the fourth power, indicating the profound effect that airway size has on the resistance to gas flow. Increasing airway size results in much lower resistance. For example, if airway size is increased from a radius of 1 to 2 cm and all other variables are held constant, resistance would be reduced to $\frac{1}{16}$ of the initial value:

$$R \approx \frac{1}{r^4}$$
$$\text{when } r = 1 \text{ cm, } R \approx \frac{1}{1^4} \approx \frac{1}{1} \text{ or } 1$$
$$\text{when } r = 2 \text{ cm } R \approx \frac{1}{2^4} \approx \frac{1}{16}$$

Conversely, when airway size decreases, airway resistance increases. If airway radius is reduced to half of its original size (e.g., from 2 to 1 cm), resistance is increased 16 times. Looked at in another way, if the airway is reduced to half of its original size, it would require 16 times more driving pressure to maintain flow. This explains why the work of breathing can become excessive with airway obstructive diseases such as asthma.

Causes of Increased Airway Resistance

Airway resistance can be altered by a variety of conditions (Box 10-3). These changes have significant effects on the ease or work of breathing and the ability to distribute gas throughout the lung. Those factors that increase airway resistance are most problematic for gas movement into and out of the lung.

Airway Diameter

Narrowed airways can be caused by a several different pathologic conditions (Fig. 10-20). Inflammation and edema of the airway wall, bronchospasm from smooth muscle

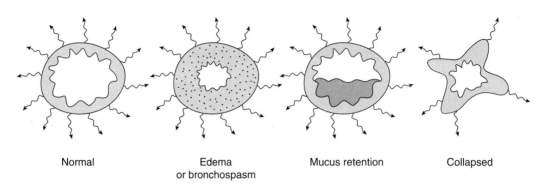

Normal   Edema   Mucus retention   Collapsed
                or bronchospasm

FIG. 10-20 Causes of airway narrowing that result in increased airway resistance.

BOX 10-3

Factors that Influence Airway Resistance

INCREASED AIRWAY RESISTANCE
Decreased airway diameter
Bronchoconstriction
Increased airway length
Increased gas viscosity
Turbulent flow
Decreased lung volume

DECREASED AIRWAY RESISTANCE
Increased airway diameter
Bronchodilation
Decreased airway length
Decreased gas viscosity ·
Laminar flow
Increased lung volume

---

constriction, mucus retention, tumor growth near or in the airway wall, and loss of outside tissue support (emphysema) lead to airway collapse and result in decreased airway diameter. As Poiseuille's law describes, a decrease in luminal diameter results in increased airway resistance.

Turbulent Flow

Ideally, flow through all the airways would be **laminar** in nature. Laminar flow exists when all the gas molecules are moving in the same direction (Fig. 10-21). The leading edge of gas flow is conical in shape because molecules in the center of the stream move slightly faster than molecules closer to the outer edge. This shape and speed difference is the result of greater friction at the outer edge of the stream. When the gas flow travels through a curved airway, a moderately distorted flow front results from the frictional interaction with the outer airway wall. During quiet breathing the laminar flow pattern normally occurs in the airways that are less than 2 mm in diameter. Laminar flow produces less friction and airway resistance because gas molecules are not interacting as much with each other and the airway wall.

In the upper and large airways, flow is generally **turbulent** in nature. Turbulent flow is a chaotic flow pattern that includes forward motion as well as streams of gas that swirl and eddy (see Fig. 10-21). The leading edge of turbulent flow is squared off. Molecular collisions are more numerous during turbulent flow, resulting in greater friction and airway resistance.

Turbulent flow can be detected by adding smoke to the gas stream and visualizing the chaotic behavior of the flow pattern. It can also be detected by determining **Reynolds' number,** a dimensionless number or ratio that describes the dynamics of fluid or gas flow.

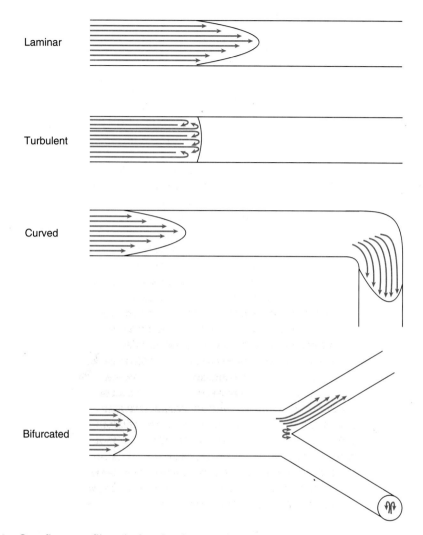

FIG. 10-21 Gas flow profiles during laminar and turbulent flow through straight, curved, and bifurcated airways.

Reynolds' number is computed with the following relationship:

$$R_e = \frac{d\dot{V}\rho}{\eta}$$

where R_e is Reynolds' number, d is the diameter of the airway, $\dot{V}$ is the flow rate of gas, ρ is the density of the gas, and η is the viscosity of the gas. Gas flow is defined to be laminar when the value of Reynolds' number is less than 2000. When Reynolds' number is greater than 2000, flow is defined as turbulent.

Turbulence occurs when flow increases, viscosity decreases, airway diameter decreases, and with irregular airway geometry. All of these factors are present in the upper airway and cause turbulent flow. During resting tidal ventilation, flow through small airways is laminar. The larger total cross-sectional diameter of these small airways and relatively low flow contribute to the formation of laminar flow. Turbulent flow can occur in small airways when gas flow increases, when airway diameter decreases, and when the airway bifurcates into two smaller airways (see Fig. 10-21).

Gas Density and Viscosity

Increased gas density or viscosity requires a greater transairway pressure gradient to move it. This is caused by greater friction that results in greater airway resistance. Narrowed airways create even greater friction when higher density or viscosity gases move through them. In those cases where narrowed airways exist, less dense gases such as helium (He) can be used to replace the nitrogen in air to reduce airway resistance. The less dense He-O_2 gas mixture (e.g., 80% He and 20% O_2) generates less airway resistance in narrowed airways and improves gas flow. This effect can be used to help uncover the presence of narrowed airways. If a subject is breathing a He-O_2 mixture and is asked to make a forceful expiratory effort, flow rates will improve in those that have narrowed or obstructive airway disease such as emphysema. Similar mixtures can be used to improve the distribution of ventilation and to reduce the work of breathing in a patient with life-threatening asthma.

Lung Volume and Transmural Pressure

The large airways, like the trachea and bronchi, have supportive cartilage in their walls that prevent their collapse. Small airways, especially those less than 2 mm in diameter, have no cartilage for support and have flexible walls. The flexible walls of these small airways are normally held open by the surrounding alveolar tissue. The elastic fibers within the alveolar walls act like numerous rubber bands that pull the airway open from all directions. This support can be altered when lung volume changes and can be enhanced or overcome when the pressure difference across the airway wall (transmural pressure) changes. As lung volume and transmural pressures change, changes in small airway diameter occur.

During slow inflation, pleural pressure decreases from -5 to -8 cm H_2O, lung volume increases by an amount equal to the tidal volume, alveolar wall tension increases, and transmural pressure (inside − outside) remains positive. This improves the outward support of the airway, maintains its diameter, and may even slightly expand the airway (Fig. 10-22). During slow exhalation, pleural pressure returns to -5 cm H_2O, lung volume drops back to the functional residual capacity, and alveolar wall tension decreases. Intraairway pressure remains positive with respect to pleural pressure (positive transmural pressure) as gas is exhaled; this supports the airway to remain open.

Small airway closure does occur in some regions of the lung when a subject is instructed to exhale completely. Significant airway closure occurs in the normal lungs of a 20-year-old subject when the lungs contain about 10% of maximal volume. This is known as the **closing volume.** Those regions most prone to closure during complete exhalation are located in the lower lobes where alveolar volume is lower. With age, alveolar wall tension declines, resulting in earlier airway closure. The closing volume in the normal 70-year-old person increases to about 40% of maximal lung volume. Increased closing volume has a significant impact on the distribution of gas in the lung during tidal ventilation when lung volume is at or below the closing volume. When the closing volume occurs during tidal ventilation, gas is brought to those regions where the airways remain open, resulting in a mismatching of regions that receive ventilation and pulmonary blood flow. The consequence of this is abnormal gas exchange.

Forceful breathing brings about greater changes in pleural pressure and transmural pressure. During forced exhalation, pleural pressure can reach values of 30 to 60 cm H_2O. This can exceed intraairway pressure and pro-

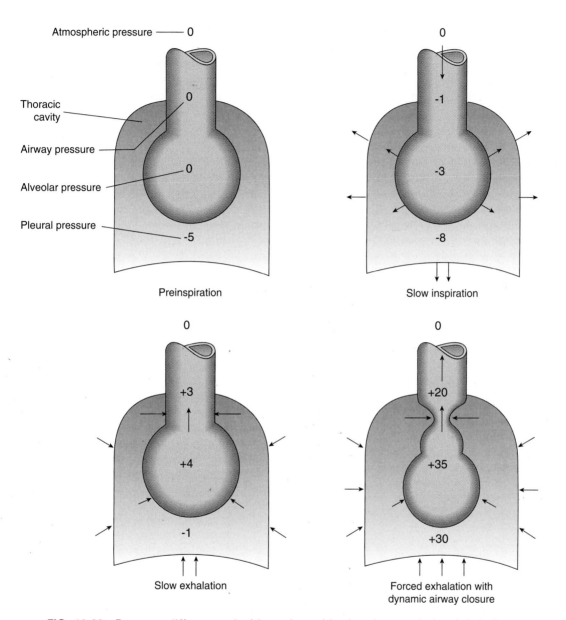

FIG. 10-22 Pressure differences inside and outside the airways during inhalation and exhalation. Dynamic airway closure occurs during forceful exhalation.

duce a negative transmural pressure. When the outside pressure exceeds inside airway pressure and transmural pressure becomes negative, **dynamic airway closure** occurs (see Fig. 10-22). This effect causes a rapid decline in the expiratory flow rate from a subject as he or she exhale forcefully and completely. The compressive effort of the accessory muscles and the recoil nature of the lungs are opposed by increasing airway resistance (secondary to declining lung volume and airway closure) and an increasing tendency of the thorax to spring outward. The combined effects of increasing airway resistance and reduced thoracic compression result in a steady decline in flow rate until the respiratory muscles are unable to compress the thorax further and flow ceases.

This process of dynamic airway closure is intensified in those who have narrowed or poorly supported airways. These individuals experience rapid closure of their small airways as they forcefully exhale and rapid declines in expiratory flow.

With forceful inhalation, the opposite occurs as pleural pressure becomes strongly negative, transmural pressure becomes positive, lung volume increases, and airway diameter increases. These effects combine to result in reduced airway resistance and relatively stable flow into the lungs. This stable flow continues until the lung's elastic recoil overcomes respiratory muscle strength and flow stops.

Nervous Control of Airway Diameter

Airway diameter is influenced by the nervous system. A variety of nerve branches penetrate the lungs and release different neurotransmitters that interact with receptors on the cell membranes of airway smooth muscle and submucosal glands (Table 10-5). Generally, the different neurotransmitters cause either inhibition or excitation of these tissues. Excitation

results in airway constriction and increased mucus production whereas inhibition results in the opposite effect. Different neurotransmitters are released from neurons of three different neural pathways. Two of these pathways arise out of the autonomic nervous system as the **parasympathetic** and **sympathetic** branches. A third pathway, called the **nonadrenergic and noncholinergic (NANC) system,** appears to control airway diameter by releasing a peptide-type neurotransmitter.

Excitation of smooth muscle and submucosal glands is brought about by activation of parasympathetic fibers. Parasympathetic fibers are supplied to the lungs from the brain stem by the vagus nerve. When active, parasympathetic fibers release the neurotransmitter **acetylcholine,** which activates **cholinergic receptors** on both smooth muscle cells and submucosal gland cells. This causes smooth muscle to develop tension and constrict the airway and submucosal glands to secrete mucus into the airway. Smooth muscle constriction and mucus secretion cause the diameter of the airway to decrease and airway resistance to increase.

Inhibition of smooth muscle tension is brought about by activation of the sympathetic nervous system. Sympathetic fibers exit from the spine as branches of the thoracic spinal nerves and penetrate the lung. When

Table 10-5   Branches of the Nervous System that Influence the Airways

Nervous Branch	Neurotransmitter Released	Receptor Activated	Action
Parasympathetic fibers	Acetylcholine	Cholinergic	Smooth muscle constriction Bronchoconstriction Mucus secretion
Sympathetic fibers	Norepinephrine	Adrenergic (β_2 receptors)	Smooth muscle relaxation Bronchodilation Reduced mucus production
NANC system fibers	VIP	VIP receptors	Smooth muscle relaxation Bronchodilation

NANC, Nonadrenergic and noncholinergic; *VIP,* vasoactive intestinal peptide.

activated, they release the neurotransmitter **norepinephrine.** However, they do not release norepinephrine directly into the airway smooth muscle and submucosal glands, but they release essentially all of their norepinephrine into the walls of the pulmonary blood vessels. From here it moves to other tissues by diffusion. **Epinephrine,** a hormone produced by the adrenal gland during sympathetic stimulation, also flows into the lungs (via pulmonary blood flow) during stressful events. Norepinephrine and epinephrine activate a type of **adrenergic receptor** called a β_2 receptor. Activation of β_2 receptors inhibits smooth muscle contraction and submucosal gland secretion of mucus. The airway dilates and less mucus fills the airway, which results in lower airway resistance.

Bronchodilating drugs carry out their action by either stimulating β_2 adrenergic receptors or by blocking cholinergic receptors, resulting in inhibition of smooth muscle activity and reduction of mucus production. Together they reduce the effort of breathing by reducing airway resistance.

The NANC system, the main pathway that inhibits smooth muscle tension, secretes a peptide hormone called **vasoactive intestinal peptide (VIP)** directly into the wall of the airway. VIP was first found to be produced in the gut. When the NANC system is activated, VIP is released, activating NANC receptors on smooth muscle. This inhibits smooth muscle tension, resulting in dilation of the airway.

The amount of activity in the parasympathetic, sympathetic, and NANC systems determines the degree of airway constriction or dilation. The system that is most active provides the dominant effect. Nervous regulation of the airway is provided by balancing the excitatory action of the parasympathetic system against the inhibitory actions of the sympathetic and NANC systems. These effects provide some level of control over the entry of substances into the lungs. Activation of the parasympathetic branches helps protect the lungs by preventing the entry of material whereas the sympathetic and NANC branches function to counteract parasympathetic activity and enhance air flow in response to stress and increased metabolism.

Regional Differences in Resistance and Compliance

Compliance and airway resistance are not uniform throughout the lungs. Some regions have higher compliance than others. The same is true for airway resistance. These differences are produced by the effects of gravity on the lungs as they "hang" within the thorax. This results in greater ventilation in some regions than others.

The regions of the lungs where compliance is greatest have alveoli that are not overinflated. The apical lung is pulled by gravity into a greater state of inflation when compared with alveoli in the lower parts of the lungs. This results in a higher compliance in the lower lung zones when compared with upper lung zones. Fig. 10-23 illustrates this by comparing pleural pressure changes, positions in the pressure-volume relationship, and degree of volume change in the two regions. The apical region experiences less volume change than the basal region despite their exposure to the same pleural pressure change of 3 cm H_2O. As a result, a greater portion of the tidal volume is distributed to the lower lung region during tidal ventilation.

Airway resistance is also different in different lung regions. The somewhat overinflated alveoli in the apical lung zone produce greater alveolar wall tension on the walls of the small airways. This greater airway opening force causes greater airway diameter and lower airway resistance. The lower lung zones have less alveolar wall tension and less small airway wall tension. As a consequence, the airways of the lower parts of the lung have a slightly smaller diameter and a greater airway resistance. This tends to enhance gas flow toward the apical lung zones. However, the

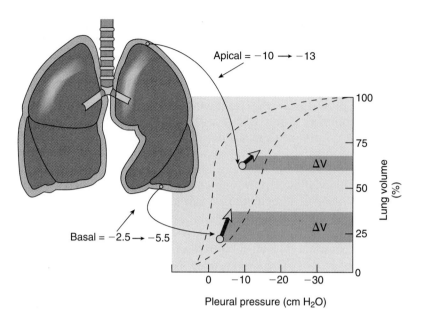

FIG. 10-23 Apical regions of the lung have a lower compliance than the basal regions. Greater amounts of volume are distributed to the lower lung regions during tidal breathing.

lower compliance of the apical lung prevents enhanced flow to this region.

These differences result in somewhat better distribution of gas volume to the lower regions of the upright lungs. The lessons from these differences can be applied to regions of the lungs that have altered lung mechanics. Those areas that have lower compliance and greater airway resistance are more difficult to ventilate.

Measuring Airway Resistance

Airway resistance is determined by simultaneous measurements of gas flow ($\dot{V}$) and transrespiratory pressure (P_{rs}):

$$R_{AW} = \frac{P_{rs}}{\dot{V}}$$

The use of an airtight cabinet called a **body plethysmograph** is the most common tool employed to make these measurements (Fig. 10-24). The subject sits within the sealed body plethysmograph and breathes through a mouthpiece equipped with a pressure sensor,

flow sensors, and an occlusive shutter. Mouth pressure, cabinet pressure, and flow are simultaneously measured. When the subject is instructed to pant through the mouthpiece, two different measurements are made to determine gas flow and transairway pressure. Initially the shutter is open and gas flow generated during the panting maneuver is measured with the flow sensor. Simultaneously, the changes in cabinet pressure are measured and both are recorded on an oscilloscope screen. The shutter is then closed and the subject is instructed to continue panting with the same force. With the shutter closed the fluctuations in pressure measured at the mouth and cabinet pressure are recorded simultaneously on the oscilloscope screen. When the shutter is closed, mouth pressure equals alveolar pressure. Cabinet pressure becomes positive as the thorax enlarges during inhalation and becomes negative during exhalation as the thorax becomes smaller. Dividing flow (during open shutter panting) and alveolar pressure (mouth pressure during closed

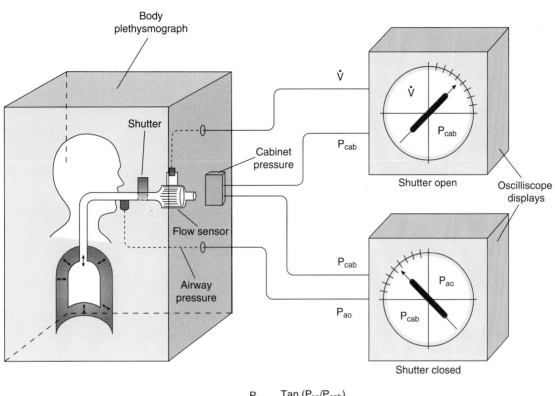

$$R_{AW} = \frac{P_{rs}}{\dot{V}} = \frac{Tan\ (P_{ao}/P_{cab})}{Tan\ (\dot{V}/P_{cab})}$$

FIG. 10-24 Airway resistance (RAW) can be determined with a body plethysmograph by measuring airway pressure (P_{ao}), cabinet pressure (P_{cab}), and flow ($\dot{V}$) during open and closed shutter panting.

shutter panting) by cabinet pressure enables these two values to be proportioned so that they approximate the magnitude they would be if they were measured simultaneously.

Airway resistance is determined with the body plethysmograph technique by using the following relationship:

$$R_{AW} = \frac{P_{rs}}{\dot{V}}$$

$$= \frac{Tan\left(\dfrac{\Delta P_{ao}}{P_{cab}}\right)}{Tan\left(\dfrac{\dot{V}}{P_{cab}}\right)}$$

The average $\Delta P_{ao}/P_{cab}$ and $\dot{V}/P_{cab}$ produced during the maneuver is determined by taking the tangent of the angles produced on the oscilloscope during open- and closed-shutter panting. This technique reveals that normal adult R_{AW} values range from 0.6 to 2.8 cm $H_2O/L/sec$.

Total airway resistance is the sum of the resistances generated in the upper airways (e.g., nose, mouth, and pharynx), large airways (e.g., trachea and bronchi), and small airways (e.g., bronchioles less than 2 mm in diameter). Because these airways are arranged anatomically in series, total airway resistance is equal to the sum of the resistance they each contribute:

$$R_{total} = R_{upper\ airway} + R_{large\ airways} + R_{small\ airways}$$

The airway resistance generated in each region of the tracheobronchial tree is shown in Fig. 10-25. Upper and large airways are responsible for about 80% of total airway resistance, and the small airways contribute the remaining 20%. The much lower resistance in airways that are the size of tiny terminal bronchioles is due to the large number of these airways and their parallel arrangement. When the cross-sectional area of all 30,000 terminal bronchioles is added up, it yields a value of about 115 cm². This is 23 times larger than the 5-cm² cross-sectional area of the trachea. The large cross-sectional diameter of the bronchioles results in much lower resistance.

Airway Conductance

Airway conductance (G_{AW}) is another approach that is used to describe the resistive properties of gas flow. Airway conductance is the reciprocal of airway resistance:

$$G_{AW} = \frac{\dot{V}}{\Delta P}$$
$$= L/sec/cm\ H_2O$$

Airway conductance defines the amount of flow generated through the airways when the transairway pressure gradient is 1 cm H_2O. The normal value of airway conductance in the adult ranges from 0.36 to 1.70 L/sec/cm H_2O.

Specific Airway Resistance and Conductance

Airway resistance and conductance changes with different lung volumes. Higher lung volumes cause the small airways to dilate. Alveolar walls are stretched with higher lung volume, and this force is applied to the outside of the airway wall. These forces, oriented in a radial pattern around the airway, pull outward on the airway wall to open it. This causes small airway dilation, which reduces airway resistance and increases airway conductance. The opposite activity occurs with low lung volume. Reduced lung volume results in lower alveolar volume and less alveolar wall stretching. Lower alveolar wall tension causes reduced radial force to be applied to the small airway. This causes these airways to partially or completely close. As a result, resistance increases and conductance decreases.

The standard technique for measuring airway resistance with the body plethysmograph assumes the subject is panting at a normal lung volume. This assumption can be wrong when the subject pants at high or low lung volume. As a consequence, the measurements can give the impression of lower or higher resistance. To improve the significance of the measurements, the value can be adjusted for the volume of gas in the lung at the time of the measurement. The adjustment entails measuring lung volume and dividing the resistance

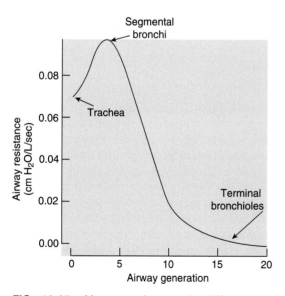

FIG. 10-25 Airway resistance in different regions of the airway.

or conductance value by the lung volume. This procedure produces the value known as **specific airway resistance (SR_{AW})** or **specific airway conductance (SG_{AW}):**

$$SR_{AW} = \frac{R_{AW}}{V_{Lung}}$$

$$SG_{AW} = \frac{G_{AW}}{V_{Lung}}$$

Average lung volume is determined during the panting maneuver and this is used to adjust R_{AW} and G_{AW}. The normal adult value for specific airway resistance ranges from 0.19 to 0.67 cm $H_2O/L/sec/L$. Normal adult specific airway conductance ranges from 0.11 to 0.40 $L/sec/cm$ H_2O/L.

Dynamic Respiratory System Compliance

The beginning of this chapter described the elastic behavior of the lungs and chest wall through the use of static inflation and determination of static compliance. A similar approach can be used to describe how the combined effects of elastic and resistive forces retard expansion when the respiratory system is dynamically filled and emptied. The amount of pressure needed to expand the lung and to overcome airway resistance can be used to determine the **dynamic compliance** of the system.

Dynamic compliance, measured during active breathing rather than during breath holding, yields pressure changes that are influenced by both elastic-resistive as well as flow-resistive properties. Dynamic lung compliance is determined by measuring the change in lung volume and pleural pressure simultaneously with the use of a flow sensor and esophageal balloon-tipped catheter. As the subject breathes, the flow sensor detects the volume change, and the esophageal balloon-catheter detects pleural pressure changes. During normal resting breathing the lung is inflated and deflated (ΔV) with a tidal volume of 0.5 L whereas the pleural

pressure varies (ΔP_{pl}) from -5 to -8 cm H_2O for a net change of 3 cm H_2O (see Fig. 10-9). The following relationship is then used to determine dynamic lung compliance ($dynC_L$):

$$dynC_L = \frac{\Delta V}{\Delta P_{pl}}$$
$$= \frac{0.5\ L}{3\ cm\ H_2O}$$
$$= 0.167\ L/cm\ H_2O\ or\ 167\ ml/cm\ H_2O$$

Note that this normal value is somewhat lower than the normal value of static lung compliance (200 ml/cm H_2O). Dynamic compliance is consistently lower than static compliance as a result of airway and pulmonary tissue resistance. The difference reflects the resistance generated during active inflation. The added resistance causes a greater change in pressure and, therefore, a lower compliance value.

Dynamic lung compliance is also effected by the respiratory rate. This sensitivity makes dynamic compliance a **frequency-dependent compliance**. The change in dynamic compliance is brought about by gas flow turbulence and incomplete emptying of various lung regions.

As a subject increases their respiratory rate, air flow increases and becomes more turbulent. In addition, the amount of time available for the ventilatory cycle decreases. Decreasing the expiratory time results in some incomplete alveolar emptying. With increasing alveolar volume, the compliance of the lung declines. The combination of increasing turbulence and decreasing alveolar compliance results in a decreased dynamic compliance.

Airway obstructive diseases (e.g., asthma and emphysema) cause greater declines in dynamic compliance when the respiratory rate increases. These conditions reveal a greater frequency-dependent compliance.

Total respiratory system dynamic compliance, measured during mechanical ventilation,

CASE STUDY FOCUS

Respiratory Distress during a Severe Asthma Attack

A 28-year-old woman was brought to the emergency room for increasing respiratory distress that had escalated over the past 6 hours. Her vital signs were as follows:

Heart rate	127/min
Blood pressure	137/89
Respiratory rate	24/min (with difficulty)
Temperature	38° C

Also, her blood oxygen levels were reduced. She had high-pitched expiratory wheezing that was audible without the use of a stethoscope and had difficulty answering questions in complete sentences without gasping for air. She said that she had developed a cold and that her asthma suddenly got worse.

The asthmatic airway is generally hypersensitive, and, during an attack or exacerbation, the medium and small airway smooth muscles constrict, the bronchial mucosa become inflamed and edematous, and large amounts of thick mucus is produced by the mucosa. These changes result in narrowing of the airway lumen, increased airway resistance, and increased work of breathing. In severe cases the airways can be narrowed to the point of complete obstruction. An asthma attack can be triggered by exposure to allergens, infections, breathing cold air, inhaling pollutants, eating certain foods, and other types of exposures.

She was instructed in the use of a peak expiratory flow meter (her peak expiratory flow was 22% of normal, which is consistent with severe airway obstruction). She was given supplemental oxygen to breathe, an intravenous line was started, and an inhalation treatment of aerosolized albuterol was given. Albuterol is a β_2 antagonist that stimulates airway smooth muscle relaxation. This was followed by a chest x-ray, which showed hyperinflation of both lungs. Over the next 40 minutes she was given two more aerosolized albuterol treatments. Shortly after the third treatment her peak expiratory flow had improved to 52% of normal and she felt that the work of breathing was less. She was discharged 6 hours later without significant dyspnea and in stable condition. She was instructed in the use of the peak flow meter, how to use it to monitor asthma, and when to better time the use of the asthma medications she has at home.

is determined by measuring the peak inflation pressure needed to move a volume of gas into the lungs at a given flow. The normal value is 70 ml/cm H_2O or about 70% of total static compliance. The value of total dynamic compliance reveals the combined effects of elasticity, surface tension, air flow resistance, and tissue resistance that must be overcome to inflate the lungs dynamically. Dynamic compliance reveals how much volume fills the lungs when a given amount of pressure is applied. This is a good indicator of the overall mechanical condition of the system and how much effort the respiratory muscles have to develop to move a certain amount of gas.

Time Constant

When the respiratory muscles work on the thorax and lungs to enlarge them and cause alveolar pressure to become negative, alveolar pressure does not instantaneously return to airway opening pressure, or 0. Instead it requires some time for gas to flow through the airways and fill the lungs. This time-dependent process is influenced by respiratory system compliance and airway resistance. For example, when the lung becomes stiff and compliance drops, the lungs take less time to distend. On the other hand, if the airways become narrow and airway resistance increases, the lungs require more time to distend. The amount of time required can be determined by calculating the **time constant.** The time constant (τ) is the product of multiplying airway resistance (R_{AW}) and compliance (C_{rs}):

$$\tau = R_{AW} \times C_{rs}$$

One time constant is the amount of time it takes to fill (or empty) 60% of a region of lung. To completely fill (or empty) a region requires three time constants. The normal time constant in the adult lung is 0.2 second. This means that it will takes 0.6 second for gas to finish flowing into a region to fill it. Stiff lungs with large airways require less time whereas highly compliant lungs with narrow airways require much more time. If the amount of time that is devoted to inflating the lungs is less than three time constants, the lungs will not completely fill. In those situations where there are less than three time constants to exhale, the lungs will not empty but will trap gas.

● RESPIRATORY MUSCLE WORK

Work of Breathing

The amount of effort the respiratory muscles exert during the ventilatory cycle is frequently described as the **work of breathing.** Respiratory muscle work must be sufficient to overcome the elastic, surface tension, resistive, and inertial properties of the lungs, chest wall, and gas. Normally, the respiratory muscles have sufficient strength and endurance to perform the amount of work necessary on an indefinite basis. In some cases, however, ventilatory failure can occur when the muscles are incapable of performing sufficient work.

The workload of the respiratory muscles can be evaluated in a number of different ways. Observation of a patient can reveal increased workload. Careful analysis of the pressure changes generated during tidal ventilation can reveal the mechanical workload.

Measurements of the amount of oxygen consumed by the respiratory muscles provide an index of the metabolic "cost" of breathing.

Bedside Indicators of Increased Work

The most common method employed to evaluate respiratory muscle work is the physical examination of a subject while he or she is breathing. Through careful inspection, palpation, and **auscultation** (listening to the chest with a stethoscope), the level of respiratory muscle activity can be assessed. During quiet breathing, the normal subject breathes at a rate of 12 to 16 times per minute while rhythmically expanding and collapsing the chest and abdominal walls in a synchronous fashion. During this cycle the chest and abdominal walls move about 1 or 2 cm in an anterior direction. The soft tissues found above the clavicle, between the ribs, and just below the inferior rib margin do not retract or bulge during the normal cycle. The amount of time devoted to the inspiratory phase is about 1 to 2 seconds whereas the expiratory phase lasts about 3 to 4 seconds. This yields a normal **inspiratory-to-expiratory** (I:E) **ratio** of about 1:3. Palpation of the neck, chest, and abdominal walls reveals little muscle tensing. Auscultation of the chest with a stethoscope discloses some faint "white" noise (the sound of sanding wood) during the inspiratory phase and relatively quiet noise during the expiratory phase.

Numerous changes can be detected that indicate increasing respiratory muscle work (Box 10-4). Increasing rate, thoracic wall movement, and inspiratory time require increased muscle activity. The most commonly encountered respiratory rhythm disturbance that indicates increasing work is rapid **(tachypnea)** and shallow **(hypopnea)** breathing with an I:E ratio that approaches 1:1. Detecting the use of accessory muscles, either by seeing or palpating increased muscle tension, is an important sign that increasing effort

Physical Findings that Indicate Increasing Respiratory Muscle Work

Increasing respiratory rate (>20 breaths/min)
Increasing tidal volume (chest and abdominal wall expansion)
Increasing inspiratory time
Rhythm changes (increased rate, tidal volume, and inspiratory time)
Soft tissue retractions
Nasal flaring
Accessory muscle use (abdominal wall muscle and sternocleidomastoid tensing)
Alternating use of diaphragm and accessory muscles (respiratory alternans)
Chest and abdominal dyssynchrony (paradoxical motion)
Adventitious breath sounds (crackles, wheezes, or rhonchi)

is needed to breathe. Nasal flaring also occurs with increased work and represents a form of accessory muscle use that results in dilation of the external nares in an attempt to reduce upper airway resistance. Often the individual mouth breathes to reduce upper airway resistance. Increasing muscle activity with low compliant lungs or high airway resistance causes pleural pressures to "swing" further with greater negative and positive pressure changes. This, in turn, causes the soft tissues between the ribs, above the clavicles, and below the lower rib margins to retract and bulge. Soft tissue retractions are significant indicators of elevated work. In rare cases the subject may alternate the use of chest muscles for a short period followed by use of the diaphragm and then a repeat of this pattern. This alternating use has been given the name **respiratory alternans** and is thought to be a strategy for resting some muscles for a short period while other muscles carry the load. Loss of chest and abdominal wall synchronous motion during the breathing cycle also signals increasing respiratory muscle work.

Occasional loss of respiratory rhythm indicates respiratory muscle fatigue. The detection of **adventitious breath sounds** (crackles, wheezes, or rhonchi) indicates increased airway resistance and added work. All of these changes are the signs of increasing respiratory muscle work and breathing discomfort commonly referred to as **dyspnea.**

Mechanical Work

Work (W) is defined mechanically as the application of force to move an object of known weight a given vertical distance:

$$W = Weight \times Vertical\ distance\ moved$$

The units used to express the amount of mechanical work done on an object are the kilogram × meter (kg × m) and the joule (J) (1 kg × m is equivalent to 10.0 J).

The concept of mechanical work can be applied to the work done by the respiratory muscles on the lungs and thorax. The respiratory muscles perform work by causing pleural pressure changes and inflation of the lungs and thorax. These changes are analogous to moving an amount of weight a given vertical distance.

Measuring the mechanical work of breathing requires simultaneous recordings of pressure and volume change. The work done on the lungs alone is determined by recording tidal volume and pleural pressure on a pressure-volume plot. The area within various parts of the pressure-volume loop corresponds to the amount of mechanical work being performed.

Fig. 10-26 illustrates a recording of a normal pleural pressure-tidal volume loop and its relationship to the normal static inflation curve. Note that the tidal breathing loop oscillates around a region of the static inflation curve where the slope of the curve is steepest and a region where static compliance is greatest.

Fig. 10-27, *A*, shows an enlargement of a normal pleural pressure-tidal volume loop. It records changes that take place during various parts of one breathing cycle: inhalation

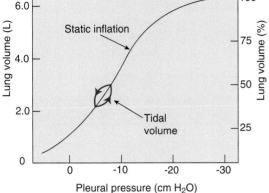

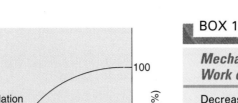

FIG. 10-26 Position of a normal pressure-volume loop generated during tidal breathing and its relationship to a normal static inflation curve.

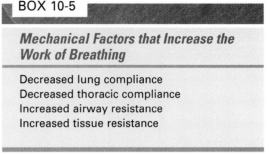

BOX 10-5

Mechanical Factors that Increase the Work of Breathing

Decreased lung compliance
Decreased thoracic compliance
Increased airway resistance
Increased tissue resistance

starts at point *A,* inhalation extends along *I* to point *B,* and exhalation begins and extends along *E* to point *A.* The shaded area, labeled *AIBCA,* represents the work done to overcome elasticity, surface tension, and the resistive properties of the lung when inflating it with a normal tidal volume. The shaded region of Fig. 10-27, *B,* labeled *ABCA,* reveals that portion of the work done during inflation to overcome the elastic and surface tension properties of the lungs. This work is stored as potential energy in the lung and released during exhalation when the respiratory muscles relax. Normally the potential energy stored in the lungs during inflation is sufficient to force gas from the lungs when the respiratory muscles relax. The unshaded region of the loop in Fig. 10-27, *B,* labeled *AIBA,* corresponds to the work done during inhalation to overcome airway and tissue resistance. All of this resistive work is not stored in the lung as potential energy. It is lost as an insignificant increase in temperature as the result of frictional resistance.

Analysis of the pressure-volume loop can reveal the effects that different types of pul-

monary disease have on the work of breathing. Fig. 10-28 shows that obstructive and restrictive pulmonary diseases increase the pleural pressure, and as a consequence, the shaded area of the loop increases when compared with a normal condition. This indicates that increased work is necessary to inflate the lung with the same volume in both conditions. Closer analysis of the loop reveals that increased work is performed in different ways. Obstructive pulmonary diseases, such as asthma or emphysema, cause increased work as a result of greater airway resistance. The respiratory muscles perform more work by generating greater pleural pressure to move gas through obstructed airways. In addition, the respiratory muscles are active during inhalation and exhalation. This causes the loop to "open up" and expand laterally. In restrictive pulmonary diseases, such as pulmonary fibrosis or reduced surfactant synthesis, greater work is caused by lower lung compliance. The respiratory muscles perform more work to generate greater pleural pressure changes to expand the stiff lungs. This causes the loop to "tip over" to the right and increases the area that indicates greater elastic tension- or surface tension-generated work. Those factors that increase the mechanical work of breathing are summarized in Box 10-5.

The area within the pressure-volume loop can be determined by planimetry or by integration of the simultaneous changes of pressure and volume with the following equation:

$$W = \Delta P_{pl} \times \Delta V$$

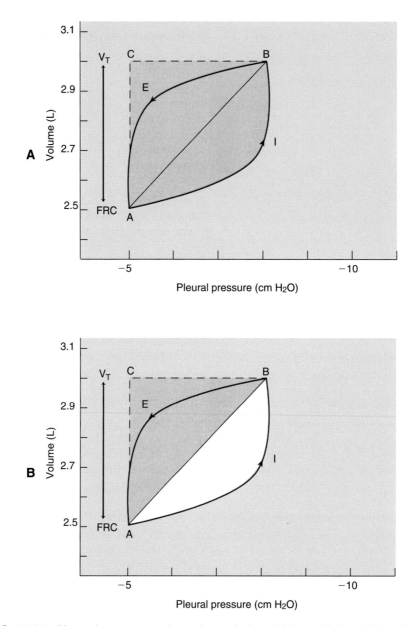

FIG. 10-27 Normal pressure-volume loop during tidal ventilation (*I,* inhalation; *E,* exhalation). **A,** Shaded area corresponds to the amount of work done to inflate the lungs and overcome the elastic, surface tension, tissue resistance, and airway resistance. **B,** Shaded area corresponds to the amount of work done to overcome only the elastic and surface tension properties of the lung (see text for further description). *FRC,* Functional residual capacity; *VT,* tidal volume.

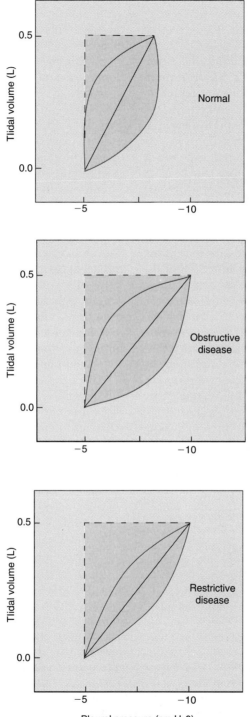

FIG. 10-28 Pressure-volume loops in a normal subject and those with obstructive and restrictive pulmonary diseases.

where W is work performed, P_{pl} is pleural pressure, and V is the volume change in the lung. When using this technique, the respiratory muscles are found to perform about 0.025 kg × m or 0.25 J of work per breath to inflate the lungs in a normal subject. To put this into perspective, a subject performs about 100 J of work per second when riding a bicycle up a steep hill. Thus the normal amount of work done by the respiratory muscles to inhale a normal tidal volume is an extremely small fraction of the total work being performed by all of the skeletal muscles when a subject is active.

Presently, there is no method for measuring the mechanical work done to move either the thorax or the total respiratory system in a spontaneously breathing subject. However, it is possible to measure the work done on the total respiratory system when a mechanical ventilator is used to inflate the lungs of a passive subject. This can be accomplished by measuring airway pressure, pleural pressure, and tidal volume. The work done on the entire system can be determined by measuring the area of the volume-airway pressure loop. Work done on the thorax can be measured by analyzing the volume-transthoracic (atmospheric-pleural) pressure loop. The work done on the lungs alone is determined by analyzing the volume-transpulmonary (airway-pleural) pressure loop.

Effects of Pulmonary Mechanics and Breathing Pattern

The following relationship shows how the mechanical work of breathing is proportional to the breathing pattern and mechanical properties of the respiratory system:

$$W \approx \times f \times V_T \times R \times E$$

where W is the total work of breathing, f is the frequency or rate of breathing, V_T is the tidal volume, R is the resistance (tissue and airway) of the system, and E is the elasticity (surface tension and elastic tissue properties) of the system. This relationship demonstrates how changes in these variables effect the work of breathing. Increases in airway or tissue resistance, rate of breathing, tidal volume, and elasticity (or decreased compliance) result in increased work of breathing. A worst-case scenario would be conditions that lead to high airway resistance, reduced lung or chest wall compliance, and deep and rapid breathing that require the greatest amount of work.

Various therapeutic approaches to reduce the work of breathing often address one or more of the previously mentioned conditions. The use of bronchodilator drugs can reduce elevated airway resistance in individuals with bronchospasm. Surfactant replacement therapy effectively reduces surface tension and improves lung compliance. Oxygen therapy is useful in reducing the rate and depth of breathing. Mechanical ventilation performs all or most of the work that the respiratory muscles would have to perform.

The normal rate and depth of breathing occurs in a combination that results in the least amount of work. Fig. 10-29 shows how changes in the rate of breathing and size of the tidal breath effect the work that is performed. Elastic work increases with the size of the tidal breath. Flow-resistive work increases with increasing flow rates as the rate of breathing increases. The total work of breathing reaches a minimum at an optimal combination of rate and tidal volume: rate = 12 to 16, tidal volume = 400 to 500 ml, and an I:E = 1:3. This normal breathing pattern reflects an unconscious economy on the part of the respiratory control center to do the least amount of work for effective gas exchange.

Shifts in the breathing pattern reflect the need to minimize the work of breathing as mechanical and gas exchange properties of the respiratory system change. Conditions that result in restrictive pulmonary disease, such as surfactant deficiencies or thoracic deformities, often cause rapid and shallow breathing. To avoid the increased elastic work brought

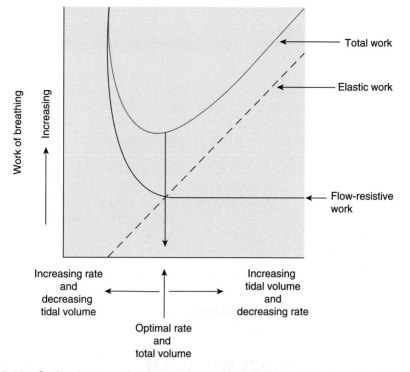

Work of breathing · Increasing →

Total work

Elastic work

Flow-resistive work

Increasing rate and decreasing tidal volume ←

→ Increasing tidal volume and decreasing rate

Optimal rate and total volume

FIG. 10-29 Optimal rate and volume of breathing is that point where the total work of breathing (elastic and flow-resistive) is at a minimum.

on with restrictive pulmonary diseases, the patient often elects to breathe with a smaller tidal breath at a faster rate. Obstructive airway diseases, such as asthma, often cause a different shift in the breathing pattern. Airway obstruction creates greater resistance in those who are breathing with higher flow rates. To compensate, these individuals tend to breathe more slowly with a deeper tidal volume. This shift reduces airway-resistive work but costs these people more elastic work as they compensate by breathing with larger tidal volumes. Although these responses to restrictive and obstructive pulmonary diseases minimize the added work of breathing, in virtually all cases, the overall work of breathing increases. These changes in the breathing pattern represent a form of partial compensation for the added work.

Metabolic Cost of Breathing

Like other skeletal muscle tissue, the respiratory muscles have a dynamic metabolic rate that changes with activity. The oxygen consumption rate of these tissues is a good indicator of their overall metabolic rate. Measuring whole body oxygen consumption during spontaneous and then during fully supported mechanical ventilation reveals a difference that results from respiratory muscle activity. At rest the difference is about 3 to 5 ml/min which represents about 1% to 2% of the total metabolic rate. This indicates that the cost of quiet breathing is low. During voluntary hyperventilation, when both rate and depth of breathing are increased to maximum, the metabolic rate of the respiratory muscles can reach 70 to 80 ml/min or about 30% of the total metabolic rate. This increase is brought about by recruiting more muscle fibers to develop greater force during both phases of breathing.

The cost of breathing can be excessive when oxygen delivery to the respiratory muscles is not sufficient to meet their metabolic needs and muscle fatigue occurs. This can happen in the patient with end-stage pulmonary disease. In this situation, poor gas exchange coupled with elevated respiratory muscle workload can be life threatening. Elevated metabolic rate and poor oxygen delivery can result in reduced respiratory muscle endurance, fatigue, and eventual ventilatory failure.

The respiratory muscles (especially the diaphragm) are well equipped for sustained use. About 55% of their muscle fibers are the highly aerobic, slow-twitch type, which gives these muscles greater endurance as long as they are supplied with an adequate blood flow and are not overloaded.

Respiratory Muscle Strength

The respiratory muscles normally have the ability to perform sufficient work to deform the respiratory system and move the tidal volume at a normal rate indefinitely, which says little about their maximal ability or strength. Maximal strength can be determined by measuring either the maximal volume that can be moved or the maximal pressure that can be generated.

The maximal volume of gas a subject can move in a single breath can be measured with a device called a **spirometer.** The single breath maximum is determined by having a subject force as much gas from the lungs as possible during one expiratory effort after completely filling the lungs. This volume of gas is called the **forced vital capacity (FVC).** The normal amount of gas that can be forced from the lungs during this effort ranges from 3 to 6 L in the adult and is largely influenced by the size of the thorax and lungs. Measurement of the FVC gives important information about how well the respiratory muscles are able to

fill and empty the lungs during a maximal effort. Reduced muscle strength results in a reduced ability to fill and exhale a normal vital capacity.

Another measure of respiratory muscle strength is the ability of the respiratory muscles to generate pressure change. Normally, the respiratory muscles cause pleural and alveolar pressure to change about 3 cm H_2O during the breathing cycle. Maximal pressure generation can be determined by blocking the upper airway and recording mouth pressure changes during maximal effort. **Maximal inspiratory pressures (P_{Imax})** generated by adults' average -114 cm H_2O in young men and -67 cm H_2O in young women. During forced expiratory efforts, **maximal expiratory pressures (P_{Emax})** average 160 cm H_2O in young men and 95 cm H_2O in young women. This means that the respiratory muscles are capable of generating more than 30 times the amount of force necessary for tidal breathing. This excess strength is in reserve for times of stress that require greater ventilation and when the respiratory system needs to be protected by an effective cough.

Respiratory muscle failure can be caused by local as well as remote defects. It can be the result of reduced signal generation in the brain, spinal cord, and peripheral nerves (e.g., injury and drug overdose). This disrupts the release of acetylcholine into the myoneural junction. At the muscle the acetylcholine receptors may be defective or blocked (e.g., myasthenia gravis). Electrolyte abnormalities and insufficient oxygen and nutrient transport to muscle fibers, can lead to actin or myosin dysfunction. All of these conditions can result in either reduced muscle tension or paralysis. The consequences could range from reduced ventilatory reserve to ventilatory failure and death. Reduced FVC and P_{max} indicate reduced respiratory muscle strength and reduced ventilatory reserve, and severe reduction can signal ventilatory failure and the need for ventilatory assistance.

CHAPTER SELF-TEST QUESTIONS

1. How do rib pairs 7 through 10 move with respect to the other ribs?
   - a. anteriorly in a bucket handle motion
   - b. laterally in a caliper motion
   - c. vertically in a pump handle motion
   - d. interiorly in a valvelike motion
2. The diaphragm enlarges the thoracic cavity by developing tension and
   - a. flattening
   - b. thickening
   - c. lengthening
   - d. constricting
3. Which of the following accessory muscles of breathing aid inspiration by enlarging the thorax?
   1. sternocleidomastoid muscles
   2. external intercostal muscles
   3. abdominal wall muscles
   - a. 1 only
   - b. 1 and 2
   - c. 2 and 3
   - d. 1 and 3
   - e. 1, 2, and 3
4. During quiet breathing, exhalation of gas from the lungs is normally propelled by the
   - a. springlike action of the thorax
   - b. compression forces developed by the accessory muscles
   - c. constricting effect of the airway smooth muscle
   - d. recoil nature of the lungs
5. The pressure difference between the mouth (airway opening) and alveolus is responsible for the movement of gas through the airways. This transorgan pressure difference is known as the
   - a. transthoracic pressure
   - b. transdiaphragmatic pressure
   - c. transmural pressure
   - d. transpulmonary pressure
   - e. transrespiratory pressure
6. Which of the following are true about the inspiratory phase of the normal ventilatory cycle?

1. about 0.5 L of gas is moved into the lungs
2. pleural pressure becomes more negative
3. alveolar pressure becomes positive
   - a. 1 only
   - b. 2 and 3
   - c. 1 and 2
   - d. 1 and 3
   - e. 1, 2, and 3
7. Which of the following changes result in reduced lung compliance?
   1. increased deposition of collagen in the alveolar wall
   2. decreasing airway diameter
   3. reduced surfactant production by the lungs
   - a. 3 only
   - b. 2 and 3
   - c. 1 and 3
   - d. 1 and 2
   - e. 1, 2, and 3
8. Which of the following are functions of surfactant?
   1. helps remove water from the alveolar surface
   2. improves lung volume for a given pleural pressure
   3. reduces the work of breathing by improving lung compliance
   - a. 2 only
   - b. 1 and 2
   - c. 1 and 3
   - d. 2 and 3
   - e. 1, 2, and 3
9. Which of the following cause the airway resistance in the lungs to increase?
   1. increased airway diameter
   2. increased gas viscosity
   3. turbulent flow
   4. decreased lung volume
   - a. 2, 3, and 4
   - b. 1, 3, and 4
   - c. 1, 2, and 3
   - d. 1, 2, and 4
   - e. 1, 2, 3, and 4

10. The mechanical work of breathing can be determined by evaluating the shape and area of a pressure-volume loop. Which of the following conditions cause the area of the pressure-volume loop to increase, indicating an increased work of breathing?
   1. increased airway resistance
   2. decreased respiratory system compliance
   3. decreased pulmonary tissue resistance
   4. increased lung surfactant
      a. 3 and 4
      b. 1 and 2
      c. 1, 2, and 3
      d. 1, 2, and 4
      e. 2, 3, and 4

For answers, see p. 475.

BIBLIOGRAPHY

1. Derenne JP, Macklem PT, Roussos C: The respiratory muscles: mechanics, control, and pathophysiology, *Am Rev Respir Dis* 118(3):581, 1978.
2. Fenn WO, Rahn H, eds: *Handbook of physiology*, vol 2, Washington, DC, 1964, American Physiologic Society.
3. Guyton AC: *Textbook of medical physiology*, Philadelphia, 1996, WB Saunders.
4. Laitinen LA, Laitinen A: Innervation of airway smooth muscle, *Am Rev Respir Dis* 136:S38, 1987.
5. Leech JA et al: Respiratory pressure and function in young adults, *Am Rev Respir Dis* 128:17, 1983.
6. Leff AR, Schumacker PT: *Respiratory physiology: basics and applications*, Philadelphia, 1993, WB Saunders.
7. Levitzky GL, Hall SM, McDonough KH: *Cardiopulmonary physiology in anesthesiology*, New York, 1997, McGraw Hill.
8. Martini FH: *Fundamentals of anatomy and physiology*, Upper Saddle River, NJ, 1998, Prentice Hall.
9. Milic-Emili J, ed: *Applied physiology in respiratory mechanics (topics in anesthesia and critical care)*, New York, 1998, Springer-Verlag.
10. Murray JF: *The normal lung: the basis for diagnosis and treatment of pulmonary disease*, ed 2, Philadelphia, 1986, WB Saunders.
11. Nunn JF: *Applied respiratory physiology*, ed 3, London, 1987, Butterworths.
12. Pierson DJ, Kacmarek RM: *Foundations of respiratory care*, New York, 1992, Churchill Livingstone.
13. Staub NC: *Basic respiratory physiology*, New York, 1991, Churchill Livingstone.
14. West JB: *Respiratory physiology: the essentials*, ed 4, Baltimore, 1990, Williams & Wilkins.
15. West JB, ed: *Bioengineering aspects of the lung*, New York, 1977, Marcel Dekker.

CHAPTER 11

Ventilation

Upon completing this chapter, you will be able to:

1 Define *ventilation*.
2 Identify the components of a breath.
3 Define *tidal volume, breathing frequency, inspiratory time,* and *expiratory time.*
4 Calculate I:E ratio, inspiratory time, expiratory time, and breathing frequency.
5 Define *minute ventilation, alveolar ventilation, anatomic dead space ventilation, alveolar dead space ventilation,* and *physiologic dead space ventilation.*
6 Calculate minute ventilation, alveolar ventilation, dead space ventilation, and dead space/tidal volume ratio.
7 List three methods for determining dead space volume.
8 Define 10 abnormal breathing patterns.
9 Describe normal and abnormal breath sounds.
10 Define the eight lung volumes and capacities.
11 Describe what a spirometer and pneumotachometer are and for what they are used.
12 Describe three methods for determining the volume of the functional residual capacity.
13 Describe the different volume and flow components of the forced vital capacity.
14 Describe the differences between restrictive and obstructive lung disease.
15 List five examples of restrictive and obstructive diseases.

Ventilation, commonly referred to as breathing, is the process of gas movement into and out of the lungs. This chapter discusses normal and abnormal breathing patterns and components as well as pulmonary function values in individuals with normal lungs and in those with pulmonary disease.

 COMPONENTS OF A BREATH

Frequency, Tidal Volume, and Inspiratory and Expiratory Time

Although each individual person is unique, when combined as a population, there are averages, or "norms." These norms are used to describe the elements of the breath and breathing pattern (Table 11-1).

There are several components of a breath. **Tidal volume (V_T)** is the amount of air inhaled or exhaled during normal breathing. To determine tidal volume, the inspired tidal volume or the exhaled tidal volume can be measured. However, they should not be measured and added together. For practical purposes the inspired tidal volume and expired tidal volume are equal if averaged over a period of time, although it should be noted that, depending

on where and how the measurement is made, the exhaled tidal volume gas warms to 37° C, thereby registering a larger volume. As gas warms, volume increases (volume is proportional to temperature if pressure is constant). Charles' law (see Chapter 1) states that gas volume is directly proportional to the gas temperature if the pressure and molecular number are held constant. The addition of moisture also increases the volume of a gas. Another factor that makes exhaled volume slightly less than inhaled volume is oxygen consumption. If oxygen is consumed at a greater rate than CO_2 production, exhaled tidal volume will be slightly less than the inhaled tidal volume. Normal spontaneous tidal volume often ranges from 6 to 10 ml/kg of ideal body weight. This range applies to children and adults. The normal value for the typical 70-kg adult is 500 ml.

Breathing frequency (f), or respiratory rate, is the number of breaths an individual takes per minute. Normal frequency is 12 to 16 breaths per minute for an adult, 16 to 20 for a child, and 20 to 40 for an infant. These normal rates are routinely observed while the individual is sedentary. During exercise and times of stress, fear, and excitement, the respiratory rate and tidal volume increases. During exercise, tidal volume normally increases first, then as exercise progresses, breathing frequency also increases.

Frequency can be divided into several components. Inspiratory time (T_I), the time it takes for inspiration, is measured from the beginning of inspiration to the beginning of expiration. The normal inspiratory time in the adult ranges from 1 to 2 seconds. An inspiratory breath hold is considered part of the inspiratory time. Expiratory time (T_E), the time spent in exhalation, is measured from the beginning of exhalation (following a breath hold if one occurs) to the beginning of the next inspiration. Routinely, toward the end of the expiratory phase an expiratory pause occurs with no air movement. The expiratory phase, normally longer than the inspiratory phase, lasts 3 to

Table 11-1 Elements of One Breathing Cycle

Element	Symbol	Normal Value
Tidal volume	V_T	7 ml/kg or 500 ml
Breathing frequency	f	12-16 breaths per minute
Inspiratory time	T_I	1-2 seconds
Expiratory time	T_E	3-4 seconds
Inspiratory/ expiratory ratio	I:E	1:3
Inspiratory/total time ratio	T_I/T_{TOT}	0.25 or 25%

4 seconds. The **I:E ratio** is the comparison of the amount of time spent during inspiratory time compared with that of expiratory time. If a patient has an inspiratory time of 1 second and an expiratory time of 3 seconds, the I:E ratio is 1:3. **Total breath time (T_{TOT})** is the time required for one breath ($T_I + T_E$). In the previous example, total breath time is 4 seconds (1 + 3). T_I/T_{TOT} is the ratio of T_I to T_{TOT} or the percent of time spent in inspiration. Using the previous example, T_I/T_{TOT} is ¼ or 25%.

The various formulas used to determine timing aspects of the breath are summarized in Box 11-1.

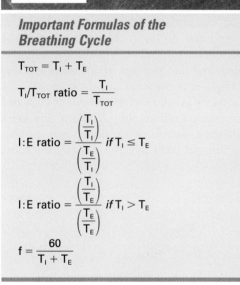

BOX 11-1

Important Formulas of the Breathing Cycle

$$T_{TOT} = T_I + T_E$$

$$T_I/T_{TOT}\ \text{ratio} = \frac{T_I}{T_{TOT}}$$

$$I:E\ \text{ratio} = \frac{\left(\dfrac{T_I}{T_I}\right)}{\left(\dfrac{T_E}{T_I}\right)}\ \text{if}\ T_I \leq T_E$$

$$I:E\ \text{ratio} = \frac{\left(\dfrac{T_I}{T_E}\right)}{\left(\dfrac{T_E}{T_E}\right)}\ \text{if}\ T_I > T_E$$

$$f = \frac{60}{T_I + T_E}$$

⬤ GAS MOVEMENT IN THE LUNGS

Minute Ventilation

Minute ventilation ($\dot{V}_E$), the amount of air moved in or out of the lungs in 1 minute, can be calculated with the following relationship:

$$\dot{V}_E = f \times V_T$$

If a patient is breathing at 12 breaths per minute and has a tidal volume of 500 ml, the minute ventilation is as follows (Fig. 11-1):

$$\begin{aligned}\dot{V}_E &= f \times V_T \\ &= 12/\text{min} \times 500\ \text{ml} \\ &= 6000\ \text{ml/min or 6.0 L/min}\end{aligned}$$

Because minute ventilation depends on both breathing frequency and tidal volume, a change

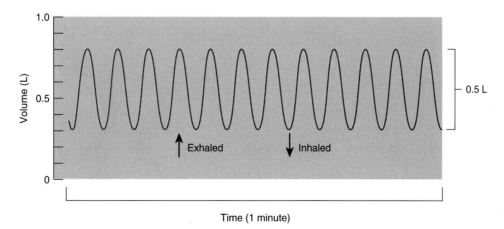

Minute ventilation = $\dot{V}_E$ = f × V_T = 12/min × 0.5 L = 6.0 L/min

FIG. 11-1 Illustration of normal tidal breathing for 1 minute with a tidal volume of 500 ml and respiratory frequency of 12 breaths per minute. Minute ventilation is 6.0 L.

in either may affect minute ventilation. For example, in the newborn infant the normal breathing frequency is 30 breaths per minute, and the tidal volume averages 20 ml. This yields a much lower minute ventilation of 600 ml/min or 0.6 L/min.

Alveolar and Dead Space Ventilation

As discussed in Chapter 9, the pulmonary system is made up of two basic types of airways: the **respiratory zone airways** (respiratory bronchioles and alveoli) and **conducting zone airways** (Fig. 11-2). The conducting zone airways extend from the nares to and including the terminal bronchioles. The respiratory zone airways have gas exchange properties and include the respiratory bronchioles to the individual alveoli. During ventilation, gas moves through these two different regions in different ways (Fig. 11-3). In the conducting zone airways gas moves by bulk flow whereas in the respiratory zone airways it moves by diffusion or diffusive flow.

During tidal ventilation, the tidal volume is divided between the respiratory zone airways and the conducting zone airways. During inspiration, that part that reaches the respiratory zone is known as the **alveolar volume (V_A)**. The **anatomic dead space volume (V_{Danat})**, the portion that remains in the conducting zone airways, does not participate in gas exchange. When the tidal volume is exhaled, the last portion of the alveolar volume remains in the anatomic dead space. This gas contains greater concentrations of CO_2 and lower concentrations of O_2. With the next breath, the anatomic dead space gas is the first to be brought back into the respiratory zone, which results in a significantly higher concen-

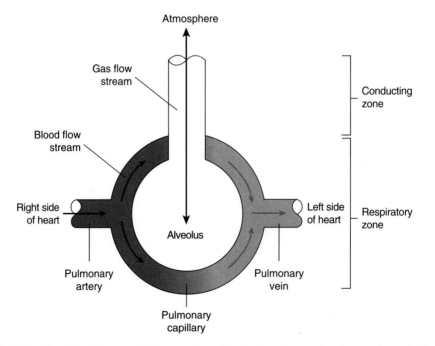

FIG. 11-2 Model of the respiratory system illustrating its conducting and respiratory zone airways. Conducting zone does not have pulmonary blood flow associated with it but does exchange gases with blood. Respiratory zone has pulmonary blood flow associated with ventilation. Gas exchange (diffusion) takes place in this zone.

tration of CO_2 and significantly lower concentration of O_2 in the respiratory zone gas when compared with atmospheric gas.

A second type of dead space occurs in regions of alveoli that are not perfused with

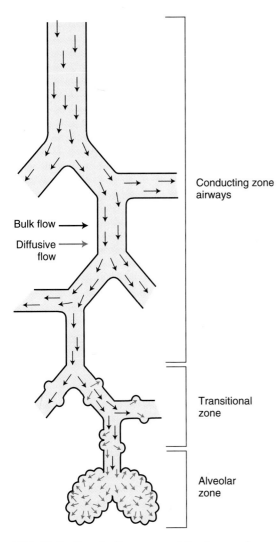

FIG. 11-3 Conducting zone of the lower airway extends from the trachea to the terminal bronchioles. Respiratory bronchioles (transitional zone) and the alveolar zone make up the gas exchange area. Gas movement in the conducting zone airways is by bulk flow whereas diffusive flow moves gas within the alveoli.

blood. These regions are known as **alveolar dead space volume (V_{Dalv})**. This dead space occurs in the normal upright lung in the apical regions. It can also be caused by a pulmonary embolus, resulting in a blockage of blood flow to alveoli that are perfused by the effected vessel.

The total amount of dead space, the combination of anatomic and alveolar dead space, is known as the **physiological dead space (V_{Dphys})**. For the purposes of simplicity, the physiological dead space will be called dead space (V_D).

An estimate of the amount of dead space (primarily anatomic) in the normal individual can be made by knowing a persons ideal body weight:

Estimated V_D = 2 ml/kg ideal body weight

If a patient has an ideal body weight of 75 kg, the estimated dead space is 150 ml.

Using this information, if a patient inhales a tidal volume of 500 ml, 150 ml of the fresh gas stays in the conducting airway and 350 ml of fresh air goes into the respiratory zone airways with the 150 ml of CO_2-rich and O_2-poor dead space gas that reenters the respiratory zone (Fig. 11-4). The 350 ml of fresh gas is the volume of air that is involved in supplying O_2 for diffusion into the blood and removing CO_2 produced by the cells.

Tidal volume can now be seen as a composite of gases that reaches the alveolar zone and that is wasted on dead space regions (anatomic plus nonfunctioning alveoli):

$$V_T = V_A + V_D$$

Dead space and alveolar volume, as described previously, are moved on a breath-to-breath basis. These volumes of gas can also be expressed and calculated, based on a minute, by multiplying them by the frequency. Alveolar ventilation ($\dot{V}_A$) is determined as follows:

$$\dot{V}_A = f \times V_A$$

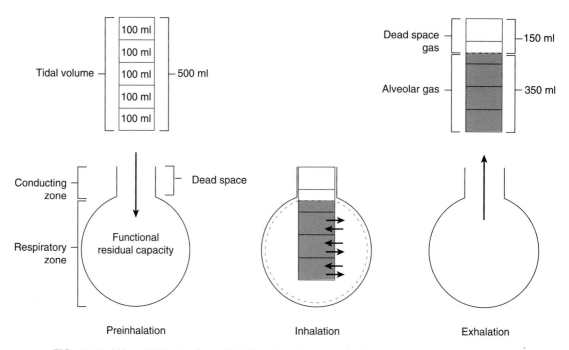

FIG. 11-4 When 500 ml of gas is inhaled, only 350 ml of that gas reaches the respiratory zone, assuming the dead space is 150 ml.

Table 11-2 Three Different Patients with the Same Minute Ventilation but Different Alveolar Ventilation

	f	V_T	V_A	V_D	V_D/V_T	$\dot{V}_E$	$\dot{V}_A$
Patient 1	14	600 ml	450 ml	150 ml	0.25	8400 ml/min	6300 ml/min
Patient 2	14	600 ml	300 ml	300 ml	0.5	8400 ml/min	4200 ml/min
Patient 3	28	300 ml	150 ml	150 ml	0.5	8400 ml/min	4200 ml/min

f, Breathing frequency; V_T, tidal volume; *VA*, alveolar volume; V_D, dead space; $\dot{V}_E$, minute ventilation; $\dot{V}_A$, alveolar ventilation.

Dead space ventilation is determined in a similar fashion:

$$\dot{V}_D = f \times V_D$$

At a frequency of 12 breaths per minute, a tidal volume of 500 ml, a dead space of 150 ml, and an alveolar volume of 350 ml, the minute ventilation is as follows:

$$\dot{V}_E = 12 \times 500 = 6.0 \text{ L/min}$$

Based on the previous information, alveolar ventilation is as follows:

$$\dot{V}_A = 12 \times 350 = 4.2 \text{ L/min}$$

and dead space ventilation is as follows:

$$\dot{V}_D = 12 \times 150 = 1.8 \text{ L/min}$$

Once tidal volume and dead space are known, the dead space/tidal volume ratio (V_D/V_T ratio) can be calculated. Using the previous values where $V_D = 150$ ml and $V_T = 500$ ml, the V_D/V_T ratio is as follows:

$$\frac{150 \text{ ml}}{500 \text{ ml}} = 0.3 \text{ (a value with no units)}$$

The normal dead space/tidal volume ratio of 0.2 to 0.4 indicates the effectiveness of ventilation. Table 11-2 compares three patients with different breathing patterns. All three patients have a minute ventilation of 8400 ml/min. Patient 1 is ventilating normally with an alveolar ventilation of 6300 ml/min that is able to maintain a normal gas exchange. Patient 2 appears to be ventilating normally but has an increased dead space that results in a reduced alveolar volume and a greatly reduced alveolar ventilation of 4200 ml/min. This patient is not ventilating effectively and is not excreting appropriate amounts of CO_2 or absorbing adequate amounts of O_2. Patient 3 has a normal dead space but a low tidal volume. The patient is trying to compensate for this abnormality by increasing his frequency to 28 so that his minute ventilation is the same as that of patients 1 and 2. This less effective ventilation results in an abnormally low alveolar ventilation of only 4200 ml/min.

Patients 2 and 3 demonstrate their ineffective breathing by their elevated dead space/tidal volume ratio. Patients with dead space/tidal volume ratios greater than 0.6 most likely require mechanical ventilation.

Measuring Dead Space and Alveolar Ventilation

The previous discussion concerns anatomical dead space volume and its estimation. The anatomical dead space can be more precisely calculated using Fowler's method. Fig. 11-5 illustrates Fowler's method and the measurement of anatomical dead space volume. To perform this test, a patient breathes into a circuit with an in-line nitrogen analyzer. The patient is instructed to exhale completely and to then take in a deep breath. During inhalation the patient receives 100% oxygen. Without holding one's breath, the patient is then

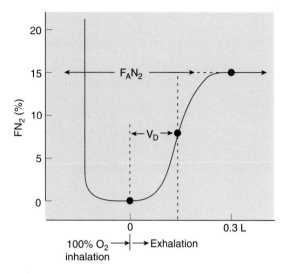

FIG. 11-5 Measurement of anatomical dead space using Fowler's method (see text for discussion).

instructed to exhale slowly at a flow rate of about 0.5 L/sec. Initially, as the patient exhales, only conducting airway gas (anatomic dead space gas) is exhaled, which contains 100% oxygen so that the nitrogen meter reads "zero." As the patient continues to exhale, a mixture of alveolar and conducting airway gas is exhaled so that the nitrogen meter reading increases. With continued exhalation, only alveolar gas is exhaled so that the slope of the exhaled nitrogen concentration becomes flat. The amount of gas exhaled from the beginning of exhalation to a point where the nitrogen concentration is 50% of the maximal exhaled concentration is the anatomical dead space volume. In Fig. 11-5 this is shown as the volume from the beginning of exhalation to the point when the exhaled nitrogen concentration equals 7.5%. In this example, the anatomical dead space is 0.15 L.

The dead space/tidal volume ratio can be calculated by using the modified **Bohr equation:**

$$V_D/V_T = \frac{P_aCO_2 - P_{\bar{E}}CO_2}{P_aCO_2}$$

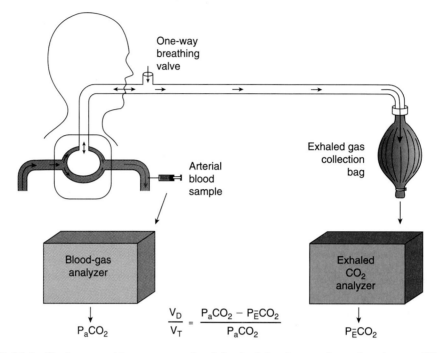

FIG. 11-6 System used to measure physiological dead space by using the modified Bohr equation.

where P_aCO_2 is the partial pressure of CO_2 in the arterial blood and $P_{\bar{E}}CO_2$ is the average exhaled CO_2. Fig. 11-6 illustrates the system for measuring dead space/tidal volume ratio. A patient may breathe room air, but all exhaled gas must be collected. Collecting gas for 1 to 3 minutes is desirable. During the collection of the exhaled gas, an arterial blood sample is taken and analyzed for P_aCO_2. After all exhaled gas is collected, the $P_{\bar{E}}CO_2$ is determined with a CO_2 analyzer. The two values are now placed into the modified Bohr equation. If the average tidal volume is known, the actual physiological dead space can be calculated by rearranging the modified Bohr equation into the following form:

$$V_{Dphys} = \frac{P_aCO_2 - P_{\bar{E}}CO_2}{P_aCO_2} \times V_T$$

Once the dead space volume is known, alveolar volume and alveolar ventilation can be determined. Alveolar volume is calculated by subtracting dead space from tidal volume:

$$V_A = V_T - V_D$$

Alveolar ventilation can also be determined in several ways. One method is to calculate the amount of minute ventilation that is reaching the alveolar region by multiplying minute ventilation by the alveolar volume/tidal volume ratio:

$$\dot{V}_E \times \frac{V_A}{V_T}$$

Another approach is to use the **alveolar ventilation equation:**

BOX 11-2

Important Formulas for Ventilation and Dead Space

Components of tidal volume	$V_T = V_A + V_D$
Minute ventilation exhaled	$\dot{V}_E = f \times V_T$
Components of minute ventilation	$\dot{V}_E = V_A + V_D$
Minute alveolar ventilation	$\dot{V}_A = f \times V_A$
Minute dead space ventilation	$\dot{V}_D = f \times V_D$
Modified Bohr equation	$\dfrac{V_D}{V_T} = \dfrac{P_aCO_2 - P_{\bar{E}}CO_2}{P_aCO}$
Alveolar volume ratio	$\dfrac{V_A}{V_T} = 1 - \dfrac{V_D}{V_T}$
Alveolar volume	$V_A = V_T - V_D$ or $V_T \times \dfrac{V_A}{V_T}$
Alveolar ventilation	$\dot{V}_A = \dot{V}_E \times \dfrac{V_A}{V_T}$
	$= \dfrac{\dot{V}CO_2 \times 0.863}{P_aCO_2}$

V_T, Tidal volume; V_A, alveolar volume; V_D, dead space; $\dot{V}_E$, minute ventilation; f, breathing frequency; V_D, dead space ventilation, $P_{\bar{E}}CO_2$, average exhaled carbon dioxide; P_aCO_2, arterial blood partial pressure of carbon dioxide; $\dot{V}CO_2$, excretion rate of carbon dioxide.

$$\dot{V}_A = \frac{\dot{V}CO_2 \times 0.863}{P_aCO_2}$$

where $\dot{V}CO_2$ is the excretion rate of CO_2 by the lungs per minute and P_aCO_2 is the arterial blood partial pressure of CO_2. The use of the alveolar ventilation equation requires precision measurement of CO_2 excretion rate and P_aCO_2.

The important equations that are used in the preceding section are summarized in Box 11-2.

NORMAL BREATHING PATTERN

Breathing rate, depth, and rhythm are the elements commonly used to describe the pattern of breathing. The control centers of the medulla oblongata (see Chapter 15) routinely control the pattern of breathing. This happens automatically without the need to control it voluntarily. However, breathing can be controlled voluntarily.

The normal values of respiratory frequency, tidal volume, and timing, all of which are influenced by age and size, are listed in Table 11-1. The breathing pattern is rhythmic and smooth with a sine wave pattern (see Fig. 11-1). The term **eupnea** refers to the normal breathing pattern.

There are many abnormal breathing patterns, some of which are seen in a health care setting. Variations in rate, depth, and timing may be encountered. Slow breathing rates, known as **bradypnea,** are often caused by such things as drug overdose, sleep, and sedation. Fast breathing rates, termed **tachypnea,** are often a response to stressful events such as fever, hypoxia, excitement, and exercise. Shallow breathing, known as **hypopnea,** is associated with respiratory center sedation. Deep breathing, termed *hyperpnea,* is caused by such things as pain and anxiety. Failure to breathe for more than 15 seconds is called **apnea.** The term **hyperventilation** refers to excessive ventilation that results in a decreased P_aCO_2 level in blood and tissues. Conversely, the term **hypoventilation** describes a condition of reduced ventilation that results in increased PCO_2 levels.

Chapter 15 discusses numerous variations in the timing of the breathing pattern.

NORMAL AND ABNORMAL BREATH SOUNDS

To the untrained person, breathing is a quiet process. With the aid of a stethoscope, the

CASE STUDY FOCUS

Respiratory Failure Caused by Skeletal Muscle Dysfunction

A 55-year-old woman was in good health when she developed flulike symptoms that included numerous fever spikes over a 4-day period. She recovered from this and then began to notice tingling and numbness in her extremities and muscle weakness that was moving up from her hands and feet 3 weeks after the flu episode. She was examined by a neurologist and was found to have generalized muscle weakness in all four extremities, reduced deep tendon reflexes, and diminished hand-grip strength. Cerebral spinal fluid was collected and was found to be clear and colorless, however, it did have an abnormally elevated protein content. The history, physical examination, and laboratory findings are consistent with the diagnosis of Guillain-Barré syndrome (GBS).

In patients with GBS, the motor and sensory nerves are attacked by the individual's own immune system. The exact cause is unknown, but it is often associated with a recent viral infection or immunization. Individuals with GBS often have increased production of immunoglobulin M and compliment-activated antibodies. The site of immune system attack is on the myelin sheath of neurons within the peripheral nerves. The resulting inflammation and demyelination by immune system attack result in reduced ability of the nerve to conduct impulses to muscles and from sensors. The demyelination proceeds up the peripheral nervous system, can result in complete paralysis, and in some cases can result in inability to breathe as a result of a loss of nerve signal conduction to the respiratory muscles.

The patient was admitted to the hospital for monitoring and support. On admission, vital signs were collected every 4 hours, a chest x-ray revealed normal anatomy, an electrocardiogram was taken and was found to be normal, and daily forced vital capacity (FVC) breathing tests were ordered to monitor her respiratory muscle function. Her FVC on admission was 2.7 L and her predicted value is 3.2 L. Over the next 5 days she developed progressive paralysis and began to have difficulty with swallowing. During this time her FVC declined daily down to 1.1 L. On the sixth day after admission she developed tachypnea and shallow breathing, her FVC was only 0.6 L, and the CO_2 levels in her blood were abnormally elevated. These indicated respiratory failure. She was sedated, intubated, and placed on mechanical ventilation. She required ventilatory support for the next 5 weeks and then began to recover. She developed sensation and motor functions gradually, was weaned from ventilatory support, underwent extensive physical therapy, and completely recovered 7 months after the onset of symptoms.

sounds of breathing can be heard and described.

Normal Breath Sounds

Normal breath sounds are divided into four categories: tracheal, bronchial, bronchovesicular, and vesicular. **Tracheal and bronchial breath sounds** are loud, high-pitched, and harsh tubular sounds that are caused by a rapid and turbulent flow of gas. They are heard over the trachea and main stem bronchi. Although bronchial breath sounds are not quite as harsh as tracheal breath sounds, both are similar in their tubular quality. **Bronchovesicular breath sounds** are heard distal to the central airways, are less intense, and are of lower pitch than tracheal and bronchial breath sounds. **Vesicular breath sounds** are the soft, breezy sounds heard primarily during inspiration over the lung periphery or parenchyma of the lung.

Abnormal Breath Sounds

Normal breath sounds become abnormal when they are heard over lung areas where they should not be heard, when they are absent, or when they are present with increased or decreased intensity. Abnormal breath sounds also include other sounds such as **crackles, wheeze, rhonchi,** and **stridor.** Together, abnormal breath sounds are referred to as **adventitious breath sounds.**

Crackles, the discontinuous sounds more often heard during mid to late inspiration, may indicate either fluid in the small airways or airways snapping open. The sound produced resembles that of Velcro being pulled apart. Crackling is more often present in the base of the lungs, especially during a deep breath. They are also much more likely to be present in a patient with a "wet" lung (increased pulmonary fluid caused by congestive heart failure).

Wheezes are high-pitched continuous sounds, whereas *rhonchi* are low-pitched continuous sounds, both of which are more often heard during expiration. The pitch is determined by the degree of airway obstruction caused by edema, spasm, mucus, or foreign object. Some recommend that the term *rhonchi* be dropped and that only the terms *high-pitched wheeze* and *low-pitched wheeze* be used.

Stridor is a high-pitched continuous sound heard over the upper airway that is caused by airway obstruction. Stridor is more common during inspiration but may also be present during exhalation. The sound is often heard in patients with croup, epiglottitis, and severe laryngitis.

⊙ DEFINING LUNG VOLUMES AND CAPACITIES

The volume of gas in the lungs can be defined in several ways. The various terms refer to the amount of gas in the lungs in different stages of inflation. Many of these terms and their normal values were developed by Hutchinson in the middle of the nineteenth century. They were the first objective measures developed in medicine for the characterization of disease.

Lung Volumes

At rest, fresh air enters the lungs and CO_2-laden air exits the lungs with each breath. This volume of gas is known as the tidal volume (Fig. 11-7). Following exhalation of the tidal volume, there is often a "rest" period before inhaling again. This resting level of breathing is known as the baseline breathing level. Under periods of stress, larger air volumes are exchanged, and pulmonary reserves above and below the baseline line can be used. Just as tidal volume can be measured and defined, so can the pulmonary reserves also be measured and defined (see Fig. 11-7).

The **inspiratory reserve volume (IRV)** is the maximum amount of air that can be inhaled following a normal inhalation or tidal volume. The **expiratory reserve volume (ERV)** is the maximum amount of air that can be exhaled (from baseline) following a normal exhalation. The **residual volume (RV)** is the amount of air left in the lungs following a maximal exhalation (after exhalation of the ERV). The RV cannot be exhaled from the lungs regardless of the force of exhalation. The residual volume can be removed from the lungs when they collapse in cases of complete pneumothorax.

Lung Capacities

Adding two or more lung volumes together yields a value known as lung capacity (Figs. 11-7 and 11-8). The **inspiratory capacity (IC)** (IC = IRV + V_T) is the maximum amount of air that can be inhaled following a normal exhalation, that is, inhaled from baseline. **Vital capacity (VC)** (VC = IRV + V_T + ERV) is the maximal amount of air that can be exhaled following a maximal inhalation. This is known as an exhaled VC, or EVC. The VC can also be defined as the maximal amount of air that can be inhaled following maximal exhalation. This

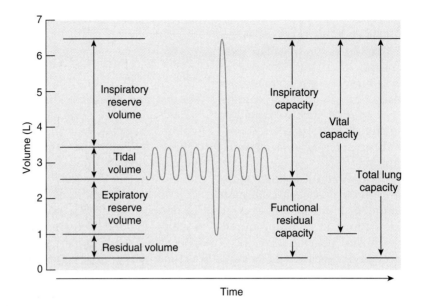

FIG. 11-7 Spirogram illustrating each lung volume and capacity (see text for definitions).

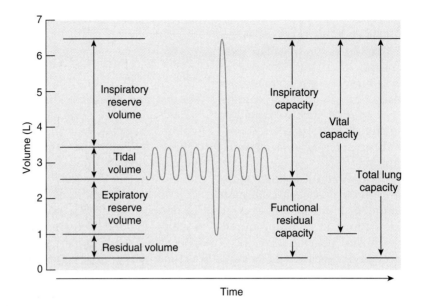

FIG. 11-8 Bar graph illustrating the relationship between the volumes and capacities.

is an inhaled VC, or IVC. The VC can also be performed as a slow maneuver (SVC) or a forced maneuver (FVC). Although easily confused, an IC and an IVC are *not* the same measurement. The **functional residual capacity (FRC)** (FRC = ERV + RV) is the amount of air left in the lungs following a normal exhalation. The FRC is the volume of air that is responsible for maintaining alveolar volume and stability. It is the volume of gas that par-

ticipates in the continuous diffusion of O_2 and CO_2 across the alveolar-capillary membrane. It is constantly replenished with O_2, and CO_2 is removed from it with each tidal breath. The **total lung capacity (TLC)** (TLC = IRV + V_T + ERV + RV) is the total amount of air contained in the lungs following a maximal inspiration.

Normal values for these different lung volumes and capacities are listed in Table 11-3. The values listed are only for purposes of reference. Actual values vary depending on an individual's age, height, gender, ethnic background, weight, and body posture.

MEASUREMENT OF LUNG VOLUMES AND CAPACITIES

The volumes and capacities change in different ways as a result of the effects of different pulmonary diseases. The ability to detect these changes is important in the diagnosis of many pulmonary diseases. A variety of devices and techniques have been developed to detect these changes.

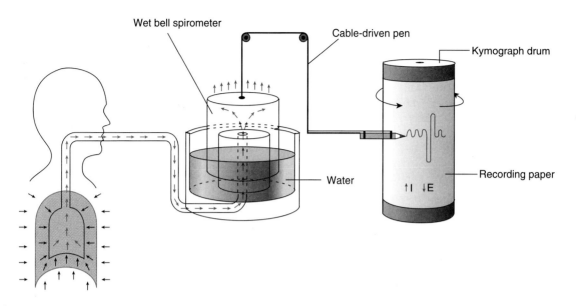

FIG. 11-9   Direct spirographic recording of lung volumes using a water seal spirometer. Because a cable and pulley system moves the pen, inspiration is recorded by the upward movement of the pen and expiration is recorded by its downward movement. Recording paper turns on the kymograph drum.

Measurement of Lung Volumes and Capacities

For measurement purposes, lung volumes and capacities can be divided into two general categories: those that are directly determined and those that are indirectly determined. Direct determination of some lung volumes is made by having a subject exhale into or inhale from a volume- or flow-measuring device. These devices record the volume as a graphic tracing, or they can be interfaced with a computer to electronically display the volume numerically. Each of the following can be directly measured: ERV, V_T, IRV, IC, and VC.

Direct Measurements of Lung Volume

A device that is used to collect and measure the amount of air that is moved by a subject is called a **spirometer.** Fig. 11-9 shows a water-sealed spirometer that collects gas in a moveable bell suspended in a water bath. A cable-driven pen records the movement of the bell on recording paper that revolves on a drum

 Table 11-3   Normal Adult Values of Respiratory Volumes and Capacities*

Parameter	Abbreviation	Value
Inspiratory reserve volume	IRV	3.0 L
Tidal volume	V_T	0.5 L
Expiratory reserve volume	ERV	1.5 L
Residual volume	RV	1.0 L
Inspiratory capacity	IC	4.0 L
Functional residual capacity	FRC	2.5 L
Vital capacity	VC	5.0 L
Total lung capacity	TLC	6.0 L

*Actual individual values vary from subject to subject depending on the individual's age, height, gender, weight, ethnicity, body posture, and effort.

assembly called a *kymograph*. Another type of water-sealed spirometer called a *Stead-Wells spirometer* has the recording pen attached to the drum itself (Fig. 11-10). This design avoids the problem of inertial dampening inherent in cable- or chain-driven pens. Both spirometers produce recordings called *spirograms*. Analysis of the spirogram reveals the various volumes and capacities; their values can be measured directly from the recording. The movement of the bell can also be detected with electromechanical transducers that produce current or voltage changes. These electrical signals can be collected and processed by a computer. The computerized spirometer can produce graphic and numeric read outs of the different volumes and capacities.

Another approach measures the amount of gas flow generated at the mouth with a device called a **pneumotachometer.** Fig. 11-11 shows a type of pneumotachometer that senses flow by detecting a pressure difference produced across a resistor. The pressure difference generated is proportional to the flow rate; greater flow causes a greater pressure gradient. The pressure gradient is detected by a pressure transducer, and the electrical signal that is produced is processed by a computer. The computer can produce volume-time, flow-time, and flow-volume spirograms with the aid of an X-Y recording device. Several other types of pneumotachometers have been developed that use hot-wire, ultrasonic, or strain-gauge types of flow sensors.

Indirect Measurements of Lung Volume

Indirect measurement of lung volumes implies that the volume or capacity cannot be measured or displayed as a spirogram but must be calculated by other means.

One method for indirect measurement of lung volumes, specifically for the FRC, is the use of the closed circuit helium dilution technique (Fig. 11-12). With this method, the sub-

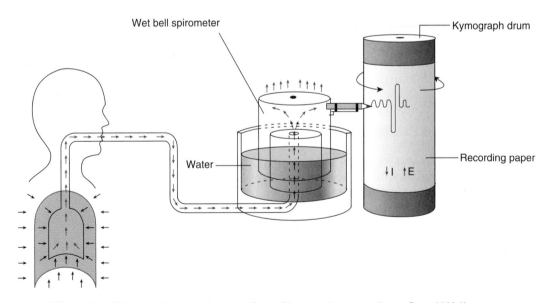

FIG. 11-10 Direct spirographic recording of lung volumes using a Stead-Wells water seal spirometer. Because no cable and pulley system is used, inspiration is recorded by the downward movement of the pen and expiration is recorded by its upward movement. This system avoids the inertial problems inherent in cable-driven pens.

ject's FRC is determined by inhaling a known concentration of helium (C_1) from a known spirometer circuit volume (V_1). While the subject breathes normally, he or she is switched from breathing air to breathing a helium-oxygen mixture (usually 10% He, 21% O_2, and 69% N_2) when their lungs only contain FRC gas. After a few minutes of breathing, the helium has equilibrated in the lungs and circuit (C_2). The final volume of the entire system (circuit and lungs [V_2]) can be calculated by using the following relationship:

$$V_1C_1 = V_2C_2$$

which is rearranged to solve for V_2 as follows:

$$V_2 = \frac{V_1C_1}{C_2}$$

This equation can then be modified to determine the FRC by subtracting the known volume of the spirometer circuit (V_1) from the circuit and lung volume (V_2) following equilibration:

$$FRC = V_2 - V_1$$

Another indirect method used to measure FRC is the open circuit multiple breath nitrogen washout test (Fig. 11-13). In this test the

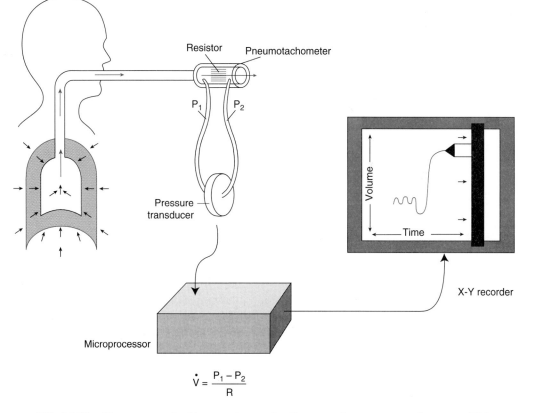

FIG. 11-11 Measurement of lung volumes by the use of a pneumotachometer. This pressure-differential type pneumotach causes a pressure drop $(P_1 - P_2)$ across a known resistor (R), which is proportional to the flow of gas $(\dot{V})$. Because time is also measured, volume can be calculated (Flow $\times$ Time = Volume). The results are displayed on an X-Y recorder or on the X-Y axis of a computer screen.

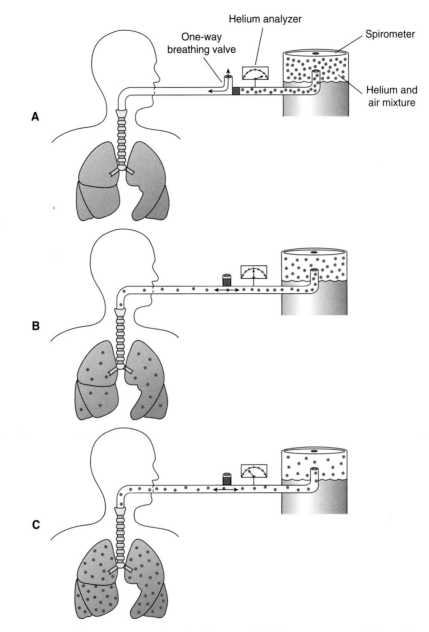

FIG. 11-12 Closed circuit helium (He) dilution test. **A,** Spirometer containing a known volume of gas (V_1) and a known He concentration (C_1) while the patient is breathing room air. **B,** Patient who was turned into the system at functional residual capacity (FRC). As the patient breathes on the system, the FRC, which contains no He, combines with the spirometer volume and dilutes the He in the system. Exhaled carbon dioxide is chemically removed from the system. The patient is given 100% oxygen (O_2) during the test to replenish the O_2 the patient consumes, keeping the total volume of the system constant throughout the test. **C,** Completed test where the He has reached equilibrium throughout the system and the patient's lungs (C_2). The spirometer volume and the patient's FRC (V_2) can then be calculated ($V_2 - \dfrac{V_1 \times C_1}{C_2}$). The FRC can then be determined by subtracting the initial spirometer volume from the equilibrium volume (FRC = $V_2 - V_1$).

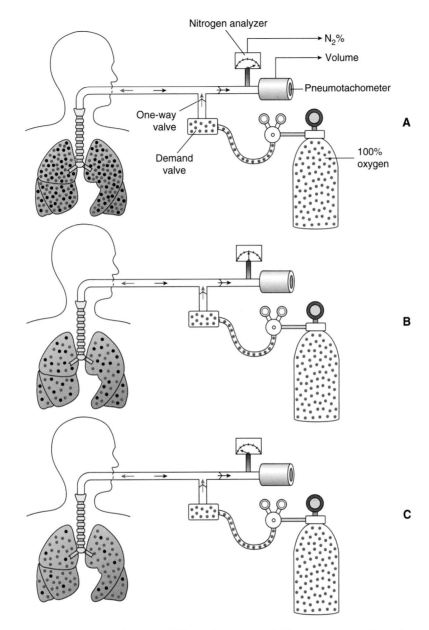

FIG. 11-13 Open circuit nitrogen (N_2) washout test. **A** illustrates a patient who was just turned into the system at functional residual capacity (FRC) and now breathes 100% oxygen (O_2); the exhaled N_2 is recorded and the exhaled volume is measured. **B** illustrates the patient halfway into the test. Breathing 100% oxygen washes the N_2 out of the lungs. **C** shows that the test is complete and that the N_2 concentration has dropped from 79% to 1.5%. FRC (V_1) is determined by measuring the initial concentration of N_2 in FRC gas (C_1), the volume of gas exhaled during the washout period (V_2), and the average concentration of N_2 in the exhaled gas (C_2). The FRC is then calculated with the equation $V_1 = \dfrac{C_2 V_2}{C_1}$.

subject breathes 100% oxygen from a one-way valve. At the beginning of the test the initial N_2 concentration in the lungs is 79% (C_1). With each breath, oxygen is inhaled and N_2-rich gas from the FRC is exhaled. This effectively washes the N_2 in the FRC gas out of the lung over several minutes until the concentration drops to about 1.5%. The volume of gas exhaled during the washout period is measured (V_2) and the average concentration of N_2 in the exhaled gas (C_2) is determined with a nitrogen analyzer. The volume of the FRC and the breathing circuit volume (V_1) can be determined with the following relationship:

$$V_1 = \frac{C_2V_2}{C_1}$$

The FRC is then determined by subtracting the known volume of the breathing circuit (V_{bc}) and corrections for the volume of N_2 excreted into the lung during the test (V_{exc}):

$$\textbf{FRC} = \textbf{V}_1 - \textbf{V}_{bc} + \textbf{V}_{exc}$$

A third method of determining lung volume is by using a body box or a **body plethysmography** to measure lung volumes (Fig. 11-14). In this technique, pressures are measured; then using Boyle's law, lung volumes can be calculated. The body plethysmograph is used to measure thoracic gas volume (V_{TG}). This volume is often measured at the level of the FRC so that thoracic gas volume equals FRC. To perform this test the patient sits in a sealed chamber and pants into a

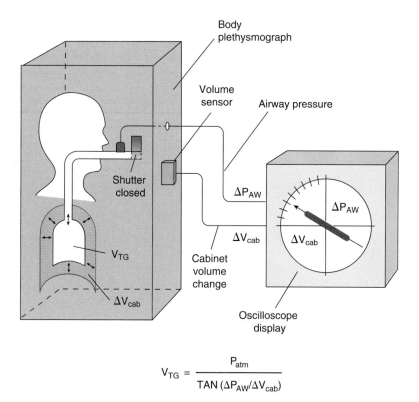

$$V_{TG} = \frac{P_{atm}}{TAN\,(\Delta P_{AW}/\Delta V_{cab})}$$

FIG. 11-14 Body plethysmograph is used to measure gas volume within the lungs (thoracic gas volume [V_{TG}]) indirectly using a modification of Boyle's law (see text for description).

pneumotachometer with a closed shutter. The chamber, which remains at a constant temperature, is calibrated so that a known pressure change in the chamber results in a known volume change. The subject's airway pressure (P_{AW}) is measured by a pressure transducer within the pneumotachometer. The measured box or cabinet pressure corresponds to volume change in the cabinet (V_{cab}). Knowing the atmospheric pressure (P_{atm}), the airway pressure, and the cabinet volume change, the change of lung volume can be calculated with the following relationship:

$$V_{TG} = \frac{P_{atm}}{TAN \, (\Delta P_{AW}/\Delta V_{cab})}$$

For each of the previously mentioned tests, the RV can be calculated by subtracting a directly measured ERV from the FRC. TLC can be calculated by adding the RV to a directly measured VC. Thus RV, FRC, and TLC are the three indirect lung volume and capacity measurements.

MEASUREMENT OF FORCED EFFORTS AND FLOW RATES

The measurement of lung volumes and capacities is a useful technique to determine the size of the lungs and the reserves of gas volume for deeper breathing. This information can then be used in the diagnosis of certain pulmonary diseases that affect the lung volume and capacity. More functional information about the lungs and airways can be obtained by measuring the ability to forcefully move gas.

Forced Vital Capacity

One of the most commonly performed and most useful pulmonary function tests is the forced vital capacity (FVC). To perform this maneuver, the subject, while breathing into and out of a spirometer, is instructed to inhale as much air as possible and then "blast" the air

out for as long and as hard as he or she can. The individual should be instructed to keep blowing for at least 6 seconds even though he or she does not "feel" any more gas is moving from the lungs. This forced expiratory maneuver, or FEVC, requires a great amount of effort and patient cooperation to perform it properly. Any submaximal efforts are not satisfactory for measuring test results.

The FEVC is routinely measured in two ways, one as a time-volume spirogram and the other as a flow-volume spirogram. The time-volume spirogram (Fig. 11-15) allows measurement of the following parameters. FVC is the total amount of air exhaled (in liters) during a forceful and complete exhalation. The FVC has been found to be one of the better predictors of long-term life span. Although it declines with age, in those who experience a more rapid drop rate, there is an association with a shortened life span. **Forced expiratory volume in 1 second (FEV$_1$)** is the amount of air exhaled in the first second of the expiratory maneuver (in liters). FEV$_1$ is most often considered a volume but because the FEV$_1$ is a volume-per-time measurement, it could be considered a type flow rate. The FEV$_1$ could be considered the average flow rate occurring during the first second of exhalation. **FEV$_1$/FVC ratio (FEV$_1$%)** is the comparison of the amount of air exhaled in 1 second to the total amount of air exhaled (expressed as a percentage). A normal adult exhales 83% of FVC in 1 second. Some authors list a value as low as 65% to 70% as acceptable for the FEV$_1$% in older persons. A value of 70% should not be considered acceptable for a young, healthy adult. Children often have an FEV$_1$% greater than 90%. The FEV$_1$% is definitely an age-related value that decreases with age. Airway obstructive defects cause the FEV$_1$% to fall below normal values. Forced exhaled volume in 2 seconds (FEV$_2$) is the amount of gas exhaled during the first 2 seconds of the FVC effort (in liters). **Forced expiratory volume in 3 seconds (FEV$_3$)** is the amount of air exhaled

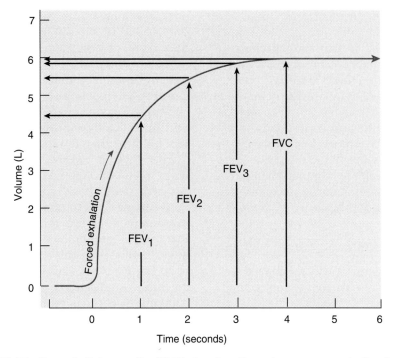

FIG. 11-15   Forced vital capacity *(FVC)* showing the values measured after 1, 2, and 3 seconds of exhalation. *FEV,* Forced expiratory volume.

after 3 seconds during the expiratory maneuver (in liters). **FEV₃/FVC ratio** (FEV$_3$%) is the comparison of the amount of air exhaled in 3 seconds to the total amount of air exhaled (expressed as a percentage). A normal adult can exhale 97% of FVC in 3 seconds. The acceptable value is ≥95%. Some authors may list lower values. Children should have a FEV$_3$% of 100%. Total expiratory time (TET) is the time (in seconds) required to completely exhale the FVC. A normal individual should be able to exhale FVC within 4 seconds. In severe airway obstructive defects the TET is often found to exceed 5 to 6 seconds.

The volume-time spirogram can also be analyzed to determine flow rates during different parts of the FVC maneuver. The greatest flow rates occur during the early part of the

effort where the spirogram line is most vertical. The flow rate in this region can be determined by measuring the slope (rise over run) of this part of the spirogram line. This maximal flow is called the **peak expiratory flow rate (PEFR).** Limitations of flow development in individuals with airway obstructive defects result in reduced PEFR. The measurement of PEFR is frequently used in the management of asthma to gauge the level of airway obstruction and the response to therapy.

Another approach is to determine the average flow during the middle portion of the FEVC. This average flow is called the **forced expiratory flow between 25% and 75% (FEF$_{25-75}$).** To calculate the FEF$_{25-75}$, the volume exhaled during the middle 50% of the FVC is determined and divided by the length of time

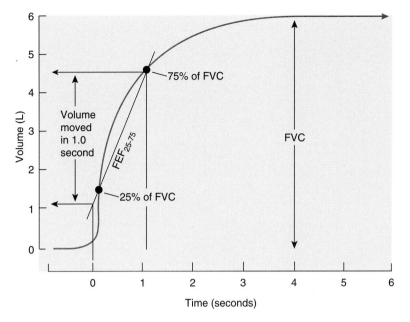

FIG. 11-16 Measurement of the forced expiratory flow between 25% and 75% *(FEF$_{25-75}$)* during the middle portion of the forced vital capacity *(FVC)*.

it took to exhale this volume. Volume divided by time equals flow rate, in this case the FEF$_{25-75}$, in liters per second (Fig. 11-16). Dots are placed at the 25% and 75% volume marks of the FVC. A line is drawn through the dots extending in both directions until it transverses 1 second. The slope (rise over run) of this line corresponds to the average flow in this region of the spirogram. The FEF$_{25-75}$, which is sensitive to small airway obstructive defects, declines with conditions such as bronchitis and asthma.

The second way the FVC can be expressed is as a flow-volume spirogram, commonly referred to as a flow-volume loop (FVL) (Fig. 11-17). The FVL allows comparison of instantaneous flows at any lung volume during maximal expiratory and inspiratory efforts. Some of the common measurements from the FVL include those described previously (e.g., FVC, FEV$_1$, and FEV$_1$%) and several other measurements that are possible only with this form of graphic presentation. These other measurements include the following. **Forced expiratory flow at 25% (FEF$_{25}$)** is the flow rate (in liters per second) at the point where 25% of the FVC has been exhaled. **Forced expiratory flow at 50% (FEF$_{50}$),** the midexpiratory flow rate (in liters per second), occurs at the point where 50% of the FVC has been exhaled. **Forced expiratory flow at 75% (FEF$_{75}$),** the flow rate (in liters per second) occurs at the point where 75% of the FVC has been exhaled. The FVL also reveals the location of PEFR and **peak inspiratory flow rate (PIFR).** Both of these flows occur at the

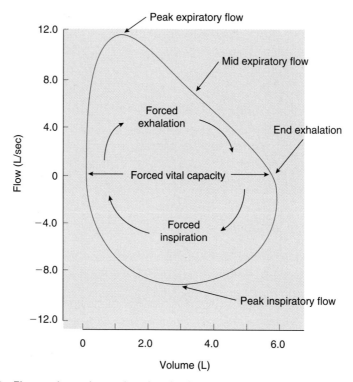

FIG. 11-17 Flow-volume loop showing both the forced inspiratory and expiratory portions of the forced vital capacity (FVC) effort. This shows the FVC and various flow rates during different parts of the FVC effort.

Table 11-4 Normal Adult Value of Forced Vital Capacity and its Components*

Parameter	Abbreviation	Value
Forced expiratory vital capacity	FEVC	5.0 L
Forced inspiratory vital capacity	FIVC	5.0 L
Forced expiratory volume in 1 second	FEV_1	4.0 L
$FEV_1/FEVC$ ratio	$FEV_1\%$	80%
Forced expiratory volume in 3 seconds	FEV_3	4.85 L
$FEV_3/FEVC$ ratio	$FEV_3\%$	97%
Peak expiratory flow rate	PEFR	10.0 L/sec
Forced expiratory flow between 25% and 75%	FEF_{25-75}	6.0 L/sec
Forced expiratory flow at 25%	FEF_{25}	9.5 L/sec
Forced expiratory flow at 50%	FEF_{50}	6.0 L/sec
Forced expiratory flow at 75%	FEF_{75}	3.0 L/sec
Total expiratory time	TET	4 seconds

*Actual individual values vary from subject to subject depending on the individual's age, height, gender, weight, ethnicity, body posture, and effort.

maximal points along the flow scale. The PEFR occurs early in the forced expiratory effort and then flow decays from this point as lung volume, airway diameter, and the force behind the expiratory effort all decline. During the inspiratory effort, PIFR is not as great, occurs in the center of the effort, and is better preserved during more of the inspiratory effort. This difference in PIFR is largely a result of the development of larger airway diameter and weaker muscle forces that occur during inspiration.

When a forced inspiratory maneuver follows the FEVC, the loop is completed. Two values are commonly measured from the inspiratory loop: the inspiratory FVC (FIVC), and the PIFR.

Modern pulmonary function systems simultaneously measure both the time-volume and flow-volume spirograms. Because of this ability, all the previously mentioned values can be measured and displayed for evaluation.

Table 11-4 summarizes the components of the forced expiratory and inspiratory vital

capacities and their normal values in the adult.

DEFINING RESTRICTIVE AND OBSTRUCTIVE PULMONARY DISEASE

Pulmonary diseases can be broadly divided into two general classifications: **restrictive pulmonary diseases** and **obstructive pulmonary diseases.** Some pulmonary diseases have components of each and are, therefore, classified as *mixed restrictive and obstructive diseases.*

Restrictive and Obstructive Pulmonary Diseases

In general, a restrictive process results in overall reduction in lung volumes and capacities while flow rates are preserved (Figs. 11-18 to 11-20). However, as restrictive diseases progress, flow rates may also decrease because of the severe reduction in lung volumes. One exception is the $FEV_1\%$. With

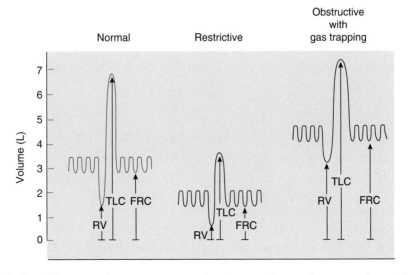

FIG. 11-18 Different spirograms comparing lung volumes for normal, restrictive, and obstructive lung disease. *RV,* Residual volume; *TLC,* total lung capacity; *FRC,* functional residual capacity.

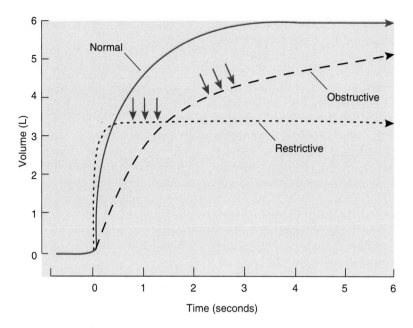

FIG. 11-19 Volume-time spirograms comparing the forced vital capacity during normal, restrictive, and obstructive lung disease.

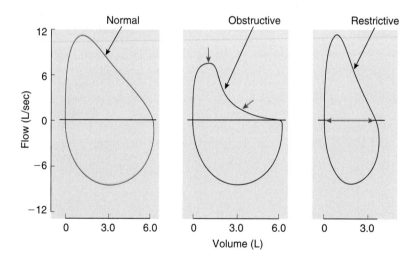

FIG. 11-20 Flow-volume loop forced vital capacity spirograms during normal, obstructive, and restrictive lung disease.

restrictive disease the $FEV_1\%$ remains normal or increases.

Diseases that produce a restrictive defect include but are not limited to neurologic disorders and neuromuscular diseases (e.g., amyotrophic lateral sclerosis, polio, Guillain-Barré syndrome, and myasthenia gravis), thoracic cage disorders (e.g., kyphoscoliosis, pectus excavatum, ankylosing spondylitis, and thoracoplasty), and diseases of the pleura and

DIAGNOSTIC FOCUS

Testing the Response to Bronchodilation Administration

A 68-year-old man was referred for pulmonary function testing to evaluate his pulmonary disease and response to aerosolized albuterol, a bronchodilator. He was diagnosed 8 years ago with asthma and has been smoking 1½ packs of cigarettes per day for the past 45 years. Recently he has developed increasing dyspnea with minor exertion. The following data were collected before and after bronchodilation in the pulmonary function laboratory:

Test	Predicted	Before Bronchodilation	After Bronchodilation
TLC (L)	6.54	7.12 (109%)*	7.04 (108%)
RV (L)	2.51	3.65 (145%)	3.59 (143%)
RV/TLC ratio (%)	40.22	51	51
FVC (L)	4.22	3.35 (79%)	3.40 (81%)
$FEV_{1.0}$ (L)	3.34	1.6 (48%)	1.7 (51%)
$FEV_{1.0}$/FVC ratio (%)	79	48	50
PEFR (L/sec)	8.34	4.1 (49%)	5.1 (61%)
FEF_{25-75} (L/sec)	3.32	1.22 (37%)	1.31 (39%)

*Values in parentheses are the percent of predicted.

These findings are consistent with gas trapping and hyperinflation (elevated TLC, RV, and RV/TLC ratio). The FVC is in the low-to-normal range. All of the flow measurements (FEV_1, FEV_1/FVC ratio, PEFR, and FEF_{25-75}) indicate significant airway obstruction. The combination of increased lung volumes and reduced flow rates is consistent with an obstructive airway disease. The smoking history and lack of response to the aerosolized bronchodilator indicate that he has emphysema rather than asthma. A patient with asthmatic airway obstruction responds to the inhalation of a broncho dilator such as albuterol. For the bronchodilator to cause significant change, the FEF_{25-75} and FEV_1 should improve more than 15%. In this case, they did not. This is more consistent with airway obstruction caused by emphysema. Emphysema that is primarily caused by chronic cigarette smoking results in destruction of alveoli, loss of small airway support to remain open, and airway inflammation. With forceful exhalation, airways collapse, air flow decreases, and gas trapping occurs. The physician decided to add aerosolized atrovent (a parasympathetic blocker) to enhance the effect of the albuterol on small and larger airways and to evaluate the patient in another month. The patient reported more relief with the addition of the atrovent inhaler.

lung parenchyma (e.g., pleural effusion, pneumothorax, atelectasis, pneumonia, pulmonary interstitial disease, and pulmonary fibrosis).

Obstructive diseases result in reduced flow rates while some lung volumes decrease (VC) and others increase (e.g., FRC and RV), demonstrating air trapping (see Figs. 11-18 to 11-20). Mixed defects have both decreased flows and volumes. Table 11-5 summarizes these differences and helps differentiate the spirometric changes that take place in restrictive and obstructive defects.

Diseases that produce an obstructive defect include but are not limited to asthma, emphysema, chronic bronchitis, bronchiectasis, and cystic fibrosis.

Table 11-5 Comparison of Lung Volumes and Flow Rates in Restrictive, Obstructive, and Mixed Pulmonary Diseases

Parameter	Mild/Moderate Restrictive	Severe Restrictive	Mild/Moderate Obstructive	Severe Obstructive	Mixed Restrictive and Obstructive
TLC	↓	↓	N	N/↑	↓
VC	↓	↓	N/↓	↓	↓
RV	↓	↓	↑	↑↑	↓
FRC	↓	↓	↑	↑	↓
FEV$_1$	N/↓	↓	↓	↓↓	↓
FEV,%	N/↑	↑	↓	↓↓	↓
FEF$_{25-75}$	N/↓	↓	↓	↓↓	↓
PEFR	N/↓	↓	↓	↓↓	↓

TLC, Total lung capacity; *N,* normal; *VC,* vital capacity; *RV,* residual volume; *FRC,* functional residual capacity; *FEV$_1$,* forced expiratory volume in 1 second; *FEV,%, FEV$_1$*/forced expiratory vital capacity; *FEF$_{25-75}$,* forced expiratory flow between 25% and 75%; *PEFR,* peak expiratory flow rate.

CHAPTER SELF-TEST QUESTIONS

1. Which one of the following patients will have the greatest alveolar ventilation?
   a. f = 12, V_T = 600 ml, V_D = 150 ml
   b. f = 24, V_T = 300 ml, V_D = 150 ml
   c. f = 18, V_T = 450 ml, V_D = 200 ml
   d. f = 12, V_T = 600 ml, V_D = 200 ml
2. What would the physiologic dead space be if a patient had a P_aCO_2 of 50 mm Hg and a $P_{\bar{E}}CO_2$ of 30 mm Hg?
   a. 0.1
   b. 0.2
   c. 0.3
   d. 0.4
3. Minute ventilation ($\dot{V}_E$) equals which of the following calculations?
   a. $\dot{V}_E = \dot{V}_A + \dot{V}_D$
   b. $\dot{V}_E = f \times V_T$
   c. $\dot{V}_E = f \times (V_A + V_D)$
   d. all of the above
4. The peak expiratory flow rate normally occurs during the _____ of the forced expiratory vital capacity.
   a. early part
   b. middle portion
   c. last third

5. Which of the following devices measure(s) the forced vital capacity?
   1. Stead-Wells spirometer
   2. pressure transducer
   3. pneumotachometer
   a. 1 only
   b. 1 and 2
   c. 2 and 3
   d. 1 and 3
6. A discontinuous sound heard more often during the middle to late inspiratory phase, especially in the lung bases, describes which of the following lung sounds?
   a. stridor
   b. rhonchi
   c. crackles
   d. bronchial
7. Total lung capacity equals which of the following?
   a. VC + RV
   b. IRV + FRC
   c. IC − ERV
   d. all of the above
8. Which one of the following cannot be measured directly?
   a. vital capacity
   b. inspiratory capacity

c. functional residual capacity
d. expiratory reserve volume

9. A body box, using the equation $P_1V_1 = P_2V_2$, uses _____ gas law to determine thoracic gas volume.
   a. Charles'
   b. Gay-Lussac's
   c. Dalton's
   d. Boyle's

10. The following findings were collected from a patient who was exposed to silica dust during a 10-year period as a cement cutter:

    FEVC = 67% of normal   TLC = 65% of normal

    FEV_1 = 55% of normal   FRC = 55% of normal

    FEV_1% = 98% of normal   RV = 49% of normal

    PEFR = 91% of normal

    These findings are most consistent with:
    a. normal lung function
    b. obstructive pulmonary disease
    c. restrictive pulmonary disease
    d. mixed obstructive and restrictive pulmonary disease

For answers, see p. 475.

BIBLIOGRAPHY

1. Fenn WO, Rahn H, eds: *Handbook of physiology,* vol 2, Washington, DC, 1964, American Physiologic Society.
2. Leff AR, Schumacker PT: *Respiratory physiology: basics and applications,* Philadelphia, 1993, WB Saunders.
3. Levitzky GL, Hall SM, McDonough KH: *Cardiopulmonary physiology in anesthesiology,* New York, 1997, McGraw Hill.
4. Martini FH: *Fundamentals of anatomy and physiology,* Upper Saddle River, NJ, 1998, Prentice Hall.
5. Milic-Emili J, ed: *Applied physiology in respiratory mechanics (topics in anesthesia and critical care),* New York, 1998, Springer-Verlag.
6. Miller WF, Scacci R, Gast LR: *Laboratory evaluation of pulmonary function,* Philadelphia, 1987, JB Lippincott.
7. Murray JF: *The normal lung,* ed 2, Philadelphia, 1986, WB Saunders.
8. Nunn JF: *Applied respiratory physiology,* ed 3, London, 1987, Butterworths.
9. Pierson DJ, Kacmarek RM, eds: *Foundations of respiratory care,* New York, 1992, Churchill Livingstone.
10. Ruppel G: *Manual of pulmonary function testing,* ed 7, St Louis, 1997, Mosby.
11. Staub NC: *Basic respiratory physiology,* New York, 1991, Churchill Livingstone.
12. Wagner J: *Pulmonary function testing: a practical approach,* ed 2, Baltimore, 1998, Williams & Wilkins.
13. West JB: *Respiratory physiology: the essentials,* ed 4, Baltimore, 1990, Williams & Wilkins.

Gas Exchange in the Lungs

CHAPTER OBJECTIVES

Upon completing this chapter, you will be able to:

1 Define *respiratory exchange ratio* and *respiratory quotient.*
2 Explain the importance of the functional residual capacity in maintaining alveolar gas concentrations.
3 Calculate P_AO_2 by using the alveolar air equation.
4 Describe those factors that influence P_AO_2.
5 List the factors that influence distribution of ventilation.
6 List the factors that influence distribution of pulmonary blood flow.
7 Differentiate between dependent and independent regions of the lung.
8 Describe the effect that lung volume has on alveolar and extraalveolar blood vessels.
9 Describe the four different zones in the lung.
10 Define $\dot{V}/\dot{Q}$ ratio.
11 Describe what an ideal lung unit, dead space unit, and shunt are in terms of $\dot{V}/\dot{Q}$ ratio.
12 List the effects that high and low $\dot{V}/\dot{Q}$ matching has on gas tensions.
13 Define $\dot{V}/\dot{Q}$ matching in the apical, middle, and base regions of upright normal lungs.
14 Define two types of pulmonary shunts and describe a shuntlike effect.
15 Explain why regions with low $\dot{V}/\dot{Q}$ ratios lead to hypoxemia.
16 Describe what effect adjustment of overall alveolar ventilation has on PO_2 and PCO_2.
17 List and explain the different tests available for the evaluation of $\dot{V}/\dot{Q}$ matching.
18 List the factors that affect gas diffusion.
19 List the barriers to diffusion in the alveolar-capillary membrane.
20 Explain why a gas is classified as either perfusion-limited or diffusion-limited.
21 Describe the single-breath carbon monoxide diffusion test.
22 List the various factors that result in either increased or decreased gas diffusion in the lungs.

The primary function of the lungs is the continuous absorption of oxygen (O_2) and the excretion of carbon dioxide (CO_2). This exchange of O_2 and CO_2 in the lungs occurs between two moving "streams" of material. One stream is alveolar gas and the other is pulmonary blood. To move from one stream to the other, these gases must cross the alveolar-capillary membrane. This chapter describes the major factors that influence the exchange of gases.

GAS EXCHANGE IN THE LUNGS

The amount of O_2 and CO_2 being exchanged in the lungs changes from minute to minute as the amount of gas exchange at the tissues changes. This occurs as the activity level and metabolic rate of the individual change. If the measurement is taken while the subject sits or lies quietly in a relaxed state, the amount of gas being exchanged in the lung stabilizes and reaches an equilibrium, with the amount of gas exchanging at the tissues. At this point, when the exchange rate in the lung and tissues is the same and relatively constant, the individual is said to be at a **steady state.**

The amount of O_2 consumed ($\dot{V}O_2$) and the amount of CO_2 excreted ($\dot{V}CO_2$) can be measured with precision flow and gas detectors. Normally, the resting $\dot{V}O_2$ is 250 ml/min and the $\dot{V}CO_2$ is 200 ml/min. These rates can increase sixfold during stressful exercise.

The ratio of $\dot{V}CO_2$ production to $\dot{V}O_2$ consumption by the lung is called the **respiratory exchange ratio (R):**

$$R = \frac{\dot{V}CO_2}{\dot{V}O_2}$$

The normal resting respiratory exchange ratio is 0.8 when the metabolism is fueled by a "normal" mixture of carbohydrates, proteins, and lipids. The value of R can shift to 1.0 when the metabolic rate is fueled by carbohydrates (e.g., glucose) and toward 0.7 when lipids are the

principal metabolic fuel source. The same ratio that is generated in the tissues is known as the **respiratory quotient (RQ).** At steady state conditions, respiratory exchange ratio equals respiratory quotient.

STABILIZATION OF ALVEOLAR GAS COMPOSITION

Stable alveolar gas partial pressures are necessary for stable gas exchange.

Tidal Volume and Functional Residual Capacity Gas Mixing

Imagine that each breath results in the complete filling of alveoli during inspiration and the complete emptying of alveoli during expiration. Oxygen-rich gas in the alveolus and blood is interfaced intermittently, resulting in cyclic up and down blood oxygenation concentration. It may be interesting to watch mucus membranes turning pink then blue when well-oxygenated and then poorly oxygenated blood flows through them. Obviously this is not the case since the alveoli are continuously held open by the volume of air normally found in the lungs at the resting level of breathing (the functional residual capacity [FRC]).

The FRC should not be considered a volume of "stale" air but a volume that is continuously being exchanged and modified by each breath. Each breath replenishes the FRC with oxygen that was removed by diffusion into the pulmonary circulation and removes CO_2 that has entered the alveoli. Some regions of the lungs have mismatched ventilation and perfusion, which results in different concentrations of O_2 and CO_2. Overall, however, the mixing of tidal volume with the FRC gas normally maintains a near constant P_AO_2 of 100 mm Hg and P_ACO_2 of 40 mm Hg in the alveoli of the respiratory zone. In disease states and other conditions where the FRC is increased (air trapping), where dead space ventilation is increased, when breathing frequency and tidal volume are decreased, or when the CO_2 production rate is increased, "ineffective ventilation" may occur. Under these conditions the FRC does not "wash out" as effectively, and the O_2 concentration decreases and the CO_2 concentration increases in the lungs and pulmonary blood stream. The opposite happens when excessive ventilation mixes with the FRC gas.

DETERMINATION OF PARTIAL PRESSURE OF OXYGEN IN ALVEOLAR GAS

Alveolar gas contains N_2, O_2, CO_2, H_2O vapor, and a variety of trace gases (Table 12-1). The amount of gas that is present can be expressed as a percentage, as a number of parts per million (ppm), or as a partial pressure. The more common method used in clinical medicine is to express the gas concentration as a partial pressure either in millimeters of mercury (mm Hg) or kilopascals (kPa). Knowing the partial pressures of gases in alveolar gas aids in the understanding of how well gases are transported within the lungs.

Alveolar Air Equation

The partial pressure of O_2 in alveolar gas can be estimated by using the **alveolar air equation.** This equation is used to estimate the average level of oxygen in the alveoli when considering the lungs as a single lung unit (i.e., one big alveolus). The alveolar air equation is derived from Dalton's law of partial pressures in which the total pressure of the system is formed by all the different partial pressures:

$$P_B = PN_2 + PO_2 + PH_2O + PCO_2 + P_{trace\ gases}$$

where P_B is the barometric or atmospheric pressure in millimeters of mercury and PN_2, PO_2, PH_2O, PCO_2, and $P_{trace\ gases}$ are the partial pressures of nitrogen, oxygen, water, carbon dioxide, and trace gases, respectively. By rearranging this equation, one can solve for the PO_2 in the gas mixture:

$$PO_2 = P_B - PN_2 - PH_2O - PCO_2 - P_{trace\ gases}$$

The expanded form of the alveolar air equation basically follows this concept by subtracting the other gases (N_2, H_2O, and CO_2) from alveolar gas to yield the partial pressure of O_2 in alveolar gas:

$$P_AO_2 = FIO_2(P_B - PH_2O) - PCO_2\left(\frac{FIO_2 + 1 - FIO_2}{R}\right)$$

where P_AO_2 is the partial pressure of O_2 in the alveoli in millimeters of mercury and FIO_2 is the percent of O_2 the patient is breathing in decimal form (40% = 0.4). Water vapor pressure is normally 47 at 37° C and 100% relative humidity (normal body temperature and pressure saturated with water vapor). Alveolar

Table 12-1 Concentration and Partial Pressures of Major Gases at Sea Level

Gas	Inhaled Dry Air		Alveolar Gas		Exhaled Air	
	Percent	mm Hg	Percent	mm Hg	Percent	mm Hg
Nitrogen dioxide	78.08	593	74.9	569	74.5	566
Oxygen	20.94	159	13.5	103	15.7	120
Carbon dioxide	0.03	0.2	5.3	40	3.6	27
Water	0	0	6.2	47	6.2	47

PCO$_2$ should be used, but arterial PCO$_2$ is frequently more available and similar enough for clinical use. The respiratory exchange ratio is normally about 0.8 in most resting, non-stressed individuals. The following is an example for a person breathing room air at sea level with a normal P$_A$CO$_2$ (the partial pressure of CO$_2$).

$$P_AO_2 = 0.21 \, (760 - 47) - 40 \left(0.21 + \frac{1 - 0.21}{0.8} \right)$$

$$= 0.21 \, (713) - 40 \left(0.21 + \frac{0.79}{0.8} \right)$$

$$= 150 - 40(1.2)$$
$$= 150 - 48$$
$$= 102 \text{ mm Hg}$$

If different FIO$_2$ values (0.21 to 1.0) and R values (0.7 to 1.0) were placed in the formula, the range of factors by which PCO$_2$ would be corrected for would vary from 1.0 to 1.34. Because the R value is often unknown and the formula is an estimate of P$_A$O$_2$, it is easier and acceptable to use the shortened version of the alveolar air equation shown below. This formula uses an R value of 0.8 where $1 \div 0.8 = 1.25$.

Using the same situation as before, the equation is as follows:

$$P_AO_2 = 0.21 \, (760 - 47) - 40 \, (1.25)$$
$$= 0.21 \, (713) - 50$$
$$= 150 - 50$$
$$= 100 \text{ mm Hg}$$

When the patient breathes a high FIO$_2$ (>60%), the value of 1.25 can be changed to 1.0. This brings the short formula more in line with the long formula when using a high FIO$_2$.

Although calculation of the alveolar air equation yields an average P$_A$O$_2$, several interesting relationships can be seen by evaluating the formula (Box 12-1).

Relationship #1: As P$_B$ increases, alveolar oxygen tension also increases. As P$_B$ decreases, alveolar oxygen tension also decreases.

This relationship is important when considering the alveolar and blood PO$_2$ changes in a patient who is either placed in a hyperbaric chamber (increased barometric pressure) or who is mountain climbing at a high altitude (decreased barometric pressure). The patient in a hyperbaric chamber breathing 100% O$_2$ at 3 atm of pressure has a P$_A$O$_2$ of more than 2000 mm Hg. The mountain climber on the summit of Mount Everest, where the FIO$_2$ is 21% and the barometric pressure is only 200 mm Hg, yields an impossible P$_A$O$_2$ of -7 mm Hg if they had a normal alveolar PCO$_2$ of 40 mm Hg. When exposed to these hypoxic conditions, the climber's respiratory center is stimulated and they compensate by hyperventilating and reducing their P$_A$CO$_2$ to about 10 mm Hg, which results in a P$_A$O$_2$ of only about 20 mm Hg. This explains why few individuals can scale Mount Everest without supplemental oxygen.

Relationship #2: As FIO$_2$ increases, alveolar oxygen tension increases. As FIO$_2$ decreases, alveolar oxygen tension decreases.

This important relationship in routine O$_2$ therapy explains why the alveolar and blood PO$_2$ values increase when gas is breathed in higher FIO$_2$ values.

BOX 12-1

Important Relationships Within the Alveolar Air Equation

$$P_AO_2 = FIO_2 \, (P_B - 47) - P_ACO_2 \, (1.25)$$

Relationship #1	↑ Barometric pressure	→ ↑ P$_A$O$_2$
	↓ Barometric pressure	→ ↓ P$_A$O$_2$
Relationship #2	↑ Inhaled O$_2$ concentration	→ ↑ P$_A$O$_2$
	↓ Inhaled O$_2$ concentration	→ ↓ P$_A$O$_2$
Relationship #3	↑ Alveolar CO$_2$	→ ↓ P$_A$O$_2$
	↓ Alveolar CO$_2$	→ ↑ P$_A$O$_2$

Relationship #3: As P_ACO_2 increases, P_AO_2 decreases. As P_ACO_2 decreases, P_AO_2 increases. Because of this relationship, hyperventilation may help compensate for a hypoxemia and moderate to severe hypoventilation can cause moderate to severe hypoxemia (if no supplemental O_2 is given). Although P_AO_2 is inversely proportional to P_ACO_2, the opposite is not true. P_ACO_2 is not directly or inversely proportional to P_AO_2. Blood and alveolar PCO_2 is determined by two basic factors: CO_2 production and alveolar ventilation (as shown in the following relationship):

$$PCO_2 = \frac{\dot{V}CO_2 \times 0.863}{\dot{V}_A}$$

where $\dot{V}CO_2$ is the rate of CO_2 production and $\dot{V}_A$ is the alveolar ventilation rate. This relationship is known as the *alveolar ventilation equation* and is rearranged here to solve for PCO_2.

● INFLUENCES OF DISTRIBUTION OF VENTILATION

Various mechanical factors influence how gas is distributed within the lung (Box 12-2). The assumption that ventilation is evenly distributed throughout the lung is inaccurate. The two factors that most influence distribution are local lung compliance and airway resistance.

Lung Compliance

Tidal volume is not distributed evenly throughout the lungs. In an upright position, a larger portion of tidal volume enters the basilar (dependent) regions of the lungs, whereas a smaller portion reaches the apical (independent) regions (Fig. 12-1). Generally, the reason for this uneven distribution is the fact that, when the lungs are at the normal FRC, the apical alveoli are more inflated and less compliant than the dependent alveoli which are less

---

BOX 12-2

Factors that Influence the Distribution of Ventilation

LOCAL COMPLIANCE
Increased with:
↑ Surfactant concentration
↓ Interstitial water
↑ Alveolar gas volume
↓ Alveolar interstitial fibers (collagen and elastin)
Decreased with:
↓ Surfactant in alveolar lining fluid
↑ Interstitial and alveolar water
↓ Alveolar gas volume
↑ Alveolar interstitial fibers (fibrosis)
Weight of local tissue

LOCAL AIRWAY RESISTANCE
Increased with:
↑ Airway wall interstitial fluid
Mucus retention
Bronchial muscle spasm
Small airway collapse
Tumor formation
Foreign body
Decreased with:
↓ Airway wall interstitial fluid
Mucus clearance
Bronchial muscle relaxation
↑ Small airway support from surrounding alveoli

---

inflated and more compliant. This allows more air to ventilate the more compliant alveolar regions in the base of the lungs. The apical alveoli are more inflated because the pleural pressure is not equal throughout the thorax. At FRC, the normal apical pleural pressure is approximately -10 cm H_2O (10 cm H_2O below atmospheric pressure) whereas the pleural pressure at the base of the lungs is only -2 cm H_2O. This phenomenon is the result of the weight of the lungs and the pull of gravity. In effect, the lungs are like an accordion that is "hanging" in the thoracic

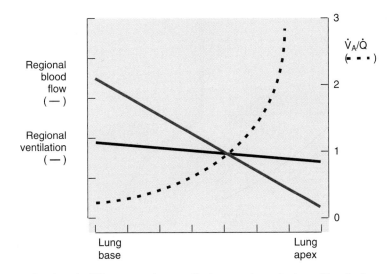

FIG. 12-1 Regional differences in ventilation and perfusion. Ventilation and pulmonary perfusion are distributed unequally throughout the lung. Lung base receives the greatest amount of ventilation and perfusion. The base receives more blood flow than ventilation and the $\dot{V}/\dot{Q}$ ratio is less than one. The apex of the lung receives more ventilation than perfusion and the $\dot{V}/\dot{Q}$ ratio is greater than one.

cavity. Having a greater transpulmonary pressure gradient at the top of the lungs results in greater distension of those alveoli. This places these alveoli higher up and on a flatter portion of the pressure-volume curve, which indicates a much lower compliance.

Airway Resistance

The flow of gas in the airways of the lungs is also uneven as a result of differences in airway resistance in different regions of the lungs. These differences in normal lungs are largely brought about by different airway diameters. Small airways in the upper lobes, where alveoli are more distended, have somewhat larger diameters. This is caused by the surrounding alveolar walls that "pull" outward (a tethering force) on the small airway wall with more force. The reverse is true in the lower lobes of the lungs. Here, where lung volume

is lower, there is less outward pulling on the small airway wall, which results in a somewhat smaller airway diameter. These differences in airway diameter contribute to the uneven flow of gas within the lungs. These differences can be made worse by airway obstructive diseases (e.g., asthma, bronchitis, emphysema, and foreign bodies) that partially block the airway (Fig. 12-2). Other factors that are external to the lungs may also affect regional ventilation (e.g., pleural effusions and paralysis of a hemidiaphragm).

INFLUENCES OF DISTRIBUTION OF PULMONARY BLOOD FLOW

Compared with the systemic circulation, the pulmonary circulation is a low-pressure, low-resistance, high-capacity system that accommodates the entire cardiac output from the

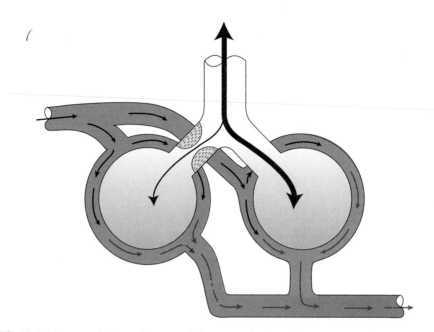

FIG. 12-2 Lung unit *A* receives much less ventilation when compared with the unobstructed lung unit *B*.

Factors that Influence the Distribution of Pulmonary Blood Flow

Gravity
Blood volume
Cardiac output
Pulmonary artery pressure
Pulmonary vascular resistance
Lung volume
Alveolar gas pressure

right side of the heart. As with air distribution, several factors determine pulmonary blood flow distribution (Box 12-3).

Gravity

Because of the pull of gravity and the low-pressure nature of the pulmonary circulation, blood flow normally goes to the dependent lung regions (normally the lung bases) (see Fig. 12-1). The dependent region changes as body position changes. When one is standing or sitting, the base of the lungs is the dependent zones. When one is lying supine, the posterior region of the lungs is the dependent zone. In a head stand position the apical region is the dependent zone.

Pulmonary Blood Volume, Pressure, and Resistance

As pulmonary blood volume and pulmonary artery pressure increase, relatively underperfused areas receive more blood flow. Because pressure rises, blood is directed into more areas of the lungs (e.g., the less dependent zones of the lungs). Because the pulmonary vessels are elastic, they are able to distend and open up some poorly perfused vessels (recruitment). Distension and recruitment

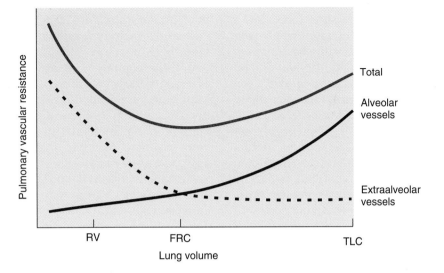

FIG. 12-3 Changes in lung volume effect pulmonary vascular resistance (PVR). Alveolar and extraalveolar blood vessels respond differently to changes in lung volume. Because of this relationship, PVR is lowest at functional residual capacity *(FRC)* and has minimal change during tidal breathing. As lung volume increases or decreases from the level of FRC, total PVR increases. *TLC,* Total lung capacity; *RV,* residual volume.

direct greater blood flow to less dependent areas of the lungs. This occurs during exercise when cardiac output increases and pulmonary artery pressure remains close to normal resting pressure. Distention and recruitment help keep pulmonary artery pressure low while being able to accommodate a large increase in blood flow.

Lung Volume

Pulmonary vascular resistance is at its lowest at FRC. Changes in lung volume toward residual volume (RV) or total lung capacity (TLC) increases resistance (Fig. 12-3). This occurs because there are two different types of vessels in the lungs: the alveolar blood vessels and the extraalveolar blood vessels. Alveolar blood vessels have a close relation to the alveoli whereas extraalveolar vessels are not in contact with alveoli. Alveolar blood vessels are compressed as lung volume increases, which causes vascular resistance to increase. When alveolar volume decreases, these vessels are not compressed and the resistance decreases. Extraalveolar vessels tend to react in the opposite way. When lung volume increases, the compression of alveolar vessels enhances blood flow toward the extraalveolar vessels, which causes them to dilate; visa versa when lung volume decreases. When examined together, lung volume at FRC results in the lowest overall vascular resistance, and any increases from FRC tend to increase vascular resistance. Thus at low lung volume greater blood flow goes toward alveolar vessels and at greater lung volume, greater blood flow goes away from them.

Alveolar Pressure: the Lung Zone Concept

Pressure in the alveoli can also influence pulmonary capillary blood flow. If alveolar pressure exceeds capillary pressure, blood has a difficult time passing through the alveolar capillaries. This, coupled with the relatively low pulmonary artery and capillary blood pressure that is influenced by gravity, can result in marked differences between blood pressure and alveolar gas pressure. Four different zones have been theorized to be present in the lungs (Table 12-2). Zone 1 occurs where alveolar pressure (Palv) is greater than pulmonary artery pressure (Ppa), which is greater than pulmonary venous pressure (Ppv) (Palv > Ppa > Ppv). This routinely occurs in the independent regions of the lungs (apical segments of upright lung). Little blood flow occurs here but some "squirting" of blood through this region occurs with the pulsatile nature of the blood pressure. Zone 2 is the area where pulmonary artery pressure is greater than alveolar and venous pressures in that order (Ppa > Palv > Ppv). This is usually the mid lung area. Blood can more easily pass through this area but is still restricted in its flow. Zone 3 is the area where pulmonary artery pressure is greater than venous and alveolar pressures (Ppa > Ppv > Palv). In this zone blood flow is unrestricted and easily passes through the alveolar capillaries. Zone 3 of the lungs receives the majority of pulmonary blood flow. This normally occurs in the base or dependent areas of the lungs. Zone 4 occurs in the most dependent area of the lungs. Because of the weight of the lungs, the alveolar capillaries can be compressed, decreasing their blood flow despite a relatively high blood pressure. Zone 4 disappears with deep inspiration because of the dilation of these vessels as lung volume increases. Lung zones are general regions that are identified according to these definitions. Zones are not fixed anatomically but change as body position, lung volume, alveolar pressure, and pulmonary artery pressure change. Some zone 2 areas will become zone 1 areas, and some zone 3 areas may become zone 2 areas, and so forth.

Regulation of Pulmonary Blood Flow

The pulmonary circulation is largely a "passive" vascular bed lacking elaborate mechanisms for autoregulation. However, several factors effect pulmonary vascular resistance (PVR) and the distribution of blood flow.

Alveolar hypoxia (low P_AO_2): Alveolar hypoxia can be local or diffuse. It causes pulmonary arteriole vasoconstriction, increased local PVR, and decreased local blood flow. This local reflex results in directing blood flow away from hypoxic areas toward regions of better oxygenation.

Acidemia (low blood pH): Acidemia causes pulmonary arteriole vasoconstriction and increased PVR (primarily in infants).

Alveolar hypercapnia (high P_ACO_2): Hypercapnia also causes pulmonary arteriole vasoconstriction and increased PVR (primarily in infants).

A number of biochemicals trigger changes in the tone of arteriolar smooth muscles. Several substances cause vasoconstriction and increased PVR. These include catecholamines (e.g., epinephrine and norepinephrine), prostaglandin F, angiotensin II, and endothelins. Substances that cause vasodilation and decreased PVR include acetylcholine, brady-

Table 12-2   Zones of the Lung

	Pressure Differences	Effects on Blood Flow
Zone 1	Palv > Ppa > Ppv	↓ ↓
Zone 2	Ppa > Palv > Ppv	↑
Zone 3	Ppa > Ppv > Palv	↑ ↑
Zone 4	Capillary compression	↓ ↓ ↓

Palv, Alveolar pressure; *Ppa,* pulmonary artery pressure; *Ppv,* pulmonary venous pressure.

kinins, prostaglandin E, nitric oxide, and prostacyclin. These chemicals can alter the perfusion of regional as well as global pulmonary capillaries. This can result in generalized increases or decreases in pulmonary artery pressure, which influence global pulmonary blood flow. At the local level, they allow the shifting of pulmonary blood flow from one region to another.

⬤ HOW MATCHING OF VENTILATION AND PERFUSION INFLUENCE GAS EXCHANGE

The action of gas exchange within the lungs is dependent on the ability to place or match two different "streams" of material: a stream of gas to and from the alveoli and a stream of blood flow to the alveolar pulmonary capillaries. Failure to match these two streams results in abnormal gas exchange. Consider the ultimate mismatch where all of the ventilation is directed into the right lung and all of the perfusion is directed into the left lung. This lethal condition results in no gas exchange.

Ventilation/Perfusion Ratio

The ventilation/perfusion ($\dot{V}/\dot{Q}$) ratio is a mathematical technique to describe the relative amounts of ventilation and perfusion. It compares the relative amount of ventilation, which goes to a given lung region and the corresponding amount of perfusion in that region. Looking only at the $\dot{V}/\dot{Q}$ ratio does not indicate absolute amounts of ventilation or perfusion but only their relative amounts. A $\dot{V}/\dot{Q}$ ratio of 1.0 is an ideal match, indicating equal amounts of $\dot{V}$ and $\dot{Q}$ are matched in a lung unit. This is illustrated in Fig. 12-4 for the

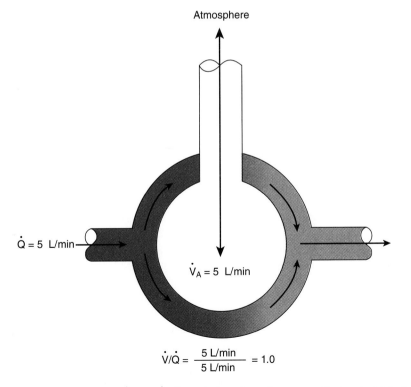

Atmosphere

$\dot{Q} = 5$ L/min

$\dot{V}_A = 5$ L/min

$$\dot{V}/\dot{Q} = \frac{5 \text{ L/min}}{5 \text{ L/min}} = 1.0$$

FIG. 12-4 Ideally matched $\dot{V}$ and $\dot{Q}$. If total alveolar minute ventilation is 5 L/min and pulmonary capillary blood flow is 5 L/min, then the overall $\dot{V}/\dot{Q}$ ratio of the lung is 1.0.

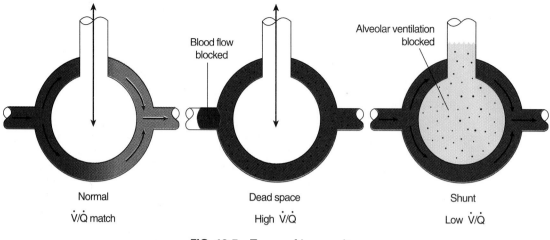

FIG. 12-5 Types of lung units.

whole lung where the alveolar ventilation is 5.0 L/min and pulmonary capillary blood flow is 5.0 L/min.

Types of $\dot{V}/\dot{Q}$ Abnormalities

Variations in $\dot{V}/\dot{Q}$ matching result in different types of lung units (Fig. 12-5). Normal lung units have well-matched ventilation and perfusion with ratios of about 0.8. Units that have excess ventilation or a deficiency of blood flow are classified as **dead space units.** These units have $\dot{V}/\dot{Q}$ ratios numerically greater than 1.0 and, in extreme cases where there is no blood flow, the values approach infinity (i.e., 0 divided into anything is an infinite number). Simply put, dead space (also known as physiological or alveolar dead space) is a region of lung that receives ventilation but lacks pulmonary blood flow. This results in wasted ventilation in regions that cannot support gas exchange. The most common cause of a dead space unit is a reduction in pulmonary blood flow brought about globally by heart failure and locally by blood clots that block blood flow to a region (e.g., pulmonary emboli).

A pulmonary **shunt** is defined as systemic venous blood that passes from the right side of circulation (right side of the heart or pulmonary arteries) directly to systemic arterial blood on the left side of circulation (left side of the heart or pulmonary veins) without the opportunity for picking up O_2. These lung units have $\dot{V}/\dot{Q}$ ratios less than 1.0. Pulmonary shunts can be classified into two types: an **intrapulmonary shunt** (also known as a capillary shunt) and an **extrapulmonary shunt** (also known as an anatomical shunt) (Fig. 12-6). Examples of an intrapulmonary shunt include alveoli that are collapsed **(atelectasis)** or fluid filled because of pulmonary inflammation and edema. An example of a right-to-left extrapulmonary anatomical shunt is an **atrial septal defect** with right atrial pressure higher than left atrial pressure. In this case, venous blood is forced to flow through the septal defect into the left atrium, causing the blood O_2 concentration leaving the left side of the heart to decrease. In both cases, blood flow is not "exposed" to ventilation and gas exchange. Normally there is minimal intrapulmonary shunting and several minor extrapulmonary shunts. The normal extrapulmonary shunts include the thebesian veins, which direct coronary venous blood into the left side of the heart, and some of the bronchial veins and mediastinal veins, which allow some blood flow into the pulmonary veins. The normal amount of blood flow through these different

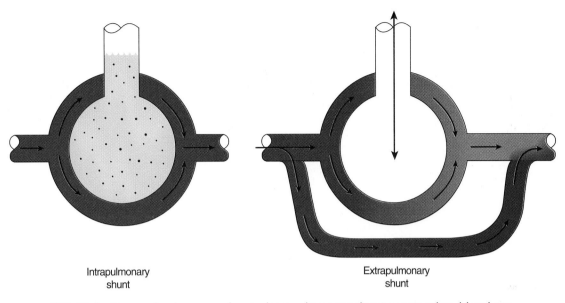

Intrapulmonary
shunt

Extrapulmonary
shunt

FIG. 12-6 Types of pulmonary shunts. Intrapulmonary shunt occurs when blood perfuses alveoli but they are not ventilated. Extrapulmonary shunt occurs when blood bypasses alveolar areas. This may occur in the lungs or elsewhere (in the heart), but the effect is the same. There is no opportunity for gas exchange, and the $\dot{V}/\dot{Q}$ ratio is 0.

pulmonary shunts is less than 2% of the cardiac output.

Regions of low $\dot{V}/\dot{Q}$ matching, which function as "shuntlike" lung units, can lead to hypoxemia. Unlike a true pulmonary shunt, hypoxemia created by low $\dot{V}/\dot{Q}$ ratio units can be corrected in most cases by delivering an elevated O_2 concentration. True shunt and shuntlike effects can all be placed together under one title called **physiological shunt** ($\dot{Q}_s$). The amount of shunted blood compared with the total cardiac output ($\dot{Q}_T$) is called the *percent shunt* ($\dot{Q}_s/\dot{Q}_T$), or **shunt fraction.** Total physiological shunt is normally 2% to 5% of cardiac output. This form of $\dot{V}/\dot{Q}$ mismatching is the most common cause of hypoxemia.

Effects of $\dot{V}/\dot{Q}$ Matching and Mismatching on Blood Gas Tension

When the $\dot{V}$ equally matches the $\dot{Q}$, yielding a ratio of 1.0, alveolar oxygen (P_AO_2) and pulmonary capillary oxygen (P_cO_2) are equilibrated at 100 mm Hg, and the alveolar carbon dioxide (P_ACO_2) and pulmonary capillary carbon dioxide (P_cCO_2) are equilibrated at 40 mm Hg as blood leaves the alveolar area. This assumes that a diffusion defect is not present. This relationship is shown in Fig. 12-7. When abnormal matching occurs in a region, PCO_2 and PO_2 stray from these normal values.

Lung conditions that produce shunting, ideal matching, and dead space are shown in Fig. 12-7 as different $\dot{V}/\dot{Q}$ relationships and as corresponding values of PO_2 and PCO_2. Lung regions that have $\dot{V}/\dot{Q}$ ratios that are greater than 1.0 have increased amounts of ventilation matched with perfusion. These conditions result in less O_2 extraction and CO_2 excretion. As a result, the P_AO_2 approaches the partial pressure of inspired oxygen (P_iO_2) levels and P_ACO_2 approaches the partial pressure of inspired CO_2 (P_iCO_2) levels. At sea level, while breathing room air, normal P_iO_2 is 150 mm Hg and P_iCO_2 is virtually 0. $\dot{V}/\dot{Q}$ mismatching of this type in the whole lungs does not lead

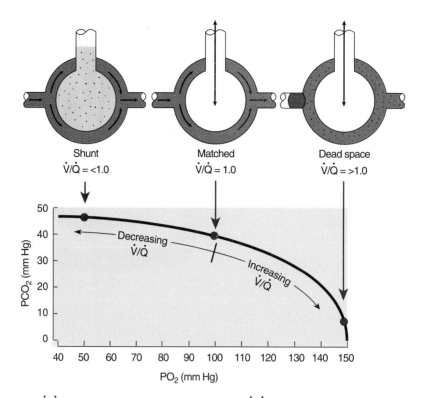

FIG. 12-7 $\dot{V}/\dot{Q}$ ratio line. In lung regions with a $\dot{V}/\dot{Q} > 1$, partial pressure of oxygen (PO₂) increases and partial pressure of carbon dioxide (PCO₂) decreases. At the extreme right end of the $\dot{V}/\dot{Q}$ line, there is ventilation without perfusion (dead space) and $\dot{V}/\dot{Q} = \infty$. In lung regions with a $\dot{V}/\dot{Q} < 1$, PO₂ decreases and PCO₂ increases. At the far left end of the $\dot{V}/\dot{Q}$ line, there is perfusion without ventilation (shunt) and $\dot{V}/\dot{Q} = 0$.

to hypoxia but instead leads to hyperventilation (decreased P_aCO_2) and hyperoxemia (increased P_aO_2). During conditions of ventilation and no perfusion, the $\dot{V}/\dot{Q}$ ratio becomes infinite. This relationship represents pure dead space ventilation ($\dot{V}_D$), which can result in reduced alveolar ventilation.

Conditions that cause greater amounts of perfusion than ventilation in a region of the lungs result in $\dot{V}/\dot{Q}$ ratios of less than 1.0. Excess pulmonary blood flow extracts move O_2 and releases more CO_2. This results in decreased PO₂ levels and increased PCO₂ levels. A region of the lungs that has blood flow and no ventilation has a $\dot{V}/\dot{Q}$ ratio of zero.

This point is defined as a true shunt. These conditions result in blood leaving the region with values of PO₂ and PCO₂ that are equal to mixed venous blood that is entering the pulmonary artery. This yields results of PO₂ = 40 mm Hg and PCO₂ = 46 mm Hg. Low $\dot{V}/\dot{Q}$ matching and true shunts are responsible for hypoxemia. Low $\dot{V}/\dot{Q}$ matching is the most common cause of hypoxemia.

Regions of $\dot{V}/\dot{Q}$ Matching in Normal Lungs

Normal lungs do not have uniform matching of $\dot{V}$ with $\dot{Q}$. Gravity causes much greater perfusion in the dependent regions of the upright

DIAGNOSTIC FOCUS

Impaired Gas Exchange Following Sudden Onset of Chest Pain

A 41-year-old woman was admitted to the hospital for gallbladder removal (cholecystectomy). She has no history of chronic diseases and takes birth control pills as a regular medication. Postoperatively, she refused to ambulate because of pain. On the third postoperative day she began complaining of shortness of breath, chest pain during inspiration, and calf pain. Her vital signs were as follows:

Heart rate	138/min
Blood pressure	105/67
Respiratory rate	28/min (with difficulty)
Temperature	39° C

The saturation of her blood with oxygen was reduced from a normal value of 97% to 88%. Her breath sounds were clear bilaterally. A 12-lead electrocardiogram (ECG) was ordered and showed a sinus tachycardia and no signs of myocardial ischemia or dysrhythmias. While breathing air, arterial blood was taken from the patient's right radial artery and was analyzed for PO_2, which was found to be 51 mm Hg (normal value is 100 mm Hg). This indicated significant hypoxemia caused by altered $\dot{V}/\dot{Q}$ matching, shunting, or a diffusion defect. The patient was given 4 L of supplemental oxygen each minute to breathe by nasal cannula. This eased her tachypnea somewhat and improved her PO_2 to 77 mm Hg. The physician suspected that the patient had developed deep vein thrombosis in her calf, that a blood clot had formed, and that one or more clots had broken free and were carried by the venous system into the lungs, resulting in a pulmonary embolism. A $\dot{V}/\dot{Q}$ scan, a test that utilizes inhaled and intravenous radioactive isotopes to "tag" the gas and blood in her lungs and a chest scanner to detect the distribution of gas and blood flow, was ordered. This showed multiple perfusion defects in the right lung. A pulmonary angiogram, which uses the injection of radiopaque material and multiple x-rays of the chest to visualize the pulmonary circulation, was then ordered. This confirmed the blockage of pulmonary blood flow in several areas in the right lung. The physical findings, relatively normal ECG, significant hypoxemia, abnormal $\dot{V}/\dot{Q}$ scan, and pulmonary angiogram indicate abnormal gas exchange that resulted from multiple pulmonary emboli that disturbed the matching of blood flow and ventilation within the lungs.

The patient continued on oxygen therapy and was started on heparin to prevent further clot formation and was gradually mobilized to improve the venous blood flow in her extremities. She was discharged 4 days later with improved oxygenation and no other complications.

---

lungs (see Fig. 12-1). This results in $\dot{V}/\dot{Q}$ ratios of about 0.6 in the base, 1.0 near the mid-lung region, and 3.0 in the apical regions. Fig. 12-8 illustrates these different regions on an O_2-CO_2 diagram. The different ratios result in different PCO_2 and PO_2 values in these different regions. These different areas can be visualized as if they have different "microenvironments" where there is an excess or a deficit of one of the streams. In the basal regions there is an excess of blood flow when compared with the apical region. These different "microenvironments" are detailed in Fig. 12-9. Only a thin slice of lung in the middle region has ideal matching. Ventilation/perfusion matching changes when the lungs are placed in a different position (e.g., supine, prone, or on one side).

The overall or average $\dot{V}/\dot{Q}$ ratio for the lungs is determined by dividing the total

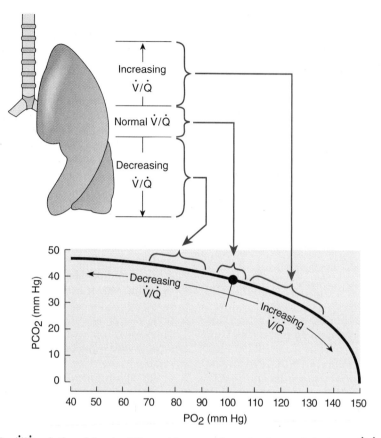

FIG. 12-8 $\dot{V}/\dot{Q}$ relationships in different lung regions. In the upright lung, $\dot{V}/\dot{Q}$ is high (>1) in the apical region, normal (=1) in the mid-lung region, and low (<1) in the lung bases.

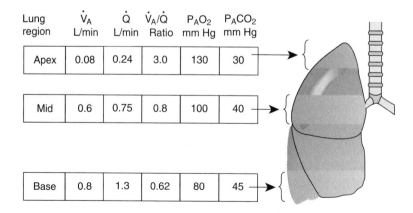

Lung region	$\dot{V}_A$ L/min	$\dot{Q}$ L/min	$\dot{V}_A/\dot{Q}$ Ratio	P_AO_2 mm Hg	P_ACO_2 mm Hg
Apex	0.08	0.24	3.0	130	30
Mid	0.6	0.75	0.8	100	40
Base	0.8	1.3	0.62	80	45

FIG. 12-9 Variations in regional alveolar ventilation $(\dot{V}_A)$ and perfusion $(\dot{Q})$ result in regional differences in alveolar oxygen pressure (P_AO_2) and alveolar carbon dioxide pressure (P_ACO_2).

alveolar ventilation (4.0 L/min) by the total pulmonary capillary blood flow (5 L/min). This yields an average $\dot{V}/\dot{Q}$ ratio of 0.8 for the entire lung. This average actually determines the PO_2 and PCO_2 in blood that leaves the pulmonary circuit and enters the aorta.

Effects on PO₂ and PCO₂ when Mixing Blood from Different Regions

As blood from all the different regions of the lung mixes together in the left heart, the O_2 and CO_2 values equilibrate, or average out. The normal gradient between venous and arterial PCO_2 levels is approximately 6 mm Hg. Because of this small V-A gradient and the manner in which CO_2 is carried in the blood, lung regions with low $\dot{V}/\dot{Q}$ ratios (shuntlike units) have a minimal affect on the overall P_aCO_2 levels. These regions can be compensated for by areas that have high $\dot{V}/\dot{Q}$ ratios. On the other hand, because O_2 is primarily carried by hemoglobin and the larger difference between venous and arterial blood PO_2, which is 60 mm Hg, blood from regions with a low $\dot{V}/\dot{Q}$ ratio can have a significant effect on overall PO_2 levels in blood leaving the lungs. This results in hypoxemia, which cannot be compensated for by regions with high $\dot{V}/\dot{Q}$ ratios. Variations in blood oxygenation are determined by analyzing the average oxygen content of blood after mixing. Once the average blood oxygen content is determined, the resulting blood PO_2 can then be determined. It is inaccurate to simply take the PO_2 of each blood sample, add them together, and divide by 2 to determine the mixed PO_2. The following examples may help illustrate this.

Example 1: Mixing blood from an ideal and a high V̇/Q̇ region

If 100 ml of blood from an ideal $\dot{V}/\dot{Q}$ region with a blood PO_2 of 100 mm Hg and blood O_2 content of 19.94 ml/dl is mixed with 100 ml of blood from a high $\dot{V}/\dot{Q}$ region with a blood PO_2 of 120 mm Hg and blood O_2 content of 20.20 ml/dl, the resulting blood O_2 content is the average of the two (19.94 + 20.20 ml/dl) ÷ 2 = 20.07 ml/dl. The resulting mixed blood PO_2 at this new blood O_2 content is 110 mm Hg. The PO_2 is determined by using the relationship between the PO_2 of blood and the resulting O_2 content shown in Table 12-3. The PO_2 that results from mixing equal volumes of blood flow from these two regions is midway between the two values. This is largely because the hemoglobin is already saturated with O_2 and the minor difference is a result of the small amount dissolved in plasma.

Example 2: Mixing blood from an ideal and a low V̇/Q̇ region

If 100 ml of blood from an ideal region with a PO_2 of 100 mm Hg and O_2 content of 19.94 ml/dl is mixed with 100 ml of blood from a region with a low $\dot{V}/\dot{Q}$ ratio (shuntlike region) with a blood PO_2 of 40 mm Hg and O_2 content of 15.18 ml/dl, the mixed content is 19.94 + 15.18 ml/dl ÷ 2 = 17.56 ml/dl.

Table 12-3 Oxygen Saturation of Hemoglobin ($S_{blood}O_2$) and Oxygen Content in Blood ($C_{blood}O_2$) at Different Blood PO_2 Values*

PO_2 (mm Hg)	$S_{blood}O_2$ (%)	$C_{blood}O_2$ (ml O_2/dl Blood)
40	74.9	15.18
50	85.0	17.24
60	90.6	18.39
70	93.8	19.06
80	95.7	19.48
90	96.9	19.75
100	97.7	19.94
110	98.3	20.07
120	98.7	20.20
130	99.0	20.29
140	99.2	20.36
150	99.3	20.41

*Assumes a hemoglobin content of 15 g/dl, O_2-binding constant of 1.34 ml/dl, blood pH of 7.40, and blood temperature of 37° C.

According to Table 12-3, the resultant mixed PO_2 is approximately 53 mm Hg.

In the first example, the hemoglobin traveling through these two regions is already loaded with O_2 so the minor differences occur largely in the amount dissolved in the plasma. When these two blood samples mix, only the plasma content of O_2 needs to equalize or average out from the two regions. This results in a midpoint PO_2 value of 110 mm Hg. In the second example, the hemoglobin saturations and content are much more different. When blood from these two regions mixes, the resulting O_2 saturation and content are much lower. This results in a PO_2 that is much lower than the average of the original two PO_2 values.

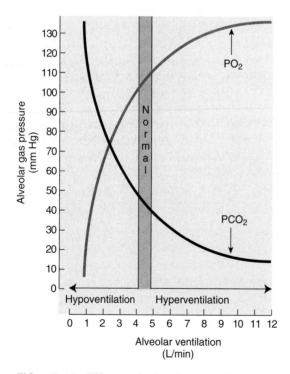

FIG. 12-10 Effects of alveolar ventilation on alveolar gas pressures. This relationship assumes a normal adult metabolic rate while breathing gas with 21% oxygen at barometric pressure of 760 mm Hg.

Example 3: Mixing blood from a high and a low $\dot{V}/\dot{Q}$ region

Using the values from the previous examples, equal amounts of blood from a region with a low $\dot{V}/\dot{Q}$ ratio whose O_2 content is 15.18 ml/dl are mixed with blood from a region with a high $\dot{V}/\dot{Q}$ ratio whose O_2 content is 20.20 ml/dl. The resulting average content is 15.18 + 20.20 ml/dl ÷ 2 = 17.69 ml/dl. This corresponds to an approximate PO_2 of 54 mm Hg (see Table 12-3). This also does not produce a blood PO_2 value at the midway point.

These examples help explain why it is difficult to improve oxygen levels in arterial blood of a patient who has significant amounts of pulmonary blood either flowing through regions of intrapulmonary shunt that are unventilated (collapsed and fluid filled) or when their blood is routed away from the pulmonary circuit and directed back to the systemic circuit via an extrapulmonary shunt. Both of these situations produce the effect of exposing blood to a region with a low $\dot{V}/\dot{Q}$ ratio.

Affects of Alveolar Ventilation on PCO_2 and PO_2

Alveolar ventilation is normally maintained at about 4.5 L/min in the adult. Adjustments of ventilation can bring about changes in the overall $\dot{V}/\dot{Q}$ ratio within the lung. Hypoventilation causes the overall ratio to decrease, resulting in a shuntlike condition. This results in increased PCO_2 and decreased PO_2. Hyperventilation results in the opposite affect. This causes an overall increase in the $\dot{V}/\dot{Q}$ ratio, producing a dead space-like affect. In turn, this results in reduced PCO_2 and increased PO_2. These relationships are shown in Fig. 12-10. It should be noted that the sum of PCO_2 and PO_2 values in Fig. 12-10 at any level of ventilation is about 150 mm Hg at sea level while breathing air with 21% O_2 with a normal metabolic rate. As ventilation increases or decreases, the PCO_2 and PO_2 within this total are altered in an inverse relationship. The extreme ends of the relationship, where ventilation is 0 L/min or 12 L/min, represent shuntlike and dead space-like effects, respectively. In the normal range of ventilation the PCO_2 stays between 35 and 45 mm Hg with the resulting PO_2 about 95 to 105 mm Hg.

HOW V̇/Q̇ MATCHING IS TESTED

A variety of techniques are available to measure the magnitude of $\dot{V}/\dot{Q}$ mismatching and to evaluate how the patient responds to treatment.

Tests of Oxygenation

The ability of the lungs to oxygenate blood that is leaving the pulmonary circuit can be analyzed and compared to an ideal ability. Abnormalities of $\dot{V}/\dot{Q}$ matching disturb this ability.

$P_{A-a}O_2$ Difference

One of the more common methods of evaluating gas exchange is to measure the alveolar-arterial PO_2 difference, or **A-a gradient** **($P_{A-a}O_2$).** The perfectly functioning lung completely equilibrates alveolar PO_2 with all of the blood leaving the lung. This results in a systemic arterial PO_2 that is identical to alveolar PO_2. The normal lung does produce a small difference as the result of shunting, $\dot{V}/\dot{Q}$ mismatching, and diffusion defects. The normal $P_{A-a}O_2$ while breathing 21% O_2 is less than 10 mm Hg. This value increases with advancing age at a rate of about 0.4 mm Hg/year after age 20. This is because of changes in $\dot{V}/\dot{Q}$ matching and diffusion with age. When an individual breathes 100% O_2 the gradient is normally less than 150 mm Hg. The larger difference that occurs with breathing 100% O_2 is thought to be the result of small changes in $\dot{V}/\dot{Q}$ matching and the effects of normal shunts on oxygenation of blood.

To measure $P_{A-a}O_2$, an arterial blood sample is collected and the P_aO_2 is determined. Simultaneously, the P_AO_2 is determined by either measuring the PO_2 that occurs during exhalation at the end-tidal exhalation point. A more common approach is to determine the P_AO_2 with the alveolar air equation and simply subtract the P_aO_2:

$$P_{A-a}O_2 = [FIO_2 (P_B - 47) - P_ACO_2 (1.25)] - P_aO_2$$

For example, a 39-year-old patient has developed pulmonary edema following rupture of an infected appendix and the development of sepsis syndrome and lung injury. The patient has the following:

FIO_2 (fraction of inhaled gas that is O_2) = 50%, or 0.5

Patm = 760 mm Hg

P_aO_2 = 73 mm Hg

P_ACO_2 = 35 mm Hg

$P_{A-a}O_2$ = [0.50 (760 − 47) − 35 (1.25)] − 73 mm Hg

= [0.50 (713) − 44] − 73 mm Hg

= [357 − 44] − 73 mm Hg

= 313 − 73 mm Hg

= 240 mm Hg

These results are highly abnormal and consistent with lung dysfunction that probably includes $\dot{V}/\dot{Q}$ mismatching, shunting, or a diffusion defect. Greater values of $P_{A-a}O_2$ indicate greater $\dot{V}/\dot{Q}$ mismatching, shunting, and diffusion defects.

P_aO_2/FIO_2 Ratio

Another approach to comparing alveolar gas and arterial blood PO_2 is the determination of the **P_aO_2/FIO_2 ratio**, or the **P/F ratio.** This is a simple technique that predicts the P_aO_2 that would be generated when breathing 100% O_2. The measured P_aO_2 from an arterial blood sample is divided by the FIO_2 of the gas being breathed. The normal value for a young adult is 476 (100 ÷ 0.21). With lung dysfunction, the value drops in proportion to the amount of dysfunction.

For example, calculate the P_aO_2/FIO_2 ratio for our 39-year-old septic patient that was described previously:

$$P_aO_2/FIO_2 = \frac{73}{0.5}$$
$$= 146$$

The value of this ratio indicates that this patient would have a P_aO_2 of only 146 mm Hg while breathing 100% O_2. This low value is consistent with severe lung dysfunction. The P_aO_2/FIO_2 ratio decreases with $\dot{V}/\dot{Q}$ mismatching, shunting, and diffusion defects. Care should be used when evaluating the P_aO_2/FIO_2 ratio from an individual who is hypoventilating and retaining CO_2. This causes the P_aO_2/FIO_2 ratio to fall also.

P_aO_2/P_AO_2 Index

A more refined technique used to compare alveolar and arterial blood PO_2 is to determine of the **oxygenation index (P_aO_2/P_AO_2)**. Instead of calculating the difference in alveolar and arterial partial pressures, the ratio is calculated. The normal value for a young adult is 0.94 to 0.96. The perfect lung would have a value of 1.0. With shunting, $\dot{V}/\dot{Q}$ mismatching and diffusion defects, the value drops in proportion to the amount of dysfunction. In the 39-year-old septic patient described previously, the oxygenation index is as follows:

$$P_aO_2/P_AO_2$$
$$= \frac{73}{313}$$
$$= 0.23$$

This low value is consistent with severe lung dysfunction. The a/A ratio is thought to be a better indicator of the amount of physiological shunting.

$\dot{Q}_S/\dot{Q}_T$

The **physiological shunt fraction**, or **venous admixture ratio** ($\dot{Q}_S/\dot{Q}_T$), is the ratio of blood flow through shunt units ($\dot{Q}_S$) to the total flow or cardiac output ($\dot{Q}_T$). It is calculated by comparing the difference between the O_2 content in blood from ideal lung units (C_iO_2) and mixed arterial blood content (C_aO_2) with the oxygen content difference between ideal units and the incoming mixed venous blood ($C_{\bar{v}}O_2$):

$$\dot{Q}_S/\dot{Q}_T = \frac{C_iO_2 - C_aO_2}{C_iO_2 - C_{\bar{v}}O_2}$$

If the patient is breathing 100% O_2, the $\dot{Q}_S/\dot{Q}_T$ ratio indicates more closely the amount of the true pulmonary shunt ($\dot{V}/\dot{Q} = 0$) rather than the effects of regions that are simply mismatched (e.g., $\dot{V}/\dot{Q} = 0.25$) or that have poor diffusion. The physiological shunt fraction calculation better reflects the shunt because breathing gas with a high concentration of O_2 helps correct the blood O_2 content that flows from regions with a moderately low $\dot{V}/\dot{Q}$ ratio and poor diffusion. The normal $\dot{Q}_S/\dot{Q}_T$ ratio in an adult is less than 2% when breathing 100% O_2 and 2% to 5% when breathing air.

To determine the $\dot{Q}_S/\dot{Q}_T$ ratio, C_iO_2 is calculated by using the alveolar PO_2 (from the alveolar air equation) to determine the O_2 content in the blood (see Chapter 13) that is leaving the ideal alveolar-capillary unit. The values of C_aO_2 and $C_{\bar{v}}O_2$ are measured by collecting arterial blood samples from a peripheral artery (e.g., radial) and mixed venous blood samples from a catheter in the pulmonary artery. The O_2 content is then determined by using the measured hemoglobin saturation and PO_2. The values are then applied to the shunt fraction equation. Shunt fractions calculated at any FIO_2 should be noted as such (e.g., 20% shunt on 40% O_2). If possible, the cardiac output should also be determined at the time of the shunt measurement. Changes in cardiac output may have an influence on both the actual amount of shunted blood and the shunt fraction. Pulmonary artery pressure and body positioning may also influence shunt fraction.

Positive End-Expiratory Pressure to Improve Gas Exchange

A 53-year-old woman has been suffering with the symptoms of the flu for the past 3 days when she developed increasing shortness of breath and was admitted to the hospital. Shortly after her arrival she was given supplemental oxygen to breathe. A chest x-ray revealed bilateral infiltrates, and sputum samples were collected and found to be free of bacteria and fungi. This is suggestive of viral pneumonia. Over the next 12 hours her respiratory rate gradually increased from 20 to 40 breaths per minute and she became increasingly confused. A sample was taken of arterial blood and, despite supplemental oxygen by mask, the PO_2 was 38 mm Hg and the PCO_2 was 31 mm Hg, indicating severe hypoxia and compensatory hyperventilation. The physician decided to sedate her, place an endotracheal tube, and support her with mechanical ventilation to improve her gas exchange. She was intubated with an 8.0-mm endotracheal tube and ventilated with 15 breaths per minute, tidal volume of 600 ml, and 100% oxygen. Arterial blood was drawn again and the PO_2 was 66 mm Hg and the PCO_2 was 42 mm Hg. The minute ventilation

being given had normalized her PCO_2, however, the PO_2 was unacceptably low despite the high level of oxygen with which she was being ventilated. This suggested that her hypoxia was being caused by $\dot{V}/\dot{Q}$ mismatching, intrapulmonary shunting, and diffusion defects. To improve the $\dot{V}/\dot{Q}$ match, to reduce the percent of blood flow being shunted, and to improve diffusion, positive end-expiratory pressure (PEEP) was programmed into the ventilator. PEEP increases the functional residual capacity (FRC) of the lungs by keeping airway pressure positive during exhalation. This results in improved gas exchange. Several different levels of PEEP were tried and the administration of 10 cm H_2O improved oxygenation but did not overinflate the lungs or compromise cardiac output. This enabled the reduction of the delivered oxygen concentration to 50% over the next 24 hours. The patient came off ventilatory support after 4 days and made a complete recovery 15 days after the initial admission. Microbiology studies of her sputum revealed that she had been infected with Influenza A.

The following example illustrates the calculation of the $\dot{Q}_S/\dot{Q}_T$ ratio in the 39-year-old septic patient with the following information:

C_iO_2 = 20.9 ml of O_2 per deciliter of blood
C_aO_2 = 19.1 ml of O_2 per deciliter of blood
$C_{\bar{v}}O_2$ = 15.2 ml of O_2 per deciliter of blood

$$\dot{Q}_S/\dot{Q}_T = \frac{20.9 - 19.1}{20.9 - 15.2}$$

$$= 1.8/5.7$$

$$= 0.315, \text{ or } 31.5\%, \text{ on } 50\% \ O_2$$

This large shunt fraction indicates that more than 30% of the cardiac output is being wasted on nonventilated or poorly ventilated alveoli.

Tests of Ventilation and Pulmonary Blood Flow

Several other tests are available to determine the extent of wasted ventilation and blood flow.

V_D/V_T and $P_{a\text{-}ET}CO_2$

The amount of ventilation that is wasted on dead space is another indicator of the degree of $\dot{V}/\dot{Q}$ matching (or mismatching). The fraction of tidal volume wasted on **anatomical dead space** was described earlier as the dead space/tidal volume ratio (V_{danat}/V_T). Normally it is about 0.3, or 30%. This can be determined with Fowler's single-breath O_2 inhalation test (see Chapter 11). **Physiological dead**

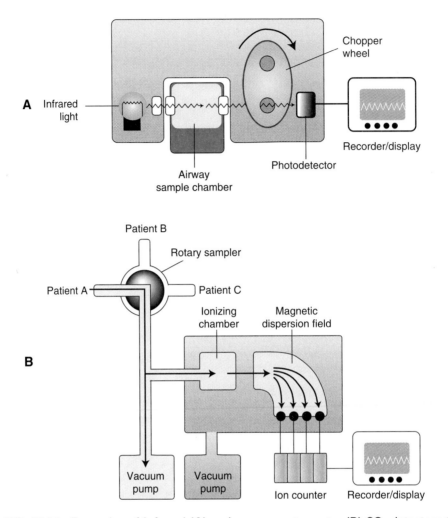

FIG. 12-11 Examples of infrared **(A)** and mass spectrometer **(B)** CO_2 detectors that measure the percent of partial pressure of CO_2 in inhaled and exhaled gas.

space (V_{Dphys}/V_T) includes both the anatomical dead space and the amount of ventilation wasted on poorly perfused alveoli (e.g., apical region of lung or regions that have their blood flow stopped by a blood clot). The modified Bohr equation (see Chapter 11) is used to determine physiological dead space:

$$V_{Dphys}/V_T = \frac{P_aCO_2 - P_{\bar{E}}CO_2}{P_aCO_2}$$

Normally the V_{Dphys}/V_T ranges around 30% ± 5%.

Another approach to measure the dead space/tidal volume ratio is to measure the P_aCO_2-end-tidal exhaled PCO_2 difference ($P_{a-ET}CO_2$). The arterial PCO_2 is measured with a blood gas analyzer, and the end-tidal PCO_2 is measured with a fast response CO_2 detector (e.g., infrared or mass spectrometer CO_2 analyzer) that is placed at the airway opening

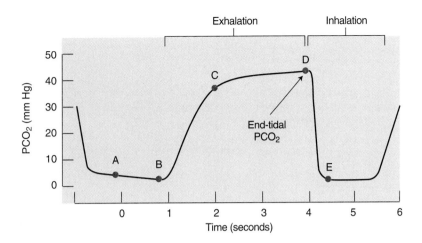

FIG. 12-12 The normal capnogram shows the partial pressure of carbon dioxide (PCO_2) in inhaled and exhaled gas. From *A* to *B*, the inspiratory phase occurs. Exhalation begins at *B*. From *B* to *C*, the subject is exhaling a mixture of gases from dead space and alveolar regions. From *C* to *D*, a more uniform emptying of alveolar gas from the lungs occurs. At *D* the PCO_2 has reached its maximum at the end-tidal exhalation. From *D* to *E*, inhalation starts.

(Fig. 12-11). Normally, the end-tidal PCO_2 is 38 to 42 mm Hg. Fig. 12-12 shows a normal **capnogram,** which is a graphic recording of inhaled and exhaled PCO_2. It shows that end-tidal PCO_2 is the maximal PCO_2 exhaled. Normally, the $P_{a\text{-}ET}CO_2$ difference is less than 3 mm Hg. With increasing dead space (anatomical or physiological) the exhaled PCO_2 is diluted with dead space gas that has no CO_2. This results in an elevated $P_{a\text{-}ET}CO_2$ gradient (e.g., 10 mm Hg).

Ventilation/Perfusion Scans Pulmonary Angiograms

The distribution and matching of ventilation and pulmonary blood flow can be visualized by giving a subject radioactive xenon (^{133}Xe) tagged gas to breathe and intravenous injection of radioactive isotopes to trace blood flow. These radioactive tracers can be detected and produce an image of the regions that are ventilated and perfused ($\dot{V}/\dot{Q}$ **scan**). Obstruction of ventilation or perfusion in any region of the lungs can be detected with this tech-

nique. Another method that can reveal some of the details of the pulmonary circuit is the **pulmonary angiography.** This test uses a radiopaque dye (contrast media) that is injected intravenously and casts a dense "shadow" of the pulmonary circulation when a standard chest x-ray is made (see Chapter 7). Obstructions of pulmonary blood flow are revealed as a loss of shadow.

Closing Volume

One of the factors that contributes to regional differences in ventilation is the tendency of unstable small airways to close during exhalation. This results in reduced ventilation of these areas with gas trapping in those alveoli beyond the point of airway closure. Those airways most susceptible to closure are those that have poor support. Small airways are supported in the open position by the surrounding alveolar tissue that pulls outward around the airway as a tethering force. Airways in the base of lung are more susceptible to early closure as the result of low lung volume and

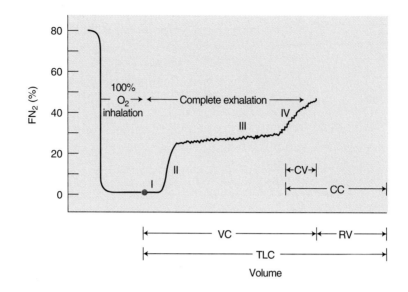

FIG. 12-13 The single-breath N_2 washout test shows the fractional concentration of N_2 *(FN_2)* in exhaled gas after inhaling 100% oxygen (O_2). Phase I gas is all anatomical dead space. Phase II gas is a mixture of dead space and alveolar gas. Phase III reveals relatively even exhalation from the alveolar regions of the lung. Phase IV reveals a sudden increase in the emptying from fewer alveoli as a result of small airway closure. The amount of gas exhaled from the onset of airway closure to the end of the vital capacity *(VC)* is known as the closing volume *(CV)* and the amount in the lungs at the beginning of airway closure is the closing capacity *(CC)*. *RV*, Residual volume, *TLC*, total lung capacity.

lower compliance. This leads to lower tethering force when compared with the airways of the mid-lung and upper lung regions. Other conditions such as emphysema, in which alveoli are destroyed, result in reduced tethering support of small airways leaving them susceptible to early closure.

The single-breath N_2 washout test evaluates this airway closure effect. In this test a subject inhales from RV to TLC a single breath of 100% O_2. They then exhale at a steady and slow rate back to RV past a rapid response N_2 analyzer, which detects the concentration of N_2 in the exhaled gas. Fig. 12-13 shows the N_2 concentration as a normal subject exhales following inhalation of 100% O_2. After exhaling the anatomical dead space gas, the N_2 concentration climbs and plateaus at about 30% N_2.

This represents stable exhalation from open airways and alveoli. Toward the end of the exhalation, a sudden rise in exhaled N_2 concentration occurs, indicating closure of some airways (normally in the lung base). The amount of gas exhaled from this point to the point of complete exhalation is known as the closing volume (CV). In the healthy young adult, the CV is normally the last 10% of the exhaled vital capacity (VC). Another approach is to determine the volume in the lungs at the time these poorly supported airways close. This volume of gas, known as the closing capacity (CC), is normally the last 30% of the TLC. CV and CC both increase with age (e.g., last 40% of VC is a normal CV in a 65-year-old person). The value of CV increases in those conditions that cause instability of small airways. Emphysema, asthma, and interstitial edema cause this type of instability.

Multiple Inert Gas Test

The most sophisticated method of determining the $\dot{V}/\dot{Q}$ match in a subject is the multiple inert gas test. This test employs six different inert gases with different blood and gas solubilities. The gases are injected intravenously until a steady state between gas elimination and injection rate is reached. Careful analysis of the rates of gas injection and exhalation is carried out with the aid of a multiple gas detection system and computer. A $\dot{V}/\dot{Q}$ distribution plot is then produced. The plot basically shows the amount of blood flow and ventilation present in lung units with different $\dot{V}/\dot{Q}$ ratios. Normally, most of the blood flow and ventilation is concentrated in units with a $\dot{V}/\dot{Q}$ ratio of 0.8.

FACTORS THAT INFLUENCE GAS DIFFUSION ACROSS THE ALVEOLAR-CAPILLARY MEMBRANE

Diffusion is the movement of gas molecules from one point to another caused by a difference in concentration of gas. In the lungs, diffusion causes the passive movement of O_2 and CO_2 to cross the alveolar-capillary membrane (Fig. 12-14).

Factors that Affect Diffusion

The diffusion of gas through the alveolar-capillary membrane is influenced by a variety of factors (Box 12-4). Several laws are used to describe these factors.

Henry's Law

Henry's law states that, at a given temperature, the amount of gas that can dissolve in a liquid is proportional to the partial pressure of the gas over the liquid. The amount of gas that

---

BOX 12-4

Factors that Affect Respiratory Gas Diffusion through the Alveolar-Capillary Membrane

Solubility of the gas in tissue and fluid
Molecular weight of the gas
Blood volume and hemoglobin concentration
Lung volume
Surface area of the membrane
Thickness and chemical composition of the membrane
Pressure gradient of gas across the membrane

---

can be dissolved in a liquid under specific conditions is known as the **solubility coefficient (C_s)**. The solubility coefficient is determined with the following relationship:

$$C_s = K \times P_{gas}$$

where C_s is the solubility coefficient, K is the solubility constant for the gas and P_{gas} is the partial pressure of the gas. The solubility coefficient for O_2 is normally stated as 0.003 ml/100 ml $\times$ mm Hg of plasma at 37° C. The solubility coefficient for CO_2 is 0.067 ml/100 ml $\times$ mm Hg of plasma at 37° C. Taking into account only the solubility coefficient of O_2 and CO_2, CO_2 should diffuse 22.3 times more rapidly than O_2 (0.067 ml CO_2/100 ml ÷ 0.003 ml O_2/100 ml = 22.3). The solubility coefficient of CO_2 can also be expressed as 0.03 ml/L $\times$ mm Hg. This form of the CO_2 solubility coefficient is frequently used when determining how much carbonic acid and bicarbonate are formed when CO_2 combines with H_2O.

Graham's Law

Graham's law states that, under the same conditions, the diffusion rate of a gas is inversely proportional to the square root of the molecular

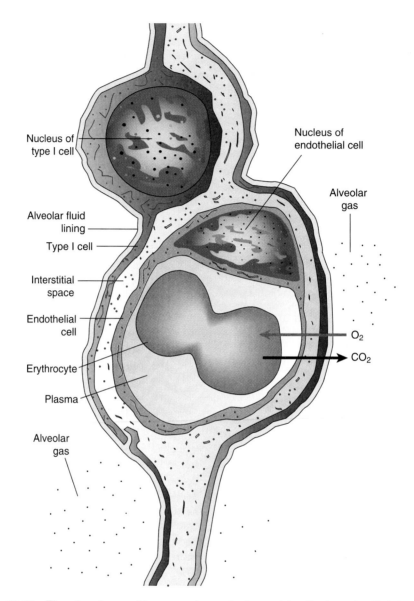

FIG. 12-14 The alveolar-capillary membrane is formed by the type I cell, interstitial space, and endothelial cell. Oxygen (O_2) and carbon dioxide (CO_2) diffuse across this membrane.

weight (or density) of the gas. The molecular weight of O_2 is 32 g/mol and the molecular weight of CO_2 is 44 g/mol. Considering only Graham's law, O_2 should diffuse faster than CO_2 by 1.17 times ($\sqrt{44} \div \sqrt{32}$). Combining Henry's law and Graham's law, the diffusion of a gas is proportional to its solubility coefficient and inversely proportional to the square root of its molecular weight:

$$C_d = \frac{C_s}{\sqrt{gmw}}$$

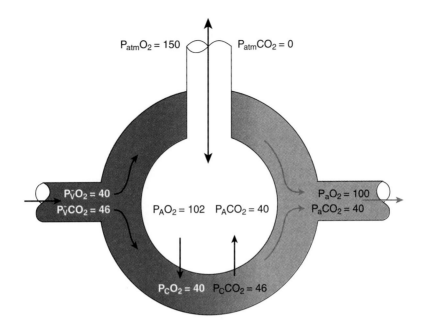

$P_{atm}O_2 = 150$ $P_{atm}CO_2 = 0$

$P_{\bar{v}}O_2 = 40$
$P_{\bar{v}}CO_2 = 46$ $P_AO_2 = 102$ $P_ACO_2 = 40$ $P_aO_2 = 100$
$P_aCO_2 = 40$

$P_CO_2 = 40$ $P_CCO_2 = 46$

FIG. 12-15 Normal PO_2 and PCO_2 values in pulmonary artery (mixed systemic venous) blood, alveolar gas, and arterial (pulmonary venous) blood supports the diffusion of oxygen *(O₂)* into and carbon dioxide *(CO₂)* out of blood.

where C_d is the **diffusion coefficient** and $\sqrt{gmw}$ is the square root of the gram molecular weight of the gas. The diffusion coefficient for O_2 is 0.003 ml/100 ml × mm Hg ÷ $\sqrt{32}$ = 0.00053. The diffusion coefficient for CO_2 is 0.067 ml/100 ml × mm Hg ÷ $\sqrt{44}$ = 0.01. When comparing the diffusion coefficient of CO_2 to that of O_2, 0.01/0.00053, the ratio is 19:1, indicating that the diffusion rate of CO_2 in plasma is 19 times faster than that of O_2.

Fick's Law

Fick's law of diffusion states that the rate of diffusion of a gas ($\dot{V}_{gas}$) is proportional to the surface area (A), the concentration gradient (ΔP), and the diffusion coefficient (C_d) but inversely proportional to the thickness (T) of the membrane:

$$\dot{V}_{gas} = A \times C_d \times \Delta P/T$$

The surface area for diffusion in the adult lungs ranges from 50 to 100 m² and averages approximately 75 m² (about the size of a singles tennis court on one side of the net). Surface area is influenced by the volume of air in the lungs: greater lung volume ≈ greater surface area for diffusion.

The concentration gradient, expressed as a partial pressure gradient across the membrane, is maintained by matching appropriate amounts of ventilation with perfusion. Fig. 12-15 illustrates the partial pressure of O_2 and CO_2 in mixed venous blood entering an average alveolar unit, the capillary blood values, alveolar gas values, and arterial blood values that are leaving the unit. Normally, the O_2 pressure gradient across the membrane is 62 mm Hg (102 − 40) and the CO_2 gradient is 6 mm Hg (46 − 40). O_2 has a ΔP that is 10 times that of the CO_2 gradient. These values of ΔP for O_2 and CO_2 are a function of the distribution of alveolar ventilation, the distribution of blood flow, and the velocity of chemical reactions (e.g., the release or binding rate of O_2 and hemoglobin). Both CO_2 and O_2 are carried as dissolved gases in the plasma and in chemical combination. O_2 combines with hemoglobin to form **oxyhemoglobin,** and CO_2 combines with hemoglobin to form **carbamino compound** and with H_2O to form HCO_3^-. The rate of these reactions influences the partial pressures of the gases and ultimately the rate of diffusion.

Barriers to Diffusion

The barriers to diffusion in the lungs for O_2 and CO_2 include the surfactant layer of the alveoli, the alveolar epithelial cell and it's basement membrane, the connective tissue of the interstitial space, the capillary endothelium and it's basement membrane, the plasma of the pulmonary capillary, the erythrocyte membrane, and the intracellular fluid of the erythrocyte (Fig. 12-16). The thickness or distance for diffusion in the lung probably averages approximately 0.5 to 1.0 μ (range is 0.3 to 2.5 μ). Changes in viscosity and chemical or cellular composition of the tissue barriers can also influence diffusion rates.

DIFFUSION- AND PERFUSION-LIMITED GASES

The actual amount of gas that crosses the alveolar-capillary membrane is influenced by the factors mentioned in Fick's Law, but it also depends on whether a gas is a **diffusion-limited gas** or a **perfusion-limited gas.**

Perfusion-Limited Gas

A perfusion-limited gas can diffuse across the membrane rather easily as long as it is carried away by an ample flow of blood. The anesthetic gas nitrous oxide (NO) is a good example of a perfusion-limited gas. It can easily diffuse across the membrane and into blood where it's partial pressure climbs to that of alveolar pressure within about $\frac{1}{10}$ of a second. When the pressure in plasma climbs to a value that is equal to that of alveolar gas pressure, diffusion stops. For diffusion to continue, a fresh volume of blood needs to flow past the membrane. This new volume of blood has a partial pressure of zero, which enables NO to continue diffusing across the membrane. Because of this need for flow blood to support diffusion, NO is said to be a perfusion-limited gas.

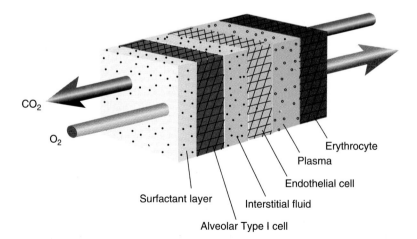

FIG. 12-16 Pathway for diffusion constitutes a barrier that is 0.3 to 2.5 μ thick. It, however, presents little challenge to oxygen *(O₂)* and carbon dioxide *(CO₂)* as they transit through the barriers in about 0.25 second.

O_2 normally acts like a perfusion-limited gas. As the pulmonary capillaries bring blood to the lungs, the partial pressure of O_2 in the pulmonary capillaries is 40 mm Hg ($P_cO_2 = 40$). Blood is in contact with the alveolar surface area for approximately 0.75 second (see Fig. 12-14). In one third of this time, or 0.25 second, O_2 diffuses into the blood from the alveoli, and the partial pressure in the capillary blood ($P_cO_2 = 100$ mm Hg) equals the driving pressure in the lung ($P_AO_2 = 100$ mm Hg), thus the concentration gradient becomes zero ($\Delta P = 0$). Although the blood still has 0.5 second of contact or reserve time with the alveoli, no more oxygen diffuses. The amount of O_2 that can dif-fuse into the blood is not normally limited by its ability to diffuse but by its dependence on the flow of blood past the alveoli; thus the diffusion of O_2 is said to be perfusion limited. In cases where the alveolar-capillary membrane is thickened or in other conditions where O_2 does not equilibrate across the membrane (e.g., when $P_cO_2 < P_AO_2$), O_2 becomes a diffusion-limited gas. CO_2, normally a perfusion-limited gas as well, may under some situations behave as a diffusion-limited gas. It moves across the alveolar-capillary membrane and equilibrates in about 0.25 second (Fig. 12-17). This is about the same amount of time that is required for O_2 to equilibrate.

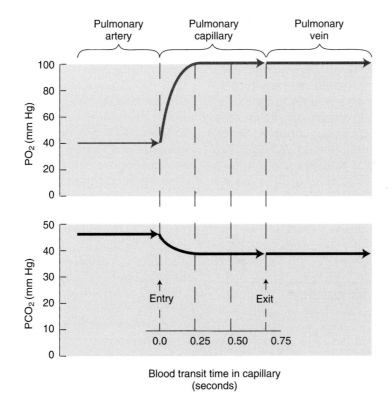

FIG. 12-17 Equilibrium time for the respiratory gases as blood passes through the alveolar capillary at rest. Blood normally spends 0.75 second in contact with the alveolar regions. In one third of that time, or 0.25 second, oxygen (O_2) and carbon dioxide (CO_2) have equilibrated across the membrane. Although CO_2 diffuses 19 times faster than O_2, the chemical reactions that CO_2 must undergo to leave the plasma "slow down" the equilibrium time for CO_2.

Diffusion-Limited Gases

A diffusion-limited gas may move through the alveolar-capillary membrane more slowly, but it is not sensitive to the need for blood flow to maintain a pressure gradient. The gas does not build up a back pressure on the downstream side of the membrane, so there continues to be a concentration gradient that is greater than zero. Carbon monoxide (CO) is such a gas. When low concentrations of CO are inhaled into the lungs, the CO in the alveolar areas continues to diffuse into the blood stream. The reason for this is that CO has an affinity or attraction for hemoglobin that is approximately 240 times the affinity that O_2 has for hemoglobin. This means that as CO crosses the membrane, it immediately attaches to hemoglobin. This effectively removes it from the dissolved state in the plasma. Once gas molecules are chemically combined with hemoglobin, they no longer exert a partial pressure in the plasma. During the time blood is in contact with the alveoli, CO continually diffuses into the blood. CO is said to be a diffusion-limited gas because the amount of CO that will crosses the alveolar-capillary membrane is determined by its ability to diffuse and not by the perfusion rate of the blood. Because of this property, CO is an excellent gas to use for diffusion tests in the pulmonary function laboratory.

⬤ MEASURING THE DIFFUSION CAPACITY OF THE LUNGS

Diffusion capacity of the lungs is an important test to determine lung health.

Carbon Monoxide Diffusion Tests

Although there are several methods used to test the diffusion capacity of the lungs, only the single-breath diffusion capacity test is discussed here. The single-breath carbon monox-

ide diffusion test of the lung ($DL_{CO}SB$) is a short procedure. The patient is asked to exhale to RV, then to inhale a special gas mixture (0.3% CO, 10% helium [He], 21% O_2, and the balance is N_2) until the lungs are filled, hold the breath for 10 seconds, then exhale at a moderate speed until told to stop. The pulmonary function machine analyzes the gas inhaled and exhaled (alveolar gas) and compares them by calculating the $DL_{CO}SB$ with the following formula:

$$DL_{CO}SB = VI_{STPD} \times \frac{He_I}{He_E} \times \frac{60}{T \times EBP} \times$$
$$Ln \times \frac{CO_I}{CO_E} \times \frac{He_E}{He_I}$$

where VI_{STPD} is the inspired VC (corrected to standard temperature and pressure that contains no water vapor), He_I is the inhaled He concentration, He_E is the exhaled He concentration, T is the actual breath hold time of the test and should be approximately 10 seconds, EBP is the effective barometric pressure, and CO_I and CO_E are the inhaled and exhaled percents of CO measured, respectively. It is recommended that the VC be at least 90% of the patient's best VC to increase accuracy. When the test gas is inhaled, then exhaled, the CO is reduced in concentration for two reasons. The inhaled CO concentration is diluted by the RV, which has no CO in it, and the CO diffuses into blood. Helium is included in the test gas mixture to determine the lung volume during the test and to determine the amount of dilution the CO experiences when the test gas is mixed with the RV. Basically, the $DL_{CO}SB$ test process determines the amount of CO that diffuses into the pulmonary circulation.

The normal $DL_{CO}SB$ for the typical adult is about 25 ml/min/mm Hg. This value varies with age, height (lung volume), and gender. Tall young males have the highest values.

CO is a good gas to use for this test for several reasons.

1. Normally there is little CO in the blood or lungs to interfere with the test. Normal metabolism and red cell destruction result in low levels of **carboxyhemoglobin (COHb)** in the blood, which can be ignored. The increased levels of COHb caused by smoking should be corrected for.
2. The affinity of CO for hemoglobin is 240 times the affinity of O_2 for hemoglobin.
3. Since the test lasts for only 10 seconds and a low concentration of CO is used (0.3%), CO behaves as a rather pure diffusion-limited gas.
4. CO has a diffusion rate similar to O_2 but actually is a little slower. The solubility coefficient for CO is 0.0023 ml/100 ml of plasma at 1 mm Hg and 37° C. Its molecular weight is 28, so its diffusion coefficient is $0.0023 \div \sqrt{28}$, or 0.000435. Comparing O_2's diffusion coefficient to that of CO (0.00053/0.000435) illustrates that O_2 diffuses 1.22 times faster than CO.

 ## CLINICAL FACTORS THAT AFFECT DIFFUSION RATES

The diffusion capacity of the lungs can change for a variety of reasons. Conditions that reduce the $DL_{CO}SB$ include anemia (less hemoglobin sites for CO attachment allow the partial pressure of CO in plasma to increase), reduced lung volume (causes a reduced surface area, pneumonectomy, pneumonia, and atelectasis), restrictive lung disease (causes decreased lung volume and thickening of membrane), loss of alveolar-capillary membrane surface area without loss of lung volume (emphysema), poor distribution of ventilation ($\dot{V}/\dot{Q}$ mismatching), increased dead space ventilation (pulmonary embolus), thickened alveolar-capillary membrane (interstitial lung disease), and highly increased P_aO_2 (O_2 competes with CO for hemoglobin-binding sites).

Causes of increased $DL_{CO}SB$ include increased pulmonary capillary blood volume (more hemoglobin-binding sites), polycythemia, supine position (better $\dot{V}/\dot{Q}$ matching), and exercise (increased surface area and improved $\dot{V}/\dot{Q}$ matching when recruitment and distention of the pulmonary capillaries occur).

Because many factors are responsible for decreasing $DL_{CO}SB$, it is desirable to try to differentiate between the causes of decreased diffusion. One such technique corrects the diffusion rate for the lung volume (D_L/V_A). Calculation of the D_L/V_A helps differentiate between the loss of lung volume, that is, loss of functional lung units and other reasons for a decreased $DL_{CO}SB$. If $DL_{CO}SB$ is decreased because of the loss of functional lung units *only*, the D_L/V_A will be normal, that is, the same as predicted. Examples include lung resection and some restrictive defects without increased thickness of the alveolar-capillary membrane. If the $DL_{CO}SB$ is decreased because of factors other than just loss of functional lung units, the D_L/V_A will be decreased, that is, lower than predicted. Examples include emphysema, pulmonary embolus, $\dot{V}/\dot{Q}$ mismatch, pulmonary fibrosis, and other interstitial lung diseases. A decreased $DL_{CO}SB$ may actually be the earliest sign of development of an interstitial lung process.

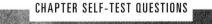

CHAPTER SELF-TEST QUESTIONS

1. Given the following information, determine the P_AO_2:
   $P_B = 747$ mm Hg
   $FIO_2 = 40\%$
   $P_ACO_2 = 60$ mm Hg
   $R = 0.8$.
   a. 185 mm Hg
   b. 195 mm Hg
   c. 205 mm Hg
   d. 225 mm Hg

2. The respiratory exchange ratio is equal to

a. $$\frac{\text{Oxygen consumed}}{\text{Carbon dioxide produced in the lung}}$$

b. $$\frac{\text{Carbon dioxide produced}}{\text{Oxygen consumed in the lung}}$$

c. $$\frac{\text{Oxygen consumed}}{\text{Carbon dioxide produced at the tissues}}$$

d. $$\frac{\text{Carbon dioxide produced}}{\text{Oxygen consumed at the tissues}}$$

3. P_AO_2 increases when
   1. barometric pressure increases
   2. P_ACO_2 decreases
   3. FIO_2 increases
      a. 3 only
      b. 1 and 2
      c. 2 and 3
      d. 1 and 3
      e. 1, 2, and 3

4. Which of the following hormone or humoral substances causes dilation of the pulmonary vasculature?
   a. nitric oxide
   b. bradykinin
   c. prostaglandin E
   d. all of the above

5. A lung region with a $\dot{V}/\dot{Q}$ ratio of 3 indicates that:
   a. there is proportionally more ventilation than perfusion present
   b. the ratio is abnormally low
   c. hypoxemia will result
   d. hypoventilation is occurring in the region

6. A $\dot{V}/\dot{Q}$ ratio of 0 indicates which of the following?
   a. anatomical dead space
   b. alveolar dead space
   c. a diffusion defect in the alveolar-capillary membrane
   d. a true shunt

7. The most common cause of hypoxemia is:
   a. increased dead space ventilation
   b. hypoventilation
   c. a $\dot{V}/\dot{Q}$ mismatch
   d. extrapulmonary shunting

8. Which of the following is *not* an example of a true shunt?
   a. thebesian vein blood flow
   b. a pulmonary embolus
   c. atelectasis
   d. pulmonary edema and alveolar flooding

9. Gas diffusion through the alveolar-capillary membrane increases when the
   1. surface area increases
   2. thickness of the membrane increases
   3. pressure gradient increases
      a. 1 only
      b. 1 and 2
      c. 2 and 3
      d. 1 and 3
      e. 1, 2, and 3

10. What is the A-a oxygen gradient in a 64-year-old patient who has a gas exchange impairment with the following information:
    $P_B = 760 \text{ mm Hg}$
    $FIO_2 = 80\%$
    $P_ACO_2 = 35 \text{ mm Hg}$
    $R = 1.0$
    a. 535 mm Hg
    b. 550 mm Hg
    c. 565 mm Hg
    d. 600 mm Hg

For answers, see p. 475.

BIBLIOGRAPHY

1. Comroe JH: *Physiology of respiration,* ed 2, Chicago, 1974, Year Book Medical.
2. Green JF: *Fundamental cardiovascular and pulmonary physiology,* ed 2, Philadelphia, 1987, Lea & Febiger.
3. Jones NL: *Blood gases and acid-base physiology,* ed 2, New York, 1987, Thieme-Stratton.
4. Leff AR, Schumacker PT: *Respiratory physiology: basics and applications,* Philadelphia, 1993, WB Saunders.
5. Levitsky MG: *Pulmonary physiology,* ed 3, New York, 1991, McGraw-Hill.
6. Levitzky GL, Hall SM, McDonough KH: *Cardiopulmonary physiology in anesthesiology,* New York, 1997, McGraw Hill.
7. Martini FH: *Fundamentals of anatomy and physiology,* Upper Saddle River, NJ, 1998, Prentice Hall.

8. Miller WF, Scacci R, Gast LR: *Laboratory evaluation of pulmonary function,* Philadelphia, 1987, JB Lippincott.
9. Murray JF: *The normal lung,* ed 2, Philadelphia, 1986, WB Saunders.
10. Pierson DJ, Kacmarek RM, eds: *Foundations of respiratory care,* New York, 1992, Churchill Livingstone.
11. Ruppel G: *Manual of pulmonary function testing,* ed 6, St Louis, 1994, Mosby.
12. Staub NC: *Basic respiratory physiology,* New York, 1991, Churchill Livingstone.
13. West JB: *Ventilation/blood flow and gas exchange,* ed 3, Baltimore, 1977, Williams & Wilkins.

CHAPTER 13

Respiratory Gas Transport

Upon completing this chapter, you will be able to:

1 List the two forms in which oxygen is carried in the blood.
2 Explain the importance of dissolved oxygen.
3 Describe the composition and basic structure of the hemoglobin molecule.
4 Describe the binding sites of oxygen and carbon dioxide on the hemoglobin.
5 Calculate oxygen capacity and total oxygen content.
6 Explain the relationship between the partial pressure of oxygen and oxyhemoglobin saturation through the use of the oxyhemoglobin dissociation curve.
7 Describe what a left and right shift of the oxyhemoglobin dissociation curve means with regard to oxyhemoglobin affinity and the P_{50}.
8 List the factors that cause increased and decreased oxyhemoglobin affinity.
9 Describe how oxygen affinities for fetal hemoglobin, methemoglobin, and carboxyhemoglobin compare with the normal adult form of hemoglobin.
10 Explain the difference between functional and fractional oxyhemoglobin saturation.
11 Describe how oxyhemoglobin saturation is measured.
12 List the normal values and describe the calculation of mixed venous and arterial oxygen content.
13 Calculate oxygen transport, consumption, and the extraction ratio.
14 List normal values for oxygen transport, consumption, and extraction.
15 List several factors that affect the amount of oxygen transported and returned to the heart.
16 List the three forms of carbon dioxide transport.
17 Calculate carbon dioxide content in blood.
18 Describe the carbon dioxide dissociation curve and how it compares to the oxyhemoglobin dissociation curve.
19 List the factors that influence carbon dioxide content in blood.
20 Define the Bohr and Haldane effects.

The storage, transport, and release of oxygen (O_2) and carbon dioxide (CO_2) by blood is a critical link between gas exchange in the lungs and tissues. Blood, a remarkable fluid that has evolved to carry out this task, provides an inner "stream" of O_2 that flows to the tissues and a second "stream" of CO_2 that flows from the tissues to the lungs. This chapter brings into focus the abilities blood has as a vehicle for the respiratory gases.

⬤ OXYGEN STORAGE AND TRANSPORT IN BLOOD

O_2 is transported in blood in two different forms: it is dissolved in plasma and it is bound to specific sites on the hemoglobin (Hb) molecule (Fig. 13-1).

Dissolved Oxygen

The amount of O_2 that is able to dissolve in blood is actually a minor amount when compared with the total that is transported. Yet it is the dissolved amount that has a partial pressure that supports the diffusion of O_2 onto Hb-binding sites and into the tissues. According to Henry's law, the volume of gas (V_{gas}) that dissolves in a liquid is proportional to its solubility coefficient (C_s) and the partial pressure of that gas (P_{gas}) over the liquid:

$$V_{gas} = C_s \times P_{gas}$$

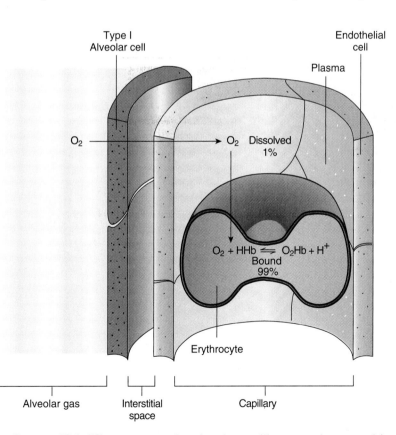

FIG. 13-1 Oxygen (O_2) diffuses across the alveolar-capillary membrane and is carried in blood in the dissolved state and bound to hemoglobin (Hb). About 1% to 2% of the total O_2 is dissolved, and 98% to 99% is bound to Hb.

As discussed in Chapter 12, the solubility coefficient for O_2 is 0.003 ml/100 ml or dl of blood. If the partial pressure of O_2 (PO_2) is 40 mm Hg, the amount of O_2 dissolved in every 100 ml of blood is 0.003×40 or 0.12 ml. This is the normal amount dissolved in systemic venous blood. If the PO_2 is 100 mm Hg, the amount of O_2 dissolved in every 100 ml of blood is 0.003×100 or 0.3 ml/dl or 3 ml/L. This is the normal amount dissolved in systemic arterial blood. If the PO_2 is 600 mm Hg, the amount of O_2 dissolved in every 100 ml of blood is 0.003×600 or 1.8 ml. This can occur in systemic arterial blood when normal lungs breathe 100% O_2. This dissolved O_2 however, makes up only 1% to 2% of total O_2 content.

If the amount of O_2 dissolved in blood was solely relied upon, the cardiac output would have to be much higher to support the O_2 needs of the tissues. With a normal O_2 consumption ($\dot{V}O_2$) of 250 ml/min and an O_2 content that is dissolved ($C_{dissolved}O_2$) of 3 ml/L, the amount of blood flow ($\dot{Q}_T$) that is necessary can be calculated with a modified form of the Fick equation that was described in Chapter 6:

$$\dot{Q}_T = \frac{\dot{V}O_2}{C_{dissolved}O_2}$$
$$= \frac{250 \text{ ml/min}}{3 \text{ ml/L}}$$
$$= 83.3 \text{ L/min}$$

This means that the heart must pump the impossible amount of 83.3 L/min to just support metabolism at rest when using just the dissolved amount of O_2.

Oxygen Bound to Hemoglobin

The need to improve the ability of blood to carry O_2 in support of metabolism leads to the evolution of the O_2-carrying molecule, Hb (Fig. 13-2). This second form of O_2 carriage in

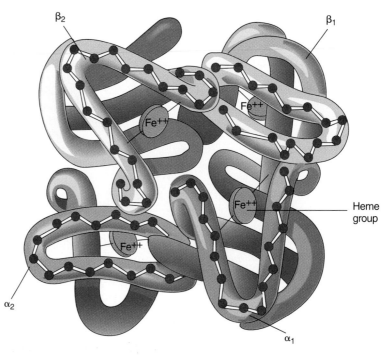

FIG. 13-2 Hemoglobin molecule is a moderately large pigmented globular protein. It is pigmented with four ferrous iron ions.

blood is characterized as a reversible chemical combination with reduced or deoxygenated Hb (Hb in this state normally has a hydrogen ion [H$^+$] bound to it, HHb) to form oxyhemoglobin (O$_2$Hb):

$$O_2 + HHb \rightleftharpoons O_2Hb + H^+$$

Hb is a globular protein molecule (see Fig. 13-2). The **globin** portion is comprised of four polypeptide (amino acid) chains (Fig. 13-3). The adult form of Hb (HbA) is formed from two α and two β polypeptides. The α chains are formed from 141 amino acids and the β chains from 146. The molecular weight of Hb is 66,500 g/mol. Each of these chains has a **heme** portion formed by a **porphyrin ring** containing an iron ion in the ferrous state (Fe^{++}). The Fe^{++} is the reversible binding site for one molecule of O$_2$ (Fig. 13-4), which means that one Hb molecule is able to combine with up to four O$_2$ molecules with the potential of being 100%, 75%, 50%, 25%, or 0% saturated with O$_2$ (S$_{blood}$O$_2$). As the Fe^{++} binding sites combine with O$_2$, Fe^{++}O$_2$ is formed and turns blood red. As the O$_2$ is released, the Fe^{++} returns to a purplish-blue.

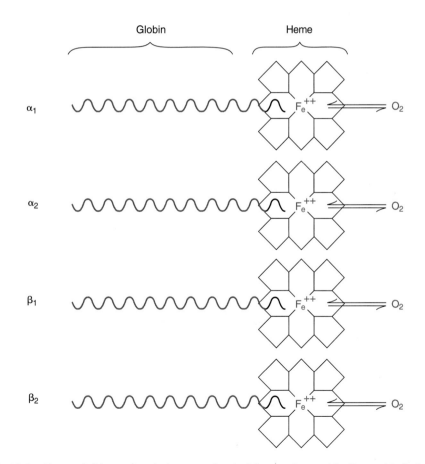

FIG. 13-3 Hemoglobin molecule is comprised of four polypeptide (2α and 2β) chains in the adult form. Each chain is attached to a porphyrin ring containing an iron ion in the ferrous state (Fe^{++}). *O$_2$*, Oxygen.

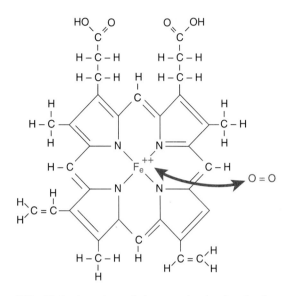

FIG. 13-4 Iron ion of the porphyrin ring is the loose binding site of oxygen.

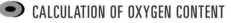

Table 13-1 Oxygen Saturation (S_aO_2) of Hemoglobin and Oxygen Content (C_aO_2) in Blood at Different Arterial Partial Pressure of Oxygen (P_aO_2) Values*

P_aO_2 (mm Hg)	S_aO_2 (%)	C_aO_2 (ml of O_2/dl Blood)
40	74.9	15.18
60	90.6	18.39
100	97.7	19.94
130	99.0	20.29
150	99.3	20.41

*Assumes a hemoglobin content of 15 g/dl, oxygen-binding constant of 1.34 ml/dl, blood pH of 7.40, and blood temperature of 37° C.

CALCULATION OF OXYGEN CONTENT

Amount Bound to Hemoglobin

The hemoglobin content in blood is commonly expressed in grams per 100 milliliters or deciliters of blood or as a gram percent. The normal concentration is 15 g/dl. Each gram of Hb is capable of carrying 1.34 ml of O_2 when 100% saturated. This is known as the **oxygen capacity** of Hb. The following relationship is used to determine the **O_2 content ($C_{blood}O_2$)** carried on the Hb molecule when the concentration of Hb is 15 g/100 ml of blood when it is saturated ($S_{blood}O_2$ = 100%):

$$C_{blood}O_2 = [Hb] \times 1.34 \times S_{blood}O_2$$

The following examples will help demonstrate this relationship:

arterial blood:

$$Hb = 15 \text{ g/100ml}$$
$$S_aO_2 = 98\% \text{ (normal arterial blood)}$$
$$15 \times 1.34 \times 0.98 = 19.7 \text{ ml of } O_2 \text{ per 100 ml}$$

venous blood:

$$Hb = 15 \text{ g/100 ml}$$
$$S_{\bar{v}}O_2 = 75\% \text{ (normal venous blood)}$$
$$15 \times 1.34 \times 0.75 = 15.08 \text{ ml of } O_2 \text{ per 100 ml}$$

hypoxia:

$$Hb = 10 \text{ g/100ml}$$
$$S_aO_2 = 90\% \text{ (anemic patient with lung disease)}$$
$$10 \times 1.34 \times 0.9 = 12.06 \text{ ml of } O_2 \text{ per 100 ml}$$

Because of the nature in which O_2 binds with Hb, Hb molecules are normally 100% saturated. A 90% Hb saturation indicates that 90% of Hb molecules are 100% saturated with O_2 and the other 10% of the Hb molecule binding sites have less O_2 attached.

Total Oxygen Content

Total O_2 content is calculated by adding the dissolved O_2 content and the O_2 content of hemoglobin. The following relationship is used:

$$\text{Total content} = \text{Dissolved} + \text{Bound}$$
$$C_{blood}O_2 = (0.003 \times PO_2) + (Hb \times 1.34 \times SO_2)$$

The following example determines the O_2 content in a normal arterial blood sample where the P_aO_2 = 100 mm Hg, Hb = 15 g/100ml, and S_aO_2 = 97%:

$$C_aO_2 = (0.003 \times 100) + (15 \times 1.34 \times 0.97)$$
$$= 0.3 \text{ ml/100 ml} + 19.5 \text{ ml/100 ml}$$
$$= 19.8 \text{ ml of } O_2 \text{ per 100 ml (or dl) of blood}$$

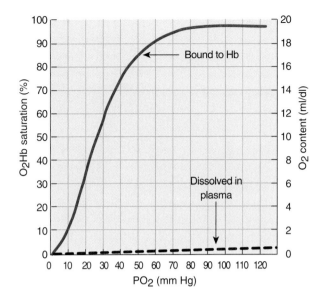

FIG. 13-5 Oxyhemoglobin (O_2Hb) dissociation curve. The solid line shows the relationship between PO_2 and O_2Hb saturation. The dotted line shows that oxygen O_2 content is dissolved in the plasma for a given PO_2. These curves are for normal arterial blood conditions (T = 37° C, pH = 7.40, PCO_2 = 40 mm Hg).

This indicates that there is 19.8 ml of O_2 in every 100 ml of blood that leaves the lungs and is pumped by the heart to the body's tissues. Table 13-1 shows the relationship between PO_2, S_aO_2, and C_aO_2 in normal blood for a variety of different levels of O_2 loading. The normal range for total C_aO_2 is 18 to 21 ml of O_2 per deciliter.

RELATIONSHIP BETWEEN THE PARTIAL PRESSURE OF OXYGEN AND OXYHEMOGLOBIN SATURATION

As described in the previous discussion, 98% to 99% of the O_2 contained in the blood is carried on the Hb molecules whereas the remaining 1% to 2% is dissolved in plasma. This does not mean, however, that the dissolved O_2 is not important. The plasma PO_2 provides the means by which O_2 is able to diffuse into the erythrocyte and attach to the Hb molecule. If O_2 could not dissolve in the plasma, how would O_2 get to the hemoglobin binding sites? Although little O_2 is contained in the dis-

solved form, it is the PO_2 of the dissolved form that is responsible for how well Hb becomes saturated with O_2. As O_2 passes from the alveoli into the dissolved form in the plasma, the PO_2 of the plasma increases. As the PO_2 increases in the plasma and cytoplasm of the erythrocyte, O_2 is "pushed" into the hemoglobin. All of the O_2 that is eventually attached to the Hb is initially in the dissolved form. The amount of O_2 that is available to attach to Hb is determined by the PO_2.

The process of unloading O_2 from O_2Hb is the reverse of the above process. Dissolved O_2 is the first to leave blood as O_2 diffuses into the tissues. With the diffusion of O_2 into the tissues, the blood PO_2 drops, which causes the O_2Hb to unload its O_2 into the plasma.

Oxyhemoglobin Dissociation Curve

The relationship between PO_2 and the saturation of Hb with O_2 is graphically expressed in the form of the **oxyhemoglobin dissociation curve** shown in Fig. 13-5. This relationship is

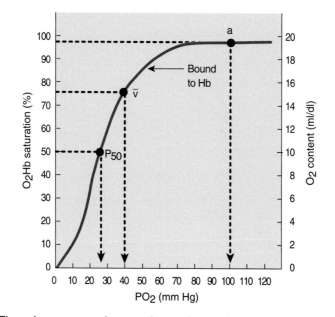

FIG. 13-6 Three important points on the oxyhemoglobin (O_2Hb) dissociation curve. Normal arterial PO_2 of 100 mm Hg results in a saturation of 97% to 98%, a normal mixed venous PO_2 of 40 mm Hg generates a saturation of 75%, and the P_{50} point normally occurs when the PO_2 of 26.5 generates a saturation of 50%.

curvilinear, which gives Hb several physiological advantages in the loading and unloading of O_2. Below a PO_2 of 60 mm Hg, the curve is "steep" and becomes "flat" at PO_2 levels greater than 90 mm Hg. On the steep portion of the curve, a small change in P_aO_2 results in a large change in saturation. This enhances the unloading and loading of O_2. On the flat portion of the curve, a large change in P_aO_2 results in a small change in saturation.

Several important points can be located on the curve (Fig. 13-6). Along the steepest portion of the curve, there is a point where the O_2Hb saturation is 50%. The normal PO_2 that is necessary to reach this saturation is 26.5 mm Hg. This point is known as the **P_{50}.** It is a useful point for the study of O_2Hb affinity. Any changes in affinity result in either a higher or lower P_{50}. Further up the steeper portion of the curve the mixed venous satura-

Table 13-2 Relationship Between Partial Pressure of Oxygen (PO_2) and Oxyhemoglobin Saturation ($S_{blood}O_2$)*

PO_2 (mm Hg)	$S_{blood}O_2$ (%)
26.5	50.0
40	74.9
50	85.0
60	90.6
70	93.8
80	95.7
90	96.9
100	97.7
130	99.0
150	99.3
500	99.9

*Assumes a pH of 7.40, PCO_2 of 40 mm Hg, temperature of 37° C, and normal adult hemoglobin.

A full-term newborn boy was delivered following uneventful labor and delivery. After the initial steps in supporting him, he demonstrated persistent tachycardia, tachypnea, cyanosis (bluish coloration of the skin, nail beds, lips, and mucous membranes), and arterial oxyhemoglobin saturation of 78% despite supplemental oxygen (O_2) delivered to him.

Cyanosis is caused by the presence of large quantities of deoxygenated hemoglobin. When the hemoglobin molecule releases its O_2, it becomes bluish purple. Generally, cyanosis occurs when more than 5 g of deoxygenated hemoglobin is present per deciliter of blood. This is approximately 30% of the total hemoglobin content. Normally less than 3% to 4% of the arterial blood hemoglobin is deoxygenated. Cyanosis can also occur peripherally and centrally. Peripheral cyanosis is the condition in which the fingers and toes are cyanotic and the face, tongue, and trunk are not. This is caused by poor peripheral blood flow that results in greater O_2 removal by the tissues of the extremities. The oxyhemoglobin saturation

within the local blood drops and the deoxyhemoglobin levels climb. Central cyanosis is a more uniform dispersal of greater quantities of deoxyhemoglobin within the arterial blood. This is caused by intrapulmonary or extrapulmonary shunting of blood away from regions of gas exchange in the lungs. This leads to greater quantities of deoxygenated blood entering the aorta.

Auscultation of the chest revealed clear breath sounds and a postsystolic cardiac murmur. A chest x-ray showed well-inflated lungs and an enlarged heart. An echocardiogram showed transposition of the great vessels (aorta attached to the right ventricle and the pulmonary artery arising from the left ventricle). This type of congenital heart defect results in cyanosis caused by poor flow of blood from one circuit to the other. The resulting type of extrapulmonary shunting causes poor gas exchange and hypoxia that does not respond to O_2 therapy. This infant was eventually taken to surgery to switch the position of the vessels to improve gas exchange.

---

tion ($S_{\bar{v}}O_2$) point can be found where a PO_2 of 40 mm Hg produces a saturation of 75%. By having the $S_{\bar{v}}O_2$ located on the steeper portion of the curve, the Hb molecule is better able to unload O_2 down to a saturation of 75% as it passes the tissues and O_2 diffuses from the blood. This enhances the diffusion of larger quantities of O_2 into the tissues. At the "shoulder" of the curve is the point where 90% saturation occurs when the PO_2 is 60 mm Hg. This is an important minimum saturation point that is used in clinical practice to guide the use of supplemental O_2 therapy. The arterial saturation (S_aO_2) point lies up on the flatter portion of the curve where a PO_2 of 100 mm Hg pro-

duces a saturation of 97%. At this point the Hb-binding sites are almost completely saturated. This indicates that the Hb loading properties have been adjusted so that the molecule is completely loaded at a normal alveolar PO_2 of about 100 mm Hg. These and several others are further summarized in Table 13-2.

SIGNIFICANCE OF AN OXYHEMOGLOBIN DISSOCIATION CURVE SHIFT

Although there is a normal relationship between PO_2 and SO_2, this relationship can be influenced by several factors. These factors are responsible for the shifting of the curve. When shifting occurs, a change in the O_2-Hb relationship occurs, which can be visualized by analyzing the O_2Hb curve for a shift in its position.

Right and Left Shifting of the Dissociation Curve

The O_2Hb dissociation curve can be shifted to the right or shifted to the left (Fig. 13-7). A right shift indicates that for any given PO_2, the SO_2 is lower than expected. The P_{50} is greater than its normal value of 26.5 mm Hg. A PO_2 of 60 mm Hg, which normally yields an SO_2 of

90%, now generates an SO_2 of less than 90%. The more the curve shifts to the right, the lower the saturation is. A shift to the right results in decreased loading of O_2 on the Hb in the lungs, lower saturation, and decreased O_2 content. On the other hand, a right shift improves unloading of O_2 at the tissues. A right shift generally indicates a decreased affinity of O_2 for Hb.

A left shift indicates that, for any given PO_2, the SO_2 is higher than expected. The P_{50} is lower than its normal value of 26.5 mm Hg in this situation. A PO_2 of 60 mm Hg, which normally yields an SO_2 of 90%, now generates an SO_2 of greater than 90%. The more the curve

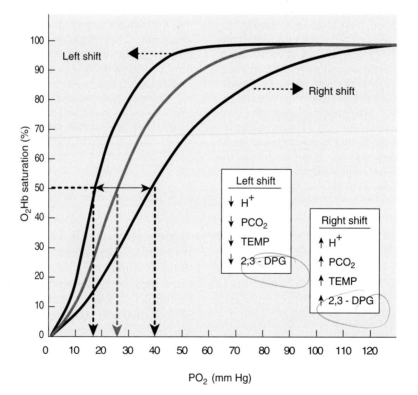

FIG. 13-7 Shifts of the oxyhemoglobin (O_2Hb) dissociation curve. The dissociation curve can be shifted away from its normal PO_2-SO_2 relationship by several factors. Notice that as the curve shifts to the right the P_{50} increases and shifts to the left, resulting in a decreased P_{50}. Although P_{50} is often used to document that the curve is shifted, changes in other PO_2-SO_2 relationships can also reveal shifts in the curve and changes in affinity.

shifts to the left, the higher the saturation. A left shift results in increased loading of O_2 on the Hb molecule at the lungs, higher saturation, and increased O_2 content, but unloading of O_2 at the tissues may be impaired. A left shift generally indicates that the affinity of O_2 for hemoglobin is increased.

Factors that Change Affinity and Shift the Curve

The O_2Hb dissociation curve is shifted and thus the affinity is altered by a variety of different factors (Box 13-1).

Effects of [H+], Temperature, and Partial Pressure of Carbon Dioxide

Changes in blood pH cause the curve to shift. A decrease in blood pH (an increase in [H+], or acidemia) causes greater hydrogen bonding within the Hb molecule. This results in a "tighter" molecular structure, which, in turn, reduces the ability to load the binding sites for a given PO_2. This causes the dissociation curve to shift to the right, indicating reduced O_2Hb affinity. Increasing blood pH (a decrease in [H+], or alkalemia) causes the molecule to "open" as the result of less hydrogen bonding, which results in a left shift of the dissociation curve and increased affinity.

Temperature changes also cause the Hb molecule to change shape and shift the dissociation curve. Increased temperature results in reduced affinity, and reduced temperature causes increased affinity.

Increased and decreased PCO_2 affects the O_2Hb affinity. As the PCO_2 in blood increases, greater amounts of CO_2 can chemically react with the amino acids of the Hb molecule. The chemical combination of CO_2 and Hb produces **carbamino compound,** also known as *carbaminohemoglobin.* This reaction also alters the structure of Hb and its affinity for O_2. Increased PCO_2 causes decreased affinity, and reduced PCO_2 causes increased affinity. This influence is known as the **Bohr effect.**

The effects of [H+], temperature, and PCO_2 on O_2Hb affinity occur as blood moves from the lung to the tissues and back. At some tissues the temperature is a little higher, PCO_2 increases as CO_2 diffuses into blood, and acids are added to the blood by the tissues. The combined effect of these changes brings about a moderate rightward shift in the dissociation curve and reduced affinity. This enhances the off-loading of O_2 from Hb to plasma and on to the tissues. The reverse occurs in the lungs as the temperature drops a small amount, PCO_2 declines as CO_2 diffuses into alveolar gas, and the pH increases as carbonic acid is converted into CO_2 and H_2O and the CO_2 is excreted. These effects improve the ability to load O_2 onto Hb by causing the curve to shift toward the left as the affinity for O_2 improves.

Effects of 2,3-Diphosphoglyceric Acid

All erythrocytes synthesize **2,3-diphosphoglyceric acid (2,3-DPG).** It is an end product

---

BOX 13-1

Factors that Alter Oxyhemoglobin Affinity

Causes of increased affinity that shift the dissociation curve to the right
Acidemia (increased [H+])
Hyperthermia
Increased carbaminohemoglobin (higher PCO_2, Bohr effect)
Decreased 2,3-diphosphoglycerate levels
Oxidation of Fe^{++} to Fe^{+++} (methemoglobinemia)
Increased carboxyhemoglobin
Hemoglobin variants: fetal Hb, Seattle, Kansas, sickle cell, Sulfhemoglobinemia

Causes of increased affinity that shift the dissociation curve to the left
Alkalemia (decreased [H+])
Hypothermia
Decreased carbaminohemoglobin (lower P_aCO_2, Bohr effect)
Increased 2,3-diphosphoglycerate levels
Hemoglobin variants: Chesapeake, Rainier, Hiroshima

of glucose metabolism. This organophosphate (as well as other intracellular phosphates such as phospholipids and adenosine triphosphate [ATP]) can bind to the Hb molecule and cause its structure to change and cause it to reduce affinity. By producing 2,3-DPG, the erythrocyte can decrease the affinity of Hb for O_2, which helps off-load O_2 to the tissues. Individuals who are chronically exposed to hypoxemia, such as those who frequently exercise, those who live at high altitudes, those with chronic anemia, and those who have chronic lung or heart disease, produce significantly greater amounts of 2,3-DPG. At first glance this appears to be counterintuitive. It would seem that this would reduce the ability to load O_2. Although this does occur to some degree,

the benefit lies in the improved ability of the Hb molecule to release greater quantities of O_2 into the tissues at reduced PO_2.

Several other conditions cause 2,3-DPG levels to decrease. Acidosis causes reduced 2,3-DPG synthesis. The combination of acidosis (that causes a decrease in O_2Hb affinity) and decreasing 2,3-DPG (that results in increasing affinity) tends to counteract each other. Storage of blood in acid-citrate and dextrose also causes reduced synthesis of 2,3-DPG. This could impair O_2 release into the tissues when large quantities (e.g., >15 units) of stored blood are transfused into a patient who is experiencing massive blood loss. The short-term and long-term effects of this, however, are unknown.

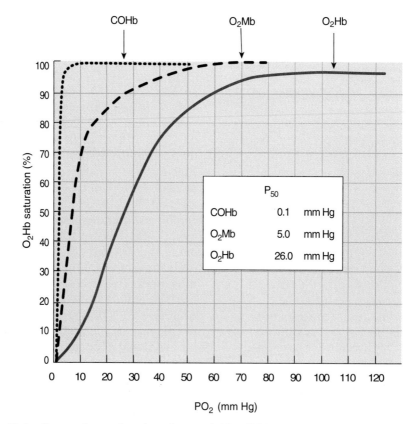

FIG. 13-8 Comparison of carboxyhemoglobin *(COHb)*, oxymyoglobin *(O_2Mb)*, and oxyhemoglobin *(O_2Hb)* dissociation curves. Note the high affinities of COHb and O_2Mb when compared with O_2Hb.

Variant Forms of Hemoglobin

Several variant forms of Hb also affect O_2Hb affinity. **Fetal hemoglobin (HbF),** the major Hb present in fetal life, is produced primarily in the liver and is chemically different in that it is comprised of two α chains and two γ chains. The γ chains have a slightly different amino acid sequence than the β chain. Its concentration decreases over the first few months of extrauterine life as the erythrocytes with the adult form (HbA) are produced in larger quantities by the bone marrow. HbF has a P_{50} of 19 to 20 mm Hg, indicating a leftward shift of its dissociation curve and improved affinity. This appears to be the result of the combined effects of a different polypeptide and reduced 2,3-DPG maintenance within the fetal erythrocyte. While in the placenta the greater affinity enhances the loading of O_2 into fetal blood, thus improving the O_2 content at the low PO_2 values in fetal blood.

Methemoglobin (Met-Hb) results when the normal ferrous state of iron (Fe^{++}) oxidizes to the ferric state (Fe^{+++}). In the ferric state, Hb has a high affinity to O_2. This means that O_2 binds to Hb but will not release until the PO_2 is low. This not only results in the O_2Hb curve being shifted to the left, but also limits the total amount of O_2 that can be released. A small amount of Met-Hb is produced normally, resulting in a normal concentration of less than 1% of the total amount of Hb. The amount of Met-Hb increases when the blood is exposed to strong oxidizing chemicals such as nitrites. This turns the blood rusty brown. For example, the vasodilator drug, nitroprusside, can cause increased Met-Hb production, limiting the amount of O_2 released into the tissues. The degree of limitation varies depending on the amount of Hb converted to Met-Hb. Methemoglobinemia can be changed back to the ferrous state by treatment with methylene blue.

Carboxyhemoglobin (COHb) results when Hb is exposed to carbon monoxide (CO), which has an affinity for Hb approximately 240 times that of O_2. This is shown in Fig. 13-8 where the COHb saturation curve is compared with O_2Hb and **oxymyoglobin (O_2Mb),** an intramuscular O_2 storage protein that has only one globin and heme complex. Thus CO is much more likely to fill or displace O_2 from binding sites on the Hb molecule when CO and O_2 are both present. Once CO attaches to Hb, it is difficult to remove and the amount of O_2 that can be carried by Hb is limited. In addition, any O_2 bound to Hb has a much greater affinity and will not release normally. Carboxyhemoglobin poisoning occurs when CO is inhaled. This condition presents a double problem of taking up the binding sites for O_2 and producing a functional form of anemia as well as limiting the release of bound O_2. Fig. 13-9 shows a normal O_2 content curve, the curve from a patient with anemia ([Hb] = 7.5 g/dl), and the curve of a patient who has

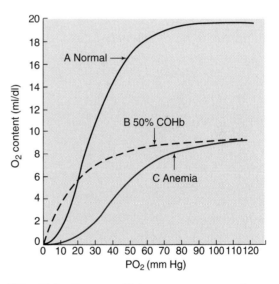

FIG. 13-9 Oxygen (O_2) content curves from three different conditions. *A,* Normal arterial blood with a normal Hb content. *B,* Arterial blood with 50% oxyhemoglobin and 50% carboxyhemoglobin *(COHb)* poisoning. The content curve of the blood with 50% COHb is not only carrying the same low content, but also it is shifted to the left, revealing that it has an abnormally high affinity that limits the ability to release O_2. *C,* Normal saturation of arterial blood with a low Hb content (7.5 g/dl).

50% of their Hb saturated with O_2 and 50% saturated with CO. Note how the O_2 content is reduced in the case of anemia and COHb poisoning and how the COHb curve is shifted to the left. This left-shifted curve signals a higher O_2Hb affinity and the reduced ability to release the bound O_2. These two effects of CO poisoning explain the profound result it has on O_2 transport to the tissues. CO not only affects the blood, but also crosses into the cells and incapacitates cytochrome enzymes within the mitochondria, resulting in reduced ability to produce ATP. CO also competes for binding sites on the myoglobin of skeletal and cardiac muscle cells and reduces the availability of O_2 within the cell.

CO poisoning is treatable. A patient with a 50% HbCO level would have half of his or her Hb filled with CO. If this patient were to breathe room air for approximately 4 hours, the COHb level would drop to 25% (Fig. 13-10). In another 4 hours the patient's COHb level would be 12.5%, etc. This illustrates that the half-life of COHb is 4 hours. That is, the COHb level is cut in half every 4 hours while breathing air. If this same patient breathes 100% O_2, the COHb level is cut in half in less than 2 hours. The increased PO_2 is better able to compete with the much more scarce but higher affinity CO, effectively "pushing" CO off the Hb. **Hyperbaric oxygen therapy (HBO),** another method for treating CO poisoning, decreases the half-life of COHb even more rapidly. Breathing 100% O_2 at 3 atm of pressure reduces the half-life to less than 30 minutes.

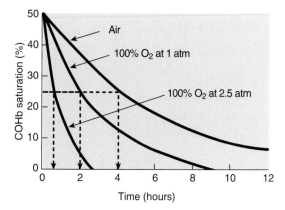

FIG. 13-10 Three situations of carbon monoxide clearance from hemoglobin. The time it takes for carboxyhemoglobin *(COHb)* level to drop to half the original value (its half-life) is illustrated by the dotted lines. The half-life for COHb is 4 hours when breathing room air, 2 hours when breathing 100% oxygen (O_2), and less than 30 minutes when treated with hyperbaric oxygen therapy.

◕ EXPRESSING OXYHEMOGLOBIN SATURATION

O_2Hb saturation readings can be determined in several ways. Two different ways are used to express the O_2 saturation of Hb. One method calculates the percent of freely available O_2 binding sites, or functional oxygen saturation, and the other determines the percentage of total sites, or fractional oxygen saturation.

Functional Versus Fractional Oxygen Saturation

Functional O_2 saturation (functional SO_2) is determined by dividing the amount of O_2Hb by the sum of the O_2Hb and deoxyhemoglobin (HHb) concentrations. No other Hb concentrations are considered in this calculation:

$$\text{Functional } SO_2 = \frac{O_2Hb}{O_2Hb + HHb}$$

Fractional O_2 saturation (fractional SO_2) is determined by dividing the amount of O_2Hb by the sum of all the different fractions of total Hb (THb) present:

$$\text{Fractional } SO_2 = \frac{O_2Hb}{THb}$$

where $THb = O_2Hb + HHb + COHb + Met-Hb +$ any other forms of hemoglobin.

Tables 13-3 and 13-4 help point out the difference between functional and fractional O_2Hb saturation.

In patient "A" the functional SO_2 and the fractional SO_2 are similar (2.2% difference) because the abnormal Hb concentrations are small. In patient "B" the functional SO_2 and the fractional SO_2 are different because the concentrations of abnormal Hb molecules are elevated. If only the functional SO_2 is evaluated, the

Table 13-3 Hemoglobin Saturation Case: Patient A

	Hemoglobin Levels	Fraction of Total Hemoglobin	Percent of Total Hemoglobin
Total hemoglobin	14.0 g	1.0	100.0
Oxyhemoglobin	13.44 g	0.96	96.0
Carboxyhemoglobin	0.14 g	0.01	1.0
Methemoglobin	0.14 g	0.01	1.0
Deoxygenated hemoglobin	0.28 g	0.02	2.0

$$\text{Functional } SO_2 = \frac{13.44}{13.4 + 0.28}$$
$$= \frac{13.44}{13.68}$$
$$= 98.2\%$$

$$\text{Fractional } SO_2 = \frac{13.44}{13.44 + 0.14 + 0.14 + 0.28}$$
$$= \frac{13.44}{14}$$
$$= 96\%$$

Table 13-4 Hemoglobin Saturation Case: Patient B

	Hemoglobin Levels	Fraction of Total Hemoglobin	Percent of Total Hemoglobin
Total hemoglobin	14.0 g	1.0	100.0
Oxyhemoglobin	11.48 g	0.82	82.0
Carboxyhemoglobin	1.4 g	0.1	10.0
Methemoglobin	0.7 g	0.05	5.0
Deoxygenated hemoglobin	0.42 g	0.03	3.0

$$\text{Functional } SO_2 = \frac{11.48}{11.48 + 0.3}$$
$$= \frac{11.48}{11.78}$$
$$= 97.5\%$$

$$\text{Fractional } SO_2 = \frac{11.48}{11.48 + 1.4 + 0.7 + 0.3}$$
$$= \frac{11.48}{14}$$
$$= 82\%$$

abnormal Hb molecules may be overlooked; the reported functional SO_2 appears to be normal when, in reality, the fractional SO_2 is low.

Measuring Oxyhemoglobin Saturation

The determination of O_2Hb saturation can be made through several different methods. One approach uses the following relationship:

$$O_2Hb\% = 100 \times \frac{Z^{2.60}}{[26.6]^{2.6} + Z^{2.6}}$$

where $Z = PO_2 \times 10^{-0.48(7.40 - pH)}$. A computer can easily carry out this calculation when given the PO_2 and the pH of the blood sample. This relationship assumes, however, that the blood being analyzed has a normal affinity ($P_{50} = 26.6$ mm Hg) and is not poisoned with CO or other hemoglobins. This may not be the case in some patients, thus this calculation could result in an erroneous estimation of O_2Hb concentration and lead to mistakes in patient care.

Another approach uses an **oximeter** to measure the percentage of O_2Hb. Oximeters use light spectrometry to determine the amount of Hb in a sample. Two general types of oximeters are commonly used. The **CO-oximeter,** a bench-top instrument, uses five or more different wavelengths of light to measure the light absorbance properties of the different forms of Hb in a blood sample. This device requires a sample of blood from the patient to be introduced into a measuring chamber. It reports the fractional amount of O_2Hb, $COHb$, HHb, etc. present in a blood sample. A variation of this technique has been developed in conjunction with fiberoptic channels in a pulmonary artery catheter, allowing the continuous measurement of mixed venous O_2Hb saturation ($S_{\bar{v}}O_2$ in the pulmonary artery.

Another approach uses two wavelengths of light that are directed into the subject's skin to analyze the color of pulsing blood in the arterioles in the dermis of the skin. This device, called a **pulse oximeter,** employs a light emitting diode and receiving sensors placed on the ear lobe, finger, or toe. By analyzing the color of pulsing blood, the percent saturation of arterial blood (S_aO_2) can be determined. This device has the advantage of being noninvasive and can be used continuously to monitor for changes in saturation over long periods. It has the disadvantage of reporting the functional saturation of O_2Hb.

Pulse oximetry should not be performed on patients with suspected CO poisoning inhalation. Since COHb is not detected, the pulse oximeter reports a falsely high S_aO_2 when COHb is elevated. This may trick the clinician into believing that the O_2 level in the blood is okay; therefore the needed supplemental O_2 goes without being recognized. In this situation the P_aO_2 can be normal despite having a significant reduction in O_2 content. Persons with suspected CO inhalation should be given 100% O_2 to breathe until their fractional S_aO_2 can be obtained by analyzing the blood in a CO-oximeter. In addition, pulse oximetry poorly indicates if the O_2Hb curve has shifted and if the O_2Hb affinity has changed.

AMOUNT OF OXYGEN DELIVERED AND CONSUMED BY TISSUES

O_2 must be transported or delivered to the tissues continuously. Failure to supply an adequate amount of O_2 to the tissues results in organ dysfunction and altered metabolism.

Oxygen Delivery to the Tissues

As previously discussed, arterial O_2 content (C_aO_2) can be calculated based on the P_aO_2, S_aO_2 (the fractional saturation), and the Hb concentration. This calculation determines the amount of O_2 carried in 100 ml of blood. Since blood flow is a dynamic process, C_aO_2 can

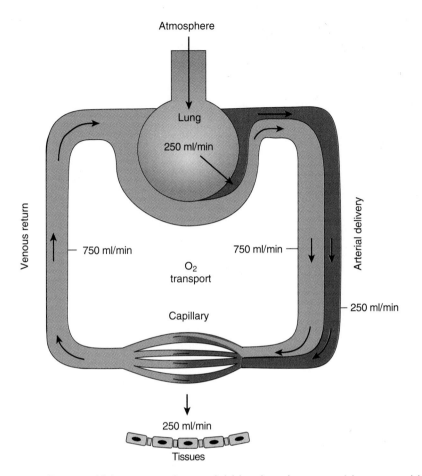

FIG. 13-11 Oxygen *(O₂)* transport in arterial blood to tissues and in venous blood back to the lungs. As venous blood reaches the lung, 250 ml of O_2 is picked up each minute and added to the 750 ml of O_2 already present in the venous blood. This 1000 ml of O_2 is transported to the systemic capillary beds where 250 ml/min is consumed by the tissues.

be thought of as the amount of oxygen delivered or transported to the tissues for every 100 ml of blood (Fig. 13-11). Normally this is about 20 ml of O_2 per 100 ml of blood. Another way to determine O_2 delivery or transport (TO₂) to the tissues is the calculation of the total amount of O_2 delivered per minute. This is done by multiplying the arterial O_2 content (C_aO_2) times the cardiac output ($\dot{Q}_T$):

$$TO_2 = C_aO_2 \times \dot{Q}_T$$

If normal C_aO_2 is 20 ml of O_2 per 100 ml of blood and normal $\dot{Q}_T$ is 5 L/min or 5000 ml/min, the normal TO₂ is calculated the following way:

$$TO_2 = \frac{20 \text{ ml of } O_2}{100 \text{ ml of blood}} \times$$
$$5000 \text{ ml of blood per minute}$$
$$= 1000 \text{ ml of } O_2 \text{ per minute}$$

TO₂ is the global amount of O_2 available for tissue consumption (Fig. 13-12). TO₂ can be increased when $\dot{Q}_T$ is increased (e.g., during

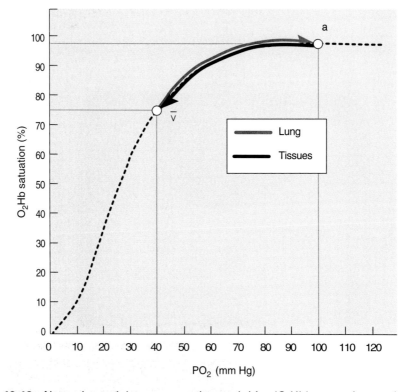

FIG. 13-12 Normal arterial-venous oxyhemoglobin *(O₂Hb)* saturation and partial pressure of O_2 *(PO₂)* differences on the dissociation curve as blood passes from the lungs to the systemic capillaries and back.

exercise) or when a low C_aO_2 is increased (e.g., when supplemental O_2 administration increases the S_aO_2). TO_2 may decrease if $\dot{Q}_T$ decreases (e.g., heart failure) or if C_aO_2 decreases (e.g., anemia, hypoxemia). When O_2 demand exceeds the current TO_2 rate, the body can compensate by increasing $\dot{Q}_T$ via sympathetic stimulation of cardiac function to better match TO_2 with $\dot{V}O_2$ by the tissues.

Oxygen Consumption by the Tissues

A certain amount of O_2 that is delivered to the tissues is consumed during oxidative metabolism. Oxygen consumption can be evaluated in several ways.

Venous Partial Pressure of Oxygen and Saturation

The O_2 levels in venous blood returning to the lungs from the tissues can reveal how well O_2 is being used (see Fig. 13-12). It is important to evaluate true mixed systemic venous blood collected or analyzed in the right ventricle or pulmonary artery. Samples collected from the superior or inferior vena cava or from the right atrium are not well mixed, reflecting the metabolic activity of the tissues from which the blood comes. The normal oxygenation values of mixed venous blood are summarized in Table 13-5. These values reflect the balance between O_2 delivery to and the consumption of O_2 by the tissues. Increased O_2 consumption

Table 13-5   Normal Oxygenation Values of Systemic Arterial and Mixed Venous Blood

Parameter	Arterial Blood	Mixed Venous Blood
Partial pressure of oxygen (mm Hg)	100	40
Oxyhemoglobin saturation (%)	97	75
Oxygen content (ml/100 ml)	20	15

BOX 13-2

Conditions that Cause Alteration in Mixed Venous Oxygenation

DECREASED $P_{\bar{v}}O_2$, $S_{\bar{v}}O_2$, AND $C_{\bar{v}}O_2$
↑ Metabolic rate (exercise, shivering, fever, and seizures)
↓ Cardiac output (heart failure and hypovolemia)
↓ Oxygen content in arterial blood
↓ P_aO_2 and S_aO_2 ($\dot{V}/\dot{Q}$ abnormality)
Anemia

INCREASED $P_{\bar{v}}O_2$, $S_{\bar{v}}O_2$, AND $C_{\bar{v}}O_2$
↓ Metabolic rate (rest, hypothermia, paralysis, and cyanide poisoning)
Peripheral shunts around tissues (sepsis and trauma)
↑ Cardiac output (cardiac stimulation)
↑ Oxygen content in arterial blood (minor influence)
Polycythemia

removes more O_2 from blood, thereby reducing the venous oxygenation. Likewise, reduced cardiac output presents the tissues with less O_2 per minute and the tissues consume about the same amount of O_2 per minute. This, again, results in reduced venous oxygenation. On the other hand, conditions that result in greater O_2 delivery to the tissues cause venous oxygenation to be increased to a point. Various conditions that cause alterations in venous oxygenation are listed in Box 13-2.

An interesting situation arises when a normal individual breathes 100% O_2. The arterial PO_2 climbs to about 550 mm Hg and the saturation increases to 100%. If a mixed venous sample of blood is collected simultaneously, the venous PO_2 will only be about 45 mm Hg and the saturation will be about 78%. The addition of little O_2 being loaded into the already well-oxygenated arterial blood results in a minor rise in venous PO_2 despite the huge increase in arterial PO_2. The saturation only increases about 2%. When this arterial blood passes the tissues, the blood equilibrates with tissue oxygenation and the small additional amount of O_2 brought about by breathing 100% O_2 is easily consumed and the saturation drops to a value close to 75% to 78%, resulting

in the PO_2 dropping to a value of about 40 to 45 mm Hg.

Arterial-Venous Oxygen Differences

Another approach expresses O_2 consumption on the basis of the amount consumed per 100 ml of blood. On average, about 5 ml of O_2 is consumed for every 100 ml of blood flowing past the tissue. The O_2 diffuses out of the blood and into the tissue where it is used in cellular metabolism to produce ATP. Different tissues have different O_2 consumption rates, but on average about 5 ml of O_2 per 100 ml of blood is consumed. If 20 ml of O_2 per 100 ml of arterial blood flows past the tissue and 5 ml of O_2 is consumed, 15 ml of O_2 remains in the 100 ml of venous blood as it leaves the tissues. The 15-ml O_2 content in venous blood ($C_{\bar{v}}O_2$) acts as a reserve form of O_2.

The amount of O_2 consumed by the tissues from 100 ml of blood represents the arterial-

---

BOX 13-3

*Causes of Increased and Decreased
Oxygen Consumption*

INCREASED CONSUMPTION
(indicated by increased arterial-to-venous
   oxygen difference and oxygen extraction
   ratio)
↑ Metabolic rate (exercise, fever, and
   seizures)
↓ Cardiac output (heart failure and
   hypovolemia)

DECREASED CONSUMPTION
(indicated by decreased arterial-to-venous
   oxygen difference and oxygen extraction
   ratio)
↓ Metabolic rate (rest, hypothermia, paralysis, and cyanide poisoning)
↑ Cardiac output (cardiac stimulation)

---

venous oxygen content difference ($C_{a\text{-}\bar{v}}O_2$),
which is also called the *a-v difference*. At rest
with normal blood flow and metabolism, the
difference is easily calculated by measuring
the O_2 content in arterial and mixed venous
blood (from pulmonary artery):

$$C_{a\text{-}\bar{v}}O_2 = C_aO_2 - C_{\bar{v}}O_2$$
$$= 20 \text{ ml}/100 \text{ ml} - 15 \text{ ml}/100 \text{ ml}$$
$$= 5 \text{ ml of } O_2/100 \text{ ml of blood}$$

Several other ways can be used to evaluate the
a-v O_2 difference. The O_2Hb saturation difference ($S_{a\text{-}\bar{v}}O_2$) between arterial and mixed
venous blood also illustrates the difference
caused by metabolism in the tissues and gas
exchange in the lungs. Normally this difference
is 97% − 75%, or about 22% (see Fig. 13-12).
The PO_2 difference can also be evaluated. Normally it is about 100 − 40 mm Hg, or
60 mm Hg (see Fig. 13-12).

The a-$\bar{v}$ O_2 difference can increase and
decrease in response to several different conditions (Box 13-3). Generally, when metabo-

lism consumes greater amounts of O_2 than is
delivered, the a-$\bar{v}$ O_2 difference increases. The
opposite occurs when O_2 delivery exceeds the
metabolic rate.

Oxygen Consumption

The third way to describe O_2 consumption is
to express it as the amount removed from the
blood and lungs per minute ($\dot{V}O_2$). O_2 consumption can be determined by evaluating
the O_2 difference in the arterial and venous
blood over a period of several minutes. O_2 consumption can be calculated in several ways:

$$\dot{V}O_2 = (C_aO_2 - C_{\bar{v}}O_2) \times \dot{Q}_T$$

If the normal a-$\bar{v}$ O_2 difference is 5 ml/100 ml
of blood and $\dot{Q}_T$ is 5000 ml of blood per
minute, the normal $\dot{V}O_2$ would be as follows:

$$\dot{V}O_2 = \frac{5 \text{ ml}}{100 \text{ ml}} \times 5000 \text{ ml/min}$$
$$= 250 \text{ ml of } O_2 \text{ per minute}$$

Another approach measures the amount of O_2
extracted from inhaled air:

$$\dot{V}O_2 = \dot{V}_E \times (FIO_2 - FEO_2)$$

With normal resting data, it is calculated using
the following relationship:

$$\dot{V}O_2 = 5000 \text{ ml/min} \times (0.21 - 0.16)$$
$$= 250 \text{ ml/min}$$

Measuring $\dot{V}O_2$ by this method also includes
the amount of O_2 consumed by the lung's tissue. This can result in a slightly greater estimate of $\dot{V}O_2$ when compared with the content
difference technique.

Oxygen Extraction Ratio

The **oxygen extraction ratio (O_2ER)**, or the
oxygen utilization coefficient (O_2UC), compares total delivered O_2 with the amount consumed. The O_2ER, a ratio of the amount
consumed to the total amount sent, can be
calculated on the basis of the ratio of extrac-

CASE STUDY FOCUS

Gastrointestinal Bleeding and Hypoxia

A 47-year-old man was brought to the emergency department because he was increasingly confused and was vomiting bright red blood (hematemesis). He has a history of consuming large quantities of 70-proof ethyl alcohol on a daily basis for the last 8 years. His vital signs were as follows:

Heart rate	142/min
Blood pressure	72/35
Respiratory rate	28/min
Temperature	36° C

His breath sounds were clear but diminished bilaterally, and an electrocardiogram revealed sinus tachycardia. Arterial blood gases showed a PCO_2 of 31 mm Hg, PO_2 of 106, arterial oxyhemoglobin saturation of 100%, hematocrit of 27%, hemoglobin content of 9 g/dl, and an arterial O_2 content of 12 ml/dl. His arterial PO_2 and oxyhemoglobin saturation were supranormal, however, he is anemic and has severely decreased O_2 content. The low PCO_2 indicates that he is hyperventilating in response to the severe hypoxia. The anemia and reduced oxygenation are a result of the bleeding. The patient was diagnosed with hemorrhagic shock from gastrointestinal bleeding. He was transferred to the intensive care unit (ICU) for further monitoring and treatment.

In the ICU the patient was given a transfusion of several units of blood and vasopressin intravenously. Vasopressin is a vasoconstrictor that reduces blood flow to the intestine, which reduces mesenteric and portal blood pressure. This reduced the frequency and amount of bloody vomiting over the next 12 hours. The next day he underwent esophageal and gastric endoscopy with a flexible fiberoptic scope. A bleeding esophageal variceal was observed just above the stomach. Esophageal varices are engorged vessels in the mucosal wall of the esophagus. They are caused by chronic ethyl alcohol abuse that leads to liver inflammation and hepatic fibrosis. This, in turn, causes portal vessel hypertension that backs blood volume up into the vessels of the esophagus and distends them.

After the patient's blood pressure and hemoglobin content were normalized with fluids and blood, the patient underwent a series of endoscopic injections of a sclerosing agent (e.g., tetradecyl sulfate) directly into the vessels to cause the vessel walls to thicken and stop bleeding. He tolerated this and was discharged 8 days later to outpatient treatment for follow-up and to start a substance abuse program.

tion per 100 ml of blood that passes by the tissues:

$$O_2ER = \frac{C_aO_2 - C_{\bar{v}}O_2}{C_aO_2}$$

With normal O_2 content data, the O_2ER is calculated in the following way:

$$O_2ER = \frac{20 - 15 \text{ ml of } O_2/100 \text{ ml}}{20 \text{ ml}/100 \text{ ml}}$$

$$= \frac{5}{20}$$

$$= 0.25, \text{ or } 25\%$$

O_2ER can also be calculated on the basis of the ratio of consumption to total delivered per minute:

$$O_2ER = \frac{\dot{V}O_2}{TO_2}$$

With normal O_2 consumption and delivery data, the O_2ER is calculated in the following way:

$$O_2ER = \frac{250 \text{ ml/min}}{1000 \text{ ml/min}}$$

$$= 0.25, \text{ or } 25\%$$

A third way to estimate O_2ER is to consider the Hb saturations. This is appropriate because Hb carries 99% of the O_2. The following equation can be used to determine O_2ER:

$$O_2ER = \frac{S_aO_2 - S_vO_2}{S_aO_2}$$

This can be performed continuously by comparing the O_2Hb saturation displayed by an arterial pulse oximeter and a pulmonary artery-equipped oximeter:

$$O_2ER = \frac{98 - 75}{98}$$
$$= \frac{23}{98}$$
$$= 0.23, \text{ or } 23\%$$

The O_2ER normally ranges from 22% to 27% in the healthy, fit individual. Values greater than 0.35 may indicate that cellular O_2 needs are not being met and values below normal indicate excessive O_2 delivery for the amount consumed. Box 13-3 lists some of the conditions that can bring about an abnormal O_2ER.

◖ CARBON DIOXIDE TRANSPORT IN THE BLOOD

When CO_2 is produced in the mitochondria of the cell during metabolism, it diffuses out of the cells and into blood. About 200 ml of CO_2 is added to the blood per minute in the capillaries that surround the tissues (Fig. 13-13). This increases the total CO_2 content in blood by about 9%. When the blood passes through the lungs, the CO_2 added to blood by the tissues is released into alveolar gas and out to the environment with breathing. CO_2 is carried in three forms in blood; dissolved, bound to protein, and bicarbonate ions (Fig. 13-14).

Dissolved Carbon Dioxide

CO_2 is dissolved in blood in two ways (see Fig. 13-14). About 5% of CO_2 added to blood dissolves in the plasma. An additional 5% is dissolved in the cytoplasm of the erythrocyte. The solubility coefficient (C_s) for CO_2 (0.03 mm/L × mm Hg) defines the ability to dissolve CO_2 in blood. To determine the amount of CO_2 carried in the dissolved form, multiply the C_s times the blood PCO_2. For arterial blood this is 0.03 × 40 mm Hg, or 1.2 mm/L.

Carbamino Compound

CO_2 also has the ability to chemically combine with amino acids of protein in the plasma and in Hb (see Fig. 13-14). This is generally known as **carbamino compound.** Less than 1% is added to the plasma in this form. About 21% of the CO_2 added to blood is bound to Hb (carbaminohemoglobin). CO_2 is able to attach to Hb but not at the same site as O_2.

Bicarbonate Ion

The third form that CO_2 takes in blood is in the form of bicarbonate (HCO_3^-) (see Fig. 13-14). About 68% of the CO_2 added to blood is in this form. As CO_2 dissolves in the blood, it may combine with water (H_2O), forming carbonic acid (H_2CO_3). Carbonic acid then dissociates to HCO_3^- and H^+:

$$CO_2 + H_2O \rightarrow H_2CO_3 \rightarrow HCO_3^- + H^+$$

In the plasma this process is slow. When CO_2 enters the erythrocyte, the intracellular enzyme **carbonic anhydrase (CA)** speeds up this reaction. This enzyme speeds up the formation of carbonic acid:

$$CO_2 + H_2O \xrightleftharpoons{CA} H_2CO_3$$

This allows a more rapid transformation of CO_2 to HCO_3^-. Once HCO_3^- forms in the erythrocyte, it diffuses out of the cell while Cl^- diffuses into the cell to take its place and maintain electrical neutrality. This process, called the **chloride shift,** was first described by the Dutch physiologist Hamburger and is therefore

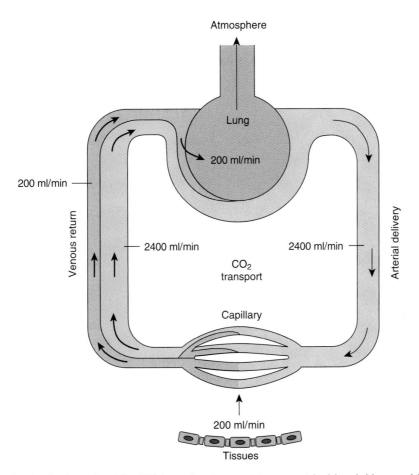

FIG. 13-13   Carbon dioxide *(CO₂)* production and transport in blood. Venous blood delivers 2600 ml of CO_2 to the lungs each minute; 200 ml of CO_2 diffuses into the lungs and is exhaled. The remaining 2400 ml/min of CO_2 transported in the blood is carried back to the systemic capillaries where another 200 ml/min of CO_2 is picked up from the cells.

sometimes called the *Hamburger phenomenon.* The H^+ formed in the erythrocyte during this reaction is buffered by the Hb molecule:

$$H^+ + O_2Hb \rightarrow HHb + O_2$$

When the blood reaches the pulmonary capillaries, the process shown in Fig. 13-14 reverses. CO_2 starts to diffuse out of the blood into alveolar gas. This small but significant

decrease in CO_2 causes the process to reverse. CO_2 leaves the Hb. HCO_3^- enters the erythrocyte and Cl^- diffuses out of the erythrocyte. Inside the erythrocyte, CO_2 is reformed by the action of CA on carbonic acid:

$$HCO_3^- + H^+ \rightarrow H_2CO_3 \rightarrow CO_2 + H_2O$$

CO_2 diffuses out of the erythrocyte and into plasma and then into the alveoli.

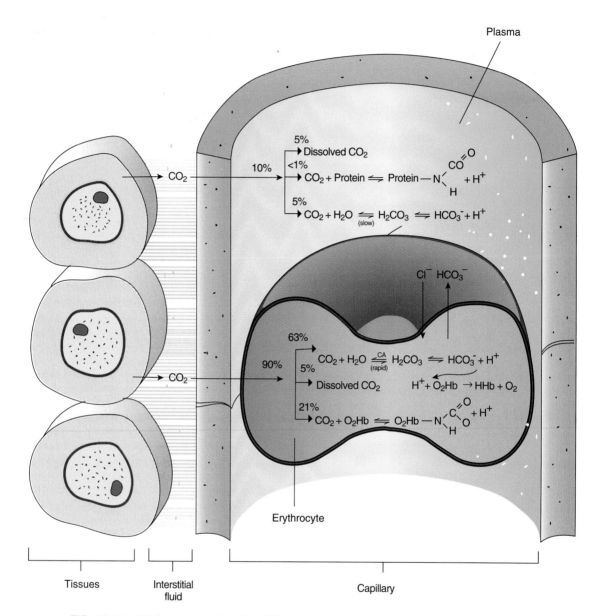

FIG. 13-14 Of the carbon dioxide *(CO₂)* that is produced by cells, 90% is processed and transported by the erythrocyte and the remaining 10% is carried in the plasma. CO_2 is transported in three primary forms: dissolved CO_2, combined with hemoglobin, and as bicarbonate *(HCO₃⁻)*. Illustrated is the process that takes place in both the plasma and in the erythrocyte as CO_2 enters blood.

HOW TOTAL CARBON DIOXIDE CONTENT IS DETERMINED

Fig. 13-14 shows the percent of incoming (or outgoing) CO_2 that is distributed to the different forms of CO_2 transport. These percentages describe the amount of CO_2 processed during loading or unloading. The actual CO_2 content distribution in blood is different. Table 13-6 shows the normal venous and arterial CO_2 transport values with the percent breakdown for each form.

Total CO_2 content can be determined by exposing a sample of blood to strong acid and measuring the amount of CO_2 that is driven out of the sample. It can also be determined by adding the three forms:

Total CO_2 content = Dissolved CO_2 +
    Carbamino compound + Bicarbonate

The amount dissolved is determined with the following relationship:

CO_2 dissolved = PCO_2 × 0.03 ml/mm Hg

The amount in the form of carbamino compound can be estimated with the following equation:

Carbamino compound = PCO_2 × [Hb] ×
    0.002 ml/mm Hg

The HCO_3^- concentration can be determined with a modified form of the Henderson-Hasselbalch equation (see Chapter 14):

HCO_3^- concentration = (Antilog pH − 6.1) ×
    PCO_2 × 0.03 ml/mm Hg

Clinically, CO_2 content is usually expressed as the sum of HCO_3^- and dissolved CO_2. The values of total CO_2 content are 52 and 48 ml of CO_2 per 100 ml blood for venous and arterial blood, respectively. This is approximately two to three times the O_2 content found in venous and arterial blood (Fig. 13-15). The large reserve of CO_2, which is primarily in the form of HCO_3^-, is an important buffer that helps maintain the pH of blood in a normal range (see Chapter 14).

Table 13-6 Normal Values of CO_2 Transport in Venous and Arterial Blood

Variable	Mixed Venous Blood	Arterial Blood
Partial pressure of carbon monoxide (mm Hg)	46	40
Total content (whole blood)		
ml/100 ml	51.8	48.0
Content distribution		
Percent dissolved	5	4
Percent carbamino compound	5	5
Percent bicarbonate	90	91

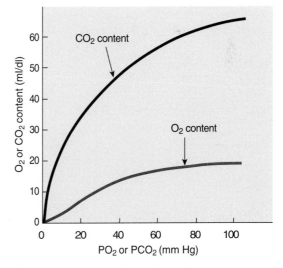

FIG. 13-15 Carbon dioxide *(CO₂)* and oxygen *(O₂)* dissociation curves. Notice that approximately two to three times as much CO_2 is carried in blood when compared with O_2 content.

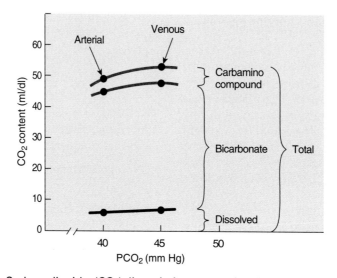

FIG. 13-16 Carbon dioxide *(CO₂)* dissociation curve showing the arterial and mixed venous blood points with the relative proportions of dissolved CO_2, bicarbonate, and carbamino compound.

FIG. 13-17 Haldane effect. As oxygen *(O₂)* leaves the hemoglobin (Hb) molecule in the systemic capillaries, carbon dioxide *(CO₂)* can more easily bind with Hb. This allows an increased CO_2 content for any given partial pressure of CO_2 *(PCO₂)* value as shown by an upward shift in the CO_2 dissociation curve.

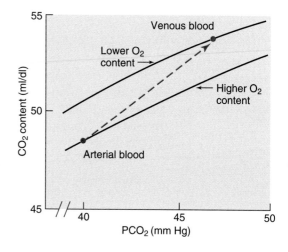

Carbon Dioxide-Hemoglobin Dissociation Curve

Total CO_2 content in blood is influenced by the PCO_2, temperature, the amount and functional status of CA, Hb content, and the saturation of O_2Hb. The CO_2 content curve is more linear than the O_2Hb curve in the physiological range of PCO_2 from 40 to 46 mm Hg (Fig. 13-16). All three forms of CO_2 trans-port change as CO_2 is loaded and unloaded. The shape and position of the curve indicates that CO_2 content remains fairly high despite the relatively low PCO_2.

When the CO_2 dissociation curve is analyzed more closely, the effects of O_2 loading and unloading on Hb become more apparent (Fig. 13-17). As O_2 leaves the Hb molecule, more CO_2 chemically binds with Hb. Therefore, at lower O_2Hb saturations, the CO_2 dissociation curve shifts upward and CO_2 content is greater at any given level of PCO_2. This enhances the removal of CO_2 from the tissues. The opposite occurs as O_2 binds to Hb and the affinity of CO_2 for Hb declines. This ability of O_2 to affect the affinity of CO_2 for Hb is known as the **Haldane effect.** The Haldane and Bohr effects interact to enhance the loading and unloading of CO_2 and O_2 on the Hb molecule as blood flows through the lungs and past the tissues.

CHAPTER SELF-TEST QUESTIONS

1. If the Hb concentration is 12 g/dl and S_aO_2 is 95%, calculate the amount of O_2 bound to Hb.
   a. 11.4 ml
   b. 12.76 ml
   c. 14.16 ml
   d. 15.28 ml
2. Which of the following sets of polypeptides forms normal adult Hb?
   a. 2 alpha and 2 gamma
   b. 2 alpha and 2 beta
   c. 2 alpha and 2 delta
   d. 2 beta and 2 gamma
3. The O_2 bound to Hb accounts for approximately what percent of the total O_2 contained in arterial blood?
   a. 2%
   b. 50%
   c. 75%
   d. 98%
4. Which of the following statements is correct concerning a rightward shift of the O_2Hb dissociation curve?
   1. it indicates an increased O_2 affinity for Hb
   2. it indicates improved release of O_2 to the tissues
   3. it results in a decreased SO_2 for any given PO_2

a. 3 only
b. 1 and 2
c. 1 and 3
d. 2 and 3
e. 1, 2, and 3

5. Each of the following Hb variants shift the O_2Hb curve to the left except:
   a. fetal Hb
   b. SulfHb
   c. COHb
   d. Met-Hb
6. A patient breathing room air has a 50% COHb level following a suicide attempt. How many hours are needed before the patient's COHb level drops to approximately 12%?
   a. 2 hours
   b. 4 hours
   c. 6 hours
   d. 8 hours
7. A patient with a total Hb of 10 g/dl has the following Hb composition in their arterial blood: 7 g/dl O_2Hb, 1 g/dl COHb, 1 g/dl Met-Hb, and 1 g/dl HHb. What is their fractional S_aO_2?
   a. 70%
   b. 80%
   c. 88%
   d. 90%
8. What is the O_2 transport to the tissues per minute in a patient who has a cardiac output of 6 L/min, a fractional saturation of 90%, a Hb concentration of 10 g/dl, and a P_aO_2 of 60 mm Hg?
   a. 684 ml/min
   b. 714 ml/min
   c. 734 ml/min
   d. 754 ml/min
9. If the $\dot{V}O_2$ is 300 ml/min, $\dot{Q}_T$ is 8 L/min, TO_2 is 900 ml/min, and the TO_2 returning to the heart is 600 ml/min, what is the O_2 extraction ratio?
   a. 0.18
   b. 0.25
   c. 0.33
   d. 0.40

10. About 90% of the CO_2 in blood is in the form of
    a. dissolved CO_2
    b. CO_2 attached to Hb
    c. HCO_3^-
    d. H_2CO_3

For answers, see p. 476.

BIBLIOGRAPHY

1. Comroe JH: *Physiology of respiration,* ed 2, Chicago, 1974, Year Book Medical.
2. Green JF. *Fundamental cardiovascular and pulmonary physiology,* ed 2, Philadelphia, 1987, Lea & Febiger.
3. Jones NL: *Blood gases and acid-base physiology,* ed 2, New York, 1987, Thieme-Stratton.
4. Leff AR, Schumacker PT: *Respiratory physiology: basics and applications,* Philadelphia, 1993, WB Saunders.
5. Levitsky MG. *Pulmonary physiology,* ed 3, New York, 1991, McGraw Hill.
6. Levitzky GL, Hall SM, McDonough KH: *Cardiopulmonary physiology in anesthesiology,* New York, 1997, McGraw Hill.
7. Martini FH: *Fundamentals of anatomy and physiology,* Upper Saddle River, NJ, 1998, Prentice Hall.
8. Miller WF, Scacci R, Gast LR: *Laboratory evaluation of pulmonary function,* Philadelphia, 1987, JB Lippincott.
9. Murray JF: *The normal lung,* ed 2, Philadelphia, 1986, WB Saunders.
10. Pierson DJ, Kacmarek RM, eds: *Foundations of respiratory care,* New York, 1992, Churchill Livingstone.
11. Ruppel G: *Manual of pulmonary function testing,* ed 6, St Louis, 1994, Mosby.
12. Staub NC: *Basic respiratory physiology,* New York, 1991, Churchill Livingstone.
13. West JB: *Respiration physiology: the essentials,* ed 4, Baltimore, 1990, Williams & Wilkins.
14. Winslow RM: New transfusion strategies: red cell sub-

14

Urinary System and Acid-Base Balance

CHAPTER OBJECTIVES

Upon completing this chapter, you will be able to:

1 List the major organs of the urinary system and describe their anatomy.
2 Describe the structure and function of the nephron.
3 Describe how the urinary system forms urine and regulates water and electrolyte balance.
4 Describe how the urinary system is controlled.
5 Define important terms and concepts in acid-base physiology.
6 Describe the importance of maintaining an optimal pH level in extracellular and intracellular fluid.
7 Describe the volatile and nonvolatile acid threats to an optimal pH level.
8 Describe the buffer systems that protect the pH level.
9 Define strong ion difference and renal adjustment of bicarbonate (HCO_3^-) concentration.
10 Describe carbon dioxide excretion by the lungs and its adjustment.
11 Describe the interaction of renal and pulmonary adjustment of the HCO_3^-/H_2CO_3 ratio.
12 Demonstrate how the HCO_3^-/H_2CO_3 ratio influences pH levels and define the normal ratio and pH level.
13 Describe how a pH-HCO_3^--PCO_2 diagram illustrates acid-base changes.
14 List the overall, respiratory, and metabolic indicators of acid-base balance and describe their normal values.
15 Describe the four different types of primary acid-base disturbances.
16 Describe the two different types of combined acid-base disturbances.
17 Define acid-base compensation and recognize its presence.
18 Perform a systematic review and interpretation of blood gas and acid-base data.

Normal organ function requires a constant supply of oxygen (O_2) and nutrients and the constant removal of carbon dioxide (CO_2), hydrogen ions (H^+), and other waste products. The lungs absorb O_2 and excrete CO_2 while the kidneys regulate blood volume, electrolyte concentration, and the excretion of metabolic waste. Both organs work together to maintain the H^+ concentration in body fluid at a precise concentration. If the H^+ concentration strays far from the normal range, cellular and organ malfunction occur and threaten the organism's homeostasis. This chapter describes the essential concepts of renal anatomy and physiology, acid-base chemistry, how H^+ concentration is regulated, and important abnormalities of acid-base balance.

URINARY SYSTEM

Ions and Electrolyte Solutions

Some molecules break up (dissociate) when added to a water-based (aqueous) solution. When this happens, charged particles called ions are formed. Ions that lose electrons during the dissociation become positively charged are called **cations.** Ions that gain electrons and become negatively charged are called **anions.** An aqueous solution that has ions dissolved in it has the ability to conduct an electrical current. This property resulted in naming it an electrolyte solution, and the ions dissolved in it are frequently referred to as **electrolytes.**

The concentration of electrolytes in blood is frequently measured to evaluate electrolyte regulation. The concentration of electrolytes in body fluid is generally expressed as a number of milliequivalents per liter (mEq/L). The mEq/L concentration is determined by dividing the number of millimoles of ions dissolved per liter (mmol/L) by the number of charges the ion has. This system is better able to account for the number of ions present in a solution such as blood.

STRUCTURES AND FUNCTIONS

Anatomy

The urinary system is comprised of two **kidneys, renal blood vessels,** two **ureters,** a **urinary bladder,** and a **urethra** (Fig. 14-1). The kidneys are dark reddish organs that are about 10 cm tall, 6 cm wide, and 2½ cm thick. They are located just below each diaphragm up against the posterior wall of the abdominal cavity in an area known as the **retroperitoneal space.** On the medial border of each kidney is the **renal hilus.** It is a fissure where blood vessels, the ureter, nerves, and lymphatic vessels enter and exit the kidney.

Each kidney receives blood from the aorta by way of a **renal artery.** Arterial blood is directed throughout the kidney through a network of arteries and arterioles. The arteriole system supplies blood to several capillary systems that participate in the filtration and reabsorption of blood plasma. Blood drains from these capillary systems through a network of venules and veins to a **renal vein** that carries blood to the inferior vena cava.

The kidney is comprised of several layers of solid tissue and a hollow inner space. The outermost layer is a connective tissue covering called the **renal capsule.** The inner functional layer, or **parenchyma,** is subdivided into an outer **renal cortex** and an inner **renal medulla.** Within the renal medulla are cone-shaped structures called **pyramids.** Each of these pyramids has an apex that ends in a structure called the **renal papilla.** Each of the renal papilla point into the hollow space, the **renal pelvis,** within the kidney. The renal pyramids are formed by dense packages of tubules that are part of the microscopic urine-forming structures called **nephrons.** Each kidney contains about 1 million nephrons.

Urine formed by the nephrons drains from the papilla of each pyramid into the renal pelvis and then to a ureter. Each ureter is about 25 cm long and is comprised of a

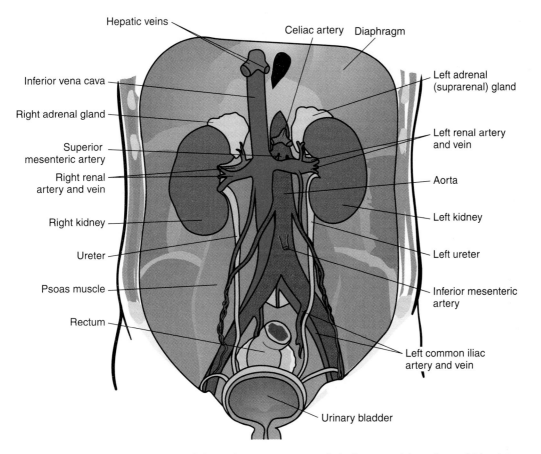

Hepatic veins

Celiac artery Diaphragm

Inferior vena cava

Right adrenal gland

Superior
mesenteric artery

Right renal
artery and vein

Right kidney

Ureter

Psoas muscle

Rectum

Left adrenal
(suprarenal) gland

Left renal artery
and vein

Aorta

Left kidney

Left ureter

Inferior mesenteric
artery

Left common iliac
artery and vein

Urinary bladder

FIG. 14-1 Components of the urinary system and their normal location within the retroperitoneal space.

mucosal inner surface, a middle layer of smooth muscle, and an outer layer of connective tissue. The proximal end of each ureter is connected to one kidney and the distal end to the posterior wall of the urinary bladder. Hydrostatic pressure of urine formation, gravity, and the peristaltic contraction of the ureter smooth muscle all propel urine to the bladder.

The bladder is a hollow organ that is located in the pelvic cavity posterior to the pubic symphysis and anterior to the rectum. The bladder wall is organized in the same way as the ureter: a transitional epithelial mucosal inner surface, a smooth muscle middle layer, and a connective tissue serosal outer surface. The flexible wall gives the bladder the ability to distend with urine to an average capacity of 700 to 800 ml. The sensation of distension begins when the bladder fills with 200 to 300 ml of urine, and stretch receptors become active and send signals to the central nervous system. Urine flows from the bladder to the external environment through the urethra. Urine flow out of the bladder to the urethra is regulated by **internal** and **external urethral sphincters** that are located at the base of the bladder. The internal sphincter is comprised of smooth muscle and is controlled subconsciously and the external sphincter is comprised of skeletal muscle that is under conscious control.

Nephron

Each of the 1 million nephrons that are located in the parenchyma of the kidney consists of two basic parts: a **renal corpuscle** and a **renal tubule and duct** (Fig. 14-2).

The renal corpuscles are all located in the cortex of the kidney and are comprised of two components: a **glomerular capillary** and a **glomerular (Bowman's) capsule** that surrounds the capillary. The glomerular capillary is a ball-like network of fenestrated capillaries that are the leakiest capillaries in the body. Blood is supplied to the glomerular capillary from an **afferent arteriole** that is supplied with blood from branches of the renal arterial system. Blood drains from the glomerulus through an **efferent arteriole.** The glomerular capsule wraps around the glomerular capillary like a water balloon that is pushed over a finger. The inner layer of the glomerular capsule is formed by epithelial cells called **podocytes.** The podocytes cover the capillary and act like a sieve. As blood flows through the glomerular capillary, water, small mole-

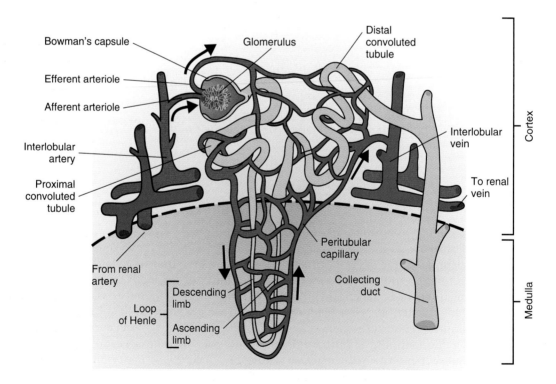

FIG. 14-2 Nephron.

cules, and ions can pass through the capillary wall and between the podocytes.

The fluid that is filtered into the capsule flows into the renal tubule. The renal tubule can be divided into three different sections: the **proximal convoluted tubule,** the **nephron loop (loop of Henle)**, and the **distal convoluted tubule.** These tubules are formed by several different types of cuboidal epithelia. The renal corpuscle and convoluted tubules all lie in the cortex of the kidney. The **descending** and **ascending limbs** of the nephron loop extend into the renal medulla. About 80% of the nephrons have relatively short nephron loops while the other 20% have longer descending and ascending limbs that extend almost to the renal papilla. The longer nephrons are more capable of concentrating the urine. The urine that flows from several distal convoluted tubules empties into a **collecting duct** that unites into several hundred **papillary ducts.** The papillary ducts, in turn, drain urine into the renal pelvis through the surface of the renal papilla.

The walls of the arterioles near the entrance and exit of the efferent and afferent arterioles that supply and drain blood from the glomerular capillary are equipped with cuffs of smooth muscle. These special smooth muscle cells are called the **juxtaglomerular cells.** They respond to changes in renal blood pressure and modify the flow and pressure of blood within the glomerular capillary network. At this location the distal convoluted tubule comes into close contact with the arterioles. A complex of cells in the wall of the distal tubule at this contact point is called the **macula densa.** The juxtaglomerular and the macula densa cells at the point of contact between the distal tubule and arterioles form the complex called the **juxtaglomerular apparatus.** The juxtaglomerular apparatus plays an important role in the regulation of blood flow and in the formation of urine. The juxtaglomerular cells regulate blood flow whereas the macula densa is equipped with sensory cells that respond to the delivery of ions and water and, in turn, regulate the production of several hormones that influence renal blood flow and ion and water reabsorption.

Physiology

The regulation of blood volume and composition by the nephrons is carried out by four different and interrelated processes: **glomerular filtration, tubular reabsorption, tubular secretion,** and **urine concentration** (Fig. 14-3). These processes result in moving certain waste products, ions, and water out of blood plasma and into urine so that the chemical composition of plasma is maintained in a "normal" range.

Glomerular Filtration

The first step in the formation of urine is the filtration of plasma across the wall of the glomerular capillaries. These capillaries are 50 times more leaky than other capillaries. The process of capillary filtration is described by **Starling's law of the capillary** (see Chapter 7). The following equation summarizes the modified form of Starling's law for determining the filtration pressure that drives fluid across the glomerular capillary wall:

$$P_{nf} = (P_{gc} - P_i) - (\pi_p - \pi_i)$$

where P_{nf} is the **net filtration pressure,** P_{gc} is the blood pressure in the glomerular capillary, P_i is the fluid pressure in the interstitial space within the glomerular capsule that opposes filtration, and π_p is the plasma oncotic pressure that is an osmotic force generated by plasma proteins (e.g., albumin). Cells and proteins are generally too large to be filtered and remain in the blood plasma. They act osmotically to attract water back into the capillary, which opposes filtration pressure, and π_i is

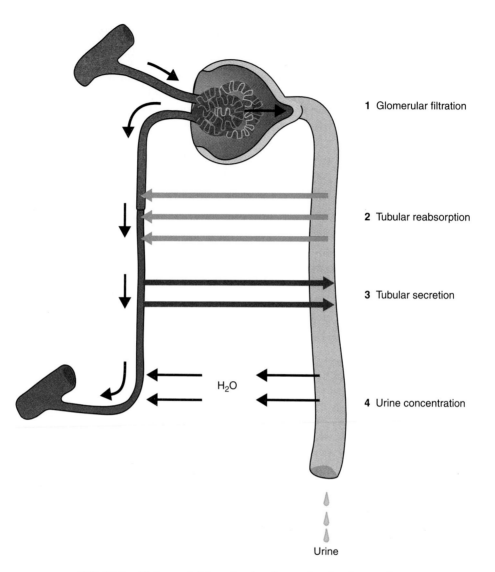

1 Glomerular filtration

2 Tubular reabsorption

3 Tubular secretion

H_2O

4 Urine concentration

Urine

FIG. 14-3 Major activities of urine formation by the nephron.

the interstitial fluid oncotic pressure generated by the few proteins that are filtered into the capsule.

The normal net filtration pressure can be calculated by using normal values for capillary blood pressure, colloid osmotic pressure, and capsular pressure:

$$P_{nf} = (55 - 16 \text{ mm Hg}) - (30 - 1 \text{ mm Hg})$$
$$= 10 \text{ mm Hg}$$

Although the normal value of 10 mm Hg seems low, it is more than enough to drive large amounts of fluid across the leaky walls of the glomerular capillary.

About 20% of the blood plasma is filtered as it passes through the glomerulus. The fluid that is filtered is called the **glomerular filtrate.** It is chemically similar to blood plasma except that it has little protein in it. The volume of filtrate that is formed over time is called the **glomerular filtration rate (GFR).** In the average adult, the GFR is about 125 ml/min or 180 L/day. This is 60 times the normal total blood plasma volume of 3 L. This is only possible by reabsorbing 99% of the filtered fluid back into blood and refiltering it over and over.

The GFR is regulated by adjusting systemic blood pressure and glomerular capillary blood flow. Systemic blood pressure is maintained at a constant mean arterial pressure of 90 mm Hg. This is carried out by adjustments of cardiac function, blood vessel tone, and blood volume, as described in Chapter 8. Generally, during stressful conditions when significant sympathetic nervous system activity occurs, renal arteriolar vasoconstriction occurs. This leads to reduced glomerular blood flow and lower GFR. Glomerular blood flow is adjusted more precisely by several other mechanisms. The kidney has the ability to maintain a constant glomerular capillary pressure and GFR despite changes in the mean systemic blood pressure. This ability is called **renal autoregulation,** a negative feedback mechanism that results in adjustments of arteriolar diameter and glomerular blood flow. When the net filtration pressure and GFR are low, the proximal convoluted tubule and nephron loop can absorb more Na^+, Cl^-, and water from the glomerular filtrate. This is detected by special chemosensory cells in the **juxtaglomerular apparatus** that are located along the distal convoluted tubule and cause (by an unknown mechanism) the afferent arteriole to dilate. This results in greater filtration pressure and GFR. As GFR increases, the amount of ions and water reaching the juxtaglomerular apparatus increases. This results

in afferent arteriolar constriction, causing relatively stable GFR despite variations in arterial blood pressure.

The kidney also uses hormones to regulate blood pressure and GFR. When GFR is reduced and less Na^+, Cl^-, and water reach the distal convoluted tubule, the juxtaglomerular apparatus secretes an enzyme called **renin.** Renin converts the plasma protein **angiotensinogen** to **angiotensin I** and, upon passing through the pulmonary circulation, a second enzyme called **angiotensin converting enzyme (ACE)** converts angiotensin I to **angiotensin II.** Angiotensin II causes generalized vasoconstriction, increased systemic blood pressure, increased glomerular blood flow, efferent arteriolar vasoconstriction, and increased GFR. In addition, **angiotensin II** stimulates the release of aldosterone, thirst, and the secretion of **antidiuretic hormone (ADH).** These effects all promote greater blood volume, renal blood flow, and GFR. Another hormone, **atrial natriuretic peptide (ANP),** is produced by the atria of the heart when distended with blood. Increased levels of ANP occur with increased blood volume. ANP is thought to increase GFR by dilating the afferent arterioles.

Tubular Reabsorption

The next step in the regulation of blood volume and composition through the formation of urine is the reabsorption of water, molecules, and ions (Fig. 14-4). As the filtrate passes through the renal tubules and collecting ducts, about 99% of it is reabsorbed and only 1% forms urine. During tubular reabsorption, water, selected molecules, and ions are passively and actively reabsorbed into blood in the **peritubular capillary** and **vasa recta** capillary systems that surround the tubules of the nephron. The molecules and ions that are selectively reabsorbed primarily include glucose, amino acids, small proteins, urea, Na^+, K^+, Ca^{++}, Cl^-, HCO_3^-, and $HPO_4^=$. These molecules and ions are reabsorbed back

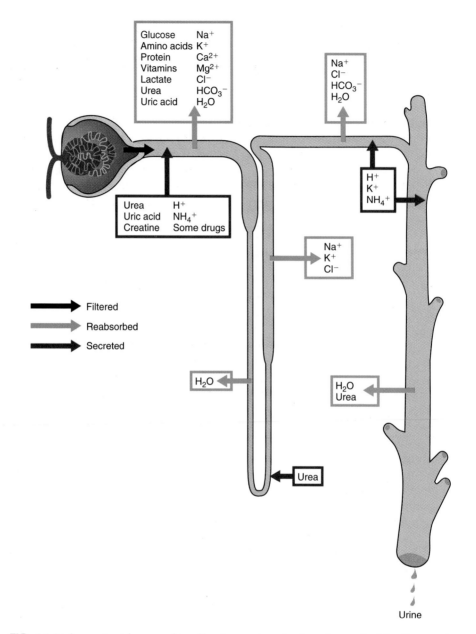

Glucose	Na⁺
Amino acids	K⁺
Protein	Ca²⁺
Vitamins	Mg²⁺
Lactate	Cl⁻
Urea	HCO₃⁻
Uric acid	H₂O

Na⁺
Cl⁻
HCO₃⁻
H₂O

Urea	H⁺
Uric acid	NH₄⁺
Creatine	Some drugs

H⁺
K⁺
NH₄⁺

Na⁺
K⁺
Cl⁻

H₂O

H₂O
Urea

Urea

Filtered

Reabsorbed

Secreted

Urine

FIG. 14-4 Important ions and molecules reabsorbed and secreted by the nephron during the production of urine.

into blood by active pumping proteins (e.g., **Na$^+$ pump proteins**), secondary active transport proteins that transport more than one molecule or ion in the same direction (e.g., Na$^+$-glucose and Na$^+$-K$^+$-Cl$^-$ **symporters**) or in opposite directions (e.g., Na$^+$-H$^+$ **antiporters**), and through channel proteins in and between the epithelial cells that form the tubules. Water is reabsorbed by osmosis as it follows the reabsorption of the molecules and ions. Approximately 65% of tubular reabsorption occurs along the proximal convoluted tubule, with the balance of the reabsorption occurring along the nephron loop and distal convoluted tubule.

Tubular reabsorption is regulated largely by the actions of **aldosterone** and ADH. Aldosterone, a steroid hormone secreted by cortical cells of the adrenal gland, stimulates cells in the wall of the distal convoluted tubule and collecting duct cells to produce more Na$^+$ pump proteins. This results in more active Na$^+$ reabsorption. Water reabsorption also increases as the result of osmosis. ADH, a protein hormone secreted by the posterior pituitary gland, stimulates the production of water channel proteins in the same cells in the wall of the distal convoluted tubule and collecting duct, which results in greater water reabsorption. During conditions of dehydration, there is greater secretion of aldosterone and ADH, which prevents excessive Na$^+$ and water loss and produces concentrated urine. With overhydration, less aldosterone and ADH are secreted. This results in less reabsorption and greater quantities of water loss as dilute urine.

Tubular Secretion

The secretion of H$^+$, K$^+$, ammonium ions (NH$_4^+$), creatinine, and some drugs (e.g., penicillin) is the third major function of the nephrons (see Fig. 14-4). Cells in the wall of the distal convoluted tubule and collecting duct actively secrete these ions into tubular fluid and, ultimately, urine. The secretion of these ions increases with elevated concen-

trations in plasma. This effectively keeps the concentration of these toxic chemicals to a minimum. Aldosterone stimulates the antiporter secretion of K$^+$ and the reabsorption of Na$^+$.

Urine Concentration

The kidney can respond to the hydration status of the body. During times of dehydration, the kidney can concentrate toxic chemicals in less urine to reduce the amount of water loss. When the individual is overhydrated, the kidney can excrete diluted urine that does not result in excess ion loss. The ability of the nephron to produce concentrated as well as dilute urine is carried out by the interaction of the **descending limbs** and the **ascending limbs** of the nephron loop and the surrounding vasa recta. Two key factors make this possible: (1) the different abilities to reabsorb solutes and water in different parts of the nephron and (2) the **countercurrent flow** of tubular fluid and blood that results from the anatomical relationship of the different parts of the nephron.

Like the convoluted tubule, the descending limb of the nephron loop and the collecting duct reabsorb water (see Fig. 14-4). The ascending limb of the loop is relatively impermeable to water and actively reabsorbs Na$^+$ and Cl$^-$. With the nephron loop and the vasa recta bent back on themselves in U-shaped structures, these different fluids can flow in the opposite directions or countercurrent flow. Water is reabsorbed along the length of the descending limb of the nephron loop and collecting duct. It is drawn into the surrounding peritubular space by osmosis. The peritubular space becomes progressively more concentrated along the longer nephrons that loop deep into the pyramids. The increased concentration is produced by the active pumping of Na$^+$ out of the ascending limb, the diffusion of urea into this space, and the removal of water by the vasa recta. The concentrations outside in the deeper nephron loops are multiplied by the countercurrent nature of the flow in the different tubules. This allows more water to be reabsorbed as more sodium and urea are concentrated just outside in the tubules of the peritubular space.

The concentration of body fluids is described with the osmotic units of milliosmoles per liter (mOsm/L). Blood plasma has a normal value of about 300 mOsm/L. The kidneys can produce urine that is about one fourth the concentration of blood plasma (e.g., 70 mOsm/L) and up to about 4 times the concentration of plasma (e.g., 1200 mOsm/L).

The amount of water reabsorbed by this mechanism is primarily regulated by the levels of ADH that are secreted by the posterior pituitary gland. ADH secretion is regulated by osmoreceptors in the hypothalamus. Dehydration is the result of osmotic movement of water out of cells. The osmoreceptors in the hypothalamus respond to this and stimulate the production of ADH. Increased ADH causes the water channels in the distal convoluted tubule and collecting duct to open, thus more water is reabsorbed by the nephron. During times of overhydration, less ADH is secreted, the water channels in the distal nephron close, and more water remains in the urine so that it is excreted.

Table 14-1 summarizes the effects that normal renal function has on water, nutrients, ions, and metabolic waste products in plasma as urine is formed on a daily basis. Note the amount of filtration compared with plasma volume, that all of the glucose and almost all of the protein and ions are reabsorbed, and that the metabolic waste products (urea and creatinine) are excreted. This activity coupled with normal ingestion of water and ions results in the maintenance of fluid and electrolyte balance. Sampling blood and analysis of the plasma electrolytes reveal how this balance is maintained. Box 14-1 lists the normal values of important ions and the normal plasma concentrations of blood urea nitrogen (BUN), which is a metabolic waste product of

---

BOX 14-1

Normal Chemical Composition of Plasma

WATER		91.5%*
PROTEIN		7.0%*
Albumin	3.5-5.0 g/dl	
Globulins	2.3-3.5 g/dl	
Fibrinogen	0.2-0.35 g/dl	
Total protein	6.0-8.0 g/dl	
OTHER SOLUTES		1.5%*
NUTRIENTS		
Total lipids	450-1000 mg/dl	
Fatty acids	190-420 mg/dl	
Cholesterol	150-220 mg/dl	
Triglycerides	40-150 mg/dl	
Glucose	70-100 mg/dl	
Amino acids	30-45 mg/dl	
ELECTROLYTES		
Cations		
Na^+	135-145 mEq/L	
K^+	3.5-5.0 mEq/L	
Ca^{++}	8.5-10.0 mEq/L	
Mg^{++}	1.5-2.5 mEq/L	
Anions		
Cl^-	100-106 mEq/L	
HCO_3^-	22-26 mEq/L	
PO_4^{3-}	0.5-1.5 mEq/L	
SO_4^{2-}	0.3-0.6 mEq/L	
WASTE PRODUCTS		
Blood urea nitrogen	10-20 mg/dl	
Uric acid	2.0-8.0 mg/dl	
Creatinine	0.6-1.5 mg/dl	
Bilirubin (total)	0.3-1.1 mg/dl	
Lactic acid	0.6-1.8 mg/dl	

*Percent of total weight.

---

amino acid breakdown, and creatinine, which is a metabolic waste product of muscle metabolism. Normally, the kidney excretes a small amount of water, ions, urea, and creatinine. In renal failure, potassium, urea, creatinine, and H^+ concentrations increase as a result of reduced excretion.

Table 14-1   Normal Amounts of Water, Ions, and Solutes in Plasma, Glomerular Filtrate, and Tubular Reabsorption and in Urine that is Produced Daily

Substances	Plasma (Total)	Filtrate (Into Tubule)	Reabsorbed (Into Blood)	Urine (Excreted)
Water (ml)	3000	180,000	178,500	1500
Glucose (g)	3	180	180	0
Proteins (g)	200	<2	1.9	0.1
Na^+ (mEq/L)	420	25,200	25,000	200
K^+ (mEq/L)	12.6	750	750	50 (secreted)
Cl^- (mEq/L)	300	18,000	17,850	150
HCO_3^- (mEq/L)	75	4500	4500	0
Urea (g)	4.8	53	28	25
Creatinine (g)	0.03	1.6	0	1.6

MAJOR CONCEPTS USED IN ACID-BASE CHEMISTRY

Acids and Bases

Chemicals that release H^+ or cause the concentration of H^+ in a solution to increase with respect to hydroxyl ions (OH^-) are called **acids.** When an acid (HA) dissociates in an aqueous solution, it releases an H^+:

$$HA \rightarrow H^+ + A^-$$

The remaining portion (A^-) has the ability to recombine with the H^+ if the reaction reverses or moves to the left. Put another way, the A^- anion is a conjugate base of HA. Hydrochloric acid (HCl) is an example of a strong acid that is produced in the stomach.

In reality, virtually all of the H^+ released into a solution does not exist as a free H^+. It combines with H_2O to form a hydronium ion (H_3O^+). To simplify the discussion presented here, the symbol H^+ will represent all H^+ and H_3O^+ ions.

A chemical that absorbs H^+ and causes the OH^- concentration to increase in an aqueous solution is known as a **base.** When a base (B) is added to a solution, it removes H^+ from H_2O molecules and produces OH^-:

$$B + H_2O \rightarrow BH^+ + OH^-$$

This results in an increased OH^- concentration and decreased H^+ concentration. In this situation, BH^+ is known as the conjugate acid and is capable of releasing H^+. Molecules that release OH^- act as bases because the OH^- can absorb H^+. Sodium hydroxide (NaOH) is an example of a strong base.

Dissociation Constant (pK)

Stronger acids, bases, and ions will dissociate more completely. Those considered weak are molecules that dissociate incompletely. Proteins act like weak acids because they have acid groups on some of their amino acids. The strength of an acid or base can be quantified by determining the amount that dissociates. This is known as a **dissociation constant** (K). The dissociation constant is a number that equals the ratio of dissociated ions to undissociated acid or base. The dissociation constant of an acid (Ka) is determined in the following way:

$$Ka = \frac{[H^+] \times [A^-]}{[HA]}$$

The dissociation constant is more frequently expressed in logarithmic terms:

$$logKa = \frac{log[H^+] + log[A^-]}{[HA]}$$

The negative logarithmic value of the dissociation constant for an acid ($-logKa$) is known as the *pKa*. A similar approach can be used to determine the dissociation constant for a base or ion.

The value of pK is proportional to the strength of the acid or base: greater values of pK indicate a stronger acid or base, and, conversely, lower values indicate a weaker acid or base.

Buffers

When a certain amount of acid or base is added to pure water, the resulting change in H^+ concentration can be predicted. A solution that has chemical **buffers** will not exhibit the same degree of change in H^+ concentration when acid or base is added. Buffers are formed from a combination of weak acids (HA) and weak bases (A^-). A buffered solution has the dual capability of releasing and absorbing H^+.

The action of a buffer solution can be shown when an acid such as HCl is added to it. HCl dissociates upon entry into the solution and releases its H^+:

$$HCl + HA + A^- \rightarrow H^+ + Cl^- + HA + A^-$$

Then the weak base A^- reacts and absorbs the excess H^+ to produce weak acid molecules and Cl^-:

$$H^+ + A^- + HA + Cl^- \rightarrow 2HA + Cl^-$$

The weak base effectively absorbs excess H^+ added to the solution and minimizes the change in H^+ concentration.

Conversely, when a base is added to a buffered solution, the change in H^+ concentration is minimized by the release of H^+ from the weak acid component of the buffer. This can be shown when NaOH is added to a buffered solution. When NaOH is added, it dissociates and releases OH^-:

$$NaOH + HA + A^- \rightarrow OH^- + Na^+ + HA + A^-$$

The OH^- is a powerful base that removes H^+ from the solution. This is countered by the action of the weak acid (HA) portion of the buffer system. The weak acid releases H^+, which reacts with OH^-:

$$OH^- + HA + Na^+ + A^- \rightarrow OH^- + H^+ + 2A^- + Na^-$$

This reaction produces water:

$$OH^- + H^+ + 2A^- + Na^- \rightarrow H_2O + 2A^- + Na^-$$

The weak acid diminishes the effect that the strong base would have had on the concentration of H^+ in the solution.

The amount of buffer in a solution determines the amount of H^+ that is absorbed and left in the solution.

Greater amounts of weak acid or lesser amounts of weak base cause the H^+ concentration to increase. Decreased H^+ concentration is produced by having a less weak acid or a weaker base. By adjusting the buffer combination in the solution, two important effects occur: (1) the ability to control H^+ concentration and (2) changes in H^+ concentration when the solution is challenged by the addition of acid or base are minimized. The body uses a number of buffers to control H^+ concentration in body fluid and to minimize changes.

H^+ Concentration and pH

The amount of H^+ present in a solution determines the overall acid-base conditions of that solution. Knowing the H^+ concentration in blood is an important first step in understanding the acid-base status in an individual. The normal H^+ concentration in blood is maintained at 0.00004 mEq/L, an extremely small quantity compared with the normal Na^+ concentration of 140 mEq/L. An alternative approach is to use the nanoequivalent per liter (nEq/L) scale. Using this system, the normal H^+ concentration in blood is 40 nM/L.

Some have argued that using this system of measurement is a straightforward arithmetic process that is more intuitive. Others have argued that it does not reflect the logarithmic behavior of many biochemical processes that occur inside and outside the cell.

An alternative system was devised by Sorensen at the beginning of the 20th century that uses a logarithmic scale. This system quantifies H^+ concentration on a **pH** scale that ranges from 0 to 14. The pH of a solution is defined as the negative log (base 10) of the H^+ concentration:

$$pH = -\log_{(10)}[H^+]$$

The relationship of H^+ concentration and pH is not an obvious one unless several different concentrations are examined. The concentration of H^+ in distilled water is 1×10^{-7} mol/L. The pH is determined in the following way:

$$
\begin{aligned}
pH &= -\log\,[H^+] \\
&= -\log(1 \times 10^{-7}) \\
&= -(-7) \\
&= 7
\end{aligned}
$$

The H^+ concentration or pH scale can be used to describe when a solution is neutral, acidic, or basic (Table 14-2). Distilled water is used to define a neutral point in the H^+ concentration and the pH scales. If a solution has an H^+ concentration equal to 1×10^{-7} mol/L or a pH equal to 7.00, it is described as a neutral solution. When the H^+ concentration in a solution is greater than 1×10^{-7} or when the pH is below 7.00, the solution is defined as being **acidic.** When H^+ concentration is less than 1×10^{-7} or when the pH is greater than 7.00 in a solution, it is said to be **basic,** or **alkalotic.** The H^+ concentration of blood is 40 nEq/L, and the pH is 7.40, making blood a slightly alkalotic solution.

In medicine and physiology the use of the pH scale is the favored way of describing overall acid-base balance in body fluids. Table 14-3 shows an expanded relationship between H^+ concentration and pH in the physiologic range around a normal blood pH of 7.40.

Henderson-Hasselbalch Equation

The pH of a solution is influenced by the amount of acid and base in the solution. This

Table 14-2 Comparison of the [H^+] and pH Scales

[H^+]*		pH
1		0
0.1		1
0.01		2
0.001	Acidic	3
0.0001		4
0.00001		5
0.000001		6
0.0000001 or 1×10^{-7}	Neutral	7
0.00000001		8
0.000000001		9
0.0000000001		10
0.00000000001		11
0.000000000001	Basic	12
0.0000000000001		13
0.00000000000001		14

*[H^+] in moles or equivalents per liter.

Table 14-3 H^+ Concentration and pH Scale in the Physiological Range of Blood

[H^+] (nEq/L)	pH
10	8.00
20	7.70
30	7.52
40	7.40 (Normal arterial blood)
50	7.30
60	7.22
70	7.15
80	7.10
90	7.05
100	7.00

can be illustrated with the following acid-base reaction:

$$HA \rightarrow H^+ + A^-$$

This reaction can be rewritten with the dissociation constant as an equilibrium equation:

$$Ka \times [HA] = [H^+] \times [A^-]$$

This equation can be rewritten to isolate the dissociation constant:

$$Ka = \frac{[H^+] \times [A^-]}{[HA]}$$

Taking the logarithm of both sides results in the following:

$$logKa = log[H^+] + log\frac{[A^-]}{[HA]}$$

This can then be rearranged to the following equation:

$$-log[H^+] = -logKa + log\frac{[A^-]}{[HA]}$$

By using the negative log relationship, the equation can be rewritten into the following form:

$$pH = pKa + log\frac{[A^-]}{[HA]}$$

This equation was developed by Hasselbalch and is based on the original work of Henderson and is named for both of them—the Henderson-Hasselbalch equation. It is an important equation for the understanding of acid-base balance. It shows that the pH of a solution is influenced by the concentration ratio of base to acid.

⬤ WHY pH IS MAINTAINED SO CAREFULLY AND THE MAJOR THREATS TO IT

Importance of pH Regulation

Cellular function is optimal when the pH of intracellular and extracellular fluid is held at a specific value. Many different cellular functions are influenced when the pH strays from a normal value. This is brought about by the profound effect that changes in H^+ concentration have on the structure and function of protein.

Protein, comprised of a chain of amino acids, coils into various shapes and is held in these shapes by the formation of hydrogen and disulfide bonds between different parts of the amino acid chain. Hydrogen bonds form when a single H^+ is shared by two nearby amino acids. Acidic and alkalotic conditions cause changes in the distribution of hydrogen bonding within the protein, causing its shape to change. Proteins, therefore, require an optimal pH for optimal shape and function.

The metabolism of every cell depends on the function of many different proteins. If the pH of the fluids inside and outside the cell strays even a small degree from the optimal value, the function of the proteins, the metabolism of the cell, and the activities of the cell are altered. The body employs a number of different mechanisms to maintain body fluids at an optimal pH. Generally, the body maintains intracellular fluid in a range near 7.00 and the extracellular fluid in a slightly alkaline range around 7.40. By maintaining the extracellular pH in a slightly alkaline range, a concentration gradient that facilitates the movement of H^+ from the intracellular to the extracellular space is established.

Threats to a Normal pH Level

The body produces and excretes a phenomenal amount of H^+ from various metabolic wastes and maintains a minuscule amount of H^+ in extracellular fluid (Fig. 14-5). More than 20 billion nEq of H^+ are produced and excreted each day. This acid load is sufficient to cause the pH of body fluid to drop into a dangerous acidosis within minutes if the buffering and excretory mechanisms fail.

Different acids are produced in different quantities on a daily basis. They can be classified on the basis of their ability to vaporize and become gaseous. Those that can vaporize easily are classified as **volatile acids,** and those that vaporize poorly are classified as **nonvolatile acids.**

Volatile Acids

The vast majority of acid produced in the body is from the oxidative metabolism of glucose and fats. This results in a continuous production of CO_2 and water (Fig. 14-6). On a daily basis the cells produce about 450 L of CO_2. CO_2 diffuses into blood, where it is transported in a variety of forms to the lungs for excretion to the external environment (see Chapter 13). Most of the CO_2 combines with water to form carbonic acid (H_2CO_3):

$$CO_2 + H_2O \rightarrow H_2CO_3$$

This reaction is accelerated by the action of **carbonic anhydrase,** an enzyme found in

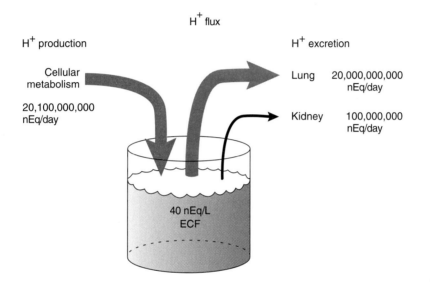

FIG. 14-5 Amount of H^+ that is produced from cellular metabolism and enters extracellular fluid (ECF) is balanced by the amount that is excreted through the actions of the lungs and kidneys. Despite this huge H^+ flux, the concentration is maintained at the incredibly small concentration of only 40 nEq/L.

$$\left.\begin{array}{l} \text{Glucose} + O_2 \rightarrow CO_2 + H_2O \rightarrow H^+ + HCO_3^- \\ \text{Fat} + O_2 \rightarrow CO_2 + H_2O \rightarrow H^+ + HCO_3^- \end{array}\right\} \begin{array}{c} 20{,}000{,}000{,}000 \\ \text{nEq/day} \end{array} \rightarrow \text{Lung}$$

$$\left.\begin{array}{l} \text{Glucose} \rightarrow \text{(Anaerobic metabolism)} \rightarrow H^+ + \text{Lactate}^- \\ \text{Cysteine} + O_2 \rightarrow H_2SO_4 \rightarrow 2H^+ + SO_4^= \\ \text{Phosphoprotein} + O_2 \rightarrow H_3PO_4 \rightarrow 2H^+ + HPO_4^= \end{array}\right\} \begin{array}{c} 100{,}000{,}000 \\ \text{nEq/day} \end{array} \rightarrow \text{Kidney}$$

FIG. 14-6 Sources of volatile acids that are excreted by the lungs and nonvolatile acids that are neutralized by buffers produced by the kidney.

erythrocytes and tubule cells of the kidney. H_2CO_3, a relatively weak acid, dissociates into H^+ and bicarbonate (HCO_3^-):

$$H_2CO_3 \rightarrow H^+ + HCO_3^-$$

From this reaction about 20 billion nEq of H^+ are produced and enter extracellular fluid. Fortunately, H_2CO_3 is a volatile acid. When blood circulates through the lungs, the reactions described previously are reversed as CO_2 diffuses from pulmonary capillary blood to alveolar gas:

$$H^+ + HCO_3^- \rightarrow H_2CO_3 \rightarrow CO_2 + H_2O$$

This makes H_2CO_3 a volatile acid because CO_2 can become gaseous and diffuse into alveolar gas and then be excreted. This is an important property that enables the body to easily rid itself of a huge source of H^+.

Nonvolatile Acids

H^+ is also produced from a variety of acids that are unable to become gaseous, making them unexcretable by the lungs. These acids, classified as nonvolatile acids, include sulfuric acid, phosphoric acid, lactic acid, and keto acids (see Fig. 14-6). Sulfuric acid is produced in small quantities from the oxidative metabolism of the amino acids cysteine and methionine, which all contain sulfur. Small quantities of phosphoric acid are produced from the metabolism of phospholipids, phosphoproteins, and nucleic acids. Lactic acid is a by-product of anaerobic metabolism of glucose. Normally anaerobic metabolism occurs at a low rate and is not a threat to pH. However, when O_2 delivery to the tissues falls to a level below what the cells need, the cells shift to anaerobic metabolism, producing large quantities of lactic acid. Keto acids (acetoacetic acid and beta-hydroxy butyric acid), which are normally produced in small quantities from the catabolism of lipids, do not threaten pH. Their production can increase when the cell does not receive enough glucose as a result of an insulin deficiency.

The total amount of nonvolatile acids produced on a daily basis is about 100 million nEq of H^+. Although this may sound like a large amount of H^+, it is only about 0.5% of the total amount produced normally. The H^+ that is released by these acids can be neutralized quickly by the large amount of buffers available inside and outside the cell. The amount of buffer consumed during these reactions is easily replaced by the actions of the kidney.

HOW pH IS MAINTAINED

The body uses a variety of mechanisms to maintain the pH of extracellular fluid in a

 Table 14-4   Major Buffers of the Body and their Dissociation Constants (pKa)

Buffer System	Reaction	pKa
INTRACELLULAR FLUID		
Protein	$HPr \rightarrow H^+ + Pr^-$	7
Bicarbonate	$H_2CO_3 \rightarrow H^+ + HCO_3^-$	6.1
Sulfate	$HSO_4^- \rightarrow H^+ + SO_4^=$	7
Organic phosphate	$H_2PO_4^- \rightarrow H^+ + HPO_4^=$	6.1
INTERSTITIAL FLUID		
Protein	$HPr \rightarrow H^+ + Pr^-$	7
Bicarbonate	$H_2CO_3 \rightarrow H^+ + HCO_3^-$	6.1
Sulfate	$HSO_4^- \rightarrow H^+ + SO_4$	7
ERYTHROCYTE		
Hemoglobin	$HHb \rightarrow H^+ + Hb^-$	8.2
Oxyhemo-globin	$HHbO_2 \rightarrow H^+ + HbO_2^-$	6.6
Bicarbonate	$H_2CO_3 \rightarrow H^+ + HCO_3^-$	6.1
Inorganic phosphate	$H_2PO_4^- \rightarrow H^+ + HPO_4^=$	6.8
BLOOD PLASMA		
Protein	$HPr \rightarrow H^+ + Pr^-$	7
Bicarbonate	$H_2CO_3 \rightarrow H^+ + HCO_3^-$	6.1
Sulfate	$HSO_4^- \rightarrow H^+ + SO_4^=$	7

slightly alkaline state with respect to the neutral intracellular pH. By keeping the extracellular fluid slightly alkaline, H^+ tends to flow out of the cell. Maintenance of extracellular fluid pH is achieved through two general mechanisms: (1) maintaining a pool of buffers through the actions of the kidney and (2) excreting CO_2 by the lungs. These mechanisms are regulated so precisely that the pH of arterial blood is maintained at 7.40 with a variance of only ±0.05 pH units.

Buffer Systems

The body maintains a large amount of buffer in both the intracellular and extracellular fluids (Table 14-4). The various buffer systems act as a first line of defense. They absorb H^+ that is released by the different acids produced from metabolism. By maintaining certain buffer combinations and regulating their concentration, the body can set a pH range and

protect it. Those buffer combinations that have a pKa close to the desired pH provide the most protection.

All of the buffer systems "work" together to minimize pH change. They do this together by absorbing or releasing H^+ simultaneously. This simultaneous activity is known as the isohydric principle. Some buffers absorb or release more H^+ than others. Those buffers with a pKa closer to the target pH provide the best buffer action.

Important Buffers in the Body

The body maintains different buffer systems in various regions of the body (Fig. 14-7). These buffers are maintained at different concentrations. The intracellular compartment possesses a wealth of buffers while the extracellular compartment has similar buffers in lower concentration.

PROTEIN. Protein is found on both sides of the cell membrane. Within the cell, it is

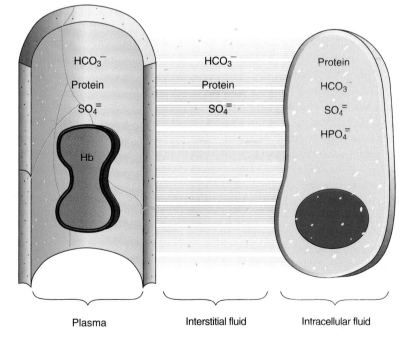

FIG. 14-7 Important buffers found in various fluid compartments in the order of their importance.

maintained at a much higher concentration. It functions as a buffer through the actions of its weak basic and acidic amino acid side chains (Pr$^-$ and HPr). It is thought that the imidazole groups of the amino acid histidine and N-terminal amino groups of several amino acids are the most important buffering groups within protein. They have dissociation constants that are close to 7.0.

Blood has a variety of extracellular and intracellular proteins that are important buffers. Blood plasma contains about 7 g of protein per deciliter, most of which is albumin. Within the erythrocyte is a large quantity of hemoglobin (Hb). Hb is an important buffer that has a buffering capability that is about six times that of the plasma proteins. Hb exists in either deoxygenated (Hb) or oxygenated (O_2Hb) states. The much greater dissociation constant of the deoxygenated form makes it much more capable of absorbing H$^+$ near a pH range of 7.40.

BICARBONATE. HCO_3^- and H_2CO_3 comprise an important buffer system that is formed from the reaction of CO_2 and H_2O and found in both the intracellular and extracellular compartments. HCO_3^- is primarily produced within the erythrocyte and tubule cells of the kidney. Most of the HCO_3^- that forms within the cell moves to the extracellular space in exchange for Cl$^-$. This exchange is known as the **chloride shift** and is performed to maintain the proper charge state on either side of the cell membrane.

The HCO_3^- buffer system is the most important buffer pair from the standpoint of its potential to be adjusted in order to maintain a desired pH. Unlike protein, which has a concentration that is maintained in response to a large variety of metabolic reactions, HCO_3^- concentration can be increased or decreased by the actions of the kidney. This makes it a useful point of control to adjust the pH to an optimal level. However, the body's ability to change HCO_3^- concentration is a relatively slow process.

SULFATE AND PHOSPHATE. Small quantities of sulfate (HSO_4^- and $SO_4^=$) and inorganic and organic phosphate ($H_2PO_4^-$ and $HPO_4^=$, glucose-6-$H_2PO_4^-$ and glucose-6-$HPO_4^=$) buffers are produced within the cell. Organic phosphate is also found within erythrocytes in the form of diphosphoglyceric acid. Sulfate and phosphate buffers are important but play a minor role as buffers in the extracellular fluid. Within the cell, they provide about one fourth of total buffering power.

Regulation of Extracellular Buffers

A certain amount of strong cations (e.g., Na$^+$, K$^+$, Mg^{++}, and Ca^{++}) and anions (e.g., Cl$^-$ $SO_4^=$, and $HPO_4^=$) are present in all body fluids. When the total amount of cations is compared with the total amount of anions, a difference is detected (Fig. 14-8). This difference is known as the strong ion difference (SID), or the **anion gap**. The SID represents the combined concentration of protein and HCO_3^- (Box 14-2). The greatest SID is found in intracellular fluid where it reaches a difference of 130 mEq/L because a large number of proteins are found within the cell. In blood plasma the SID totals 42 mEq/L where a little more than half of it is in the form of HCO_3^-.

The SID represents the amount of anion necessary to balance the number of cations (primarily Na$^+$) to maintain electrical neutrality. SID is regulated by the amount of renal reabsorption of Na$^+$. Greater Na$^+$ reabsorption yields a greater SID and visa versa. Although total protein concentration in any of the compartments is an important buffer, it is not regulated with respect to maintenance of ion or acid-base balance. HCO_3^- ion is adjusted up or down to balance the difference. Thus by adjusting the SID through the action of renal Na$^+$ reabsorption, the body can regulate the amount of HCO_3^- being reabsorbed and formed. By doing this, the body maintains a plasma HCO_3^- concentration of 22 to 26 mEq/L.

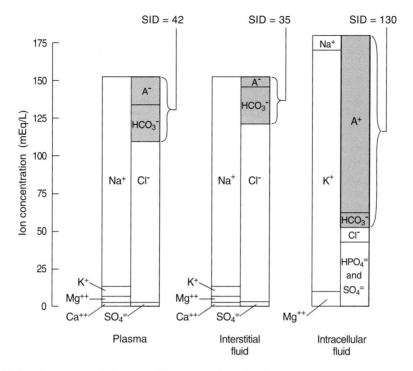

FIG. 14-8 Strong ion difference *(SID)* in various body fluids represents the amount of anions that are in the form of bicarbonate *(HCO$_3$$^-$)* and protein *(A$^-$)*.

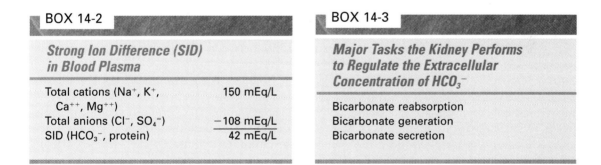

BOX 14-2	
Strong Ion Difference (SID) in Blood Plasma	
Total cations (Na$^+$, K$^+$, Ca^{++}, Mg^{++})	150 mEq/L
Total anions (Cl$^-$, SO$_4$$^=$)	−108 mEq/L
SID (HCO$_3$$^-$, protein)	42 mEq/L

BOX 14-3
Major Tasks the Kidney Performs to Regulate the Extracellular Concentration of HCO$_3$$^-$
Bicarbonate reabsorption
Bicarbonate generation
Bicarbonate secretion

Renal Regulation of Bicarbonate

The role of the kidney in acid-base balance centers on its ability to regulate the concentration of extracellular buffers. It does this by changing the SID through adjustment of Na$^+$ reabsorption into blood. By adjusting the SID up or down, more or less HCO$_3$$^-$ can be placed into blood.

The kidney performs three different tasks to regulate the HCO$_3$$^-$ concentration (Box 14-3). First, the kidney must reabsorb HCO$_3$$^-$ that is filtered out of blood during the initial step in the formation of urine. If this were not done, the body would lose more than 4000 mEq of HCO$_3$$^-$ per day. The process of reabsorbing HCO$_3$$^-$ from tubular fluid as shown in

Fig. 14-9, *A,* is an indirect process that requires conversion to CO_2 for diffusion into the renal tubular cell, conversion back into H_2CO_3 with the help of intracellular carbonic anhydrase, and reabsorption with Na^+ into blood.

Bicarbonate generation by the kidney is the second task performed. The kidney carries out this task to form about 100 mEq of HCO_3^-. This is the amount lost in the process of neutralizing the nonvolatile acids that enter the system on a daily basis. This process also results in the acidification of urine. To form excess HCO_3^- and absorb it, the kidney uses ammonia and phosphate to trap H^+ in the urine. Fig. 14-9, *B* and *C* shows the absorption of H^+ by phosphate ions ($HPO_4^=$) and ammonia (NH_3), the generation of HCO_3^-, and the movement of HCO_3^- with Na^+ into blood. This HCO_3^- generation mechanism can be increased or decreased to adjust the HCO_3^- concentration in extracellular fluid. Some tubule cells have the capability to secrete H^+ into the tubular fluid while they reabsorb K^+. This process, coupled with the ammonia and phosphate excretion mechanisms, results in the acidification of urine.

Some of the tubule cells of the kidney can perform the third task of bicarbonate secretion. Some tubule cells have the capability to reabsorb Cl^- into blood and secrete HCO_3^- into tubular fluid. This mechanism is active at a minor rate but can become more active during conditions of alkalosis when the body needs to decrease the total amount of base in extracellular and intracellular fluid.

Carbon Dioxide Excretion

The lung plays a vital role in the maintenance of extracellular and intracellular pH through the excretion of CO_2. When CO_2 is produced and enters blood, it combines with water (under the influence of carbonic anhydrase) to form H_2CO_3, which dissociates H^+ and HCO_3^-. The H^+ that enters blood from this reaction is buffered by the proteins in blood, and the pH of systemic venous blood drops to

7.35. When blood enters the pulmonary capillaries, these reactions are reversed, the buffers release the H^+, CO_2 reforms and diffuses to the alveolar gas, and the pH of blood leaving the lung increases to 7.40. This process prevents the accumulation of about 20,000,000,000 nEq of H^+ in the system on a daily basis. Despite the large quantity of CO_2 added to the system and then excreted, the buffers are capable of minimizing large changes in pH.

The lung only excretes about 8% of the total amount of CO_2 present in the blood. The amount of CO_2 in blood can be determined by measuring the PCO_2. The PCO_2 in blood depends on the amount of CO_2 added to blood ($\dot{V}CO_2$) and the alveolar PCO_2 to which it is exposed. Alveolar PCO_2 is inversely related to the rate of alveolar ventilation ($\dot{V}_A$). Since arterial blood and alveolar PCO_2 become equilibrated following gas exchange in the lung, it can be stated that the $PaCO_2$ is directly related to $\dot{V}CO_2$ and inversely related to $\dot{V}_A$ as shown in the following relationship:

$$PaCO_2 \approx P_ACO_2 = K \frac{\dot{V}CO_2}{\dot{V}_A}$$

where K is a constant. This relationship shows that the $PaCO_2$ is determined by the ratio between metabolic rate and alveolar ventilation.

Changes in the amount of ventilation or the rate of CO_2 production can bring about rapid changes in the PCO_2 in both venous and arterial blood. Unlike the kidney, which requires several days to make changes in the buffering system, the respiratory system can cause changes in the $PaCO_2$ in just several minutes.

Respiratory Regulation of pH

Normally the PCO_2 in arterial blood is maintained at 40 ± 5 mm Hg by adjusting the alveolar ventilation in such a way as to result in excretion of just enough CO_2 to match the amount that was added by the tissues. This is carried out by the respiratory control system and chemoreceptors that are sensitive to CO_2 and H^+ (see Chapter 15). The control center

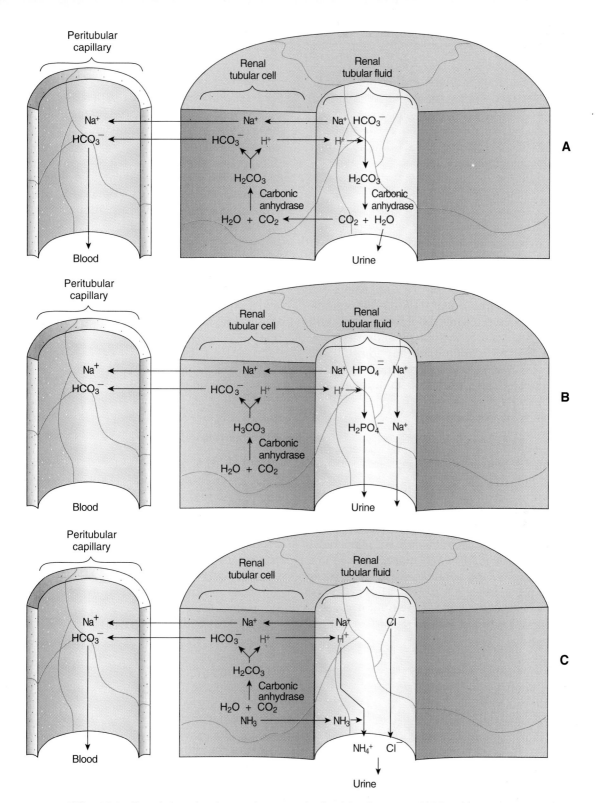

FIG. 14-9 Renal mechanisms that result in bicarbonate (HCO_3^-) production. A, HCO_3^- absorption from urine. B, Phosphate absorption of hydrogen ions (H^+). C, Ammonia formation.

adjusts the activity of the respiratory muscle, which, in turn, adjusts the alveolar ventilation. The entire system is set to maintain a PaCO₂ of 40 mm Hg. By doing so, the pH of blood is maintained at 7.40 and the pH of intracellular fluid is maintained at 7.00.

Renal and Pulmonary Interaction

The lungs and kidneys interact to maintain a precise extracellular fluid pH by manipulating different aspects of the CO_2 and H_2O equilibrium reaction (Fig. 14-10). This is carried out by the lung's regulation of CO_2 content and the kidney's adjustment of HCO_3^- concentration. By doing this, the amount of H_2CO_3 and HCO_3^- that are formed can be adjusted. The pH of extracellular fluid is set by adjusting the concentrations of this buffer pair. The Henderson-Hasselbalch relationship shows this:

$$pH = pKa + \log \frac{[HCO_3^-]}{[H_2CO_3]}$$

At a normal body temperature, the equation can use a pKa = 6.1:

$$pH = 6.1 + \log \frac{[HCO_3^-]}{[H_2CO_3]}$$

The concentration of HCO_3^- in blood and interstitial fluid is influenced by renal function, production of nonvolatile acids, and to a small degree the amount of CO_2 the lungs allow to remain in the system. The concentration of H_2CO_3 in extracellular fluid is primarily influenced by the amount of CO_2 that is present.

HCO_3^-/H_2CO_3 Ratio and pH

The concentration of H_2CO_3 that forms in extracellular fluid is influenced by the PCO₂ as shown in the following relationship:

$$[H_2CO_3] = PCO_2 \times 0.0301 \text{ mEq/L/mm Hg}$$

This relationship can be introduced into the Henderson-Hasselbalch equation as follows:

$$pH = 6.1 + \log \frac{[HCO_3^-]}{PCO_2 \times 0.0301}$$

Normally, the kidneys maintain an HCO_3^- concentration of 24 mEq/L and the lungs maintain a PCO₂ of 40 mm Hg. These values can be introduced into the Henderson-Hasselbalch equation to determine the resulting pH:

$$\begin{aligned} pH &= 6.1 + \log \frac{24 \text{ mEq/L}}{40 \text{ mm Hg} \times 0.0301} \\ &= 6.1 + \log \frac{(24 \text{ mEq/L})}{1.2 \text{ mEq/L}} \\ &= 6.1 + \log(20:1) \\ &= 6.1 + 1.3 \\ &= 7.4 \end{aligned}$$

Thus a normal pH is produced when the HCO_3^- concentration and PCO₂ are maintained at normal values.

The Henderson-Hasselbalch equation also demonstrates that a normal pH is generated when the HCO_3^-/H_2CO_3 ratio is 20:1. The maintenance of this ratio at 20:1 produces a pH of 7.40 (Fig. 14-11). When the $HCO_3^-/$

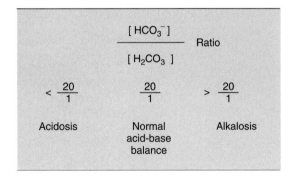

FIG. 14-11 Changes in the HCO_3^-/H_2CO_3 ratio cause acid-base changes.

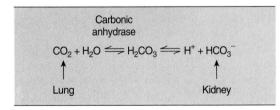

FIG. 14-10 Lungs and kidney adjust different aspects of the CO_2-H_2CO_3-HCO_3^- reaction.

H_2CO_3 ratio is not equal to 20:1, the pH will not be 7.4. Ratios of less than 20:1 result in a lower pH or acidosis. For example, a ratio of 10:1 causes the pH to change in the following manner:

$$pH = 6.1 + \log(10:1)$$
$$= 6.1 + 1.0$$
$$= 7.0$$

In this example a pH of 7.0 is a relative acidosis when compared with normal blood pH of 7.40. This situation can be brought about by either a decrease in the concentration of HCO_3^- or an increase in the concentration of H_2CO_3.

Ratios that are greater than 20:1 result in a greater pH or alkalosis. For example, a ratio of 30:1 causes the pH to change in the following manner:

$$pH = 6.1 + \log(30:1)$$
$$= 6.1 + 1.48$$
$$= 7.58$$

Conditions that bring about an increased ratio include greater concentrations of HCO_3^- or lower concentrations of H_2CO_3. Thus the renal regulation of HCO_3^- and the pulmonary adjustment of PCO_2 result in the regulation of the HCO_3^-/H_2CO_3 ratio and pH.

"Seeing" Normal Acid-Base Balance

Several different approaches to illustrating acid-base balance have been developed, all illustrating the Henderson-Hasselbalch equation as some form of pH-HCO_3^--PCO_2 diagram. The most popular was developed by Davenport in the 1950s. In the Davenport diagram the pH is shown in Fig. 14-12, *A*, as a horizontal scale. In Fig. 14-12, *B*, the HCO_3^- concentration is added as a vertical scale. A diagonal line runs through this diagram and illustrates the effect that changes of HCO_3^- concentration have on pH when the PCO_2 is maintained at 40 mm Hg. It is a direct relationship: increasing amounts of HCO_3^- result in an increased pH and vice versa. The effect that

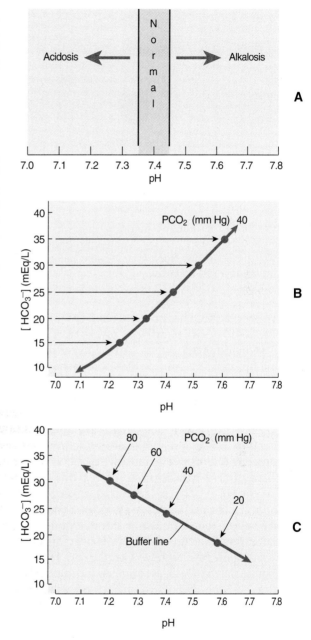

FIG. 14-12 Development of the Davenport diagrams. **A,** The pH scale of extracellular fluid. **B,** Effect on pH when changes in bicarbonate *([HCO_3^-])* concentration occur during a constant partial pressure of carbon dioxide *(PCO_2)* of 40 mm Hg. **C,** Changes in PCO_2 (shown as individualized points known as isobars) bring about changes in both [HCO_3^-] concentration and pH.

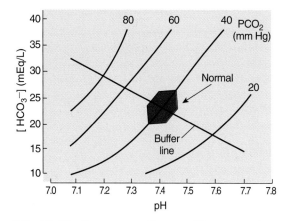

FIG. 14-13 Davenport diagram illustrates the relationship that [HCO$_3^-$] concentration and PCO$_2$ have on pH. Normal acid-base balance is shown as a red polygon.

changes in PCO$_2$ has on the system is shown in Fig. 14-12, *C*. Different PCO$_2$ levels are shown as individualized points. All of these points line up on a straight line that depicts how the pH and HCO$_3^-$ concentration change as the PCO$_2$ increases or decreases. This line is known as the *buffer line* of extracellular fluid.

These different elements are brought together in Fig. 14-13. The red polygon in the center of the diagram represents the normal range of acid-base balance. Within this polygon the HCO$_3^-$/H$_2$CO$_3$ ratio is at or very close to 20:1. Abnormal ratios generate abnormal pH values that lie outside the polygon. The buffer line that runs through the normal acid-base region reveals how the pH and HCO$_3^-$ change as the PCO$_2$ is adjusted up or down from 40 mm Hg. Each particular value of PCO$_2$ is defined by a line that is referred to as an **isobar.** In this example only four PCO$_2$ isobars represent the values of 20, 40, 60, and 80 mm Hg. Many more could be drawn. Each isobar represents a constant PCO$_2$ value and how variations of HCO$_3^-$ concentration would affect the pH along that line.

By looking at this diagram, the pH for various combinations of PCO$_2$ and HCO$_3^-$ con-

centration can be predicted. For example, if the PCO$_2$ is 80 mm Hg and the HCO$_3^-$ is 28 mEq/L the pH could be found by locating these values on the diagram, finding where they intersect, and reading down to the resulting pH. In this case it would be 7.19. Once this is done, the necessary action to correct the situation and return the pH to a normal value can also be seen. In this example, reduction of the PCO$_2$ to 40 mm Hg returns the pH along the buffer line to the normal region.

● HOW ACID-BASE BALANCE IS DESCRIBED

Indicators of Acid-Base Balance and Their Measurement

Normal acid-base balance is typically described by evaluating several different variables. The major elements of the Henderson-Hasselbalch equation (pH, PCO$_2$, and HCO$_3^-$) are the most commonly used. By sampling blood and measuring these variables, the acid-base conditions of an individual can be described. In addition to these three variables, several others have been developed and have been found to be useful. All of the different variables can be organized under three main headings: overall indicators, respiratory indicators, and metabolic indicators (Table 14-5).

Overall Indicators

The overall indicator of acid-base balance is the pH with a normal value in arterial blood of 7.35 to 7.45.

The pH of blood is commonly measured with a pH electrode system, which consists of two half-cells: a measuring half-cell and a reference half-cell. The measuring half-cell has a silver/silver chloride anode that reacts with the blood specimen housed on one side of pH-sensitive glass. The reference half-cell consists of a mercury/mercury dichloride calomel cathode. When blood is placed in the sample chamber, it completes an electrical circuit

● Table 14-5   Types of Acid-Base Indicators and their Normal Values in Blood

	Arterial Blood	Mixed Venous Blood
OVERALL INDICATORS		
[H^+]	35-45	40-50 nEq/L
pH	7.35-7.45	7.30-7.40
RESPIRATORY INDICATOR		
PCO_2	35-45	41-50 mm Hg
METABOLIC INDICATORS		
Total CO_2	24-29	26-30 mmol/L
Plasma HCO_3^-	24-26	26-28 mEq/L
Standard HCO_3^-	24-26	26-28 mEq/L
Base excess	−2-2	−1-3 mEq/L
Strong ion difference	40-44	42-46 mEq/L

between the two half-cells. The amount of H^+ present in the sample causes a certain voltage change between the two half-cells. This voltage change can be measured and compared with that produced by a known standard solution. Based on the comparison, the pH of the blood sample can be determined with considerable accuracy to a level of ±0.005 pH unit.

Respiratory Indicator

The respiratory indicator is the PCO_2 in blood. The PCO_2 in arterial blood in an individual with alveolar ventilation that is appropriate for his or her metabolic rate is 35 to 45 mm Hg. It is called the *respiratory indicator* because of its link to the level of gas exchange in the tissues and the lungs.

A PCO_2 electrode, the most common device used to make this measurement, is a modified pH electrode that has a CO_2-permeable membrane that covers the portion of the electrode that is exposed to blood. Between the membrane and electrode surface is an HCO_3^- and H_2CO_3 buffer solution. CO_2 molecules diffuse from the blood specimen, through the membrane and into the buffer solution where they react with the buffer solution. The addition of CO_2 to the solution results in the production of H_2CO_3, which dissociates into HCO_3^- and H^+, causing the solution to become acidic in proportion to the amount of CO_2 that is in the blood sample. The pH change that is detected by the electrode is compared with the known change that occurs when the electrode is exposed to a calibrating gas with a known PCO_2. By comparing the voltage change brought about by the blood sample with that which occurs with a known calibrating gas, the PCO_2 in the blood sample can be determined with an accuracy of ±2 mm Hg.

Metabolic Indicators

Several variables have been developed to determine the concentration of buffers in blood. These different variables are classed together as the metabolic indicators. Because the buffers all react together when acid or base is added to a solution and because they all remain in an equilibrium concentration with one another (the isohydric principle), determining the concentration of one buffer gives sufficient information about the state of the other buffers in the solution. Considerable effort has been made over the past 70 years to find a variable that more purely reflects the status of the buffer system in response to metabolism and not respiratory changes.

TOTAL CARBON DIOXIDE. One of the early approaches was the determination of the **total CO_2** per liter of blood. By determining the total CO_2, one could get some appreciation for the status of the buffering system since about 68% of the CO_2 is in the form of HCO_3^-. The normal value in arterial blood is 24 to 29 mmol/L.

Total CO_2 can be determined by adding strong acid to a sample of blood, which causes all of the CO_2 to be converted to the gaseous form. The volume that forms can then be measured and converted to the millimole per liter scale. Later an alternative method was developed that allowed the mathematical determination based on the following relationship:

Total CO$_2$ = [HCO$_3^-$] + [CO$_2$ protein] + [CO$_2$ dissolved]

Increases and decreases in total CO$_2$ reflect changes in the amount of HCO$_3^-$ and protein that are present in blood. It is, however, sensitive to PCO$_2$ changes and this makes it an impure variable to evaluate just the metabolic influences on the buffer system.

PLASMA HCO$_3^-$. The most popular metabolic indicator of acid-base balance is the plasma HCO$_3^-$ concentration. Its normal value in arterial blood is 22 to 26 mEq/L. This value is not measured with a detector but determined with a variation of the Henderson-Hasselbalch equation:

$$HCO_3^- = 0.03107 \times PCO_2 \times 10^{(pH-6.1)}$$

By measuring the pH and PCO$_2$ in a sample and "plugging" these values into this equation, the plasma HCO$_3^-$ concentration can be determined, with reasonable accuracy, to a level of ±0.5 mEq/L. Plasma HCO$_3^-$ concentration is, however, not a pure indicator of metabolic influence on the concentrations of the buffers. When CO$_2$ reacts with water it produces a small amount of HCO$_3^-$ when H$_2$CO$_3$ dissociates. As a consequence, changes in PCO$_2$ bring about small changes in plasma HCO$_3^-$ concentration. For example, if individuals decrease their ventilation and their PCO$_2$ acutely increases from 40 to 50 mm Hg, the plasma HCO$_3^-$ concentration increases 2 mEq/L. This change can be seen when examining the slope of the buffer line in the Davenport diagram (see Fig. 14-13). This change, however, is not being brought about by metabolic changes but by a respiratory change. This makes the plasma HCO$_3^-$ concentration less reliable as an indicator of pure metabolic change.

STANDARD BICARBONATE. An attempt to reduce the influence that PCO$_2$ changes have on the HCO$_3^-$ concentration gave rise to the development of the **standard HCO$_3^-$ concen**tration concept. Standard HCO$_3^-$ concentration is calculated in the same way that plasma HCO$_3^-$ concentration is calculated but with one exception—it uses the measured pH and substitutes a normal PCO$_2$ of 40 mm Hg into the equation instead of the actual value. This helps reduce the impact that changes in PCO$_2$ have on the calculated HCO$_3^-$ concentration. This produces a purer determination of the effect that various metabolic activities are having on the buffer system. A normal value in arterial blood is 22 to 26 mEq/L.

BASE EXCESS. Another approach to determining the amount of base present in blood led to the development of the **base excess (BE)** calculation. This approach looks at the amount of increase or decrease in total buffers relative to a normal mid-point value (Fig. 14-14). This makes BE a more robust variable that is sensitive to many more changes in buffering. The normal range of base excess is −2 to 2 mEq/L. Positive values reflect excess base whereas negative values show an actual **base deficit.**

Base excess can be determined by the analysis of the pH-HCO$_3^-$-PCO$_2$ diagram shown in Fig. 14-15. The vertical distance that an individual data point lies from the buffer line corresponds to the excess or deficit amount of base that is present in blood. It is more frequently determined with the following equation:

$$BE = (1 - 0.0143Hb)[(HCO_3^-) - (9.5 + 1.63Hb)(7.4pH) - 24]$$

The concept of base excess allows the clinician to better recognize pure metabolic acid-base derangements and calculate the total amount of excess or deficit buffer that is present in the entire blood volume. Once knowing this, the clinician can then calculate the amount of base or acid to give the patient to correct metabolic abnormalities.

STRONG ION DIFFERENCE. A more modern approach judges the status of the buffering system by determining the SID. As described earlier, SID is equal to the difference between

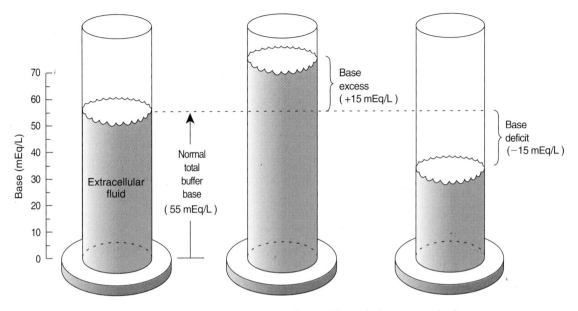

FIG. 14-14 Amount of surplus or shortage in total base is known as the base excess and deficit.

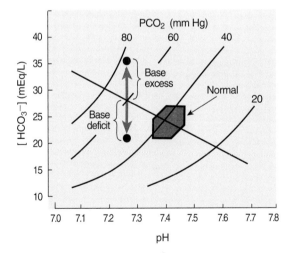

FIG. 14-15 Base excess and base deficit are determined by analyzing the vertical distance that an acid-base data point lies above or below the buffer line.

the sum of major cations (e.g., Na^+, K^+, Ca^{++}, Mg^{++}) and the sum of major anions (e.g., Cl^-, $SO_4^=$). This difference is comprised of HCO_3^- and protein. The normal SID in arterial blood is 40 to 44 mEq/L. It is a relatively pure metabolic variable of acid-base status. It is determined by measuring the major cations and anions and simply calculating the difference. It does not require the determination of PCO_2 or pH.

Siggaard-Anderson Nomogram

Most of the metabolic indicators can be graphically determined with an alignment nomogram (Fig. 14-16). This nomogram was developed by Siggard-Anderson in the early 1960s for the manual determination of various metabolic indicators. For example, locate a normal PCO_2 of 40 mm Hg and pH of 7.40. Extend a straight line through these two points and on through the other scales. The line should pass through a total CO_2 of 25 mmol/L, plasma HCO_3^- of 24 mEq/L, and base excess (using a normal Hb of 15 g/100 ml) of 0 mEq/L. The nomogram can also be used to show the impact that different combinations of PCO_2 and HCO_3^- concentration have on the pH. Modern day blood gas analyzers perform all of these different calculations and report the values.

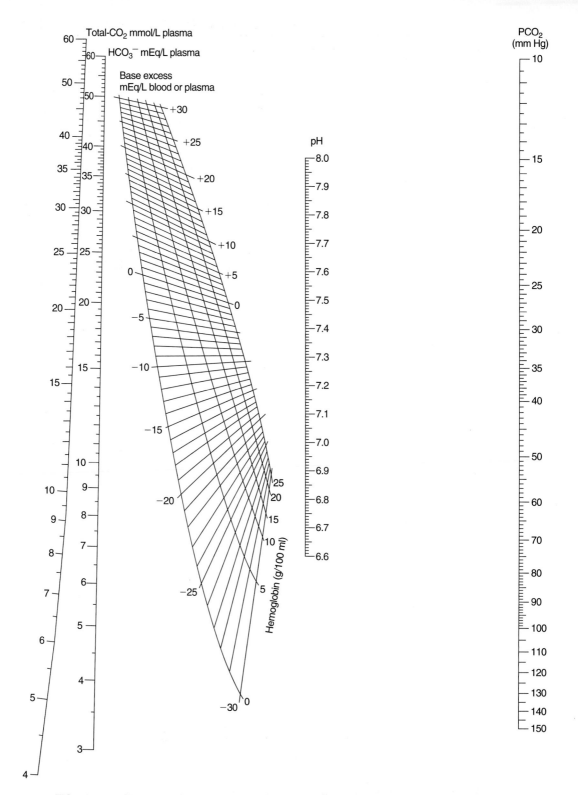

FIG. 14-16 Siggard-Anderson alignment nomogram can be used to determine the total CO_2, plasma HCO_3^-, and base excess by placing a straight line through measured PCO_2 and pH values.

ACID-BASE BALANCE DISORDERS

Primary Acid-Base Disturbances

Various conditions cause an acid-base imbalance by disturbing the rate of acid addition or by disturbing the amount of buffers in the system. When this occurs the HCO_3^-/H_2CO_3 ratio is altered from a value of 20:1 and the pH becomes abnormal.

The ratio normally remains at a value of 20:1 through independent adjustment of PCO_2 by the lungs and HCO_3^- concentration by the kidneys. Normal PCO_2 and HCO_3^- concentration brings about a normal balance and normal pH (Fig. 14-17). The ratio can be dis-

turbed when the lungs fail to maintain the PCO_2 at an appropriate level or when the kidneys fail to maintain the HCO_3^- at an appropriate concentration. Acid-base abnormalities brought about by an abnormal PCO_2 are termed *respiratory disturbances,* and those caused by abnormal HCO_3^- concentrations are termed *metabolic disturbances.* These two general types of disturbances can be further subclassified into four types of primary acid-base disturbances. They include **respiratory acidosis, respiratory alkalosis, metabolic acidosis,** and **metabolic alkalosis.** The conditions that define these primary disturbances are listed in Table 14-6.

Table 14-6   Types of Primary Acid-Base Disturbances

	pH	PCO$_2$ (mm Hg)	Plasma [HCO$_3^-$] (mEq/L)	Standard [HCO$_3^-$] (mEq/L)	BE (mEq/L)	SID (mEq/L)
Normal	7.35-7.45	35-45	22-24	22-24	−2-2	40-44
Respiratory acidosis	↓	↑	LC	LC	NC	NC
Respiratory alkalosis	↑	↓	LC	LC	NC	NC
Metabolic acidosis	↓	NC	↓	↓	↓	↓
Metabolic alkalosis	↑	NC	↑	↑	↑	↑

BE, Base excess; *SID,* strong ion difference; *LC,* little change; *NC,* no change.

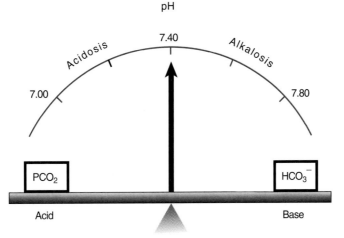

FIG. 14-17 Normal partial pressure of carbon dioxide *(PCO$_2$)* and bicarbonate *(HCO$_3^-$)* concentration results in a normal "balance" that results in a normal pH.

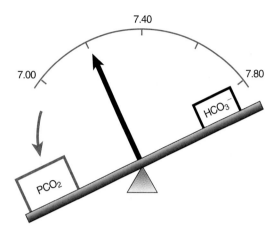

FIG. 14-18 Increased partial pressure of carbon dioxide *(PCO₂)* results in a respiratory acidosis. *HCO₃⁻,* Bicarbonate.

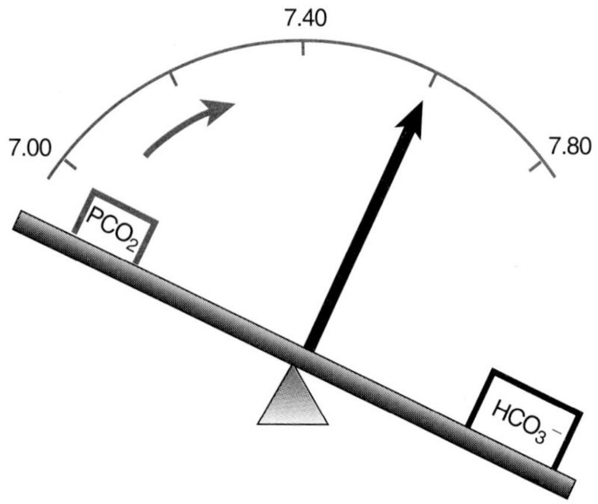

FIG. 14-19 Decreased partial pressure of carbon dioxide *(PCO₂)* results in a respiratory alkalosis. *HCO₃⁻,* Bicarbonate.

BOX 14-4

Causes and Mechanisms of Hypoventilation and Respiratory Acidosis

Drug overdose	↓ Respiratory control center activity
General anesthesia	↓ Respiratory control center activity and muscle paralysis
Brain damage	Respiratory control center activity dysfunction
Neuromuscular disease	Peripheral nerve and muscle failure
Morbid obesity	Chest wall and diaphragmatic compression
Lung disease	Airway obstruction, reduced compliance, $\dot{V}/\dot{Q}$ mismatching and hypoventilation

Respiratory Acidosis

The defining abnormality in a respiratory disturbance is a change in PCO_2. Respiratory acidosis is indicated by an elevated PCO_2. This situation is caused by different conditions that result in alveolar hypoventilation (Box 14-4). Alveolar hypoventilation leads to CO_2 retention and an elevated PCO_2. Increased PCO_2 increases the formation of H_2CO_3, causing the HCO_3^-/H_2CO_3 ratio to drop below 20:1, which lowers the pH into acidosis (Fig. 14-18). The metabolic indicators generally remain normal (see Table 14-6). Respiratory acidosis can be corrected by either increasing alveolar ventilation with a mechanical ventilator or by decreasing the metabolic rate and reducing CO_2 production.

Respiratory Alkalosis

Respiratory alkalosis, indicated by a reduced PCO_2, is caused by various conditions that stimulate the respiratory center and excessive alveolar ventilation (Box 14-5). Excessive alveolar ventilation results in greater CO_2 excretion, which produces less H_2CO_3. As a result, the HCO_3^-/H_2CO_3 ratio is increased above 20:1 and the pH increases into an alkalosis (Fig. 14-19). During a pure respiratory alkalosis, the metabolic indicators generally remain normal (Table 14-6). The correction for this problem is the reduction of excessive alveolar ventilation.

CASE STUDY FOCUS

Drug Overdose-Induced Acid-Base Imbalance

A 63-year-old man was despondent after the death of his wife and intentionally ingested an overdosage of barbiturates and ethyl alcohol. He slipped into a coma, was discovered by his daughter, and was brought to the hospital by paramedics. On admission to the emergency department, an arterial blood sample was collected from the radial artery while he was breathing 60% O_2 by mask and the following was found:

pH = 7.18
PCO_2 = 62 mm Hg
PO_2 = 133 mm Hg
HCO_3^- = 14 mEq/L
Base excess = 0 mEq/L
Creatinine = 1.5 mg/dl

Na^+ = 137 mEq/L
K^+ = 3.8 mEq/L
Ca^{++} = 8.7 mEq/L
Cl^- = 103 mEq/L
Blood urea nitrogen = 18 mg/dl

These findings show hyperoxia, although the calculation of the PaO_2/FIO_2 is 222 and is much lower than the normal value of 500, indicating $\dot{V}/\dot{Q}$ mismatching, diffusion defect, or shunting. The $PaCO_2$ indicates hypoventilation and the pH, HCO_3^-, and base excess indicate uncompensated respiratory acidosis. The electrolyte concentrations are all within normal limits. To correct the respiratory acidosis, the patient was intubated and ventilated. A repeat blood gas showed normalization of the PCO_2 and pH. He was transferred to the medical intensive care unit for further stabilization and was weaned from ventilatory support 20 hours later. He was discharged following psychiatric consultation and follow-up 4 days after admission.

BOX 14-5

Causes and Mechanisms of Hyperventilation and Respiratory Alkalosis

Anxiety, pain, and fever
Stimulant drugs (amphetamines)
Progesterone (pregnancy)
Brain inflammation
High altitude (hypoxia)
Lung disease (hypoxia and dyspnea)
Heart disease (hypoxia)

} Respiratory control center stimulation

Pure respiratory disturbances that result in a sudden or acute change in alveolar ventilation cause the PCO_2 to change, which has a minor influence on the plasma HCO_3^- concentration. Fig. 14-20 illustrates how the HCO_3^--pH-PCO_2 relationship changes during acute changes in ventilation. During alveolar hypoventilation or alveolar hyperventilation, the PCO_2 increases or decreases along the buffer line respectively. This results in pH as well as HCO_3^- concentration changes. Nor-

mally, the pH changes 0.006 unit for a change of 1 mm Hg in the PCO_2. For example, if the PCO_2 increases from 40 to 60 mm Hg, the pH drops to 7.28. The plasma $[HCO_3^-]$ changes at a rate of 0.12 mEq/mm Hg.

A sudden decrease in alveolar ventilation produces **acute respiratory acidosis.** The opposite occurs during alveolar hyperventilation and the development of **acute respiratory alkalosis.** The changes in plasma HCO_3^- concentration that are brought about by a change

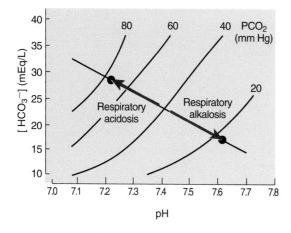

FIG. 14-20 Acute changes in ventilation cause either respiratory alkalosis or respiratory acidosis. Changes in partial pressure of carbon dioxide *(PCO₂)* cause changes in pH and bicarbonate *([HCO₃⁻])* that parallel the buffer line.

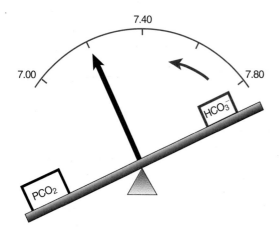

FIG. 14-21 Decreased bicarbonate *(HCO₃⁻)* results in a metabolic acidosis. *PCO₂,* Partial pressure of carbon dioxide.

in the PCO_2 reveal the weakness of using plasma HCO_3^- concentration as an indicator of metabolic status. Standard HCO_3^- concentration, base excess, and SID are not influenced as much by acute changes in PCO_2. These variables help in defining if a metabolic

> # BOX 14-6
>
> ## *Causes and Mechanisms of Metabolic Acidosis*
>
> | | |
> |---|---|
> | Circulatory failure | Hypoxia-driven lactic acid production |
> | Renal failure | ↓ HCO_3^- formed and H^+ excreted |
> | Uncontrolled diabetes | Keto acids formed |
> | Alcohol toxicity | Keto acids formed |
> | Aspirin overdose | ↑ Salicylic acid enters system |
> | Uncontrolled diarrhea | ↑ HCO_3^- loss |

component is present during an acid-base disturbance.

Metabolic Acidosis

Metabolic acidosis indicates the presence of **reduced plasma HCO_3^-**, standard HCO_3^-, or **BE.** Generally, SID decreases in a metabolic acidosis. Metabolic acidosis is caused by abnormal production of nonvolatile acids, failure to form HCO_3^-, or an excessive loss of HCO_3^-. All of these situations result in reduced HCO_3^- concentration, which causes a reduction in the HCO_3^-/H_2CO_3 ratio. Accordingly, the pH drops because of the disproportionately greater PCO_2 driven formation of H_2CO_3 (Fig. 14-21).

A variety of conditions can produce a metabolic acidosis (Box 14-6). The most common cause of this is circulatory failure and insufficient blood flow to the tissues, which results in a metabolic shift toward anaerobic reactions and the production of greater quantities of lactic acid. Renal failure, which also produces metabolic acidosis, results from the reduced ability to excrete H^+ and produce HCO_3^-. Severe insulin deficiency during uncontrolled diabetes can also result in metabolic acidosis. In this situation, the cells are unable to utilize glucose and they shift their metabolism to the

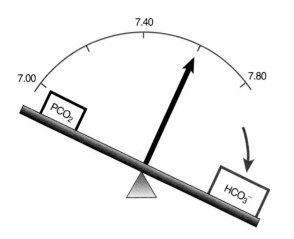

FIG. 14-22 Increased bicarbonate (HCO_3^-) results in a metabolic alkalosis. PCO_2, Partial pressure of carbon dioxide.

Causes and Mechanisms of Metabolic Alkalosis

HCO_3^- ingestion/ administration	↑HCO_3^- put into the system
Excess vomiting	↑Acid (HCl) loss
Diuretic therapy	↑Cl^- excretion, HCO_3^- retention, and H^+ excretion
Hypokalemia	↑H^+ movement into the cells and excreted by kidney
Excessive steroid therapy	Na^+ retention, ↑strong ion difference, and ↑HCO_3^- formation

oxidation of lipids, resulting in the production of keto acids (acetoacetic acid and beta-hydroxybutyric acid). In all of these situations, the HCO_3^- concentration drops as it interacts with the H^+ that these acids release. H_2CO_3 is formed and converted to CO_2 and H_2O. In the lung the CO_2 is excreted, resulting in a net loss of HCO_3^-. Conditions such as the failure of the kidney to form HCO_3^- or the loss of pancreatic-produced HCO_3^- during uncontrolled diarrhea are direct losses of Na^+ and HCO_3^- that can result in metabolic acidosis with a normal SID. The acute care for severe metabolic acidosis is the replacement of base through the administration of intravenous HCO_3^- infusion.

Metabolic Alkalosis

Increased plasma HCO_3^-, standard HCO_3^-, BE, and SID concentration all indicate the presence of metabolic alkalosis. Metabolic alkalosis occurs when the concentration of base increases, resulting in a greater concentration of HCO_3^- in proportion to the PCO_2, a greater than normal HCO_3^-/H_2CO_3 ratio, and an increased pH (Fig. 14-22).

There are various causes of metabolic alkalosis (Box 14-7). They can be organized into two general categories: excess addition of base to the system (e.g., accidental overadministration of HCO_3^- to correct an acidosis) or excess acid loss from the system (e.g., excessive gastric fluid vomiting or suction via nasogastric tube aspiration). Severe metabolic alkalosis can be corrected by slow intravenous infusion of a dilute acid.

A pure metabolic disturbance occurs when the PCO_2 is normal. Fig. 14-23 illustrates the way a metabolic acidosis and metabolic alkalosis affects the HCO_3^--pH-PCO_2 relationship. In both cases the changes occur along the 40-mm Hg PCO_2 isobar. The magnitude of pH change brought about by the change in HCO_3^- concentration can be determined by examining the slope of this isobar. Normally, the pH changes about 0.015 unit for each milliequivalent change in the HCO_3^- concentration.

Combined Disturbances

Some individuals who have an abnormal blood pH also have a combined acid-base disturbance (Table 14-7). In these situations the respiratory and metabolic changes combine to force the pH into an abnormal condition. Fig. 14-24 shows how a combined metabolic acidosis and respiratory acidosis and a combined respiratory alkalosis and metabolic alkalosis affect the HCO_3^--pH-PCO_2 relationship. In these situations the pH changes to a greater degree. Take, for example, the combined acidosis. If the only change was in the PCO_2 from 40 to 60 mm Hg, the pH would drop to 7.28. If the only change was in the HCO_3^- concentration from 24 to 17 mEq/L, the pH would drop to 7.30. When these two

conditions combine, they force the pH to a much lower value of 7.1.

A combined metabolic acidosis and respiratory acidosis is produced by a low HCO_3^- and **elevated PCO_2**. The most common cause of combined metabolic acidosis and respiratory acidosis is cardiopulmonary failure or arrest. In this situation there is failure to deliver sufficient O_2 and failure to excrete sufficient quantities of CO_2. CO_2 accumulates and cells shift to anaerobic metabolism, which produces larger quantities of lactic acid. These combined effects cause a severe drop in the HCO_3^-/H_2CO_3 ratio, which results in a severe acidosis.

Table 14-7   Types of Combined Acid-Base Disturbances

	pH	PCO₂ (mm Hg)	Plasma [HCO₃⁻] (mEq/L)	Standard [HCO₃⁻] (mEq/L)	BE (mEq/L)	SID (mEq/L)
Normal	7.35-7.45	35-45	22-24	22-24	−2-2	40-44
Respiratory and metabolic acidosis	↓↓	↑	↓	↓	↓	↓
Respiratory and metabolic alkalosis	↑↑	↓	↑	↑	↑	↑

BE, Base excess; *SID,* strong ion difference.

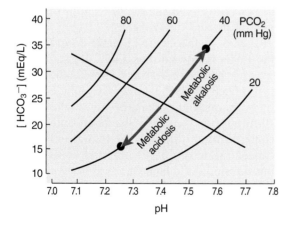

FIG. 14-23 Acute changes in bicarbonate *([HCO₃⁻])* along the normal partial pressure of carbon dioxide *(PCO₂)* isobar cause a pure metabolic acidosis or metabolic alkalosis.

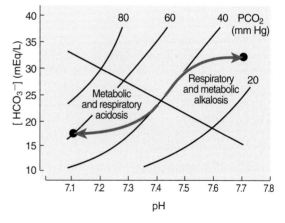

FIG. 14-24 Combined disturbances cause greater changes in pH (see text for discussion). *[HCO₃⁻],* Bicarbonate; *PCO₂,* partial pressure of carbon dioxide.

Combined respiratory and metabolic alkalosis is much less frequently encountered. It is caused by a low PCO_2 concentration and a high HCO_3^- concentration. Excessive mechanical ventilation and administration of HCO_3^- could be the cause. These two conditions result in greater quantities of HCO_3^- and a lower PCO_2. As a consequence, the HCO_3^-/H_2CO_3 ratio increases, causing the pH to increase.

Acid-Base Compensation

When a primary acid-base disturbance occurs, the body rarely sits idle. It responds by attempting to correct the pH back to a more normal value. This response is termed *compensation*. The body compensates in different ways when presented with different primary disturbances. Primary respiratory disturbances are corrected by metabolic compensation, and metabolic disturbances are corrected by respiratory compensation (Table 14-8). This results in the development of mixed acid-base disturbances.

Metabolic Compensation for Respiratory Disturbances

When the lungs suddenly fail to excrete CO_2 at an appropriate rate, the body rapidly retains CO_2, the PCO_2 increases, and acute respiratory acidosis occurs. To compensate for this acidosis, the body produces more HCO_3^- to return the HCO_3^-/H_2CO_3 ratio to 20:1. This process, however, requires time for it to occur. During prolonged CO_2 retention and chronic respiratory acidosis, which persists for several days, the pH gradually returns toward normal. This gradual increase in pH occurs as a result of a gradual increase in HCO_3^-. All of the metabolic indicators show this increase (see Table 14-8), and this signifies metabolic compensation for chronic respiratory acidosis. The increase in base can bring the pH all the way back to a normal range in a fully compensated respiratory acidosis, but this rarely occurs. More often, the metabolic variables show some compensation, but the pH is not in the normal range; this condition is termed a *partially compensated respiratory acidosis*.

 Table 14-8   Types of Combined Acid-Base Compensation

	pH	PCO₂ (mm Hg)	Plasma [HCO₃⁻] (mEq/L)	Standard [HCO₃⁻] (mEq/L)	BE (mEq/L)	SID (mEq/L)
Normal	7.35-7.45	35-45	22-24	22-24	−2-2	40-44
Compensated respiratory acidosis	N	↑	↑	↑	↑	↑
Partially compensated respiratory acidosis	<7.35	↑	↑	↑	↑	↑
Compensated respiratory alkalosis	N	↓	↓	↓	↓	↓
Partially compensated respiratory alkalosis	>7.45	↓	↓	↓	↓	↓
Compensated metabolic acidosis	N	↓	↓	↓	↓	↓
Partially compensated metabolic acidosis	<7.35	↓	↓	↓	↓	↓
Compensated metabolic alkalosis	N	↑	↑	↑	↑	↑
Partially compensated metabolic alkalosis	>7.45	↓	↑	↑	↑	↑

BE, Base excess; *SID*, strong ion difference; *N*, normal.

Fig. 14-25 shows how the HCO_3^--pH-PCO_2 relationship changes during compensation for respiratory acidosis. The initial change is an increase in PCO_2 and a decrease in pH. Metabolic compensation is triggered, HCO_3^- concentration increases, and the pH increases toward normal. Metabolic compensation is produced by greater retention and production of HCO_3^- and excretion of Cl^- by the kidney and greater release of HCO_3^- from bone. The rate of compensation is shown in Fig. 14-26. This plot shows that most of the change in plasma and cerebral spinal fluid HCO_3^- concentration occurs in the first 2 days and that maximal compensation is achieved in about 5 to 6 days.

Metabolic compensation for chronic respiratory alkalosis also occurs. In this situation chronic alveolar hyperventilation results in sustained respiratory alkalosis. Metabolic compensation occurs through diminished renal retention and formation of HCO_3^- and greater retention of Cl^-. This results in less total base, as indicated by all of the metabolic indicators (see Table 14-8), and a reduction in the HCO_3^-/H_2CO_3 ratio toward 20:1. This results in decreasing the pH toward normal. The renal release of HCO_3^- may result in fully **compensated respiratory alkalosis** when the pH returns to a normal range or in partially compensated respiratory alkalosis if the pH does not return to the normal range. The rate of HCO_3^- change during compensation for respiratory alkalosis also requires several days.

Respiratory Compensation

The body reacts much more quickly when metabolic acidosis develops. The body "senses" the acidosis with chemoreceptors located in the brain stem and along the carotid artery. This "sensation," in turn, stimulates the respiratory control center within the brain stem (see Chapter 15), resulting in greater alveolar ventilation, increased CO_2 excretion, and a lower PCO_2. The lower PCO_2 signals the presence of hyperventilation and respiratory com-

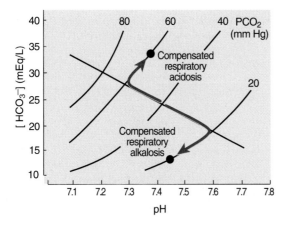

FIG. 14-25 Compensatory changes in bicarbonate ($[HCO_3^-]$) concentration for chronic respiratory alkalosis and acidosis. Initially the partial pressure of carbon dioxide (PCO_2) changes. Compensation follows with a gradual change in $[HCO_3^-]$ concentration and improvement in pH.

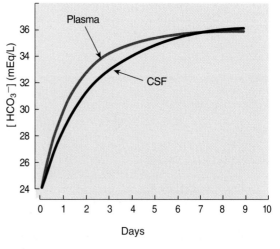

FIG. 14-26 Rate of compensatory changes in bicarbonate ($[HCO_3^-]$) concentration in plasma and cerebrospinal fluid (CSF) during chronic respiratory acidosis.

DIAGNOSTIC FOCUS

Postoperative Renal Failure

A 51-year-old woman was admitted to the intensive care unit following surgical removal of a length of necrotic bowel that lost its perfusion when a blood clot formed in the mesenteric artery. Two days later she developed a fever, had difficulty breathing, and was increasingly confused. Her vital signs were as follows:

Heart rate	127/min
Blood pressure	90/48
Respiratory rate	26/min with difficulty
Temperature	39° C
Arterial oxyhemoglobin saturation	91% while breathing air

Microscopic examination of her drawn blood revealed gram-rods, indicating septicemia. Her renal function was also abnormal with a urine output of 16 ml/hr rather than a normal value of 80 ml/hr. Arterial blood was then taken for electrolyte and acid-base balance and renal function maker analysis. The following were the results:

pH = 7.21	Na^+ = 142 mEq/L
PCO_2 = 25 mm Hg	K^+ = 5.7 mEq/L
PO_2 = 62 mm Hg	Ca^{++} = 7.7 mEq/L
HCO_3^- = 14 mEq/L	Cl^- = 97 mEq/L
Blood urea nitrogen = 54 mg/dl	Creatinine = 4.2 mg/dl

The arterial blood gases reveal moderate hypoxia, hyperventilation, and partially compensated metabolic acidosis. The sodium, calcium, and chloride were within normal limits, but the potassium concentration was elevated. In addition, the blood urea nitrogen and creatinine were significantly elevated. These findings are consistent with acute renal failure, probably produced by septicemia and hypotension. Normally, renal function is capable of excreting H^+, potassium ions, urea, and creatinine while reabsorbing HCO_3^- ions. In acute renal failure, the most common electrolyte and acid-base imbalance is a hyperkalemic metabolic acidosis. The hypoxia was produced by hypoperfusion related to $\dot{V}/\dot{Q}$ mismatching.

The patient was treated with O_2 therapy to correct the hypoxia, intravenous fluids and dopamine to improve the blood pressure, antibiotics for the septicemia, and continuous dialysis to correct the fluid and electrolyte imbalance. Over the next 6 days her pulmonary, cardiovascular, and renal function improved, and she tolerated the gradual withdrawal of support. She had no further complications and was discharged home.

pensation (see Table 14-8). A lower PCO_2 causes the HCO_3^-/H_2CO_3 ratio to return toward 20:1 and the pH to increase.

When compensation fully corrects the pH to the normal range, the condition is termed *compensated metabolic acidosis* (Fig. 14-27). More often, though, the pH is corrected part way back to the normal range. This condition is known as a partially compensated metabolic acidosis.

Respiratory compensation for metabolic alkalosis also occurs. Increased PCO_2 indicates

the presence of respiratory compensation (see Table 14-8). When metabolic alkalosis is present, the respiratory control center receives less stimulation from the chemoreceptors that are sensitive to acidosis. This results in alveolar hypoventilation, retention of CO_2, and increased PCO_2. The HCO_3^-/H_2CO_3 ratio decreases toward 20:1, and the pH returns toward the normal range. When the PCO_2 increase causes the pH to return to the normal range, compensated metabolic alkalosis occurs (see Fig. 14-27). More often, the pH is

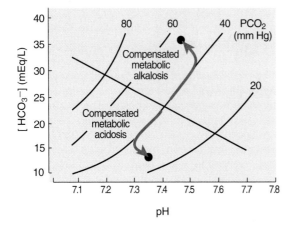

FIG. 14-27 Compensatory changes in partial pressure of carbon dioxide *(PCO₂)* for metabolic acidosis and metabolic alkalosis. Initially the bicarbonate *([HCO₃⁻])* changes. Compensation occurs rapidly with a change in PCO₂ and improvement in pH.

Variations in Acid-Base Indicators with Temperature Change

Temperature	25° C	37° C	41° C
pH	7.60	7.40	7.35
PCO₂ (mm Hg)	22	40	48

incompletely corrected and the condition is called partially compensated metabolic alkalosis.

Respiratory compensation occurs quickly and becomes maximal within minutes rather than in several days. Some controversy has existed about the degree of respiratory compensation for metabolic alkalosis. Recent studies support the concept that both metabolic acidosis and metabolic alkalosis cause proportional changes in respiratory control center activity and the resulting level of PCO₂ in blood. In these studies it was found that a loss or gain of 1 mEq/L in HCO₃⁻ concentration that is brought about by a metabolic disturbance is compensated for by a gain or loss of about 0.7 to 1 mm Hg in the PCO₂.

Effects of Temperature

If a sample of blood is cooled or warmed in a sealed syringe (no addition or loss of CO_2) and the electrodes that are used to measure pH and PCO₂ are also cooled or warmed to the

same temperature, variations in pH and PCO₂ will be found. Box 14-8 lists changes over a range of 25 to 41 C. The general pattern is one of declining pH (−0.016 pH unit/° C) and increasing PCO₂ (1.4 mm Hg/° C) with increasing temperature and vice versa with cooling. The change in PCO₂ occurs as a result of the direct relationship between pressure and temperature (Charles' law [see Chapter 1]). The pH change occurs as the result of the changes in the dissociation constants of various acids and bases within blood.

Much concern over these changes has been expressed when samples of blood from hypothermic or hyperthermic patients are to be analyzed with electrodes in the typical clinical laboratory that are maintained at 37° C. Several different approaches have been devised to mathematically correct the values measured at 37° C to values that occur at a different temperature, but this led to the problem of defining what was normal during these "abnormal" temperatures. Studies by Rahn and coworkers on the acid-base balance in various ectothermic animals (e.g., amphibians, reptiles, and fish) and in different regions of the body (e.g., cool skin and hot exercising skeletal muscle) have revealed that these apparent changes in acid-base indicators are normal conditions. These studies also reveal that it is the OH⁻/H⁺ ratio and relative alkalinity (not a stable pH) that are maintained at different temperatures. To avoid the confusion, these temperature corrections should not

Table 14-9 Domains and Indicators of Arterial Blood Gas and Acid-Base Balance

	Units	Normal	Hypoxemia	Hyperoxemia
OXYGENATION				
PaO_2	mm Hg	80-100	<80	>100
$P(A-a)O_2$	mm Hg	<10*		
SaO_2	Percent	95-98	<95	>98
[Hb]	g/dl	12-15	<12	>15
CaO_2	ml/dl	17-21	<17	>21
	Units	Normal	Hyperventilation	Hypoventilation
VENTILATION				
$PaCO_2$	mm Hg	35-45	<35	>45
	Units	Normal	Acidosis	Alkalosis
ACID-BASE BALANCE				
pH		7.35-7.45	<7.35	>7.45
$PaCO_2$	mm Hg	35-45	>45	<35
Plasma $[HCO_3^-]$	mEq/L	22-26	<22	>26
Standard $[HCO_3^-]$	mEq/L	22-26	<22	>26
Base excess	mEq/L	-2-2	-2	>2

Values >10 indicate diffusion defects, $\dot{V}/\dot{Q}$ mismatch, and shunting.

be used, but the data produced by the analyzer should be used. The data should then be compared with normal values and interpreted in the normal way.

SYSTEMATIC INTERPRETATION OF BLOOD GAS AND ACID-BASE DATA

The data from analysis of blood gases, Hb saturation, and acid-base indicators can be confusing, leading to erroneous interpretation. A systematic approach to interpreting the data and "seeing" interconnected relationships improves one's understanding. A popular approach is to break the data down into three different domains: the statuses of oxygenation, ventilation, and acid-base balance. The indicators for these different domains are listed in Table 14-9.

Step 1: Describing the Status of Oxygenation

The state of oxygenation is revealed by evaluating the PaO_2, $P(A-a)O_2$ gradient, SaO_2, Hb concentration, and CaO_2. Normal values for these various indicators are found in Table 14-9. **Hypoxemia** is indicated by **abnormally low values.** The severity of hypoxemia can be defined on the basis of the decline in PO_2. Values from 60 to 80 mm Hg are defined as slight hypoxemia, values from 40 to 60 mm Hg are described as moderate hypoxemia, and those below 40 mm Hg are consistent with severe hypoxemia. Hyperoxemia is defined by **abnormally high values.**

The $P(A-a)O_2$ indicates the ability of the respiratory system to exchange O_2 across the alveolar-capillary membrane. Normal exchange results in a gradient of less than 10 mm Hg. Diffusion defects, $\dot{V}/\dot{Q}$ mismatching, or shunting result in an elevated gradient.

Hypoxemia is often caused by combinations of these defects.

Step 2: Describing the Status of Ventilation

When alveolar ventilation is appropriate for the amount of CO_2 produced, a normal PCO_2 of 35 to 45 mm Hg is present. Abnormal alveolar ventilation causes an inverse change in the $PaCO_2$. **Hyperventilation** causes the $PaCO_2$ to drop, and **hypoventilation** causes it to climb.

Step 3: Describing the Status of Acid-Base Balance

Overall Acid-Base Balance

Describing the acid-base status begins with evaluating the overall acid-base status. An overall normal acid-base balance exists when the pH is in the normal range of 7.35 to 7.45. Values below this indicate some type of **acidosis,** and values above this indicate some type of **alkalosis.**

Primary Cause of an Acid-Base Disturbance

The next step is to determine the cause of acidosis or alkalosis, if present. Respiratory disturbances are signaled by abnormal PO_2 values. Values less than 35 mm Hg indicate the presence of respiratory alkalosis whereas values greater then 45 mm Hg reveal the presence of respiratory acidosis. Normal values for metabolic indicators indicate pure respiratory disturbances.

The most common metabolic indicators include the plasma HCO_3^-, standard HCO_3^-, and BE. Normal HCO_3^- concentrations of 22 to 26 mEq/L and BE of -2 to 2 mEq/L indicate that a normal concentration of buffers is present in the extracellular fluid. Metabolic acidosis is indicated when these values fall below the normal range, and the presence of metabolic alkalosis is determined when these values are greater than normal.

Combined respiratory alkalosis and metabolic alkalosis or metabolic acidosis exists when PCO_2, HCO_3^-, and BE concentrations show that both respiratory and metabolic causes are forcing the pH into alkalotic or acidotic ranges.

Presence of Compensation

After determining the primary cause of the acid-base disturbance, the last step is to determine if any compensation by the other system is present. Respiratory disturbances are counterbalanced by metabolic compensation. Metabolic disturbances are counteracted by respiratory compensation.

Interpretation

The following examples illustrate systematic interpretation.

Example 1

A 28-year-old male in the emergency department is suspected of taking a drug overdose. He is breathing spontaneously, is comatose, and is receiving supplemental O_2 with an FIO_2 of 60%. An arterial blood specimen is collected from the radial artery and analyzed. The following is found:

PaO_2	72 mm Hg
$P(A-a)O_2$	356 mm Hg
SaO_2	94%
[Hb]	14 g/dl
CaO_2	17.7 ml/dl
$PaCO_2$	61 mm Hg
pH	7.27
Plasma [HCO_3^-]	26.5 mEq/L
Standard [HCO_3^-]	22.0 mEq/L
BE	-2 mEq/L

OXYGENATION. These findings indicate that the patient has slight hypoxemia as indicated by the slightly low PaO_2, SaO_2, and CaO_2 despite the use of substantial supplemental O_2. His $P(A-a)O_2$ gradient is highly abnormal and indicates the presence of a diffusion defect, $\dot{V}/\dot{Q}$ mismatching, or shunting. It was later determined that the patient had aspirated gastric fluid into his lungs, which resulted in an acute lung injury.

VENTILATION. The $PaCO_2$ is elevated, indicating hypoventilation secondary to respiratory central control suppression by the drug overdose.

ACID–BASE BALANCE. There is a primary respiratory acidosis caused by the acute hypoventilation and CO_2 retention. No metabolic compensation is present.

It was determined that the patient had overdosed with heroin and was treated with a narcotic antagonist drug that promptly reversed his coma and respiratory depression.

Example 2

A 73-year-old woman is in the coronary care unit for exacerbation of congestive heart failure. She is being treated with diuretic drugs to remove excess water and breathing room-air when she suddenly becomes confused and agitated and exclaims, "I can't catch my breath." An arterial blood specimen is collected from the radial artery and the following is found:

PaO_2	46 mm Hg
$P(A-a)O_2$	122 mm Hg
SaO_2	80%
[Hb]	15 g/dl
CaO_2	16.2 ml/dl
$PaCO_2$	28 mm Hg
pH	7.69
Plasma [HCO_3^-]	34 mEq/L
Standard [HCO_3^-]	38 mEq/L
BE	14 mEq/L

OXYGENATION. These findings show the patient to be moderately to severely hypoxemic. The predicted PaO_2 for an individual of this age is about 85 to 90 mm Hg. Her SaO_2 is higher than predicted as a result of the alkalotic blood pH effects on the oxyhemoglobin affinity. Her $P(A-a)O_2$ is elevated, indicating that her lungs are not normal and that a diffu-

sion defect, $\dot{V}/\dot{Q}$ mismatching, or shunting is present. Her most recent chest x-ray shows some pulmonary edema and scattered regions of alveolar collapse (atelectasis).

VENTILATION. The $PaCO_2$ is low, which is consistent with hyperventilation.

ACID–BASE BALANCE. The abnormal pH is being caused by a combined respiratory and metabolic alkalosis. The metabolic component is a result of the diuretic therapy, which is causing excess Cl^- excretion and HCO_3^- retention. The respiratory alkalosis is being caused by hypoxemia and anxiety. These two abnormalities have led to severe alkalosis. Both systems are forcing the pH into an alkalotic state and there is no possibility for compensation.

The patient was given supplemental O_2 to improve her PaO_2 and O_2 content and a small amount of sedation to reduce the anxiety. Her intravenous fluids and diuretic therapy were adjusted to reduce the metabolic alkalosis.

Example 3

A 61-year-old man with a history of chronic obstructive pulmonary disease from a 40-year history of smoking is being seen in the emergency room for intensifying shortness of breath. He appears to be unable to complete sentences when asked to describe his condition and is receiving supplemental O_2 with an FIO_2 of 30%. An arterial blood sample was taken and the following results were found:

PaO_2	33 mm Hg
$P(A-a)O_2$	181 mm Hg
SaO_2	68%
[Hb]	17 g/dl
CaO_2	15.6 ml/dl
$PaCO_2$	68 mm Hg
pH	7.31
Plasma [HCO_3^-]	35 mEq/L
Standard [HCO_3^-]	31 mEq/L
BE	7 mEq/L

OXYGENATION. Severe hypoxemia is present despite O_2 therapy. The elevated Hb concentration (polycythemia) suggests that the hypoxemia is a chronic condition and that the bone marrow is compensating by producing more erythrocytes. The elevated $P(A-a)O_2$ indicates that a diffusion defect, $\dot{V}/\dot{Q}$ mismatching, or shunting is present. Hypoxemia is caused by the existing lung disease and more recent changes brought about by pneumonia.

VENTILATION. The $PaCO_2$ is elevated, indicating hypoventilation.

ACID-BASE BALANCE. A partially compensated respiratory acidosis is present. The abnormal pH is caused by a primary respiratory acidosis. The metabolic indicators are elevated, indicating some compensation. The pH is not corrected into the normal range, indicating partial compensation. These changes are consistent with chronic alveolar hypoventilation in end-stage lung disease.

The patient's supplemental O_2 was increased to improve the SaO_2 to a target of 88% to 90%. This is a tolerable target saturation that avoids excessive oxygenation. Intensive bronchodilator therapy and steroid therapy were begun to improve gas exchange and reduce the work of breathing. A bacterial pneumonia was found to be the cause of the exacerbation, so antibiotics were prescribed.

CHAPTER SELF-TEST QUESTIONS

1. Which one of the following reactions does carbonic anhydrase catalyze?
   a. $CO_2 + H_2O \rightleftharpoons H^+ + HCO_3^-$
   b. $H_2CO_3 \rightleftharpoons 2H^+ + CO_3^=$
   c. $CO_2 + H_2O \rightleftharpoons H_2CO_3$
   d. $H_2CO_3 \rightleftharpoons H^+ + HCO_3^-$
2. How many nanoequivalents of H^+ are produced from the combination of volatile and nonvolatile acid on a daily basis?
   a. 1000
   b. 20,000
   c. 100,000
   d. 100,000,000
   e. 20,000,000,000

3. What is the relative pH of blood if the HCO_3^-/H_2CO_3 ratio in it is 20:1?
   a. basic
   b. normal
   c. acidic
4. Which of the following indicators is/are directly determined with an electrode and not calculated?
   1. PCO_2
   2. BE
   3. pH
   a. 3 only
   b. 1 and 3
   c. 2 and 3
   d. 1 and 2
   e. 1, 2, and 3
5. Which of the following disturbances would cause an alkalosis?
   1. $\uparrow PCO_2$
   2. $\uparrow BE$
   3. $\uparrow$ Plasma HCO_3^- concentration
   a. 1 only
   b. 2 only
   c. 3 only
   d. 1 and 3
   e. 2 and 3

Use the following information to answer questions 6 to 8:

A 48-year-old male on the general medicine ward is being treated for acute renal failure. He is breathing air spontaneously and is appropriately responsive to questions. An arterial blood specimen is collected from the radial artery and analyzed. The following is found:

PaO_2	94 mm Hg
$P(A-a)O_2$	19 mm Hg
SaO_2	90%
[Hb]	9 g/dl
CaO_2	11.1 ml/dl
$PaCO_2$	37 mm Hg
pH	7.18
Plasma [HCO_3^-]	13.0 mEq/L
Standard [HCO_3^-]	13.5 mEq/L
BE	-14 mEq/L

6. How would you describe his oxygenation?
   a. normal
   b. moderate to severe hypoxemia
   c. moderate hyperoxemia
7. How would you describe his ventilation?
   a. hyperventilation
   b. normal or appropriate
   c. hypoventilation
8. How would you describe his acid-base status?
   a. respiratory acidosis
   b. metabolic acidosis
   c. combined respiratory and metabolic acidosis
   d. partially compensated respiratory acidosis
   e. partially compensated metabolic acidosis

Use the following information to answer questions 9 to 11:

A 23-year-old female is being treated in the emergency department for an acute asthma attack. She is breathing air spontaneously and receiving inhaled bronchodilators. An arterial blood specimen is collected from the radial artery and analyzed. The following is found:

PaO_2	54 mm Hg
$P(A-a)O_2$	47 mm Hg
S_aO_2	81%
[Hb]	14 g/dl
CaO_2	15.4 ml/dl
$PaCO_2$	49 mm Hg
pH	7.25
Plasma [HCO_3^-]	20.5 mEq/L
Standard [HCO_3^-]	17.5 mEq/L
BE	−7 mEq/L

9. How would you describe her oxygenation?
   a. normal
   b. moderate hypoxemia
   c. moderate hyperoxemia
10. How would you describe her ventilation?
    a. hyperventilation
    b. normal or appropriate
    c. hypoventilation

11. How would you describe her acid-base status?
    a. respiratory acidosis
    b. metabolic acidosis
    c. combined respiratory and metabolic acidosis
    d. partially compensated respiratory acidosis
    e. partially compensated metabolic acidosis

For answers, see p. 476.

BIBLIOGRAPHY

1. Cohen JJ et al: *Acid base*, Boston, 1982, Little, Brown.
2. Davenport HW: *The ABCs of acid-base chemistry*, ed 6, Chicago, 1974, The University of Chicago Press.
3. Guyton AC: *Textbook of medical physiology*, Philadelphia, 1996, WB Saunders.
4. Leff AR, Schumacker PT, eds: *Respiratory physiology: basics and applications*, Philadelphia, 1993, WB Saunders.
5. Levitzky GL, Hall SM, McDonough KH: *Cardiopulmonary physiology in anesthesiology*, New York, 1997, McGraw Hill.
6. Martini FH: *Fundamentals of anatomy and physiology*, Upper Saddle River, NJ, 1998, Prentice Hall.
7. Miller WF, Scacci R, Gast LR: *Laboratory evaluation of pulmonary function*, Philadelphia, 1987, JB Lippincott.
8. Murray JF: *The normal lung: the basis for diagnosis and treatment of pulmonary disease*, ed 2, Philadelphia, 1986, WB Saunders.
9. Nunn JF: *Applied respiratory physiology*, ed 3, London, 1987, Butterworths.
10. Pierson DJ, Kacmarek RM: *Foundations of respiratory care*, New York, 1992, Churchill Livingstone.
11. Staub NC: *Basic respiratory physiology*, New York, 1991, Churchill Livingstone.
12. Stewart PA: *How to understand acid-base: a quantitative acid-base primer for biology and medicine*, New York, 1981, Elsevier.
13. Van De Graaff KM, Fox SI: *Human concepts of anatomy and physiology*, Dubuque, Iowa, 1995, Wm C Brown.
14. West JB: *Respiratory physiology: the essentials*, ed 4, Baltimore, 1990, Williams & Wilkins.

CHAPTER 15

Control of Breathing

Upon completing this chapter, you will be able to:

1 Describe the feedback loop of breathing control.

2 Define the *respiratory control set point*.

3 Describe the location and neural interactions of the control centers for automatic and voluntary breathing.

4 Describe the nervous connections between the breathing controller and the effectors of gas exchange.

5 Describe the location and sensitivities of the central and peripheral chemoreceptors.

6 Define the respiratory response to carbon dioxide, oxygen, and acid-base imbalance.

7 Describe the pulmonary and thorax irritant, stretch, and congestion receptors and the types of breathing pattern changes they cause.

8 List the types of tests that are used to evaluate the activity of the respiratory control center system.

9 Describe how the control of breathing changes during sleep and exercise.

10 Define *sleep apnea, central apnea,* and *obstructive apnea*.

11 Describe the various types of normal and abnormal breathing patterns.

The rhythmic pattern of breathing is a process that begins during fetal development before birth and continues nonstop until death. The rhythmic pattern repeats over 500 million times during the average life time. It is adjusted during exercise or stress and overridden by conscious decisions. This has given rise to the understanding that two general regulatory mechanisms are at work to set and adjust the breathing pattern: automatic control and voluntary control. Automatic control, an unconscious process, maintains a breathing pattern that results in the maintenance of oxygen (O_2) and carbon dioxide (CO_2) exchange. Voluntary control, a conscious process, adjusts the breathing pattern during talking, breath holding, playing breath-powered musical instruments, and a variety of emotional states. This chapter describes these two different control mechanisms, the various elements of these systems, and abnormal control of breathing.

ORGANIZATION OF THE DIFFERENT ELEMENTS OF BREATHING CONTROL

General Control Theory

At a basic level, the automatic control of breathing is carried out by the same elements that are present in many other control systems (e.g., cardiovascular control of blood pressure [see Chapter 8]). These include a control center, or **controller,** that issues instructions about how often, how long, and how deep the breath should be; a number of **effectors** that physi-

cally cause breathing; and a variety of **sensors** that react to the breathing. These elements are interconnected into a **negative feedback loop** that allows ongoing adjustment of the system as conditions change (Fig. 15-1).

The respiratory controller is located in the brain and includes regions of the cerebrum and brain stem and extensions into the spinal cord. The effectors include the respiratory muscles, the airways, pulmonary blood vessels, and the alveolar-capillary membrane where gas exchange occurs. The sensors of breathing include the **chemoreceptors** that detect the levels of CO_2, O_2, and H^+ in various body fluids and **mechanoreceptors** that detect physical changes in the lungs, respiratory muscles, and chest wall. The activities of these different structures are interconnected in a feedback loop that produces a stable breathing pattern (Fig. 15-2).

The voluntary control of breathing is less well understood. The control center in this case is located in higher regions of the brain. When these areas become active, they stimulate different parts of the automatic control center or directly stimulate certain respiratory muscles.

Respiratory Set Point

Like the cardiovascular control system, the automatic respiratory control system is organized to maintain a certain target, or **set point.** The goal of the system is to generate an efficient breathing pattern that is able to maintain effective gas exchange. The target breathing pattern is that pattern that requires the least amount of work to maintain a set point of gas exchange. The primary set point that the effectors of gas exchange are directed to maintain is an arterial partial pressure of CO_2 (P_aCO_2) of 40 mm Hg (Fig. 15-3). By maintaining this set point, oxygenation of blood reaches close to a maximal value, and the kidneys can easily adjust the extracellular concentration of bicarbonate (HCO_3^-) to normalize the pH. Abnormal breathing patterns that result in either

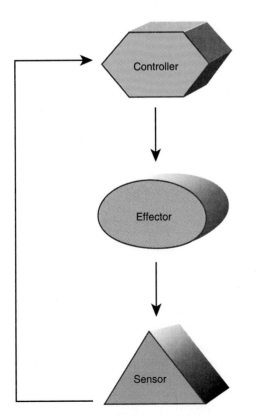

FIG. 15-1 Elements of a control feedback loop.

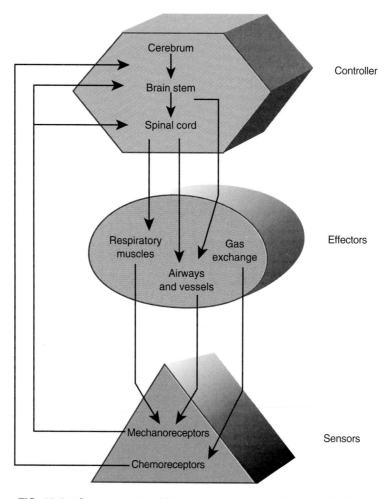

FIG. 15-2   Components of the respiratory control feedback loop.

hyperventilation or hypoventilation cause the P_aCO_2 to deviate from this set point.

RESPIRATORY CONTROLLER

Automatic Control Centers

During the 1790s the French revolution was in full swing with the people's courts handing out capital punishment in the form of beheadings. At this time a French biologist by the name of Legallois was present at some of these executions and noted that the torso stopped breathing after separation from the head and that on occasion the facial muscles of the head would cause a gasping expression as if the head was attempting to breathe. From these observations and further work in the laboratory, Legallois concluded that the control center for automatic breathing is located in the brain stem and not in the thorax, as was believed before this time.

The brain stem is that part of the brain that

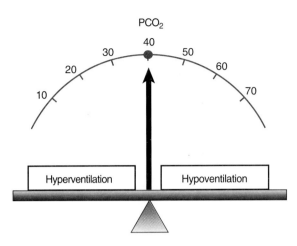

FIG. 15-3 Set point for the regulation of ventilation is a PCO_2 of 40 mm Hg. Hyperventilation and hypoventilation are abnormal breathing patterns that cause the PCO_2 to deviate from this set point.

connects the midbrain and the upper brain with the cerebellum and spinal cord. It is comprised of the **pons** and the **medulla oblongata.** This region of the brain is a relatively old embryological structure that appears with about the same complexity in all vertebrate animals. The automatic control center for breathing is located here along with the cardiovascular control center (see Chapter 8) and centers for vomiting, gagging, and coughing. In this region, cranial nerves VIII through XII connect to the central nervous system and function to carry motor signals out to various skeletal and smooth muscle groups and glands as well as carry sensory signals back to the brain from various regions of the body.

The neurons that are active in the automatic control of breathing were once believed to concentrate in centers in the brain stem. It is more generally accepted now that the neurons are arranged in a more dispersed network throughout the brain stem. Fig. 15-4 shows a more modern understanding of where these groups, or "pools," of neurons are generally located.

Medulla Oblongata

One collection of neurons, termed the *inspiratory neuron pool*, is located in both the sides and posterior region of the medulla oblongata (also known as the **dorsal respiratory group**). These neurons appear to receive excitatory impulses from other regions of the brain as well as from chemoreceptors via the glossopharyngeal (ninth cranial) and vagus (tenth cranial) nerves. The inspiratory neuron pool extends axons down the spinal cord to activate motor neurons that exit the spinal cord in the cervical and thoracic regions. These axons are organized into nerves that innervate the diaphragm and accessory muscles of breathing. When active, the inspiratory neuron pool causes the contraction of the diaphragm and accessory muscles that result in enlargement of the thorax and the act of inspiration.

Exhalation is carried out by inhibiting these inspiratory neurons. This is accomplished by the activation of an expiratory neuron pool that lies on both sides of the upper portion of the medulla oblongata in the anterior region (also known as the **ventral respiratory group**). When the expiratory pool of neurons becomes active, they inhibit the activity of the inspiratory neuron pool, resulting in relaxation of the respiratory muscles, which stops inspiration and allows exhalation.

The basic interaction of these two different pools of neurons is responsible for most of the

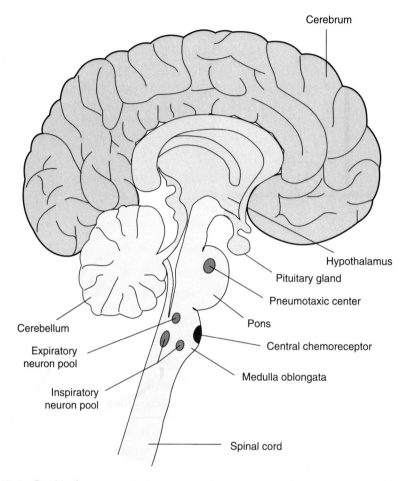

Cerebrum

Hypothalamus

Pituitary gland

Pneumotaxic center

Pons

Central chemoreceptor

Medulla oblongata

Cerebellum

Expiratory
neuron pool

Inspiratory
neuron pool

Spinal cord

FIG. 15-4   Pools of neurons that control automatic breathing are dispersed throughout the medulla oblongata and pons.

automatic pattern of rhythmic breathing. This was demonstrated by Legallois when a laboratory animal's brain down to and including the pons was severed from the medulla oblongata. The animal maintained rhythmic breathing. When the medulla was severed from the spinal cord, breathing stopped.

Pons

The expiratory pool of neurons is also activated by a group of neurons that are located within the pons and higher up in the brain. The pontine group of neurons, also known as the **pneumotaxic center** (see Fig. 15-4), is stim-

ulated by lung and thorax stretch receptors that send signals to the pons via the vagus nerves. When the pneumotaxic pool is active, it sends excitatory signals to the expiratory neuron pool in the medulla oblongata, resulting in the inhibition of the inspiratory neuron pool and aiding in the slowing or stopping of inspiration. This allows the pattern of breathing to be smoothed by the influence of the pons.

Respiratory Center Neuron Pool Interaction

The rhythmic pattern of breathing that is "driven" by these different pools of neurons

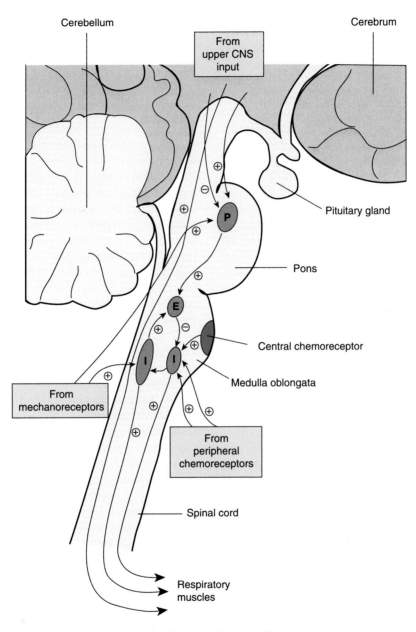

FIG. 15-5 Stimulatory (+) and inhibitory (-) interactions, sensory inputs, and motor output signals to the respiratory muscles by the various neuron pools of the brain stem that control the automatic breathing pattern (see text for further discussion). *CNS,* Central nervous system; *P,* pneumotaxic center; *E,* expiratory neuron pool; *I,* inspiratory neuron.

is the result of their interaction (Fig. 15-5) and intermittent activity. The inspiratory neuron pool is active and further activated by the input from various chemoreceptors that respond to hypercapnia and hypoxia. This results in activation of the respiratory muscles and inspiration. Inspiration continues until the expiratory pool of neurons in the ventral respiratory group of the medulla becomes more active, inhibiting the inspiratory pool. The activity of the expiratory pool is something like an inspiratory cut-off switch that stops inspiration. The activity of the pneumotaxic pool of neurons enhances the activity of the expiratory neuron pool in the medulla, smoothing out the breathing pattern. This results in exhalation and a short pause. Activity in the inspiratory pool gradually increases and is further stimulated by chemoreceptor activity. As the inspiratory pool becomes more active, inspiration begins again and the pattern starts all over. The automatic control of breathing is viewed as primarily an inspiratory activity interrupted periodically to allow exhalation.

Voluntary Controllers

The center for voluntary control over the breathing pattern is generally located in upper regions of the brain. Areas of the cerebral cortex are responsible for voluntary changes such as forceful inspiration, breath holding, and forceful exhalation. These areas are also involved in other voluntary adjustments that occur during speaking, laughing, and swallowing. The thalamus, a region involved with sensory and emotional behavior, influences the breathing pattern during fear, anger, rage, sorrow, and other intense emotions. These various centers are either connected to the neural pools of the pons and the medulla oblongata, or they are directly connected to the motor neurons of the spinal cord that innervate the respiratory muscles.

HOW CONTROLLERS ARE CONNECTED TO EFFECTORS

The effectors of breathing that influence gas flow to and in the lungs include the diaphragm, the accessory muscles of breathing, and the smooth muscles in the airway (see Chapters 9 and 10). The nervous controllers in the brain send nerve fibers to these different muscles from different regions of the central nervous system (Fig. 15-6).

The diaphragm is innervated by the left and right phrenic nerves. The phrenic nerves are formed by neural fibers that leave as branches from spinal nerves C3, C4, and C5. These fibers enter the cervical plexus and form the phrenic nerves. The accessory muscles (e.g., intercostal muscles, sternocleidomastoid muscles, scalene muscles, and abdominal wall muscles) are innervated by low cervical, intercostal, and lumbar spinal nerves.

Airway diameter and, therefore, the distribution of gas flow are controlled by the tension of smooth muscle in the airway. Smooth muscle tension is under the control of the parasympathetic and sympathetic branches of the autonomic nervous system. The parasympathetic fibers arise from the brain stem as the vagus nerve while the sympathetic fibers arise from the thoracic spinal nerves.

Spinal cord injuries that result in severing the cord at or above C5 usually result in loss of all or almost all innervation of the respiratory muscles. Injuries below C5 and above T2 result in diaphragmatic function and the ability to breathe automatically. However, injuries in this region result in loss of almost all accessory muscles and reduced ability to modify the breathing pattern in a voluntary way. For example, the ability to breathe deep and cough is dramatically reduced. High spinal cord injuries also result in loss of sympathetic innervation of the airways. This results in greater parasympathetic innervation, greater airway smooth muscle tension, and greater airway resistance to breathing and mucus production.

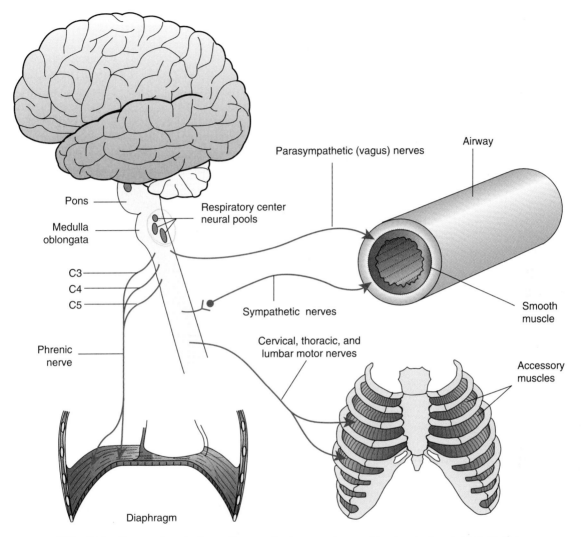

FIG. 15-6 Nerve signals from the respiratory center and brain stem are sent to the diaphragm by the left and right phrenic nerves, to the accessory muscles by numerous spinal motor nerves, and to the smooth muscle of the airway by the parasympathetic and sympathetic nerves.

TYPES OF SENSORS USED TO MONITOR BREATHING

The body is equipped with different types of chemical and mechanical sensors that monitor the activities of breathing and send information to the brain stem (Fig. 15-7). Most of the sensations are subconscious in nature and influence the automatic control of breathing. In some conditions, however, the sensations can be intense enough to reach the level of consciousness and result in the uncomfortable sensation of breathlessness, or **dyspnea.**

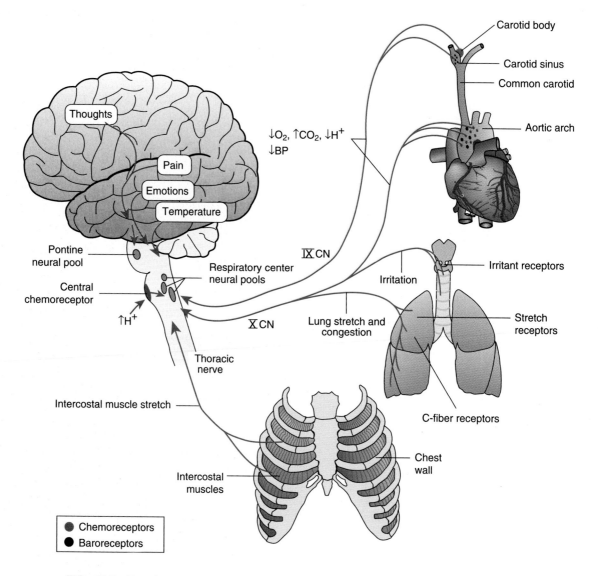

FIG. 15-7 Respiratory center receives input signals from higher brain regions in response to various emotional states and from sensors located along great vessels, the airways, and lungs and from the chest wall.

⬤   **Table 15-1**   Respiratory Chemoreceptor Location and Sensitivity

Type	Location	Stimulus
Central	Anterior surface of medulla oblongata	Cerebrospinal fluid pH changes caused by PCO_2 changes
Peripheral	Carotid bodies of common carotid artery	Blood PO_2, PCO_2, and pH

Chemoreceptors

The most important stimulation for breathing is caused by changes in the concentrations of CO_2, O_2, and H^+. These changes are detected by specialized cells or neurons that are called *chemoreceptors*. Chemoreceptor cells are located in the brain stem (central chemoreceptors) and along major systemic arteries (peripheral chemoreceptors) and respond to changes that occur in blood or extracellular fluid that surround them (Table 15-1).

Central Chemoreceptors

An increase in PCO_2 is the most powerful stimulant for breathing. The chemoreceptor most responsive to PCO_2 changes is located just below the surface on the anterior side of the medulla oblongata. Because this chemoreceptor is located near the respiratory control neurons, this group of sensitive cells is referred to as the *central chemoreceptor*. This chemoreceptor reacts to changes that take place in the surrounding extracellular fluid of brain tissue. The chemical composition of this fluid is influenced by the metabolic activity of brain cells and cerebral blood and by the chemical composition of cerebral spinal fluid (CSF). Of these, CSF has the greatest influence on extracellular fluid PCO_2.

Central chemoreceptor cells are not directly stimulated by increases in PCO_2 but actually by decreasing pH. The pH of CSF is 7.34, making it slightly acidic when compared with arterial blood. CO_2 enters CSF from cerebral blood and from brain cells (Fig. 15-8). To enter CSF from blood, CO_2 must cross through the blood brain barrier that is formed by glial cells that wrap the microcirculation of the brain. CO_2 combines with water to form carbonic acid, which dissociates and releases H^+. With increasing PCO_2, more H^+ is released, causing the pH to drop, which results in stimulation of the central chemoreceptor neurons. These cells, in turn, stimulate the inspiratory pool of neurons and increase inspiratory muscle activity.

Like other body fluids, the pH of CSF is regulated by adjusting the strong ion difference (SID) in it (see Chapter 14). CSF lacks cells and most protein. This results in the SID being almost entirely comprised of HCO_3^-, making it the primary buffer in CSF. By adjusting the SID up or down, the concentration of HCO_3^- can be adjusted and the pH of CSF is adjusted accordingly. This is accomplished by ion pumps that move the strong ions (Na^+ and Cl^-) across the blood brain barrier. HCO_3^- ions are also moved actively across the blood brain barrier to fill the SID (see Fig. 15-8). This results in a normal HCO_3^- concentration of 21.5 mEq/L. When the SID decreases, less HCO_3^- moves into CSF and vice versa. Just as in blood and other body fluids, the adjustment of HCO_3^- concentration results in setting the pH of CSF according to the Henderson-Hasselbalch relationship.

The sensitivity of the central chemoreceptors can be adjusted by changing the buffering

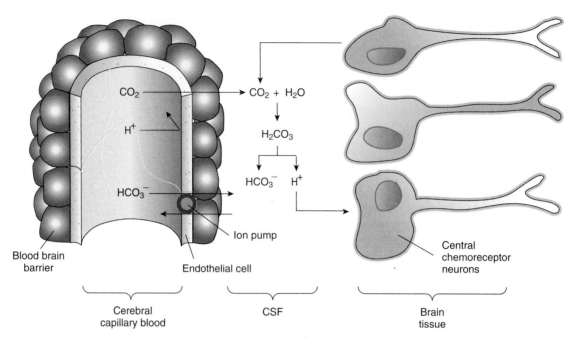

FIG. 15-8 Central chemoreceptor cells are stimulated by increasing hydrogen (H^+) concentration in cerebral spinal fluid (CSF). The major cause of CSF acidosis is the diffusion of carbon dioxide (CO_2) into it from cerebral blood and tissues. H^+ ions are unable to diffuse through the blood brain barrier. The pH of CSF can be modified over time by the activity of a bicarbonate (HCO_3^-) ion pump in the blood brain barrier.

characteristics of CSF, which, in turn, changes the buffering capacity of the brain's extracellular fluid. A greater HCO_3^- concentration results in a higher CSF pH and less pH change when CO_2 or other acids enter CSF. This effectively resets chemoreceptor activity to respond to a higher PCO_2. The increased HCO_3^- concentration occurs in conditions of chronic CO_2 retention, resulting in chronic alveolar hypoventilation. This occurs commonly during end-stage chronic obstructive pulmonary disease. In these patients, hypoxia occurs and becomes an important stimulant for breathing.

The opposite occurs when HCO_3^- concentration falls and the central chemoreceptors become more responsive to lower PCO_2 levels. This occurs during conditions of chronically low PCO_2. The most common cause of this situation is chronic hyperventilation that occurs in response to chronic hypoxia. Living at high altitudes for more than several days results in this condition. The chronic hypoxia stimulates other chemoreceptors, resulting in chronic hyperventilation and a reduced PCO_2. To correct the pH, the ion pumps decrease the SID, resulting in a lower CSF HCO_3^- concentration. This effectively resets central chemoreceptor sensitivity to a lower PCO_2. When chronic hypoxia is corrected by returning to sea level, the CSF HCO_3^- concentration returns to normal and the central chemoreceptor resets to maintain a normal PCO_2.

Peripheral Chemoreceptors

Alveolar ventilation increases with the sudden development of hypoxemia and acidemia. However, the central chemoreceptors do not respond to these changes. The chemoreceptor cells that do respond to these changes are located in bodies along the carotid artery and

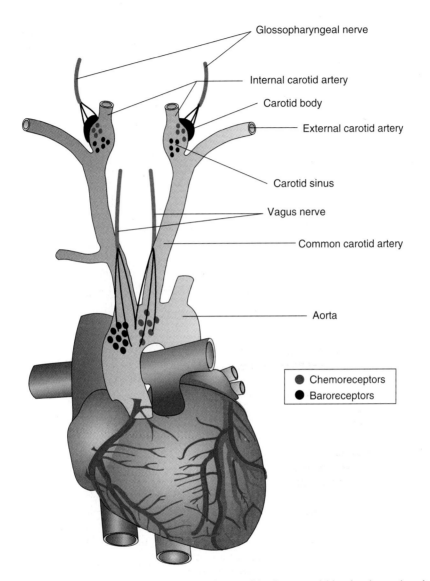

Glossopharyngeal nerve

Internal carotid artery

Carotid body

External carotid artery

Carotid sinus

Vagus nerve

Common carotid artery

Aorta

● Chemoreceptors
● Baroreceptors

FIG. 15-9 Peripheral chemoreceptors are located in the carotid body along the sinus at the bifurcation of the common carotid artery and in the wall of the aortic arch along with the baroreceptors that monitor blood pressure.

aortic arch and are known as the peripheral chemoreceptors (Fig. 15-9).

The carotid bodies are located along the sinus just beyond the bifurcation of the common carotid artery. This is the same site where baroreceptors that respond to blood pressure are found. Within the carotid sinus and extending into the carotid bodies are certain nerve endings that respond to low PO_2, elevated PCO_2, and decreased pH. These nerve signals are carried by the glossopharyngeal (ninth cranial) nerve to the brain stem, where they stimulate the inspiratory neuron pool.

The principal stimulant of the carotid body chemoreceptors is a low PO_2 in the arterial blood that is flowing through this region. A low O_2 content brought about by low hemoglobin content does not stimulate these receptors very much as long as the PO_2 is near normal. The carotid body receptors do respond to increases in PCO_2, but it is believed that they contribute only 30% of the total CO_2 stimulus to respiratory center. The balance, or 70%, of the PCO_2 response is carried out by the central chemoreceptor. The peripheral chemoreceptor also responds to a low blood pH brought about by metabolic acid-base disturbances.

Carotid body chemoreceptors can become adapted to chronic hypoxemia, reducing their stimulation of the respiratory center. It is believed that this occurs through the action of glomus cells that are found in the carotid bodies. These cells are capable of releasing the neurotransmitter dopamine, which can inhibit the neurons that carry the signals into the glossopharyngeal nerve. The prevailing theory suggests that these cells become more active during chronic hypoxia; this helps explain why an individual who is chronically hypoxic does not have the same response to hypoxia that worsens compared with normal subjects.

Response to Carbon Dioxide and Oxygen

The PCO_2 of blood, normally held at 40 mm Hg, does not change by more than +2 to −2 mm Hg throughout the day and night. This illustrates the remarkable sensitivity and responsiveness of the sensor, controller, and effector system.

The response of the system can be determined by having an individual breathe different concentrations of CO_2 while measuring the minute ventilation (Fig. 15-10). The response to a PCO_2 below 30 mm Hg is minimal. This helps explain the improved ability to hold one's breath after hyperventilating. As the PCO_2 climbs to and above the 30- to 40-mm Hg range, minute ventilation increases. The increase in ventilation brought on by a PCO_2 above 40 mm Hg is relatively linear at a rate of about 2 to 3 L/min for each 1-mm Hg increase in PCO_2.

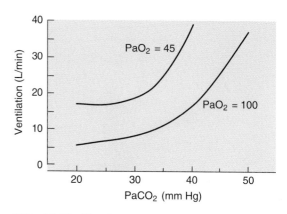

FIG. 15-10 Ventilatory response to changes in arterial PCO_2. With normal PaO_2, minute ventilation increases significantly when PCO_2 exceeds 30 to 40 mm Hg. During hypoxic conditions (PaO_2 = 45 mm Hg), ventilation is further increased.

Both the rate of breathing and the tidal volume increase with increasing CO_2. This response illustrates the set point defense by the system to maintain a PCO_2 of 40 mm Hg.

Hypoxia increases the sensitivity to CO_2. When the PO_2 is decreased the response to increasing PCO_2 occurs sooner and results in a greater minute ventilation response (see Fig. 15-10).

The normal response to CO_2 is blunted during chronic hypoventilation, during sleep in some subjects, with increasing age, and in some with racial and genetic differences. Central nervous system depressing drugs such as anesthetics, narcotics, and barbiturates also reduce the response to CO_2 and depress the respiratory center. In excessive dosages, respiratory center activity drops and the patient hypoventilates and can stop breathing **(apnea).**

When a subject breathes gas with a progressively lower O_2 concentration, the rate of breathing generally increases after the O_2 concentration drops sufficiently. Fig. 15-11 shows the response to hypoxemia and hypercapnia. Ventilation increases when the inspired O_2 concentration drops to about 7%. This corresponds to an arterial PO_2 of about 50 mm Hg.

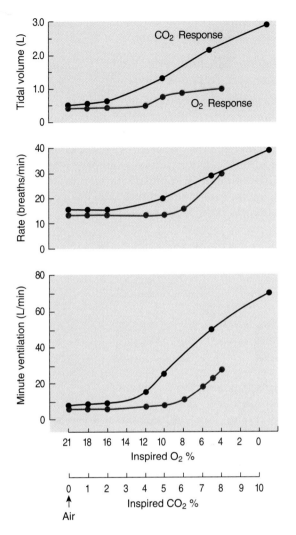

FIG. 15-11 Changes in breathing pattern (tidal volume, frequency, and minute ventilation) when breathing increasing carbon dioxide *(CO$_2$)* and decreasing oxygen *(O$_2$)* concentrations (see text for discussion).

DIAGNOSTIC FOCUS

Breathing Pattern Changes during a Diabetic Crisis

An 18-year-old woman was admitted to the emergency department after losing consciousness. She presented with normal blood pressure and heart rate. She was tachypneic and breathing deeply and had an unusual fruity smelling breath. Arterial blood was sampled and the following blood gases and acid-base balance were found:

pH	7.08
PCO$_2$	21 mm Hg
PO$_2$	15 mm Hg
HCO$_3^-$	6 mEq/L
Base excess	−24 mEq/L

These results reveal a partially compensated metabolic acidosis, significant hyperventilation, and a normal PO$_2$ when hyperventilating while breathing air. Further blood analysis revealed a markedly elevated blood glucose of 810 mg/dl and ketones in her urine. These are all consistent with a diabetic ketoacidosis that is stimulating changes in her breathing pattern consistent with Kussmaul breathing (deep and rapid). The patient was treated with intravenous fluids, HCO$_3^-$, and insulin and was monitored. Over the next 12 hours she became conscious, her glucose returned to near-normal levels, and her breathing pattern normalized. Repeat blood gas analysis showed normalization of her acid-base status.

The response is primarily brought about by an increase in respiratory rate and a minor increase in tidal volume. Peripheral chemoreceptors respond to the declining arterial PO$_2$ by stimulating the respiratory center. The response to hypoxia decreases with increasing age and long-term exposure to hypoxic environments (e.g., high altitude).

Fig. 15-11 also shows the response to inhaled CO$_2$. Increasing CO$_2$ causes an increase in both tidal volume and breathing frequencies.

Response to Acid-Base Imbalance

Reduced blood pH results primarily in peripheral chemoreceptor stimulation and increased minute ventilation. The response becomes pronounced when the pH drops below 7.20. This situation frequently occurs in subjects who are exercising to a point where O_2 delivery is insufficient to meet the demands. When this occurs, the subject shifts to anaerobic metabolism and produces greater quantities of lactic acid. This results in a metabolic acidosis that triggers increased ventilation via peripheral chemoreceptor stimulation. The response is usually a combination of increased tidal volume and respiratory rate.

Interaction during Gas Exchange Failure and Acid-Base Imbalance

Various gas exchange and acid-base disturbances cause stimulation of the chemoreceptors and alterations in breathing. Fig. 15-12 illustrates how different gas exchange and acid-base abnormalities interact with the chemoreceptors, stimulate the respiratory center, alter ventilation, and change gas exchange and acid-base back toward normal.

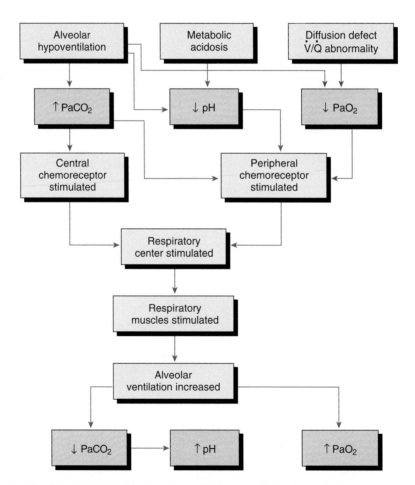

FIG. 15-12 Interconnected response of the respiratory system to various gas exchange and acid-base abnormalities.

Conditions that cause alveolar hypoventilation result in CO_2 retention, respiratory acidosis, and hypoxemia. Severe hypoxemia, circulatory failure, and a variety of metabolic derangements can cause acidosis. Diffusion defects and $\dot{V}/\dot{Q}$ abnormalities generally cause hypoxemia. These abnormalities stimulate the chemoreceptors, which, in turn, cause stimulation of the respiratory center (an example of negative feedback). Respiratory muscle activity increases, resulting in greater alveolar ventilation. Increased alveolar ventilation reduces PCO_2 and increases pH and PO_2. As the adjustments produce normalization, the stimulation of both chemoreceptors decreases and the increase in alveolar ventilation moderates toward a value that maintains the PCO_2, PO_2, and pH in a more normal range. These changes illustrate how the system can respond and help correct a gas exchange problem. The system can perform these adjustments if all the various components are functioning; in some cases, though, they do not, leading to sustained or worsening respiratory failure and acid-base imbalance.

Airway, Lung and Chest Wall Receptors

The lungs and airways have a variety of receptors that react to mechanical and chemical stimuli (Table 15-2). When these receptors are activated, they cause adjustments in the breathing pattern.

Lung Stretch Receptors

Deep breathing has an inhibitory, or negative feedback, effect on the respiratory center. Within the smooth muscles of the airway are nerve endings that become active when the airway wall is stretched during lung inflation. These **stretch receptors** are slow adapting sensors that produce greater numbers of impulses as the lung inflates. The impulses are carried to the brain stem by the vagus nerve and cause activation of the pneumotaxic and expiratory pool of neurons. This results in the inhibition of inspiratory neuron activity and reduction of inspiratory effort. In addition, the nearby cardioinhibitory centers are activated, resulting in bradycardia and diminished cardiac contractility.

When these receptors are activated by lung inflation, further inflation is inhibited and the rate of breathing slows down. This is known as the **Hering-Breuer inflation reflex,** which is most active in human subjects when the tidal volume is greater than 1.0 L. At lower tidal volumes, this reflex is not believed to be active. It appears to be more active in the newborn infant during resting ventilation and in

Table 15-2   Breathing Receptors of the Lungs, Airways, and Chest Wall

Type	Stimulus	Response
Lung stretch receptors in airway wall	Lung inflation	Inhibits deep inflation and slows breathing (Hering-Breuer reflex)
Chest wall stretch receptors in upper airway	Thorax inflation	Appears to be associated with dyspnea
Irritant receptors along upper airway	Dust, rapid gas flow, cold gas, manipulation	Coughing, sneezing, laryngeal spasm, bronchospasm, mucus production, bradycardia, hypotension
C-fiber receptors in alveolus	Alveolar congestion, chemical injury, microemboli	Rapid and shallow breathing, bradycardia, mucus secretion

the adult during exercise when tidal ventilation increases.

Muscle and Chest Wall Stretch Receptors

The diaphragm and intercostal muscles contain muscle spindles that respond to muscle stretch when the thorax is sufficiently inflated. Impulses from these sensors are sent to ascending tracts in the spinal cord where they travel up to the brain. Although it is not exactly clear what effect these signals have on the pattern of breathing, it has been suggested that they may play a role in the sensation of dyspnea. It is thought that the dyspnea experienced by those individuals with advanced chronic obstructive pulmonary disease (COPD) is, in part, a result of the chronically hyperexpanded condition of the lungs and the thorax. COPD is thought to produce persistent activation of these stretch receptors and the resulting sensation of dyspnea.

Irritant Receptors

The epithelial lining of the upper airway has rapid-adapting, free nerve endings that act as **irritant receptors.** Concentrated in the nasal cavity, larynx, trachea, and large bronchi, these receptors react to inhaled dust particles (e.g., smoke), rapid gas flow, cold gas, mechanical stimulation of the larynx and airways, and a variety of irritating chemicals (e.g., carbon dioxide, sulfur dioxide, nitrogen dioxide, and ammonia). Usually more than one of these different receptors are activated, resulting in a vagal nerve-mediated irritant reflex. This reflex response can cause coughing, sneezing, laryngeal spasm, bronchospasm, increased mucus production, bradycardia, and hypotension. It is often seen when an individual's upper airway is manipulated with a scope or suction catheter. It has also been suggested that these receptors are responsible for intermittent deep breathing, or sighing, which results in the redistribution of surfactant at the alveolar lining. The rapid adapting nature of these receptors results in their becoming less reactive to frequent irritation (e.g., chronic cigarette smoke exposure).

C-Fiber Receptors

The alveolar walls, small conducting airways, and blood vessels are supplied with an extensive network of free nerve endings that react to certain chemicals and mechanical stimulation. These receptors are generally known as *C-fibers* (those around the alveolar capillaries are also known as **J receptors**). They are stimulated by fluid accumulation and several chemicals (e.g., bradykinin) released during lung injury. The activation of these receptors is thought to result in dyspnea, bradycardia, and rapid and shallow breathing. In severe cases it is thought to result in apnea. Irritant and C-fiber sensory activity does not appear to play a role during normal automatic control of breathing.

Baroreceptors

Changes in blood pressure can cause changes in the breathing pattern. Increased blood pressure stimulates the carotid and aortic baroreceptors (see Fig. 15-9). Impulses from these receptors sent to the brain stem by the glossopharyngeal and vagus nerves cause alteration in respiratory neural activity. Two different responses are frequently observed. During hypertension an individual may decrease the rate and depth of breathing and have short periods of apnea. Hypotension generally causes a faster rate and during severe hypotension the breathing pattern can become irregular.

● MEASURING RESPIRATORY CENTER ACTIVITY

Tests of Breathing Control

A variety of different tests are available to evaluate the control of breathing (Box 15-1). These range from simply observing the

Tests of Respiratory Center Activity

Breathing pattern
Inspiratory flow rate
Mouth occlusion pressure
Response to hypercapnia
Response to hypoxia
Diaphragmatic electromyography
Phrenic electroneurography

Elements of the Normal Breathing Pattern

f	10 to 20 breaths/min
V_T	0.4-0.6 L
f/V_T	<50
T_I	1.0-2.0 seconds
I:E	1:3-1:4
T_I/T_{TOT}	0.2-0.25

breathing pattern to more sophisticated tests of respiratory center activity. These tests reveal the respiratory "drive," or strength, of neural signals for breathing. Some of these tests reflect both respiratory center drive and respiratory muscle performance, making them less able to indicate pure respiratory center activity.

Breathing Pattern

The normal breathing pattern is a rhythmic series of breaths with a normal frequency, tidal volume, and timing components. These are summarized in Box 15-2. Variations from this pattern, such as breathing fast and shallow or slow and deep, indicate variations in the control of breathing in response to various stimuli or conditions. Respiratory pattern change is often produced as an attempt to subconsciously reduce the work of breathing to a minimum. Generally, excessive rates (>30/min) and depths (>1.0 L) of breathing indicate abnormally increased respiratory drive.

Determining the ratio of frequency to tidal volume (f/V_T) is a useful method of looking at the pattern of breathing. By combining these two factors, excessive work can readily be determined. Values greater than 50 (i.e., fast and shallow) suggest increasing work and inefficient gas exchange. Values greater than 100 are suggestive of imminent respiratory failure.

Spontaneous Inspiratory Flow

The flow of gas into the lungs during inspiration is an important indicator of the strength of respiratory center activity, the strength of the respiratory muscles, and the general mechanical condition of the lungs and airway. The flow of gas can be measured with a pneumotachograph (see Chapter 11) or can be determined with the following relationship:

$$\frac{V_T}{T_I}$$

where V_T is the tidal volume and T_I is the length of the inspiratory phase. This ratio yields an average inspiratory flow. Normally, the typical value during resting inspiration is 0.5 L/sec. Increased flow indicates increased respiratory center drive. Caution is necessary with this measurement, however. Conditions that cause increased airway resistance or respiratory muscle fatigue reduce gas flow for a given amount of effort. These situations make this test an unreliable indicator for respiratory center drive when comparing individuals. If the airway resistance and respiratory muscle strength are stable, flow of gas can be used to trend changes in respiratory drive in the same individual.

Mouth Occlusion Pressure

The strength of the respiratory signal for inspiration can be evaluated by measuring the

Carbon Dioxide Retention during Treatment of a Chronic Obstructive Pulmonary Disease Patient

A 71-year-old man with end-stage chronic obstructive pulmonary disease was admitted to the emergency department for increasing dyspnea. His arterial blood gas and acid-base balance shortly after admission while he was breathing air were as follows:

pH	7.30
PCO_2	73 mm Hg
PO_2	41 mm Hg
HCO_3^-	35 mEq/L
Base excess	6 mEq/L

These findings reveal significant hypoxia, alveolar hypoventilation, and a partially compensated respiratory acidosis. He was given supplemental oxygen to breathe with a mask set to deliver 60% oxygen. Thirty minutes later the patient became hard to arouse, his breathing pattern was more relaxed, and another arterial blood sample was collected and the following was found:

pH	7.18
PCO_2	95 mm Hg
PO_2	117 mm Hg
HCO_3^-	35 mEq/L
Base excess	3 mEq/L

This shows improved oxygenation, progressing hypoventilation, and respiratory acidosis. The progressing hypoventilation was probably caused by the combining of further $\dot{V}/\dot{Q}$ abnormalities brought about by pulmonary vessel dilation and decreased hypoxic stimulation of breathing. Both of these can be caused by excessive oxygen therapy. It was decided to use positive pressure ventilatory support with a tight fitting mask to improve his alveolar ventilation and to use 35% oxygen to improve his PO_2. Repeat arterial blood gas and acid-base analysis 30 minutes after starting ventilatory support revealed improved oxygenation, acceptable levels of alveolar hypoventilation, and partially compensated respiratory acidosis. The patient was transferred to the medical intensive care unit where he further stabilized and was weaned from ventilatory support without incident. Over the next several days his dyspnea improved and he was transferred to a skilled nursing care facility for further care.

---

amount of negative pressure that is generated in the early part of inspiration. This is accomplished by having a subject breathe through a mouthpiece and, without notifying the subject, blocking the inspiratory supply of gas with a valve. When the subject starts to inhale, the amount of negative pressure generated at the mouthpiece is rapidly recorded. The amount of pressure generated during the first 0.1 second or 100 milliseconds (P_{100}) is a good indicator of respiratory drive supplied to the respiratory muscles. The short recording period avoids the confusion about the state of the respiratory muscles. Normal respiratory drive generates −4 to −6 cm H_2O. Respiratory

center depression results in reduced values, whereas increased drive results in the development of greater negative pressure.

Respiratory Gas Response

The response to increasing PCO_2 and decreasing PO_2 can be measured by exposing the subject to different gas mixtures and recording the change in the breathing pattern. By looking at the slope of the line defined by the simultaneous recording of minute ventilation and inhaled CO_2 concentration, the response can be determined. The normal response to increasing PCO_2 begins at a PCO_2 of about 30 mm Hg (see Figs. 15-10 and 11). The slope of this recording in the normal population ranges from 2 to 5 L/min/mm Hg increase in PCO_2. The response to hypoxia begins at a PO_2 of about 50 mm Hg with progressive hypoxia producing a slope of about 0.8 to 1 L/min/mm Hg drop in PO_2 (see Fig. 15-11). Depressed chemoreceptor or respiratory center activity results in a reduced response.

Respiratory Electromyography

The careful use of surface electrodes over the diaphragm and phrenic nerve and the use of signal filters enable the electrical activity in these structures to be recorded to determine the "strength" of activity. Electromyography is a noninvasive approach to recording the signals from the medulla oblongata. This technique is useful in comparing changes in activity during different conditions in the same individual. However, it is not useful for the comparison of an individual's recording to some "normal" amount of activity. For this reason, this technique remains largely a research tool for the evaluation of respiratory control. Developments in the techniques used to record activity in the respiratory muscles and phrenic nerves will undoubtedly continue to the point of clinical use in the future.

 HOW BREATHING CONTROL IS ADJUSTED DURING SLEEP AND EXERCISE

Recent investigations into the control of breathing during sleep and exercise reveal several differences when compared to resting breathing in the awake state.

Breathing Control during Sleep

Sleep is not one state of mental activity but actually several that cycle through the night about every 90 minutes. Two distinct states of sleep have been identified during the cycle: active and quiet sleep. During these two different phases the breathing pattern frequently changes.

During quiet sleep the individual displays four different stages that become progressively deeper. During the first two lighter stages the breathing pattern is being controlled by the automatic control center, often with an irregular pattern and frequent periods of short-term apnea that last less than 15 seconds. In the subsequent deeper two stages of quiet sleep, the breathing pattern is still under the control of the automatic center but becomes more regular. During these stages the minute ventilation decreases to the point where PCO_2 climbs about 5 mm Hg and PO_2 declines about 7 mm Hg, indicating a lowered response to CO_2 during the deeper periods of sleep. This suggests a less responsive system with deepening sleep.

The depression of the arousal centers of the brain (reticular activating system) during sleep is thought to cause most of the rhythm disturbances. Without the input from the arousal center and a decrease in the responsiveness to hypercapnia and hypoxia, the automatic control center appears to be less responsive to the point of rhythm disturbances.

Some individuals experience **sleep apnea** during the quiet sleep phase. Sleep apnea can be caused by two different mechanisms. During the early stages of quiet sleep, when the breathing pattern is irregular, some individuals experience apneic events that are caused by failure of the respiratory center. These individuals make no effort to breathe for more than 15 or 20 seconds. This form of sleep apnea is known as *central sleep apnea*. Another form of sleep apnea also occurs in some as the result of airway obstruction during the early stages of quiet sleep. In these early stages there is a general decrease of motor nerve activity to the hypoglossal and pharyngoglossal muscles. This results in relaxation of these muscles and narrowing of the pharynx to the point of producing snoring in some. Relaxation of these muscles and narrowing of the pharynx can lead to airway obstruction in those individuals who have an already narrowed or partially obstructed airway (more frequently in men with large tongues, short necks, and who snore). This situation can progress to complete airway obstruction. Despite making breathing efforts, the airway obstruction prevents air movement. This form of sleep apnea, known as obstructive sleep apnea, can result in declines in oxygenation to the point of stressful arousal. This phenomenon can repeat over and over in some to the point of producing sleep deprivation and hypertension.

During active sleep an individual displays **rapid eye movement (REM).** It is during this period that most dreaming occurs. During REM sleep the pattern of breathing can shift between regular and irregular rhythms. The number of apneic events declines, however, the breathing response to hypoxia is diminished during this stage. The breathing pattern becomes most irregular when there are bursts of REM activity and active dreaming. It is thought that the voluntary control centers in the upper brain are active, causing this irregular breathing pattern.

Control during Exercise

Of the many mysteries of ventilatory control, the exact mechanism that regulates breathing during exercise continues to be debated. The problem centers on the ability of the system to respond so well that there is no detectable change in PCO_2 as one warms up, reaches steady-state exercise, and cools down. Hypoxia is not the stimulus. In fact, the PO_2 actually increases with increased ventilation during exercise. Conventional descriptions of chemical control of breathing suggest that there should be a significant increase in PCO_2 to cause the increase in ventilation that is observed, but the usual observation is that the PCO_2 remains stable at 40 mm Hg or even decreases.

During the early warm-up stages, the breathing pattern is altered by sensory information from exercising muscles, proprioceptors in and around joints, and anticipatory stimuli. Lifting, jumping, and other intermittent bursts of activity are often accompanied by breath holding, which is under voluntary control. During increasing, steady-state, and decreasing exercise, CO_2 production is varied and ventilation is adjusted to maintain a normal PCO_2. The ability to maintain PCO_2 at a normal value despite variations in metabolic rate is best explained by a respiratory center/chemoreceptor system that is responsive to small increases in PCO_2. The ability to detect a small increase (<1 mm Hg) in PCO_2 above the set point and a quick reaction by the control center appear to be the primary mechanisms at work to regulate ventilation. The increased ventilation and pulmonary perfusion during exercise is often better matched; in some, this yields a greater PO_2 than at rest.

Increased levels of ventilation and O_2 consumption are common findings after exercise. This change in breathing pattern persists for about 20 to 30 minutes in most normal individuals. The increased O_2 consumption that occurs during the postexercise period is known as the **oxygen debt** of exercise. The major stimulus for postexercise hyperventilation is a metabolic acidosis that is the product of muscle hypoxia, a shift to anaerobic metabolism, and the formation of lactic acid. The hyperventilation is a compensatory action by the control center in response to peripheral chemoreceptor stimulation by low pH. The length of time it takes for the individual to return to resting ventilation levels indicates how fit the individual is. Well-trained athletes have short-term hyperventilation, whereas sedentary subjects tend to have prolonged periods of hyperventilation. Individuals with cardiopulmonary disease have prolonged and more intense postexercise hyperventilation.

The excess lactic acid is converted by the liver and heart back to glucose. This process of glucose creation is an aerobic process that results in an elevated rate of O_2 consumption. When all the excess lactic acid is converted to glucose, the increased O_2 consumption and acidosis subside and the breathing pattern returns to normal.

ABNORMAL BREATHING PATTERNS

The breathing pattern changes in response to a variety of conditions. Some of these patterns are normal responses to stress, whereas others represent abnormal control of breathing. Normal breathing, also known as **eupnea,** and abnormal patterns of breathing are shown in Figs. 15-13 and 15-14.

Variations in Rate and Depth of Breathing

The normal rate of breathing ranges from 10 to 20 breaths per minute. Rates in excess of 20/min are termed **tachypnea** (see Fig. 15-13). Tachypnea is a normal response to exercise or other conditions that result in increased metabolic rate. Tachypnea is not a normal event when a patient is at rest. In this situation, some type of abnormal condition is stimulating the respiratory center. Hypoxia, acidosis, low blood pressure, brain injuries, fever, pain, and anxiety all cause tachypnea. Rates less than 10/min are called **bradypnea** (see Fig. 15-13). The most common cause of bradypnea is the effect that anesthetic and other central nervous system depressant drugs (e.g., narcotic or barbiturate drug overdose) have on the brain stem.

The normal tidal volume in the adult ranges from 0.4 to 0.6 L. When an individual is breathing with an excessive volume, this condition is called *hyperpnea* (see Fig. 15-13). Hyperpnea, which occurs during exercise, is thought to be the result of increased CO_2 pro-

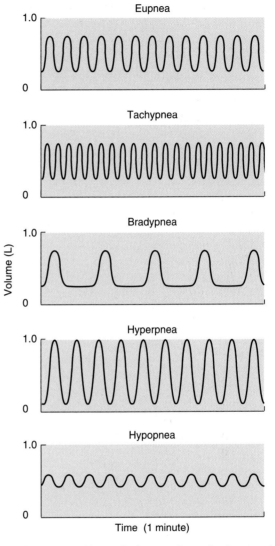

FIG. 15-13 Normal (eupnea) and abnormal breathing patterns (see text for descriptions).

duction and central chemoreceptor stimulation. Breathing with a reduced tidal volume is known as **hypopnea** (see Fig. 15-13); this normally occurs during stages of deep sleep. However, it is generally an abnormal finding that occurs in those with a neuromuscular

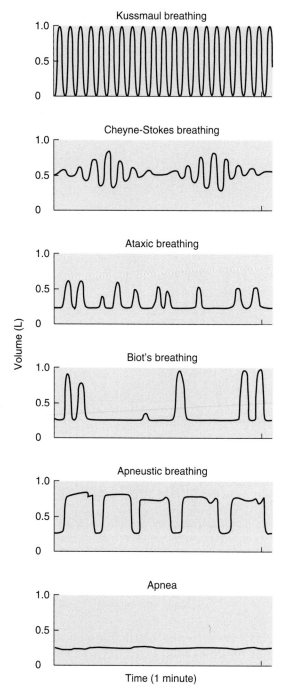

FIG. 15-14 Abnormal breathing patterns (see text for descriptions).

disease (e.g., Guillain-Barré syndrome and end-stage multiple sclerosis) and during conditions of severely reduced lung or chest wall compliance (e.g., pulmonary fibrosis). Often a compensatory tachypnea occurs to increase alveolar ventilation.

The patient in out-of-control diabetic acidosis often demonstrates a rapid and deep breathing pattern known as **Kussmaul breathing** (see Fig. 15-14). This pattern normally occurs during and shortly after severe exercise.

Periodic Breathing

Some patients who are severely hypoxic or who are in cardiac failure display a bizarre pattern of breathing that results in gradual increasing and decreasing tidal volume. A short apneic period usually occurs as the tidal volume drops to a minimum. This form of periodic breathing with waxing and waning tidal volume is known as **Cheyne-Stokes breathing** (see Fig. 15-14). It is thought that severe hypoxia and severe cardiac failure both result in reduced cardiac output, prolonging the circulation time between the lung and the chemoreceptors. This lengthens the time it takes for the effect of gas exchange in the lung to reach the chemoreceptors and stimulate the brain. The delay enables the respiratory center to underreact and overreact as different blood PCO_2 values are presented to the chemoreceptors. However, not all cases of Cheyne-Stokes breathing can be explained by this mechanism.

Highly irregular tidal volume and respiratory rate rhythm, known as **ataxic breathing** (see Fig. 15-14), can be seen during respiratory muscle fatigue and impending respiratory failure. It is an important finding in someone who is in respiratory failure, suggesting that ventilation and gas exchange will probably continue to deteriorate.

A more ominous form of ataxic breathing is the highly irregular pattern that has frequent periods of apnea and irregular tidal volume. This pattern, known as **Biot's breathing** (see Fig. 15-14), represents highly abnormal ventilatory control that is unable to maintain normal gas exchange.

Injuries to the brain stem can lead to a highly abnormal pattern of breathing known as **apneustic breathing** (see Fig. 15-14). This pattern has a prolonged inspiratory phase that results in a reversed I:E ratio. The cause is frequently associated with injuries to the pons or expiratory neuron pool of the medulla. In either case, the inspiratory pool is not inhibited and the pattern is dominated by an abnormal inspiratory phase. This pattern can be elicited for short periods by sudden immersion in cold water (e.g., the cold shower effect).

The absence of breathing, known as *apnea* (see Fig. 15-14), is caused by total failure of the respiratory center (central sleep apnea, brain injury, or drug overdose), failure of respiratory signals to reach the respiratory muscles (spinal cord injury at C3), respiratory muscle failure (end-stage multiple sclerosis), or airway obstruction (obstructive sleep apnea).

CHAPTER SELF-TEST QUESTIONS

1. The set point for control of breathing is a
   a. PO_2 of 100 mm Hg
   b. pH of 7.40
   c. lung inflation of 1.0 L
   d. PCO_2 of 40 mm Hg
2. The pool of neurons that "drives" inspiration during the automatic control of breathing is located in the
   a. cerebellum
   b. medulla oblongata
   c. hypothalamus
   d. pons
   e. spinal cord

3. The neuron pool in the pons acts to
   a. stimulate inflation during automatic breathing
   b. inhibit the cough reflex
   c. inhibit inspiration during automatic breathing
   d. stimulate the gag reflex that results in glottic closure
4. The control center that is responsible for performing the forced vital capacity maneuver is located in the
   a. cerebral cortex
   b. brain stem
   c. thalamus
   d. pons
5. What is the most powerful stimulant for breathing?
   a. elevated levels of PCO_2
   b. lower levels of PO_2
   c. decreased SaO_2
   d. increased CSF pH
   e. lung inflation
6. The primary site for hypoxia sensation is/are the
   a. central chemoreceptor
   b. alveolar walls
   c. carotid sinus bodies
   d. pulmonary arterioles
7. What level of PO_2 results in significant sensor stimulation, respiratory center activity, and increased ventilation?
   a. 80 to 100 mm Hg
   b. 65 to 80 mm Hg
   c. 50 to 60 mm Hg
   d. 30 to 50 mm Hg
8. Metabolic acidosis stimulates the _____ and this causes a compensatory _____.
   1. central chemoreceptor
   2. peripheral chemoreceptor
   3. hypoventilation
   4. hyperventilation
      a. 1 and 3
      b. 1 and 4
      c. 2 and 3
      d. 2 and 4

9. Stimulating the upper airway with inhaled dust, cold air, increased flow, noxious gases, or mechanical stimulation can result in:
   1. coughing
   2. laryngospasm
   3. bronchospasm
      a. 3 only
      b. 1 and 2
      c. 2 and 3
      d. 1 and 3
      e. 1, 2, and 3

10. Which of the following findings indicate increased respiratory center drive?
    1. f = 33 breaths/min
    2. $V_T/VI = 1.5$ L/sec
    3. $P_{100} = 2$ cm H_2O
       a. 1 only
       b. 1 and 2
       c. 2 and 3
       d. 1 and 3
       e. 1, 2, and 3

For answers, see p. 476.

BIBLIOGRAPHY

1. Caruana-Montaldo B, Gleeson K, Zwillich CW: The control of breathing in clinical practice, *Chest* 117:205, 2000.
2. Comroe JH, Jr: *Physiology of respiration,* ed 2, Chicago, 1974, Year Book Medical.
3. Guyton AC: *Textbook of medical physiology,* ed 8, Philadelphia, 1991, WB Saunders.
4. Hornbein TF, ed: *Regulation of breathing,* parts I and II, vol 17, New York, 1981, Marcel Dekker.
5. Leff AR, Schumacker PT: *Respiratory physiology: basics and applications,* Philadelphia, 1993, WB Saunders.
6. Levitsky MG: *Pulmonary physiology,* ed 3, New York, 1991, McGraw Hill.
7. Levitzky GL, Hall SM, McDonough KH: *Cardiopulmonary physiology in anesthesiology,* New York, 1997, McGraw Hill.
8. Martini FH: *Fundamentals of anatomy and physiology,* Upper Saddle River, NJ, 1998, Prentice Hall.
9. Miller WF, Scacci R, Gast LR: *Laboratory evaluation of pulmonary function,* Philadelphia, 1987, JB Lippincott.
10. Mitchell RA, Burger AJ: *Neural regulation of respiration, Am Rev Respir Dis* 111:206, 1975.
11. Murray JF: *The normal lung,* ed 2, Philadelphia, 1986, WB Saunders.
12. Staub NC: *Basic respiratory physiology,* New York, 1991, Churchill Livingstone.
13. West JB: *Respiratory physiology,* ed 4, Baltimore, 1990, Williams & Wilkins.
14. West JB, ed: *Best and Taylor's physiological basis of medical practice,* ed 12, Baltimore, 1990, Williams & Wilkins.

*Pulmonary and Cardiovascular Symbols and Abbreviations

PRIMARY SYMBOLS

Primary symbols are capitalized and indicate the nature of the variable. They can be modified by the addition of a dot that indicates movement of this variable per minute or the flow of some substance (e.g., "$\dot{V}$" indicates gas flow). The primary symbols can be organized into several different groups.

Gas Exchange Group

C	concentration of a substance in a liquid
D	diffusion capacity
f	breathing frequency
F	fraction or decimal concentration of a particular gas within a gas mixture
P	pressure, partial or total
Q	blood volume
$\dot{Q}$	perfusion, blood flow per minute, cardiac output
R	gas exchange ratio
RQ	respiratory quotient
S	saturation
V	gas volume
$\dot{V}$	ventilation of the lungs per minute

Respiratory Mechanics Group

C	compliance
E	elastance
f	frequency of breathing
G	conductance
P	pressure, partial or total
R	resistance

---

*Modified from recommendations of the American Physiologic Society and the ACCP-ATS Committee on Pulmonary Nomenclature.

T	time
V	gas volume
W	work

QUALIFYING SYMBOLS

The primary symbols are further defined by the use of qualifying symbols. Qualifying symbols follow the primary symbol and are subscripted. They describe the location or physical phase of the primary variable. Gas phase variables are expressed as upper case symbols while liquid phase variables are expressed as lower case symbols. They can be modified by the addition of a bar over them to indicate an average or mixed variable (e.g., "$\bar{v}$" indicates mixed venous blood and "$\bar{E}$" indicates mixed expired gas).

a	arterial blood
A	alveolar gas
ab	abdominal
ao	airway opening
aw	airway
B	barometric or ambient
bs	body surface
c	capillary blood
D	dead space
di	diaphragmatic
dyn	dynamic
E	expired
es	esophageal
I	inspired
L	lung
max	maximum
pa	pulmonary artery
pl	pleural
pv	pulmonary vein
rs	total respiratory system

S	shunt
st	static
T	total or tidal
tm	transmural
tot	total
v	venous
$\bar{v}$	mixed venous
w	chest wall or thorax

SELECTED CARDIOVASCULAR AND PULMONARY ABBREVIATIONS AND SYMBOLS IN COMMON USE

Regional Pulmonary Anatomy

LLL	left lower lobe
LUL	left upper lobe
RUL	right upper lobe
RLL	right lower lobe
RML	right middle lobe

Lung Volumes

CV	closing volume
CC	closing capacity
ERV	expired reserve volume
FRC	functional residual volume
IC	inspiratory capacity
IRV	inspiratory reserve volume
RV	residual volume
TLC	total lung capacity
VC	vital capacity
V_D/V_T	dead space-to-tidal volume ratio
V_D	dead space volume
V_T	tidal volume
V_{TG}	thoracic gas volume

Spirometry

FEF_x	forced expiratory flow at a given percentage (x) of the expiratory FVC
FEV_x	forced expiratory volume for a given amount of time (x) in seconds
FIF_x	forced inspiratory flow at a given percentage of the inspiratory FVC
FIFR	forced inspiratory flow rate
FVC	forced vital capacity
MVV	maximum voluntary ventilation
PEFR	peak expiratory flow rate
SVC	slow vital capacity

Ventilation

f	breathing frequency
$\dot{V}_A$	alveolar ventilation per minute
$\dot{V}_D$	dead space ventilation per minute
$\dot{V}_E$	exhaled minute ventilation
$\dot{V}_I$	inhaled minute ventilation

Pulmonary Mechanics

C_{dyn}	dynamic compliance of respiratory system (lungs and thorax)
C_L	lung compliance
C_{rs}	respiratory system compliance
C_{st}	static compliance of respiratory system
C_W	chest wall compliance
E_{rs}	respiratory system elastance
G_{aw}	airway conductance
P_A	alveolar pressure
P_{ao}	pressure at airway opening
P_{aw}	airway pressure
P_B	barometric, ambient, or body surface pressure
P_{es}	esophageal pressure
P_L	transpulmonary pressure
P_{pl}	pleural space pressure
P_{rs}	transrespiratory or transairway pressure
P_W	transthoracic pressure
PE_{max}	maximal expiratory pressure
PI_{max}	maximal inspiratory pressure
R_{aw}	airway resistance to gas flow
R_E	expiratory phase resistance to gas flow
R_I	inspiratory phase resistance to gas flow
WOB	work of breathing

Diffusing Capacity

D_LCO	diffusing capacity of the lungs
D_LCO_{sb}	single breath holding diffusion capacity of the lungs
D_LCO_{ss}	steady state diffusing capacity of the lungs
D_LCO/V_L	diffusing capacity for a given gas volume of the lungs

Gas Exchange

$\dot{Q}_s/Q_T$	shunt fraction, ratio of shunted blood flow to total blood flow
$\dot{V}_A/Q_C$	alveolar ventilation fraction, ratio of alveolar ventilation to alveolar capillary blood flow
$\dot{V}CO_2$	carbon dioxide production per minute
V_D/V_T	dead space fraction, ratio of dead space volume to tidal volume
$\dot{V}O_2$	oxygen consumption per minute
$\dot{V}O_{2max}$	maximum oxygen consumption per minute

Blood Gas and Acid-Base Balance

C_aO_2	content of oxygen in arterial blood
$C_{(a-\bar{v})}O_2$	content difference of oxygen between arterial and mixed venous blood
C_cO_2	content of oxygen in the pulmonary end-capillary blood
$C_{\bar{v}}O_2$	content of oxygen in mixed venous blood
$[HCO_3^-]$	bicarbonate concentration
P_ACO_2	partial pressure of carbon dioxide in alveolar gas
P_aCO_2	partial pressure of carbon dioxide in arterial blood
P_cCO_2	partial pressure of carbon dioxide in capillary blood
$P_{\bar{E}}CO_2$	partial pressure of carbon dioxide in mixed exhaled gas
$P_{ET}CO_2$	partial pressure of carbon dioxide in exhaled gas at the end-tidal point
$P_{\bar{v}}CO_2$	partial pressure of carbon dioxide in mixed venous blood
P_AO_2	partial pressure of oxygen in alveolar gas
$P_{(A-a)}O_2$	partial pressure difference of oxygen between alveolar gas and arterial blood
P_aO_2	partial pressure of oxygen in arterial blood
P_aO_2/P_AO_2	partial pressure ratio between arterial blood and alveolar gas
$P_{(a-\bar{v})}O_2$	partial pressure difference of oxygen between arterial and mixed venous blood
P_cO_2	partial pressure of oxygen in capillary blood
P_cO_2	partial pressure of oxygen in pulmonary end-capillary blood
$P_{\bar{v}}O_2$	partial pressure of oxygen in mixed venous blood
pH	negative log of hydrogen ion concentration
S_aO_2	oxyhemoglobin saturation in arterial blood
$S_{\bar{v}}O_2$	oxyhemoglobin saturation in mixed venous blood

Cardiovascular Anatomic Regions

LA	left atrium
LV	left ventricle
RA	right atrium
RV	right ventricle

Hematologic Variables

Hb	hemoglobin
HTC	hematocrit
RBC	red blood cell
WBC	white blood cell

Cardiovascular Pressures, Blood Flow, and Other Mechanics

BP	blood pressure
CI	cardiac index
CO	cardiac output
CVP	central venous pressure
DBP	diastolic blood pressure
EDV	end diastolic volume
EF	ejection fraction
HR	heart rate
LAP	left atrial pressure
LVP	left ventricular pressure
LVSW	left ventricular stroke work
MAP	mean arterial pressure
PAP	pulmonary artery pressure
PAWP	pulmonary artery wedge pressure
PCWP	pulmonary capillary wedge pressure
PVR	pulmonary vascular resistance
Q	blood volume
$\dot{Q}$	blood flow or cardiac output per minute
RAP	right atrial pressure
RVP	right ventricular pressure
RVSW	right ventricular stroke work
SBP	systolic blood pressure
SV	stroke volume
SVR	systemic vascular resistance

GENERAL MEASUREMENT SYMBOLS AND ABBREVIATIONS

A	age
ATPS	gas conditions that are at ambient temperature, ambient barometric pressure, and saturated to 100% humidity
BSA	body surface area
BTPS	gas conditions that are at normal body temperature (37° C), one atmosphere of pressure (760 mm Hg), and saturated to 100% humidity
f	frequency of a repeating event (cycles per minute)
H or Ht	height
STPD	gas conditions that are at standard temperature (0° C), one atmosphere of pressure (760 mm Hg), and dry conditions with 0% humidity
T	temperature
W or Wt	weight

APPENDIX B

Selected Cardiopulmonary Formulas

CARDIOVASCULAR RELATIONSHIPS

Maximum heart rate	$HR_{max} = 220 - Age$
Stroke volume	$SV = \dot{Q}_T/HR$
Stroke index	$SI = SV/BSA$
Cardiac output	$\dot{Q}_T$ or $CO = SV \times HR$
Fick's method of determining cardiac putput	$\dot{Q}_T = \dot{V}O_2/(CaO_2 - C\bar{v}O_2)$
Cardiac index	$CI = CO/BSA$
Cardiac reserve	$CR = CO_{max} - CO_{rest}$
Ventricular ejection fraction	$EF = SV/EDV$
Mean arterial blood pressure	$MAP = (SBP + 2 \times DBP)/3$
Systemic vascular resistance	$SVR = (MAP - CVP/\dot{Q}_T) \times 80)$
Pulmonary vascular resistance	$PVR = (MPAP - PAWP/\dot{Q}_T) \times 80$
Double product	$DP = HR \times SBP/100$
Left ventricular stroke work index	$LVSWI = SI \times MAP \times 0.0136$
Right ventricular stroke work index	$RVSWI = SI \times MPAP \times 0.0136$
Left cardiac work index	$LCWI = CI \times MAP \times 0.0136$
Right cardiac work index	$RCWI = CI \times MPAP \times 0.0136$

PULMONARY RELATIONSHIPS

Transthoracic pressure	$P_w = P_{pl} - P_B$
Transpulmonary pressure	$P_L = P_{AW} - P_{pl}$
Transairway pressure	$P_{rs} = P_A - P_{ao}$
Transdiaphragmatic pressure	$P_{di} = P_{pl} - P_{abd}$
Static compliance of the respiratory system	$C_{stL} = \Delta V/\Delta P_A$
Specific lung compliance	$SpC_L = (\Delta V/V_L)/\Delta P_A$
Airway resistance	$R_{AW} = P_{rs}/\dot{V}$
Airway conductance	$G_{AW} = \dot{V}/P_{rs}$
Dynamic respiratory system compliance	$dynC_l = \Delta V/\Delta P_{pl}$

Selected Cardiopulmonary Values in a Normal Adult at Rest and During Exercise

Variable	Units	Resting	Exercise
HEMATOLOGIC			
Hematocrit	%	45	45
Erythrocyte count	per mm³	5,000,000	5,000,000
Hemoglobin	g/dl	15	15
Leukocyte count	per mm³	7000	7000
Thrombocyte count	per mm³	250,000	250,000
CARDIOVASCULAR			
Heart rate	beats/min	70	140
Stroke volume	ml/beat	80	120
Stroke volume index	ml/m²	50	75
Ventricular ejection fraction	%	65	80
Cardiac output	L/min	5	15
Cardiac index	L/min/m²	3.5	10.5
Systemic arterial blood pressure			
systolic/diastolic	mm Hg	120/80	130/85
mean	mm Hg	90	95
Resting double product		100	
Central venous pressure	mm Hg	5	7
Pulmonary artery blood pressure			
systolic/diastolic	mm Hg	25/10	40/20
mean	mm Hg	15	30
Pulmonary artery wedge pressure	mm Hg	10	15
Systemic vascular resistance	dyne × sec × cm⁻⁵	1000	470
Pulmonary vascular resistance	dyne × sec × cm⁻⁵	100	80
Left ventricular stroke work index	g × m/beat/m²	50	97
Right ventricular stroke work index	g × m/beat/m²	8	37
Left cardiac work index	kg × m/min/m²	4	14
Right cardiac work index	kg × m/min/m²	0.6	4

Continued.

Variable	Units	Resting	Exercise
LUNG VOLUME			
Total lung capacity	L	6	6
Vital capacity	L	5	5
Functional residual capacity	L	2.5	2.5
PULMONARY MECHANICS			
Respiratory rate	breaths/min	12	35
Tidal volume	L/breath	0.5	2.0
Static compliance of the respiratory system	ml/cm H_2O	100	125
Airway resistance	cm H_2O/L/s	1	1.5
Airway conductance	L/sec/cm H_2O	1	0.75
Dynamic respiratory system compliance	ml/cm H_2O	75	65
GAS EXCHANGE AND BLOOD GASES			
Carbon dioxide production	ml/min	200	1500
Oxygen consumption	ml/min	250	1500
Respiratory exchange ratio	ratio	0.80	1.0
pH		7.40	7.45
$PaCO_2$	mm Hg	40	35
HCO_3^-	mEq/L	24	23
PaO_2	mm Hg	100	105

D

Gas Volume and Flow Correction for Selected Ambient Temperatures to BTPS Conditions (Volume or Flow at BTPS Conditions = Volume or Flow at Ambient Temperature × Correction Factor)*

Ambient Temperature (° C)	Correction Factor
20	1.102
21	1.096
22	1.091
23	1.085
24	1.080
25	1.075
26	1.068
27	1.063
28	1.057
29	1.051
30	1.045
31	1.039
32	1.032
33	1.026
34	1.020
35	1.014
36	1.007
37	1.000

*Correction factors for constant barometric pressure.

Pressure Conversions (Starting Pressure × Factor = Converted Pressure)

Conversion	Factor
lb/in^2 to mm Hg	51.71 mm Hg/lb/in^2
mm Hg to cm H_2O	1.359 cm H_2O/mm Hg
cm H_2O to mm Hg	0.7355 mm Hg/cm
mm Hg to kPa	0.1333 kPa/mm Hg
kPa to mm Hg	7.50 mm Hg/kPa
cm H_2O to kPa	0.1812 kPa/cm H_2O
kPa to cm H_2O	5.519 cm H_2O/kPa

Regression Equations for Predicting Normal Adult Pulmonary Function Values

These equations are a representative sample of the various equations available for use in the pulmonary function laboratory. To use these equations, the height (H) in centimeters (cm = inches × 2.54), age (A) rounded to the nearest whole year, body surface area (BSA) in square meters, and weight (W) in Kg of the subject are employed to predict the normal value of the variable in question.

Variable		Regression Equation	Reference
TLC (L)	Males	$0.094\ H - 0.015\ A - 9.167$	1
	Females	$0.079\ H - 0.008\ A - 7.49$	
FRC (L)	Males	$0.0810\ H - 1.792\ A - 7.11$	1
	Females	$0.0421\ H - 0.00449\ A - 3.825$	
RV (L)	Males	$0.027\ H + 0.017\ A - 3.447$	1
	Females	$0.032\ H + 0.009\ A - 3.9$	
RV/TLC (ratio)	Males	$0.343\ A - 16.7$	1
	Females	$0.265\ A - 21.7$	
VC (L)	Males	$0.058\ H - 0.025\ A - 4.24$	2
	Females	$0.0453\ H - 0.024\ A - 2.852$	
FVC (L)	Same as VC prediction		
FEV_1 (L)	Males	$0.052\ H - 0.027\ A - 4.203$	3
	Females	$0.027\ H - 0.021\ A - 0.794$	
$FEV_{1\%}$ (%)	Males	$103.64 - 0.087\ H - 0.14\ A$	3
	Females	$107.38 - 0.111\ H - 0.109\ A$	
FEV_3 (L)	Males	$0.063\ H - 0.031\ A - 5.245$	3
	Females	$0.035\ H - 0.23\ A - 1.633$	
PEFR (L/s)	Males	$0.0567\ H - 0.024\ A + 0.225$	4
	Females	$0.0354\ H - 0.018\ A + 1.13$	
$FEF_{50\%}$ (L/s)	Males	$0.069\ H - 0.015\ A - 5.4$	3
	Females	$0.035\ A - 0.013\ A - 0.444$	
$FEF_{25\%-75\%}$ (L/s)	Males	$0.0185\ H - 0.045\ A + 2.513$	2
	Females	$0.0236\ H - 0.03\ A + 0.551$	

Continued.

Variable		Regression Equation	Reference
MVV (L/min)	Males	$1.19\ H - 0.816\ A - 37.9$	4
	Females	$0.84\ H - 0.685\ A - 4.87$	
MIP or P_{Imax} (cm H_2O)	Males	$143 - 0.55\ A$	5
	Females	$104 - 0.51\ A$	
MEP or P_{Emax} (cm H_2O)	Males	$268 - 1.03\ A$	5
	Females	$170 - 0.53\ A$	
Static Crs (ml/cm H_2O)	Males	$0.00516\ H + 0.0024\ A - 0.677$	6
	Females	$0.0039\ H + 0.0019\ A - 0.471$	
CV/VC (%)	Males	$0.357\ A + 0.562$	7
	Females	$0.293\ A + 2.812$	
CC/TLC (%)	Males	$0.496\ A + 14.878$	7
	Females	$0.536\ A + 14.42$	
P_aO_2 (mm Hg)	Supine	$103.5 - 0.42\ A$	8
	Sitting	$104.2 - 077\ A$	
$P_{A-a}O_2$ (mm Hg)	Supine	$0.42\ A$	8
	Sitting	$0.27\ A$	
$D_LCO_{single\ breath}$ (ml/min/mm Hg)			
	Males	$0.0984\ H - 0.177\ A + 9.93$	9
	Females	$0.112\ H - 0.177\ A + 7.72$	
Resting $\dot{V}O_2$ (ml/min)			
	Males	$1.98\ W + 0.72\ H - 0.97\ A + 9.6$	10
	Females	$1.37\ W + 0.266\ H - 0.67\ A + 9.4$	
Maximum $\dot{V}O_2$ (ml/min)			
	Males	$4.2 - 0.032\ A$	11
	Females	$2.6 - 0.014\ A$	

BIBLIOGRAPHY

1. Goldman HI, Becklake MR: Respiratory function tests: normal value at median altitude and predictions of normal results, *Am Rev Respir Dis* 76:457, 1959.
2. Morris JF, Koski A, Johnson LC: Spirometric standards for healthy non-smoking adults, *Am Rev Respir Dis* 103:57, 1971.
3. Knudson RJ et al: The maximal expiratory flow volume curve normal standard variability and effects of age, *Am Rev Respir Dis* 113:587, 1976.
4. Cherniack RM, Raber MD: Normal standards for ventilatory function using an automated wedge spirometer, *Am Rev Respir Dis* 106:38, 1972.
5. Black LF, Hyatt RE: Maximal respiratory pressures: normal values and relationship to age and sex, *Am Rev Respir Dis* 99:696, 1969.
6. Permutt S, Martin HB: Static pressure-volume characteristics of the lungs, *J Appl Physiol* 42:111.1977.
7. Buist SA, Ross BB: Predicted values for closing volumes using a modified single breath nitrogen test, *Am Rev Respir Dis* 111:405, 1975.
8. Bates DV, Macklem PT, Christie RV: *Respiratory function in disease,* ed 2, Philadelphia, 1971, WB Saunders.
9. Gaensler EA, Wright GW: Evaluation of respiratory impairment, *Arch Environ Health* 12:146, 1966.
10. Altman PL, Dittmer DS: *Respiratory and circulation,* Baltimore, 1971, Federation of American Societies for Experimental Biology.
11. Jones NL, et al: *Clinical exercise testing,* ed 2, Philadelphia, 1983, WB Saunders.

Answers to Chapter Self-Test Questions

1. c   5. c   8. b
2. d   6. c   9. a
3. b   7. c   10. d
4. c

1. e   5. c   8. d
2. b   6. c   9. b
3. b   7. e   10. d
4. c

1. c   5. d   8. d
2. a   6. b   9. a
3. b   7. a   10. a
4. e

1. c   5. a   8. b
2. a   6. d   9. c
3. d   7. a   10. b
4. a

1. a   5. d   8. a
2. d   6. b   9. a
3. b   7. d   10. e
4. a

1. a   5. c   8. b
2. c   6. d   9. c
3. d   7. e   10. a
4. a

1. d   5. d   9. b
2. c   6. c   10. c
3. b   7. d   11. a
4. d   8. e

1. a   5. d   8. b
2. d   6. e   9. b
3. b   7. b   10. a
4. a

1. b   5. d   8. c
2. a   6. b   9. c
3. a   7. c   10. d
4. d

1. a   5. e   8. e
2. a   6. c   9. a
3. b   7. c   10. b
4. d

1. a   5. d   8. c
2. d   6. c   9. d
3. d   7. a   10. c
4. a

1. c   5. a   8. b
2. b   6. d   9. d
3. e   7. c   10. a
4. d

CHAPTER 13

1. d	5. b	8. c
2. b	6. d	9. c
3. d	7. a	10. c
4. d		

CHAPTER 14

1. c	5. e	9. b
2. e	6. b	10. c
3. b	7. b	11. c
4. b	8. b	

CHAPTER 15

1. d	5. a	8. d
2. b	6. c	9. e
3. c	7. c	10. b
4. a		

Glossary

A-a gradient ($P_{A-a}O_2$) the difference between the alveolar and arterial oxygen partial pressure; an index or measure of the lung's ability to oxygenate blood

a/A ratio (PaO_2/PAO_2) the ratio of arterial to alveolar oxygen partial pressure; an index or measure of the lung's ability to oxygenate blood

absolute humidity the actual amount of water vapor in a given amount of air

acetylcholine a neurotransmitter released by selected neurons in the central nervous system; motor neurons that innervate the skeletal muscles and the neurons of the parasympathetic nervous system

acid a chemical substance with the ability to release hydrogen ions into a solution

acidemia a blood condition in which there is an excessive number of hydrogen ions resulting in a pH less than 7.35

acidic a condition of increased hydrogen ion concentration (low pH)

acidosis a general body fluid condition in which an excessive number of hydrogen ions results in a pH that is lower than normal

actin a contractile protein within muscle cells that interacts with myosin to result in twitching and tension development

action potential a rapid reversal in the membrane potential that occurs in nerve and muscle cells that is caused by a change in the membrane permeability for sodium and potassium ions

active transport the energy requiring movement of ions or molecules by carrier proteins through a membrane from a region of lower concentration to one of higher concentration

acute metabolic acidosis a condition of low blood pH brought about by a sudden decrease in buffers (e.g., HCO_3^-)

acute metabolic alkalosis a condition of high blood pH brought about by a sudden increase in buffers (e.g., HCO_3^-)

acute respiratory acidosis a condition of low blood pH brought about by sudden hypoventilation and elevated PCO_2

acute respiratory alkalosis a condition of high blood pH brought about by sudden hyperventilation and reduced PCO_2

adenosine a nucleotide that contains adenine and ribose

adenylate cyclase an enzyme that catalyzes the conversion of adenosine triphosphate to cyclic adenosine monophosphate

adrenergic a term used to describe the actions of epinephrine, norepinephrine, or other molecules with similar activity

adult respiratory distress syndrome (ARDS) a progressive form of pulmonary edema that results in respiratory failure; caused by numerous types of lung injury

adventitious breath sounds sounds within the lungs that are added as the result of spasmic or inflamed airways (wheezes), small airways that pop open during inhalation (crackles), and the bubbling sounds that air makes during passage through airways that are partially filled with secretions (rhonchi)

aerobic a type of tissue metabolism that relies on oxygen for the normal synthesis of adenosine triphosphate

aerosol a suspension of solid or liquid particles in a gas

afferent the movement of impulses or fluid toward a central point; afferent nerve impulses travel toward the brain and spinal cord

affinity the tendency of a drug or chemical to bind to a receptor

477

afterload the vascular resistance against which a ventricle pumps

agglutinate when antibodies in blood bind to antigens on the surface of a foreign protein or cell

agglutinins a specific kind of antibody whose interaction with antigen manifests as clumps

agglutinogens any antigenic substance that causes agglutination by the production of agglutinin

agonist a drug or other substance having a specific cellular affinity that produces a predictable response

agranulocytes white blood cells that do not contain cytoplasmic granules; specifically lymphocytes and monocytes

AIDS abbreviation for acquired immunodeficiency syndrome

airway conductance (G_{AW}) a measure of the ease of gas flow through an airway

airway resistance (R_{AW}) a measure of the resistance to gas flow through an airway

alkalemia a blood condition in which a reduced number of hydrogen ions results in a pH greater than normal

alkalotic a condition of decreased hydrogen ion concentration (high pH)

alpha-1 antitrypsin a chemical substance that inhibits the action of the proteolytic enzyme trypsin and that is associated with a form of destructive emphysema

alveolar air equation a mathematical relationship used to determine the partial pressure of oxygen in alveolar gas

alveolar dead space (V_{Dalv}) the amount of gas that fills the alveoli of the lungs that are not perfused by the pulmonary circulation; a form of ineffective lung volume

alveolar pressure (P_A) the total gas pressure exerted within the alveoli

alveolar ventilation ($\dot{V}_A$) the amount of air brought to the alveolar region of the lungs per minute

alveolar ventilation equation the product of the constant 0.863 and the ratio of CO_2 production divided by the partial pressure of alveolar CO_2

alveolar volume (V_A) that part of the tidal volume that reaches the alveolar region of the lungs; normally about 70% of the tidal volume

alveoli the terminal saclike structure of the lungs that is the location of gas exchange

ambient of or referring to the surrounding environmental conditions

ambient temperature and pressure, saturated (ATPS) the surrounding conditions of temperature and pressure that is saturated with water vapor

anaerobic a metabolic process that does not require oxygen for the synthesis of adenosine triphosphate

anatomical dead space includes all the airways from the nose and mouth through the terminal bronchioles; these airways do not have alveoli and do not participate in gas exchange

anatomical dead space volume (V_{Danat}) the volume of gas that fills the conducting airways of the respiratory system that does not participate in gas exchange with the blood; includes all the airways from the nasal cavity to and including the terminal bronchioles of the lungs

anemia a condition of reduced numbers of erythrocytes or hemoglobin

aneurysm a localized dilation of the wall of a blood vessel

angina pectoralis an attack of severe chest pain associated with reduced coronary blood flow and myocardial hypoxia; the pain commonly radiates into the neck, jaw, left shoulder, and left arm

angiogram a visual record of the blood flow within an artery produced by placing a radiopaque dye in the blood and taking a series of x-ray scans

angioplasty the surgical repair of an artery; balloon dilation of an artery

angiotensin II a powerful vasoconstrictor and a stimulator of aldosterone secretion from the adrenal cortex that is secreted as an inactive form by the liver and converted to an active form in the lungs

anion a negatively charged ion

anion gap the difference in the total number of cations and anions in blood plasma.

annulus fibrosus a connective tissue plate located between the atria and the ventricles that houses the valves of the heart

antagonist a substance that acts in opposition to another substance

antecubital fossa in front of the elbow; at the bend of the elbow

antiarrhythmic of or pertaining to a procedure or substance that prevents or corrects an abnormal cardiac rhythm

antidiuretic hormone (ADH) a hormone secreted by the posterior pituitary that stimulates water reabsorption along the distal tubule of the nephron

aorta   the major systemic vessel of the arterial system of the body; emerges from the left ventricle

aortic regurgitation   backflow of blood from the aorta into the left ventricle, indicating an incompetent valve

aortic semilunar valve   a valve in the heart between the left ventricle and the aorta

aortic trunk   the superior left bend of the aorta between the ascending and descending portions; also known as the aortic arch

aortic valve stenosis   a cardiac anomaly characterized by a narrowing or stricture of the aortic valve

apical   of or pertaining to the summit, peak, or apex

aplastic anemia   a condition of reduced blood cell numbers in blood that is caused by failure of the bone marrow to form new cells

apnea   an absence of spontaneous breathing

apneustic breathing   a pattern of respirations characterized by a prolonged inspiratory phase followed by a short expiratory phase

ARDS   abbreviation for adult (or acute) respiratory distress syndrome

arrhythmia   absence of rhythm of the heartbeat; irregular heartbeat

arteriole   a small-diameter artery that carries blood to a capillary bed

artery   a vessel that carries blood away from the heart to the tissues

ascites   an abnormal intraperitoneal accumulation of a fluid containing large amounts of protein and electrolytes

asphyxia   cessation of ventilation leading to acute hypoxia and hypercapnia

asthma   an airway disorder caused by airway smooth muscle spasm, mucosal inflammation, and excessive mucus secretion; causes increased airway resistance and wheezing

asynchronous breathing   an abnormal breathing pattern in which the rib cage and abdomen do not move outward

asystole   the absence of a heartbeat

ataxic breathing   a respiratory pattern marked by disorder or irregularity

atelectasis   an abnormal condition characterized by the collapse of lung tissue preventing gas exchange

atherosclerosis   an arterial disorder characterized by the deposit of plaques of cholesterol, lipids, and cellular debris in the inner layers of the walls of arteries

atrial fibrillation   irregular and rapid contractions of the atria working independently of the ventricles

atrial flutter   very rapid atrial contractions

atrial "gallop"   an S_4 heart sound that resembles the gait of a running horse and indicates atrial contraction into a stiff ventricle

atrial natriuretic peptide (ANP)   a hormone secreted within the atrium that inhibits sodium reabsorption by the kidneys, thus increasing sodium and water excretion in the urine

atrial septal defect   an abnormal opening in the interatrial septum that allows blood to flow from one atrium to the other

atrioventricular block   an abnormality of the cardiac conduction system that results in slowing or complete blockage of the impulse as it travels through the atrioventricular node and causes abnormal lengthening of the PR interval

atrioventricular node   a microscopic aggregation of specialized cardiac fibers located in the interatrial septum of the heart; part of the conduction system of the heart

atrioventricular sulcus   a shallow grove that runs horizontally around the heart between the upper and lower chambers

atrium   either of the two superior chambers of the heart that receives venous blood

atropine   a parasympathetic cholinergic receptor-blocking drug used to speed up the heart rate

auscultation   the act of listening for sounds within the body to evaluate the condition of the heart, lungs, pleura, intestines, and other organs or to detect the fetal heart sounds

automaticity   a property of neuron and muscle cells that allows self-activation, such as the cells found in the sinoatrial node of the heart

auto-PEEP (occult-PEEP)   an abnormal condition that produces pressure within the lungs at end-exhalation caused by trapped gas not exhaled as the result of insufficient time for exhalation

autoregulation   the ability to self-regulate a mechanical or physiological system

AV   abbreviation for atrioventricular

B cells   lymphocytes that can be transformed by antigens into plasma cells that secrete antibodies

band cells   immature neutrophils

barometric pressure (P_B)   the total pressure exerted by the atmosphere on the surface of the body

baroreceptors   a pressure-sensitive nerve ending found within the walls of the atria, vena cava, aorta, and sinus of the carotid artery

base   any substance that absorbs hydrogen ions

base deficit   the drop below normal in the amount of total buffers within the blood

base excess (BE)   the rise above normal in the amount of total buffers within the blood

basic   a condition of decreased hydrogen ion concentration (high pH)

basophils   a granular leukocyte that readily stains with basophilic dye

bicarbonate (HCO₃⁻)   an anion that acts as an important base in intracellular and extracellular fluid

bicuspid valve (mitral valve)   a two-leafed valve that allows blood to flow from the left atrium into the left ventricle and prevents backward blood flow into the left atrium from the left ventricle

bigeminy   literally "an association in pairs"; commonly refers to the cardiac arrhythmia characterized by paired premature ventricular contractions

Biot's breathing   an abnormal respiratory pattern characterized by irregular breathing with periods of apnea; symptomatic of meningitis or increased intracranial pressure

blood vessel tone   the comprehensive tension the smooth muscle cells develop in the wall of a vessel

blood-brain barrier (BBB)   a covering of glial cells around the brain's capillaries that prevents various chemicals from entering the brain tissue and causing dysfunction

body plethysmography   a device for studying alveolar pressure, lung volume, and airway resistance

body temperature and ambient pressure, saturated (BTPS)   the conditions of 37° C, one atmosphere of pressure and saturated with water vapor

Bohr effect   the impact of variations in blood pH on the affinity of hemoglobin for oxygen

Bohr equation   the equation used to determine the dead space/tidal volume ratio

brachiocephalic artery (innominate artery)   the first artery on the arch of the aorta, which gives rise to the right common carotid and subclavian veins

bradycardia   an abnormal condition characterized by a heart rate of less than 60 beats per minute

bradykinin   a nine-amino acid peptide that causes vasodilation

bradypnea   an abnormally slow rate of breathing (less than eight breaths per minute)

bronchitis   an acute or chronic inflammation of the mucous membranes of the tracheobronchial tree

bronchoconstriction   narrowing of a bronchus caused by the contraction of smooth muscle

bronchodilation   the opening or dilation of an airway (reverse of bronchoconstriction) usually via sympathetic stimulation

bronchorrhea   the excessive discharge of respiratory tract secretions

bronchovesicular breath sounds   breath sounds heard distal to the central airways that are less intense and of lower pitch than tracheal-bronchial breath sounds

Brownian motion   the random movement of molecules within a mass of molecules

bruit   an abnormal sound heard on auscultation of the heart or large vessels caused by turbulence or obstruction

buffer   a molecule in a chemical solution that minimizes fluctuations in pH

bundle branches   a segment or network of specialized muscle fibers that conduct electrical impulses within the heart

bundle of His   a bend of fibers in the myocardium through which the cardiac impulse is transmitted from the atrioventricular node to the ventricles

canals of Lambert   intercommunicating channels between terminal bronchioles and the alveoli that are 30 μm in size and appear to remain open even when bronchiolar smooth muscle is contracted

capillary   a microscopic blood vessel that connects an arteriole and a venule; the functional unit of the circulatory system

capillary action   a physical phenomenon whereby a liquid in a small tube tends to move upward against the force of gravity because of both adhesive and surface tension forces

capnogram   a recording of the proportion (partial pressure or percent) of carbon dioxide in expired air

capnography   the process of obtaining a tracing of the proportion of carbon dioxide in expired air using a capnograph

captopril   a drug that inhibits the action of angiotensin-converting enzyme

carbamino compound   a chemical compound consisting of carbon dioxide combined with one or more free amino groups (NH_2) of a protein molecule

carbonic anhydrase (CA) an enzyme found in erythrocytes and the tubule cells of the kidney that catalyzes the reaction of water with carbon dioxide to form carbonic acid

carboxyhemoglobin (COHb) an abnormal form of hemoglobin that has carbon monoxide bound to it

cardiac center a nerve center in the medulla oblongata that controls the activities of the heart

cardiac cycle a complete heartbeat of systole and diastole of both atria plus systole and diastole of both ventricles

cardiac jelly a loose connective tissue matrix within which the embryonic heart forms

cardiac output the volume of blood pumped per minute by either the right or left ventricle

cardiac output index (CI) a standardized measure of cardiac performance equal to a person's cardiac output in liters per minute divided by the body surface area in square meters

cardiac reserve the maximum percentage that cardiac output can increase above normal

cardiac skeleton a plate of fibrous connective tissue within which the valves of the heart are imbedded

cardiac tamponade compression of the heart caused by excessive fluid or blood in the pericardial sac that could result in cardiac failure

cardiac veins large veins that drain the myocardium and converge into a venous channel on the posterior surface of the heart called the *coronary sinus*

cardiac work index (CWI) a standardized measure of cardiac performance equal to a patient's cardiac work per minute divided by the body surface area in square meters

cardiogenic pertains to caused by or arising from the normal function of the heart

cardiogenic shock shock that results from low cardiac output

cardiomegaly hypertrophy of the heart caused most frequently by pulmonary hypertension; also occurs in arteriovenous fistula, congenital aortic stenosis, ventricular septal defect, patent ductus arteriosus, and Paget's disease

cardiomyopathy any disease that affects the myocardium; frequently leads to cardiogenic shock

cardiovascular center groups of neurons scattered within the medulla that regulate heart rate, force of contraction, and blood vessel diameter

carina any structure shaped like a ridge or keel such as the carina of the trachea, which projects from the lowest tracheal cartilage

carotid bodies receptor on or near the carotid sinus that responds to alteration in blood levels of oxygen, carbon dioxide, and hydrogen ions

carotid sinus reflex a reflex that causes a decrease in the heart rate from pressure on or within the carotid artery at the level of its bifurcation

catecholamines any one of a group of sympathomimetic compounds comprised of a catechol molecule and the aliphatic portion of an amine

cation a positively charged ion

CBC abbreviation for complete blood count

central venous pressure (CVP) the blood pressure in the large veins of the body

cephalad toward the head

C-fiber receptors sensors around the capillaries of the alveoli that respond to fluid accumulation

chemoreceptor receptor outside the central nervous system on or near the carotid and aortic bodies that detects the presence of chemicals

chemotaxis the movement of cells, such as white blood cells, toward a chemical

Cheyne-Stokes breathing an abnormal breathing pattern characterized by alternating periods of apnea and periods of rising then falling tidal volumes that is associated with central nervous system abnormalities and cardiac failure

CHF abbreviation for congestive heart failure

chloride shift an exchange of chloride ions in red blood cells in peripheral tissues in response to the PCO_2 of blood; the shift reverses in the lungs

cholinergic of or pertaining to nerve fibers that secrete acetylcholine at the myoneural junctions

chordae tendineae tendonlike, fibrous cords that connect the heart valves with the papillary muscles

chronotropic state refers to the heart rate and the factors that influence it

circumflex arteries a branch of the left coronary artery that supplies blood to the lateral and posterior aspects of the left ventricle

closing capacity (CC) the volume of air remaining in the lungs when small airway closure occurs during a maximal exhalation

clotting cascade a series of chemical reactions between various clotting factors that culminates in the production of a fibrin clot

clubbing bulbous swelling of the distal phalanges of the hands and feet caused by chronic hypoxia and the hormones produced by certain types of cancer

CO abbreviation for cardiac output

collagen an inelastic protein fiber consisting of reticular fibrils; forms tendons and is deposited during scar formation

collateral vessels secondary vessels that supply blood to the same region as the primary vessels

colloid osmotic pressure (oncotic pressure) the hydrostatic pressure that equals the osmotic attractive force of proteins in a fluid on one side of a semipermeable membrane

colloidal oncotic pressure the osmotic pressure generated across a membrane by the proteins within a solution

complement a group of 20 or more plasma proteins that participates in nonspecific body defense through cytolysis and triggers inflammation

complete blood count (CBC) the number of red cells, white cells, and platelets in a cubic millimeter of blood

compliance the relationship between volume and distending pressure for a hollow organ; the lungs and cardiovascular system expand with a certain volume of air or blood when exposed to a given distending pressure

conductance the ratio between flow and driving force of electricity, gas flow, and liquid flow; the reciprocal of resistance; the ease of flow through a system

conducting zone the zone comprised of the airways of the lungs that extend from the nose and mouth to the terminal bronchioles; these airways do not participate in respiratory gas diffusion with pulmonary blood

congestive heart failure (CHF) a condition of left ventricular failure resulting in pulmonary hypertension and congestion

contractility the strength of muscle contraction

controller the element in a physiologic feedback loop that regulates the activity of the effector tissue or organs

CO-oximeter a device that uses optical colorimetry to measure the percent of different forms of hemoglobin in a blood sample (e.g., HHb, O_2Hb, COHb)

COPD abbreviation for chronic obstructive pulmonary disease

cor pulmonale right ventricular enlargement and failure caused by chronic pulmonary hypertension secondary to chronic pulmonary parenchymal or vascular disease

coronal plane a plane that divides the body into front (anterior) and back (posterior) portions; also called the frontal plane

coronary arteries vessels that supply blood to the heart

coronary artery bypass graft (CABG) a surgical procedure in which a portion of a blood vessel is removed from another part of the body and grafted onto a coronary artery to bypass an obstruction in the coronary artery

coronary atherosclerosis a process in which fatty substances are deposited in the vessels of coronary arteries

coronary perfusion pressure the pressure difference between the mean aortic blood pressure and the right atrial blood pressure that determines the amount of coronary blood flow

coronary sinus a wide venous channel on the posterior surface of the heart that collects the blood from the coronary circulation and returns it to the right atrium

costophrenic angle the region of the thorax where the chest wall meets with the diaphragm

Coumadin a drug that inhibits the coagulation of blood and depresses synthesis of vitamin K-dependent coagulation factors (II, IIV, IX, and X)

CPAP abbreviation for continuous positive airway pressure

CPFT abbreviation for certified pulmonary function technologist

crackles abnormal adventitious breath sounds that sound like the high-pitched popping sound made by the parting of Velcro that are primarily heard during the inspiratory phase and are associated with pulmonary edema

cricoid cartilage a circular cartilage found below the thyroid cartilage

cricothyrotomy an emergent surgical opening into the cricothyroid membrane to provide an open airway

cusps leaves of the cardiac valves

cyanosis an abnormal blue coloration caused by increasing concentrations of deoxygenated hemoglobin in blood

cyanotic heart disease an abnormal blue coloration caused by intracardiac shunting that results in reduced pulmonary blood flow and hypoxemia

cystic fibrosis a homozygous recessive genetic condition of chromosome 7 that results in the formation of a defective Cl^- transport pump and results in chronic pancreatic insufficiency and chronic bronchiectasis in children

cytokine   a growth factor produced by activated lymphocytes and other cells that acts as an autocrine or paracrine with various roles in immunity and blood cell development

Dalton's law   the total pressure exerted by a gas mixture is equal to the sum of the partial pressures exerted by each of the gases in the mixture

dead space   the portion of inhaled gas volume that does not participate in gas exchange; may be anatomic, alveolar, or mechanical

defibrillation   the termination of ventricular fibrillation by delivering a direct electric countershock to the patient's precordium

dependent lung zone   the field of the lungs being bottom-most relative to the earth's gravitational field

depolarization   the reduction of a membrane potential to a less negative value by the influx of sodium ions; in cardiac fibers, this results in the release of calcium ions into the myofibril and activates the contractile process

dew point   the temperature at which the water vapor content of air reaches the saturation point and water begins to condense into a liquid state

dextrocardia   the rare location of the heart in the right hemithorax as a result of either displacement by disease or congenital defect

diapedesis   the movement of white blood cells through the wall of the capillary toward the surrounding tissues

diastole   the filling or relaxation phase of the cardiac cycle

dicrotic notch   a notch on the descending limb of the systemic arterial pressure tracing that occurs as a result of aortic valve closure

differential blood count   an examination and enumeration of the distribution of leukocytes in a stained blood smear; the different kinds of white cells are counted and reported as a percentage of the total examined

diffusion   the process that molecules within a liquid or gas move from an area of higher concentration toward an area of lower concentration

diffusion coefficient   the diffusion property of a gas in a substance determined by the solubility of the gas in the substance and the molecular weight of the gas

diffusion limited   any limitation of alveoli-capillary diffusion caused by pathological changes in any of the structures of the alveoli-capillary membrane; results in fewer molecules of oxygen crossing the membrane

digitalis   a cardiac glycoside that is given in some cases of heart failure to improve the strength of contraction and reduce the heart rate

diphosphatidylchole (DPPC)   the most abundant type of phospholipid in surfactant

2,3-diphosphoglyceric acid (2,3-DPG)   a substance in the erythrocyte that affects the affinity of hemoglobin for oxygen; the chief end product of glucose metabolism and a link in the biochemical feedback control system that regulates the release of oxygen to the tissue

disseminated intravascular coagulation (DIC)   a grave coagulopathy resulting from the overstimulation of the body's clotting and anticlotting processes in response to disease or injury

dissociation constant (K)   the numerical value that describes the degree of separating into parts or sections; the ratio of base divided by acid

dissociation curve   the graphic presentation of the relationship between blood PO_2 and oxyhemoglobin saturation

distensibility   of or pertaining to the ease of inflation or compliance

diuretic   a chemical that inhibits sodium reabsorption and reduces antidiuretic hormone concentration causing diuresis

dive reflex   an automatic change in the cardiovascular system that occurs when the face and nose are immersed in the water

dopamine   a naturally occurring sympathetic nervous system neurotransmitter; a cardiac stimulant used to improve blood pressure and cardiac output

dorsal respiratory group   a group of neurons in the posterior aspect of the medulla oblongata that stimulates the respiratory muscles to cause inspiration

Dubois' formula   a logarithmic method of calculating the body surface area by multiplying the height in centimeters, the weight in kilograms, and the constant 0.007184

duty cycle   the length of time for one complete cycle of a repetitive event; the length of one cardiac or ventilatory cycle

dyspnea   a subjective sensation of difficult or labored breathing

dysrhythmia   any disturbance or abnormality in a normal rhythmic pattern

dysynchrony pertaining to ventilatory support, a situation in which interaction between the patient and the machine is poorly coordinated, causing the patient extra effort and discomfort

ECG abbreviation for electrocardiogram

ECMO abbreviation for extracorporeal membrane oxygenation

ectopic beats heartbeats that arise from regions that are outside the sinoatrial node

edema a local or generalized condition caused by the buildup of excessive amounts of fluid in the extracellular space characterized by swelling

effector that which produces an effect; that part of a mechanical or physiological system that acts to create a specific condition or change

efferent carrying or conducting impulses away from the central nervous system

ejection fraction (EF) the ratio of cardiac stroke volume to end diastolic volume

elasticity the ability of tissue to regain its original shape and size after being stretched, squeezed, or otherwise deformed

elastin a fibrous protein found in many tissues that has the properties of stretch and elastic recoil

electrocardiogram (ECG) the recording of the electrical activity of the heart

electromechanical dissociation (EMD) a condition in which the electrical events of the heart are not followed by the mechanical pumping events

embolization the process by which an embolus forms and lodges in a branch of the vasculature

embolus a foreign object, a quantity of air or gas, a bit of tissue or tumor, or a piece of thrombus that circulates in the bloodstream until it becomes lodged in a vessel

EMD abbreviation for electromechanical dissociation

emphysema a destructive process of the lung parenchyma leading to permanent enlargement of the distal air space; classified as either centrilobular, which mainly involves the respiratory bronchioles, or panlobular, which can involve the entire terminal respiratory unit

end-diastolic volume (EDV) the volume of the blood, about 120 ml, remaining in a ventricle at the end of its diastole

endocarditis inflammation of the endocardium and heart valves

endocardium the layer of the inside of the heart wall that is comprised of endothelial and smooth muscles

endoscopy the visualization of the interior of organs and cavities of the body with an endoscope

endothelial cells simple squamous epithelial cells that line the cavities of the heart, blood vessels, and lymphatic vessels

endothelial-derived relaxant factor (EDRF) a factor (probably nitric oxide) produced in the local region of a capillary causing precapillary sphincter dilation

endothelin a group of peptides produced by endothelial cells that cause vasoconstriction

endothelium the layer of simple squamous epithelium that lines the cavities of the heart, blood vessels, and lymphatic vessels

end-systolic volume (ESV) the volume of the blood, about 40 ml, remaining in a ventricle following systole

eosinophilia an increase in the number of eosinophils in the blood that accompanies many inflammatory conditions

eosinophils a type of white blood cell characterized by granular cytoplasm readily stained by eosin

epicardium the thin outer layer of the heart wall comprised of serous tissue and mesothelium

epiglottis a large, leaf-shaped piece of cartilage lying on the top of the pharynx

epiglottitis an acute and often life-threatening infection of the upper airway caused primarily by *Haemophilus influenzae* that causes severe obstruction secondary to supraglottic swelling

epinephrine a catecholamine hormone secreted by the adrenal medulla that produces actions similar to those that result from sympathetic stimulation

erg a unit of energy in the centimeter-gram-second system that is equal to the work done by a force of 1 dyne through a distance of 1 cm

erythrocytes red blood cells

erythropoiesis the process by which the erythrocytes are formed

erythropoietin a hormone released by the kidneys that stimulates erythrocyte production

esophageal varices a complex of distended superficial veins in the lower third of the esophagus caused by portal hypertension that is susceptible to hemorrhage

eupnea normal, quiet breathing

evaporation the change of state of a substance from its liquid to its gaseous form that occurs below its boiling point

exosphere the outermost layer of Earth's atmosphere, found beyond an elevation of 300 km

expiratory reserve volume (ERV) the total amount of gas that can be exhaled from the lungs following a quiet exhalation

expiratory time (TE) the amount of time for exhalation during the ventilatory cycle; from the end of inspiration to the start of the next inspiration

external elastic lamina a portion of the outer layer of a blood vessel that contains elastin fibers and other elastic proteins

extrapulmonary shunt systemic blood that bypasses the pulmonary circuit and flows directly to the aorta; a ventricular septal defect allows blood to flow from the right ventricle to the left ventricle; also known as an anatomical shunt

f abbreviation for respiratory frequency or rate of breathing per minute

facilitated diffusion the diffusion of molecules through a membrane with the aid of carrier molecules or channel proteins

feedback loop an interconnected series of elements that control a particular physiological variable; includes a controller, sensor, and effector

fetal hemoglobin (HbF) the type of hemoglobin formed in the fetus by the liver; has a slightly different amino acid sequence

FEV1/FVC ratio (FEV$_{1\%}$) the ratio of the amount of air forcefully exhaled in the first second to the total amount exhaled

FEV3/FVC ratio (FEV$_{3\%}$) the ratio of the amount of air forcefully exhaled in the first 3 seconds to the total amount exhaled

fibrin an insoluble protein formed during blood clotting that is formed from fibrinogen by the action of thrombin

fibrinolysis a continual process of fibrin decomposition by fibrinolysin that is the normal mechanism for the removal of small fibrin clots

fibrous pericardium the inelastic portion of the pericardium that forms the bulk of the pericardial sac

Fick's principle the flow of blood through an organ or the entire organism can be determined by dividing the amount of oxygen consumed by the arterial-to-venous oxygen concentration difference

filtration the separation of molecules as they are forced through a membrane; some pass through, whereas others do not

fissure a groove, fold, or slit that may be normal or abnormal

folate-deficiency anemia a reduced number of red blood cells that results from a B$_9$ deficiency in the diet that results in lower blood cell formation

foramen ovale an opening in the fetal heart in the septum between the right and left atria

forced expiratory flow at 25% (FEF$_{25}$) the flow rate at the point of exhaling 25% of the forced vital capacity

forced expiratory flow at 50% (FEF$_{50}$) the flow rate at the point of exhaling 50% of the forced vital capacity

forced expiratory flow at 75% (FEF$_{75}$) the flow rate at the point of exhaling 75% of the forced vital capacity

forced expiratory flow between 25% and 75% (FEF$_{25-75}$) the average flow during the middle half of the forced vital capacity

forced expiratory vital capacity (FEVC) the maximum volume of gas forcefully exhaled after completely filling the lungs

forced expiratory volume in 1 second (FEV$_1$) the volume of gas exhaled in the first second of a forced vital capacity measurement

forced expiratory volume in 3 seconds (FEV$_3$) the volume of gas exhaled in the first 3 seconds of a forced vital capacity measurement

forced inspiratory vital capacity (FIVC) maximum volume of gas that can be inhaled after emptying the lungs

forced vital capacity (FVC) the maximum amount of air that can be moved forcefully

Frank-Starling's law of the heart the force of muscular contraction is determined by the length of the cardiac muscle fiber; within limits, the greater the length of the stretched fiber, the stronger the contraction

FRC abbreviation for functional residual capacity

functional residual capacity (FRC) the total amount of gas left in the lungs after a resting expiration that is produced by the balance between the desire of the lungs to collapse and the chest wall to spring out

FVC abbreviation for forced vital capacity

gap junction a type of connection between cells that allows molecules and ions to flow from one cell to another; in cardiac cells, this allows the electrical events to flow from one cell to the next

glial cell a supportive cell that surrounds the neurons in the central nervous system

globin the portion of hemoglobin that is comprised of four polypeptide (amino acid) chains

glomerular filtration rate (GFR) the rate at which fluid is filtered through the renal nephrons' glomerular capillaries in the first step in urine formation

glossopharyngeal nerve one of the cranial nerves that innervates the tongue, larynx, and carotid body

gram molecular weight the weight in grams of a mole, or 6.02×10^{23} molecules

granulocytes one of white blood cells characterized by the presence of cytoplasmic granules when stained

Hagen-Poiseuille's law a mathematical relationship that describes how driving pressure, tube inner radius, tube length, and liquid or gas viscosity influence the flow of matter through a tube

Haldane effect the influence of hemoglobin saturation with oxygen on the binding of carbon dioxide on hemoglobin

Hb abbreviation for hemoglobin

HbCO abbreviation for carboxyhemoglobin, hemoglobin saturated with carbon monoxide

HbO$_2$ abbreviation for oxyhemoglobin, hemoglobin saturated with oxygen

HCT abbreviation for hematocrit

hematocrit a measure of the packed cell blood volume obtained by centrifugation of a blood sample

heme an iron-containing porphyrin ring; nonprotein portion of the hemoglobin molecule

hemidiaphragm pertaining to the left or right dome of the diaphragm

hemithorax pertaining to either the right or left side of the thorax

hemocytoblasts stem cells in the bone marrow; primitive blood cells

hemolysis the escape of hemoglobin from the interior of the red blood cell into surrounding medium that results from the disruption of the integrity of the cell membrane by toxins or drugs, freezing or thawing, or hypotonic solutions

hemolytic anemias a disorder characterized by the premature destruction of red blood cells

hemophilia a hereditary blood coagulation disorder caused by deficiency of coagulation factor XIII that is transmitted as an x-linked recessive trait

hemopneumothorax an accumulation of blood and air in the pleural space, usually the result of trauma

hemopoiesis blood cell production occurring in the red marrow of bone

hemoptysis coughing up of blood from the respiratory tract

hemorrhage the escape of blood from the vascular system

hemorrhagic anemia most common form of reduced red blood cell numbers in blood; occurs from either acute blood loss following trauma and surgery or chronic loss from a gastrointestinal ulcer

hemorrhagic shock a shock brought about by sudden and rapid loss of significant amounts of blood

hemostasis the termination of bleeding by mechanical or chemical means or by the complex coagulation process of the body

hemothorax an accumulation of blood and fluid in the pleural space

heparin a naturally occurring mucopolysaccharide that acts in the body as an antithrombin factor or to prevent intravascular clotting

hepatic portal vein a large vein that empties blood into the heart from the liver

hepatic veins a network of veins in the liver

hepatomegaly abnormal enlargement of the liver

Hering-Breuer inflation reflex an inflation reflex mediated via the lung's stretch receptors that appears to limit further spontaneous inflation and slows breathing

Hertz (Hz) a measure of frequency or cycles per unit time; 1 Hz is equal to 1 cycle per second

HFO abbreviation for high-frequency oscillation

HHb abbreviation for unoxygenated or reduced hemoglobin

hilum a depression in any organ in which blood vessels and nerves enter or exit; pertains to the "root" of the lungs

histamine a substance found in many cells (especially mast cells, basophils, and platelets) that is released when the cells are injured; results in vasodilation, increased permeability of blood vessels, and bronchiole constriction

homeostasis the condition in which the body's internal environment remains relatively constant within physiological limits

humidity content the amount of water vapor that actually exists in a volume of gas

humoral of or pertaining to the body fluid

hydrostatic fluid pressure the pressure exerted by a fluid on the walls of its container

hyperbaric oxygen therapy (HBO)   the therapeutic application of oxygen at pressures greater than one atmosphere

hypercalcemia   a condition of elevated blood calcium ion concentration

hypercapnia   the abnormal presence of excess amounts of carbon dioxide in the blood

hyperglycemia   an abnormal condition of having a glucose concentration in blood that is above the normal range of 70 to 110 mg/dl

hyperinflation   a condition of maximal inflation pertaining to artificial ventilatory support, the application of volumes greater than normal to reinflate collapsed alveoli

hyperkalemia   a condition of elevated potassium ion concentration in blood

hypernatremia   a condition of abnormally high sodium ion concentration in blood

hyperoxia   a condition of abnormally high oxygen tension in the blood

hypertension   persistently high blood pressure

hypertonic   having a greater concentration of solute than another solution, hence exerting more osmotic pressure than that solution

hyperventilation   ventilation in excess of that necessary to meet metabolic needs that is signified by a PCO_2 less than 35 mm Hg in the arterial blood

hypervolemia   an increase in extracellular fluid, particularly in the volume of circulating blood or its components

hypobarism   a condition of being exposed to atmospheric pressure less than the pressure normally experienced at sea level

hypocalcemia   a condition of reduced calcium ion concentration in blood

hypocapnia   the presence of lower-than-normal amounts of carbon dioxide in the blood

hypoglycemia   an abnormal condition of having a glucose concentration in blood that is below the normal range of 70 to 110 mg/dl

hypokalemia   a condition of reduced blood potassium ion concentration

hyponatremia   a condition of reduced sodium ion concentration in blood

hypopharynx   beneath the pharynx

hypopnea   shallow breathing

hypotension   persistently low blood pressure

hypotonic   a condition of solute concentration in a liquid that results in it being less concentrated than another liquid

hypoventilation   ventilation less than necessary to meet metabolic needs signified by a PCO_2 more than 45 mm Hg in the arterial blood

hypovolemia   an abnormally low circulating blood volume

hypoxemia   an abnormal deficiency of oxygen in the arterial blood

hypoxia   an abnormal condition in which the oxygen available to the body cells is inadequate to meet their metabolic needs

hysteresis   the failure of the two associated phenomena to coincide, as in the observed difference between the inflation and deflation volume-pressure curves of the lungs

ICP   abbreviation for intracranial pressure

I:E ratio   the ratio of inspiratory time to expiratory time during breathing; by convention, the ratio is always reduced so that the numerator equals 1 (e.g., 1:4 or 1:2.5)

immunoglobulin (Ig)   an antibody synthesized by plasma cells derived from B lymphocytes in response to the instruction of an antigen

in situ   in the natural or usual place

in vitro   a biological reaction occurring in a laboratory apparatus; in glass

in vivo   a biological reaction occurring in a living organism

inert   refers to a substance that does not take part in a chemical reaction or cause a pharmacological action

innominate artery   the older name for the brachiocephalic artery found on the arch of the aorta

inotropy   pertains to the force of muscular contraction

inspiratory capacity (IC)   the maximum volume of gas that can be inhaled from the resting expiratory level

inspiratory reserve volume (IRV)   the maximum volume of gas that can be inspired from the end-tidal inspiratory level

inspiratory time (T_I)   the length of time devoted to the inspiratory phase of breathing; the length of time from the start of inflation to the end of inflation

interatrial septum   the septum between the right and left atria

intercalated disk   an irregular transverse thickening of sarcolemma that contains desmosomes that hold cardiac muscle cells together and gap junctions that aid in conduction of muscle action potentials

intercostal of or pertaining to the space between two ribs

intercostal muscle of or pertaining to the muscle located between adjacent ribs, designated as external or internal; functions as secondary ventilatory muscles

interferon a cellular protein that is produced during viral infections and causes other cells to produce antiviral proteins which block the development of more viruses

interleukins 15 different proteins (IL-1 through IL-15) that are secreted by lymphocytes and cause a variety of reactions such as inducing fevers, stimulating or inhibiting other lymphocytes, stimulating blood cell production, and activating neutrophils during inflammation

internal elastic lamina a portion of the inner layer of a blood vessel that contains elastin fibers and other elastic proteins

interstitial fluid the portion of extracellular fluid that fills the microscopic space between the cells of tissues; the internal environment of the body

interstitial space pertains to the space between cells; also known as the extracellular space

interventricular septum the septum between the left and right ventricle

interventricular sulci grooves that run down the anterior and posterior surfaces of the heart from the base to the apex of the heart

intracellular pertains to the region within cells

intracranial pressure (ICP) pressure that occurs within the cranium

intrapulmonary shunt a condition of perfusion without ventilation within the lungs; also known as a capillary shunt

intravenous within a vein; usually describing a method for infusing fluid and drugs

invasive refers to the use of diagnostic or therapeutic methods requiring access to the inside of the body

inotropic state pertains to the strength of muscular contraction

iron-deficiency anemia reduced red blood cell numbers and hemoglobin content as a result of inadequate amounts of iron in the diet

irritant receptors sensors that respond to various types of stimuli that are experienced as an unpleasant sensation (e.g., coughing, gagging, and sneezing)

ischemia decreased blood supply to a body organ or part

isobar a line connecting points of equal pressure on a graph, as lines connecting points of equal carbon dioxide tension on a pH-bicarbonate diagram

isoproterenol a synthetic adrenergic drug that stimulates beta receptors on heart and airway smooth muscle cells

isotonic having equal tension or tone; having equal osmotic pressure between two different solutions or between two elements in a solution

isovolumic having the same volume

J receptors a juxtacapillary sensor; a type of congestion sensor found in the region around the capillaries of the alveoli

joule a measure of energy or work in the meter-kilogram-second system of measurement, equal to 1×10^7 or 1 watt second

ketoacidosis a metabolic acidosis caused by the accumulation of excess ketones in the body that results from faulty carbohydrate metabolism as can occur in certain forms of diabetes

kinetic energy the energy a body processes by virtue of its motion

Korotkoff's sounds sounds heard during the taking of blood pressure when using a sphygmomanometer and a stethoscope

Kussmaul breathing an abnormally deep and very rapid breathing pattern that is characteristic of diabetic acidosis

kyphoscoliosis an abnormal condition characterized by an anteroposterior curvature and a later curvature of the spine, often associated with cor pulmonale

laminar a condition of bulk flow where all of the molecules are moving in the same direction through a tube

laminar flow a type of flow state of liquids and gases in which the molecules all move in a parallel motion with each other and with the wall of the tube

Laplace's law a principle in physics that describes that the collapsing pressure exerted by a liquid bubble is equal to the surface tension divided by the radius of the bubble times 4

laryngitis inflammation of the larynx

laryngoscope a device used to visually inspect the larynx

laryngospasm an involuntary laryngeal muscular spasm that results in partial or complete closure of the larynx

lateral refers to a position away from the body's midline

left common carotid artery   a major vessel in the neck that carries blood from the aortic arch to the left side of the head and to the brain

leukemia   an abnormal condition of excessive white blood cells brought about by a malignant group of leukocytes

leukocytes   refers to an abnormally high number (greater than $10,000/mm^3$) of white blood cells in blood

leukopenia   refers to an abnormally low number (less than $5000/mm^3$) of white blood cells in blood

ligate   to tie off

lingula   segments in the left upper lobe of the lung that correspond to the right middle lobe

lobectomy   the surgical removal of a lobe

lobule   a small lobe; the primary lobule of the lung is a cluster of alveoli supplied with gas by a single terminal respiratory bronchiole; the secondary pulmonary lobule is the smallest cluster of primary lobules that are divided from each other by connective tissue

lumen   the cavity within a hollow organ; the passage way within a tube or vessel

LVSW   abbreviation for left ventricular stroke work

lymph nodes   solid nodules of lymph tissue (primarily lymphocytes and macrophages) that receive lymph fluid from a series of lymph vessels

lymph vessels   vessels that drain lymph fluid away from the interstitial space of tissue and toward lymph nodes

lymphatic ducts   large lymph vessels that carry lymph fluid from the lymph nodes to the subclavian veins

lymphocytes   a type of white blood cell that can become sensitized to produce antibodies or that can become special killer or regulator cells of the immune system

lymphokine   a general term that refers to chemicals that are released by T-lymphocytes

lysis   the process of breaking apart or decomposing

macrophage   a wandering phagocytic cell that is part of the nonspecific defenses of the body

main stem   refers to the first branch of airways from the trachea

mast cells   a secretory cell that can become sensitized, releasing various chemicals that stimulate inflammation

maximum inspiratory force or pressure (MIP or P_{IMAX})   the maximum pressure that can be generated at the mouth during forceful inspiration

mean circulatory filling pressure   the average pressure exerted by the blood volume within the cardiovascular system

mechanoreceptors   types of sensor cells that respond to physical disturbance (stretch or pressure)

mediastinum   the region between the lungs that contains the heart and other organs

medulla oblongata   a region in the brain stem that contains a variety of automatic control centers

metabolic acidosis   an acidic condition caused by a buffer deficiency

metabolic alkalosis   an alkaline condition caused by a buffer excess

metarterioles   small vessels that carry blood directly from arterioles to venules

methemoglobin (MetHb)   an abnormal condition of hemoglobin in which the iron is oxidized from the ferrous state to the ferric state

minute ventilation ($\dot{V}_E$)   the total amount of gas being moved into or out of the lungs per minute

mitral regurgitation   the backward flow of blood through the bicuspid valve

mitral stenosis   a narrowing and stiffening of the bicuspid valve

mitral valve   the valve that prevents blood from flowing backward from the left ventricle to the left atrium (also called the bicuspid valve)

mitral valve prolapse   a backward opening of one or more cusps of the bicuspid valve during systole

monocyte   a rare form of white blood cell that can move into the tissues and become a macrophage

mucociliary   refers to the layer of epithelial tissue that has cilia and secretes mucus that lines the respiratory tract

mucokinesis   refers to the movement of mucus

mucolysis   refers to the breakdown of liquefaction of mucus

mucosa   refers to the mucous membrane of a hollow organ

muscarinic   refers to the effect that acetylcholine has on the parasympathetic receptors and organs that have these receptors

myocardial infarction   blockage of a coronary artery that results in cardiac muscle cell death

myocarditis   an inflammatory condition of the heart muscle brought about by an infection of virus, bacteria, or fungi

myocyte   a cardiac muscle cell

myofilaments   the contractile proteins actin and myosin

myoglobin   the iron-containing protein of cardiac and skeletal muscle that serves as an intracellular oxygen storage site

myosin   a contractile protein found in muscle cells

nares   the external openings of the nose into the nasal cavity

nasal flaring   dilation of the alar nasi on inspiration; a sign of increased ventilation and respiratory muscle work

nasogastric   refers to the pathway between the nose and the trachea; a nasotracheal tube passes through the nose and into the trachea

negative feedback   a mechanical, electrical, or physiological control scheme that results in the opposite action of an effector on a variable when a sensor of a variable is stimulated (e.g., increasing blood pressure [variable] stimulates a set of baroreceptors [sensors], which results in decreasing heart rate [effector] and contraction strength to lower blood pressure)

neonatal   refers to the period from the time of a baby's birth to 28 days of age

nephron   the microscopic structure that is the functional unit of the kidney that includes the glomerular capillary housed within Bowman's capsule, renal tubule, and associated peritubular capillaries

neutrophil   the most common leukocyte found in blood that contains granules in its cytoplasm and a multilobulated nucleus; an important phagocytic defense cell

nifedipine   a calcium ion, channel-blocking drug that prevents the inflow of calcium ions into cardiac muscle cells, reduces myocardial metabolism, and prevents coronary artery spasm

nitric oxide (NO)   a nitrogen-oxygen molecule that is gaseous under BTPS (body temperature, pressure and saturated with water vapor) conditions and that has vasodilating properties at low levels (30 ppm) in blood and tissues

nitrite   an ester of nitrous acid; a vasodilator useful in the treatment of coronary vasospasms that produce angina pectoris that can cause formation of methemoglobin; includes amyl nitrite and sodium nitrite

nitroglycerin   a vasodilator frequently used to improve coronary blood flow and to relieve angina pectoris

nitroprusside   a vasodilating drug that results in reduced vascular resistance and cardiac work

nomogram   a graphic presentation of a numerical relationship between two or more variables

noninvasive   a diagnostic or therapeutic procedure that does not require penetration of the skin or entrance into a body cavity

nonvolatile acid   a type of acid that is poorly converted from a dissolved state to a gaseous state

norepinephrine   a neurotransmitter commonly released by the neurons of the sympathetic nervous system that stimulates adrenergic receptors found on the surface of some cells

normal sinus rhythm (NSR)   a normal cardiac electrical conduction rhythm that starts in the sinoatrial node and passes throughout the conduction system with a frequency of 60 to 100 times per minute

normoblast   the nucleated precursor cell normally found in bone marrow that differentiates into a mature erythrocyte

normovolemic   a state of having a normal fluid (e.g., blood) volume

nosocomial   pertaining to or originating in a hospital (e.g., a bacterial infection)

NSR   abbreviation for normal sinus rhythm

nuchal   refers to the back or posterior region of the neck

O_2 content ($C_{blood}O_2$)   the total amount of oxygen found dissolved and bound to hemoglobin in blood

O_2Hb   abbreviation for oxyhemoglobin

oblique   angled away from being straight up and down

obstructive pulmonary disease   a pulmonary disease characterized by some form of airway obstruction

obtunded   insensitive to pain and other noxious stimuli as the result of reduced consciousness

oliguria   reduced urine formation

oncotic pressure   the amount of force exerted by dissolved molecules to attract water molecules across a semipermeable membrane; also known as osmotic pressure

Ondine's curse   a condition of apnea that results from failure of the automatic control of breathing derived from the name of a fabled water nymph who placed a curse on a mortal man for being unfaithful

oropharynx   the middle anatomic divisions of the pharynx that lie behind the oral cavity and between the nasopharynx and the laryngopharynx

orthopnea   an abnormal condition that is characterized by difficult breathing when lying down

orthostatic hypotension a condition of abnormally low blood pressure that is brought about when moving to a standing or upright position

osmotic pressure the hydrostatic pressure that is equal to the force necessary to stop the osmotic movement of water through a membrane

oximeter a photoelectrical device used to determine the oxygen saturation of hemoglobin in blood

oxygen debt the amount of oxygen consumed above resting levels during the period following exercise

oxygen extraction ratio (O_2ER) the decimal amount of percent of oxygen consumed compared to the amount delivered

oxygen toxicity a pathological response of the body to long-term exposure to an elevated partial pressure of oxygen; pulmonary changes include airway and alveolar edema, inflammation, and congestion

oxygenation index (P_aO_2/P_AO_2) the ratio of arterial-to-alveolar partial pressure of oxygen; a measure or index of the ability of the lungs to oxygenate blood

oxyhemoglobin (O_2Hb) the form of hemoglobin that has oxygen bound to its ferrous binding sights

oxyhemoglobin saturation (S_aO_2) the percent of ferrous binding sights in hemoglobin loaded with oxygen

oxymyoglobin (O_2Mb) the form of myoglobin, an intracellular pigmented protein, that has oxygen bound to its ferrous binding site

P wave the first portion of the electrical cycle of the heart that is recorded in the electrocardiogram that represents atrial electrical activity

P/F (P_aO_2/FIO_2) ratio the ratio of the arterial partial pressure of oxygen to the fraction of inspired oxygen concentration

P_{50} the partial pressure of oxygen that results in 50% saturation of the hemoglobin

P_{100} or $P_{0.1}$ the pressure at the airway opening at 100 msec after the start of an occluded inspiratory effort; an indicator of the output of the respiratory center

PAC abbreviation for premature atrial contraction

palatine pertaining to the palate or roof of the mouth

pallor an unnatural paleness or absence of color in the skin

papillary muscles small bulblike extensions of myocardial muscle that provide tension to the cordea tendinea

paranasal refers to a region alongside or near the nose

parasympathetic refers to the craniosacral branch of the autonomic nervous system that primarily releases acetylcholine

parenchyma the functional tissue portion of an organ

parietal pleura the serous membrane that lines the inner surface of the chest wall

partial compensation incomplete action to correct some condition

partial pressure that portion of the total pressure exerted by a particular gas

patent open, as in an airway

patent ductus arteriosus an abnormal condition in which the ductus arteriosus artery, which connects the pulmonary artery trunk to the aorta, remains open after birth

PAWP abbreviation for pulmonary artery wedge pressure

PCWP abbreviation for pulmonary capillary wedge pressure

peak expiratory flow rate (PEFR) maximum flow generated during forceful exhalation

peak inspiratory flow rate (PIFR) maximum flow generated during forceful inhalation

pectoriloquy voice sounds transmitted to the lungs and heard through the chest wall

pectus carinatum chicken or pigeon chest; an unusual condition of anterior projection of the sternum

pectus excavatum funnel chest; an unusual indentation of the sternum

PEEP abbreviation for positive end-expiratory pressure

PEFR abbreviation for peak expiratory flow rate

pendelluft back and forth motion; abnormal flow of gas from one lung or lung region to another lung or lung region

percent body humidity (%BH) the amount of water vapor in gas that is expressed as a percent of the amount in saturated gas at body temperature (43.8 mg/L)

percutaneous through the skin

perfusion blood flow in a region

perfusion limited the movement of gas or ions from one region to another depends on the blood flow in that region

perfusionist a person who operates blood-pumping equipment such as a heart/lung machine

pericardial fluid a colorless fluid found in the space around the heart that is formed by the pericardial sac

pericarditis inflammation of the outer membranes of the heart

pericardium the outer membranes of the heart that are largely formed from connective tissue and serous membranes

peritubular nearby or adjacent tubules (e.g., the peritubular capillaries of the nephron)

pernicious anemia a condition of reduced red blood cells caused by a vitamin B_{12} deficiency, which results in fewer, larger, and more fragile red blood cell formation

pH an acid-base scale that ranges from 0 to 14; the negative log (base 10) of the H^+ concentration in a solution

pharynx the space in the posterior part of the mouth that extends from the posterior nasal cavity to the larynx

phenylephrine an alpha-sympathetic stimulating drug that results in vasoconstriction

phonocardiogram visual recording of the heart sounds

phospholipid organic molecules that have long chain lipids and phosphorous ions on one end; commonly found in the cell membrane and in surfactant

phrenic nerve the motor nerve that innervates the diaphragm and begins as right and left portions of spinal nerves C3, C4, and C5 and travels down through the mediastinum and onto each hemidiaphragm

physiological dead space (V_{Dphys}) the portion of the tidal volume delivered to both the conducting airways and nonperfused alveoli

physiological shunt blood flow that is not being exposed to ventilated regions of the lungs and results in lower oxygen and higher carbon dioxide levels in blood

physiological shunt fraction the percent of cardiac output that is not being exposed to ventilated regions of the lungs

plasma the nonliving clear yellow liquid matrix of blood

plasmin a plasma protein that has a clot-dissolving activity

platelet aggregation the binding of platelets together or onto a surface

platypnea difficult breathing while in the upright or standing position

plethysmograph an instrument designed to measure the volume changes of an organ or an entire organism

pleural effusion an abnormal collection of fluid in the pleural space around the lungs

pleural space pressure (P_{pl}) the pressure within the pleural space

pleurisy an abnormal deposition of fibrinous material on the pleural surface of the lung; a painful condition brought on by deep breathing; often associated with infectious pneumonia and lung cancer

plexus a network of intersecting nerves or blood vessels

PMI abbreviation for point of maximal impulse

pneumocyte a lung cell

pneumonectomy removal of an entire lung

pneumonitis inflammation of the lung; pneumonia

pneumotachometer an instrument to measure gas flow

pneumotaxic center a region in the pons of the brain stem that takes part in the automatic control of breathing and stimulates exhalation

pneumothorax an abnormal collection of air in the pleural space

point of maximal impulse (PMI) a region of the anterior chest wall just below the left nipple where cardiac motion can be felt

polycythemia abnormal elevation of red blood cells in blood

polymorphonuclear leukocytes (PMN) a neutrophil

polysomnography the act of recording a variety of physiological events such as air flow, brain waves, and chest motion during sleep; used in the diagnosis of sleep disturbances and sleep apnea in particular

pons a region in the upper portion of the brain stem that is important in the rhythm of automatic control of breathing that connects the brain with the cerebellum

pores of Kohn openings in the alveolar membrane that are 5 to 15 μm in diameter that allow direct movement of gas from one alveolus to another

porphyrin ring an organic pyrrole ring that can contain iron or magnesium ions

positive end-expiratory pressure (PEEP) pressure during the expiratory phase of the breathing cycle that is above atmospheric pressure

potential energy the energy an object has by virtue of its position

ppm abbreviation for parts per million

P-R interval the portion of the electrical cycle of the heart that starts at the beginning of the P wave and extends to the W wave that represents atrial electrical activity

precapillary sphincters donut-shaped rings of smooth muscle that surround small arterioles and control the flow of blood into capillary beds

precordium the external anatomical region over the heart

preload the filling pressure of a ventricle exerted by venous return

preload pressure the blood pressure in the atria responsible for filling and stretching the ventricle before contraction

premature atrial contraction (PAC) a premature contraction of the heart stimulated by an irritable site of cardiac tissue located within the atria

premature ventricular contraction (PVC) a premature contraction of the heart stimulated by an irritable site of cardiac tissue that is located in the ventricles

pressure-time index (PTI) the ratio of mean to maximum transdiaphragmatic pressure difference times the length of the respiratory cycle (duty cycle); an indicator of the breathing work load on the diaphragm

propranolol a beta-sympathetic receptor-blocking drug used to slow and reduce the force of cardiac contraction

prostacyclin (PGI$_2$) a naturally occurring prostaglandin that inhibits platelet aggregation, inhibits the vasoconstrictive action of angiotensin, and stimulates the synthesis of renin

prostaglandins 20-carbon organic chemicals produced by cells from arachidonic acid; prostaglandin E causes relaxation of bronchial smooth muscle and F$_{2\alpha}$ causes bronchial constriction

prothrombin a plasma protein synthesized by the liver that can be converted by thromboplastin and calcium to thrombin, which is necessary for blood clotting

pseudostratified the appearance of being falsely layered; pseudostratified epithelium

PTI abbreviation for pressure-time index

pulmonary angiogram a visual recording of the pulmonary arteries by placing a radiopaque dye in the pulmonary artery and recording the image with x-ray and x-ray sensitive film

pulmonary artery wedge pressure (PAWP) the pressure generated at the tip of a pulmonary artery catheter with its balloon inflated; an accurate measurement of the pulmonary capillary, left atrial and preload pressures of the left ventricle

pulmonary capillary wedge pressure (PCWP) the pressure generated at the tip of a pulmonary capillary catheter with its balloon inflated; an accurate measurement of the capillary, left atrial, and preload pressures of the left ventricle

pulmonary circuit the system of vessels that carries blood from the right ventricle to and through the lungs and back to the left atrium

pulmonary edema an abnormal collection of fluid in the lung tissue and air spaces

pulmonary embolism a blood clot that lodges in a portion of the pulmonary circulation

pulmonary fibrosis an abnormal condition with scarring of the lungs; characterized by the widespread deposition of collagen and other fibers in the tissues of the lungs

pulmonary hypertension abnormally elevated blood pressure in the pulmonary circuit of the lungs

pulmonary oxygen toxicity lung inflammation and edema brought about by exposure to excessive concentrations (>60%) of oxygen in the air being breathed

pulmonary (or pulmonic) semilunar valve a tricuspid valve that directs blood flow from the right ventricle to the trunk of the pulmonary arteries

pulmonary shunt blood that passes from the right side of circulation (venous blood [right side of the heart or pulmonary artery]) to the left side of circulation (arterial blood [left side of the heart or pulmonary veins]) without the opportunity for gas exchange in the lungs

pulmonary trunk a short vessel that carries blood flow from the right ventricle to the bifurcation of the left and right pulmonary arteries

pulmonary vascular resistance (PVR) the numerical ratio of the pressure drop across the pulmonary circuit (mean pressure in the pulmonary artery minus left atrial pressure) to the total pulmonary blood flow; the ratio is very low when compared with the vascular resistance in the systemic circuit

pulse oximeter a device that noninvasively measures the oxyhemoglobin percent saturation in arterial blood

pulsus alternans an unusual cycling of the systolic pressure from higher to lower values

pulsus paradoxus an abnormal decrease in the systolic pressure during the inspiratory phase of breathing

Purkinje fibers a network of specialized cardiac muscle fibers that carries the conduction impulse of the heart from the bundle branches into the ventricles

PVC abbreviation for premature ventricular contraction

PVR abbreviation for pulmonary vascular resistance

QRS complex the portion of the cardiac cycle recorded on the electrocardiogram that represents ventricular depolarization and atrial repolarization

radiolucent pertaining to a substance or tissue that allows x-rays to pass through

radiopaque pertaining to a substance or tissue that will not allow x-rays or other forms of radiation to pass through

rapid eye movement (REM) cyclic movement of closed eyes during sleep

RCP abbreviation for respiratory care practitioner

reduced hemoglobin (HHb) the form of hemoglobin not bound with oxygen

referred pain pain felt in a region of the body that is not responsible for the pain (e.g., left arm pain felt during a myocardial infarction)

relative body humidity (RBH) the humidity content of a gas that is expressed as a percentage of the maximum a gas can hold at a normal body temperature of 37° C

renin a proteolytic enzyme that is produced by the juxtaglomerular apparatus of the renal nephrons and acts to convert angiotensinogen to angiotensin I

repolarization the return to a potential or voltage difference between two regions or poles

residual volume (RV) the air remaining in the lungs after a maximal exhalation

respiratory acidosis an acidic condition caused by carbon dioxide retention from hypoventilation

respiratory alkalosis an alkaline condition caused by reduced levels of carbon dioxide from hyperventilation

respiratory alternans the alternating use of respiratory muscles during conditions of increased work of breathing

respiratory exchange ratio (R) the ratio of carbon dioxide production to oxygen consumption in the lungs

respiratory failure the condition of reduced ability to excrete carbon dioxide and to absorb oxygen

respiratory quotient (RQ) the ratio of carbon dioxide production to oxygen consumption in the tissues or for the whole body

respiratory zone the airways that participate in gas exchange with pulmonary blood

respirometer an instrument used to measure a volume of gas

resting membrane potential the voltage difference across the cell membrane when the cell is not actively signaling (in neurons) or contracting (in muscles)

restrictive pulmonary disease a condition that results in reduced ability to move normal volumes of gas in and out of the lungs

retrosternal the region behind the sternum

Reynolds' number a numerical value that describes the state of flow as it passes through a tube that is equal to two times the radius of the tube times the average velocity of the gas times the density of the gas divided by the viscosity of the gas

rhonchi abnormal, adventitious, high-pitched breath sounds that are primarily heard during the expiratory phase as the result of partial airway obstruction caused by inflammation, bronchoconstriction, or mucus retention that is also known as wheezing and is commonly associated with asthma

RPFT abbreviation for registered pulmonary function technologist

RRT abbreviation for registered respiratory therapist

RV abbreviation for residual volume

RVSW abbreviation for right ventricular stroke work

S_1 the first heart sound ("lubb"), which is produced during closure of the mitral and tricuspid valves

S_2 the second heart sound ("dupp"), which is produced during closure of the aortic and pulmonic semilunar valves

sagittal a sectional plane of the body that is vertical and oriented anterior to posterior; the midsagittal plane passes through the head vertically between the eyes

S_aO_2 abbreviation for oxyhemoglobin saturation in arterial blood

sarcomere the functional unit of a striated muscle cell

semilunar valves the three-cusped outflow valves of the ventricles; aortic and pulmonic valves

sensor the component of a physiological control feedback loop that senses change in the concentration of the substance or condition that is being controlled

serotonin a naturally-occurring derivative of tryptophan found in platelets, neurons of the brain, and selected cells of the intestine; a potent vasoconstrictor

serous pericardium the portion of the pericardial membranes that secretes pericardial fluid into the pericardial sac

set point the desired value or range of concentration of a substance or condition that is being controlled by a physiological control system

shock a condition where blood flow to tissues is inadequate to support the metabolic needs of those tissues

shunt blood flow that bypasses a functional region of tissue or an organ

shunt fraction ($\dot{Q}_S/\dot{Q}_T$) the ratio of blood flow that shunts around a tissue or organ to the total amount of blood flow in the organ; an index of the ability to match blood flow with the tissues of an organ

SI abbreviation for stroke index

sickle cell anemia a genetic disorder that alters the amino acid sequence of a protein in hemoglobin; low oxygen levels cause the hemoglobin in sickle cell disease to change into a sickle-shaped structure that can increase the breakdown rate of the erythrocytes leading to anemia

SID abbreviation for strong ion difference

SIDS abbreviation for sudden infant death syndrome

sinoatrial node a specialized bundle of cardiac tissue in the right atrium that acts as a pacer for the heart

sleep apnea a condition of apnea that occurs during sleep that can be caused by central neurological failure of the respiratory center or airway obstruction

sliding filament theory the description of the interaction of actin and myosin proteins within muscle cells that results in twitching and development of muscle tension

solubility coefficient (C_s) the amount of gas that can be dissolved in a liquid under specific conditions

sphygmomanometer a device that includes an inflatable cuff and pressure gauge that is used in the noninvasive measurement of blood pressure

spinal shock a condition of reduced blood pressure and flow brought on by spinal cord paralysis or injury and loss of sympathetic innervation of the blood vessels

spirometer an instrument used to measure gas flow and volume moving into or out of the lungs

splanchnic pertains to the liver, spleen, and intestines

S_pO_2 the symbol for oxyhemoglobin saturation determined with a pulse oximeter

sputum a mixture of respiratory tract secretion and saliva

ST segment that portion of the cardiac cycle recorded in the electrocardiogram that represents the period between ventricular depolarization and repolarization; ST segment elevation indicates abnormally low coronary blood flow

standard HCO_3^- concentration the concentration of bicarbonate in plasma that would exist if the partial pressure of carbon dioxide was normal (40 mm Hg)

standard temperature and pressure, dry (STPD) the conditions of 0° C, one atmosphere of pressure, and saturated and no water

steady state a condition of stability that often refers to a stable metabolic rate

stenosis a condition of narrowing

stretch receptors a type of mechanoreceptor that produces nervous signals when stretched to critical length

stridor an abnormal adventitious breath sound that is a harsh, high-pitched sound heard primarily during the inspiratory phase as a result of partial upper airway obstruction

stroke a neurological injury that results from loss of blood flow to a region of the brain

stroke index (SI) the ratio of the stroke volume to body surface area

stroke volume (SV) the amount of blood pumped during a single ventricular contraction; 80 ml in adults

stroke work index (SWI)   the amount of work being done by one ventricle during one contraction

strong ion difference (SID)   the numerical difference between total anion and cation concentration in a body fluid

subclavian arteries   the arteries found below the clavicles that carry blood from the aorta to the arms

supraglottic   referring to a region above the vocal cords

surface tension   the force generated at the surface of a liquid that results from the cohesive interaction of the molecules making up the liquid

surfactant   a collection of chemicals (primarily phospholipids) produced by the type II pneumocyte that results in reduction of alveolar surface tension

SV   abbreviation for stroke volume

SVR   abbreviation for systemic vascular resistance

Swan-Ganz catheter   an inflatable balloon-tipped catheter placed through the right side of the heart and into a branch of the pulmonary artery that is used to measure pulmonary artery pressure including the wedge pressure

SWI   abbreviation for stroke work index

sympathetic nervous system   the thoracic branch of the automatic nervous system that releases norepinephrine and stimulates adrenergic receptors in various tissues; activation results in stimulation of the heart, bronchodilation, and inhibition of gastrointestinal activity

syncytium   a group of interconnected cells that share cytoplasm

systemic circuit   the vessels that carry blood from the left ventricle to the tissues of the body and back to the right atrium

systemic vascular resistance (SVR)   the numerical ratio of the blood pressure drop across the systemic circuit (mean pressure in the aorta minus central venous pressure) to the total systemic blood flow; the ratio is higher when compared to the vascular resistance in the pulmonary circuit

systole   the contractile phase of the cardiac cycle; the period between mitral valve closure and mitral valve opening in the cardiac cycle

T cells   a group of lymphocytes that matures in the tissues and is responsible for the control of the immune response; T cells act as killer cells and function as memory cells

T wave   the portion of the cardiac cycle recorded in the electrocardiogram that represents the period of repolarization of the ventricles

tachycardia   a rapid heart rate; >100/minute in adults

tachypnea   a rapid breathing rate; >20/minute in adults

tamponade   stopping blood flow to a region, organ, or tissue by the use of pressure or compression

tangent   a straight line that is parallel to a portion of a curved line

thermistor   a device that reacts to temperature change

thoracentesis   a perforation through the chest wall with a needle for the aspiration of pleural fluid or air

thoracotomy   surgical opening of the chest wall

thrill   an abnormal sound produced by turbulent blood flow

thrombocytes (platelets)   cellular fragments that adhere to each other and to the surface of an injured blood vessel as part of the blood clotting process

thrombocytopenia   an abnormal condition of reduced numbers of platelets

thrombophlebitis   inflammation of and blood clot formation within a vein

thrombosis   the formation of a blood clot

thrombus   a blood clot

tidal volume (V_T)   the volume of gas that is inhaled or exhaled during a single breath

time constant   the mathematical product of airway resistance times compliance; the length of time required to inflate a region of lung tissue to 60% of its maximal value

titration   the gradual adjustment of some activity while its effects are evaluated until the desired effect is reached

TLC   abbreviation for total lung capacity

tomogram   a focused x-ray scan of a structure at a particular depth in the body

total breath time (T_{TOT})   the length of time it takes to complete one cycle of breathing; inspiratory time plus expiratory time

total CO_2   the total amount of carbon dioxide found in blood plasma in all its different forms; the sum of the amount dissolved, the amount bound to protein, and the amount in the form of bicarbonate

total expiratory time (TET)   the length of time it takes to exhale

total lung capacity (TLC)   the amount of gas within the lungs after completely filling the lungs with a maximum effort

t-PA   the abbreviation for tissue plasminogen activator

trabeculae carneae   fibers that extend from the papillary muscle within the ventricles to the cusps of the bicuspid and tricuspid valves and helps prevent prolapse of the cusps of the bicuspid and tricuspid valves

tracheal and bronchial breath sounds   loud, high-pitched, harsh tubular sounds caused by the rapid and turbulent flow of gas

tracheoesophageal   refers to the region or tissue between the trachea and esophagus

tracheostomy   a surgical opening made in the tissues of the anterior neck and trachea

transairway pressure   refers to the pressure difference from the airway opening to the alveolus

transbronchial   refers to the crossing through the bronchial wall

transcutaneous   to cross through the skin

transducer   a device capable of converting one form of energy or activity into another form of energy or activity

transect   to cut through

transmural pressure   the pressure difference between the inner and outer pressures of blood vessels, airways, and any hollow organ

transpulmonary pressure   the difference between alveolar and pleural pressures

transthoracic pressure   the difference between pleural and body surface pressure

Trendelenburg position   a position in which the head is lower than the body and limbs

tricuspid valve   the valve that directs blood flow from the left atrium to the left ventricle

troposphere   the innermost layer of the Earth's atmosphere that extends to an elevation of 8 to 10 km

T$_{TOT}$ symbol for the ventilatory cycle time

tunica externa   the outer layer of the blood vessel

tunica interna   the inner layer of the blood vessel

tunica media   the middle layer of the blood vessel

turbulent   a condition of bulk flow in which the molecules are moving in swirls and eddies in varying directions through a tube; a chaotic flow pattern

turbulent flow   a flow condition in which the gas or liquid molecules move in a chaotic pattern resulting in eddying, increased friction, and increased flow resistance

turgor   the normal resilience of the skin caused by the outward pressure of the fluid within and outside the cells

Type A blood   blood that has erythrocytes with type *A* agglutinogens on their surface and has anti-*B* agglutinins in the plasma

Type AB blood   blood that has erythrocytes with type *B* agglutinogens on their surface and has anti-*A* agglutinins in the plasma

Type B blood   blood that has erythrocytes with types *A* and *B* agglutinogens on their surface and has no anti-*A* or anti-*B* agglutinins in the plasma

Type O blood   blood that has **neither** types *A* nor *B* agglutinogens on its surface and has **both** anti-*A* and anti-*B* agglutinins in the plasma

unperfused   a condition in which a region of tissue lacks blood flow

V̇/Q̇ mismatch   a condition that results when the distribution of ventilation and blood flow in the lung are not matched

V̇/Q̇ scan   a nuclear medicine procedure that uses radioactive isotopes to visualize the regions of the lungs that receive blood and ventilation

vagal (vasovagal) reflex   activation of the vagus nerve that results in parasympathetic stimulation of the heart and lungs and results in bradycardia, hypotension, bronchoconstriction, and increased mucus production

vagotomy   cutting of the vagus nerve

vagus nerve   the tenth cranial nerve that carries both motor and sensory nerve signals; the primary route of parasympathetic fibers to the organs of the thorax and most of the abdomen

Valsalva maneuver   a breathing maneuver that includes taking a deep breath and breath holding with compression of the thorax by the abdominal muscles and intercostal muscles; intrapulmonary pressures increase significantly

vascular resistance   the numerical ratio of the blood pressure drop across the vascular circuit to the total blood flow in the circuit

vasoconstriction   the decrease of blood vessel diameter by the tensing of the smooth muscle in the tunica media

vasodilation the increase of blood vessel diameter by the combination of relaxation of the smooth muscle in the tunica media and the internal blood pressure

vasomotor center the region within the medulla oblongata involved with regulation of blood vessel constriction and dilation

vasopressin an antidiuretic hormone produced by the posterior lobe of the pituitary gland that stimulates the nephrons of the kidney to retain water and reduce urine production

vasopressor a chemical agent that stimulates vessel constriction

V_D/V_T abbreviation for dead space/tidal volume ratio

$\dot{V}_E$ abbreviation for minute ventilation

vein a vessel that carries blood back toward the heart

vena cava large veins that carry systemic blood to the right atrium (inferior and superior)

venous admixture the mixing of systemic venous blood that has low oxygen content with arterialized blood that leaves the lung with a higher oxygen content and that results in lower arterial blood oxygen content

venous return the amount of blood that returns to the atria and fills the ventricles

ventilatory cycle (T_{TOT}) the length of time it takes to inhale and exhale one breath

ventral respiratory group a pool of neurons in the anterior region of the medulla oblongata that stimulates respiratory muscles, causing inspiration

ventricle a hollow cavity; the pumping chamber of the heart; one of the fluid-filled cavities within the brain

ventricular compliance the volume-filling characteristic of a ventricle for a given amount of pressure

ventricular fibrillation a lethal form of disorganized electrical activity of the heart that produces ineffective pumping of blood

ventricular flutter a rapid heart rate that results from an abnormal pacer within the ventricular myocardium

ventricular "gallop" abnormal cardiac sound produced by turbulent blood flow and a rapid heart rate

ventricular septal defect (VSD) a congenital heart defect that results in a perforated interventricular septum

ventricular tachycardia a rapid heart rate that results from an abnormal pacer within the ventricular myocardium

venule a small vessel that drains blood from a capillary bed

Verapamil a cardiac and vascular calcium ion channel-blocking drug used to slow and reduce cardiac contraction

vesicular breath sounds the soft, breezy sounds heard primarily during inspiration over the lung periphery or parenchyma of the lungs

visceral pericardium the portion of the pericardial membrane that is found in direct contact with the myocardium of the heart

visceral pleura a serous membrane that covers the outer surface of the lung

viscosity the internal resistance that opposes the flow and mixing of a fluid or gas

vital capacity (VC) the maximum volume of air that can be exhaled after a maximal inspiration

volatile acid an acid that can become gaseous and evaporate

V_T abbreviation for tidal volume

V_T/T_I abbreviation for average inspiratory flow, which is used to assess the drive of breathing

watt a unit of power that equals the work done at a rate of 1 joule per second

wheeze an abnormal, adventitious, high-pitched breath sound that is primarily heard during the expiratory phase as the result of partial airway obstruction caused by inflammation, bronchoconstriction, or mucus retention and is commonly associated with asthma

xiphoid process the bone at the inferior end of the sternum

Index

Page references followed by f indicate figures, t indicate tables, and b indicate boxes.